Practical Guide to
Catheter Ablation
of Atrial
Fibrillation

Practical Guide to Catheter Ablation of Atrial Fibrillation

SECOND EDITION

EDITED BY

Jonathan S. Steinberg, MD

Director, Arrhythmia Institute, The Valley Health System
Professor of Medicine (adj), University of Rochester School of Medicine & Dentistry
New York, NY and Ridgewood, NJ, USA

Pierre Jaïs, MD

CHU de Bordeaux, Hopital Cardiologique Haut Leveque, Pessac, France
Université de Bordeaux, IHU LIRYC, Bordeaux, France

Hugh Calkins, MD

Professor of Medicine, Division of Cardiology, Department of Medicine
Johns Hopkins University School of Medicine, Baltimore, MD, USA

WILEY Blackwell

This edition first published 2016 © 2016 by John Wiley & Sons Ltd
Previous edition: © Lippencott, Williams & Wilkins

Registered office: John Wiley & Sons, Ltd, The Atrium, Southern Gate, Chichester, West Sussex, PO19 8SQ, UK

Editorial offices: 9600 Garsington Road, Oxford, OX4 2DQ, UK
      The Atrium, Southern Gate, Chichester, West Sussex, PO19 8SQ, UK
      111 River Street, Hoboken, NJ 07030-5774, USA

For details of our global editorial offices, for customer services and for information about how to apply for permission to reuse the copyright material in this book please see our website at www.wiley.com/wiley-blackwell

Library of Congress Cataloging-in-Publication Data

Practical approach to catheter ablation of atrial fibrillation.
   Practical guide to catheter ablation of atrial fibrillation / edited by Jonathan S. Steinberg, Pierre Jais,
Hugh Calkins. – Second edition.
      p. ; cm.
   Preceded by A practical approach to catheter ablation of atrial fibrillation / editors, Hugh Calkins, Pierre Jais,
Jonathan S. Steinberg. c2008.
   Includes bibliographical references and index.
   ISBN 978-1-118-65850-5 (cloth)
   I. Steinberg, Jonathan S., editor. II. Jais, Pierre, 1964- , editor. III. Calkins, Hugh, 1956- , editor. IV. Title.
   [DNLM: 1. Atrial Fibrillation–surgery. 2. Catheter Ablation–methods. WG 330.5.A5]
   RD598.35.C39
   617.4′120592–dc23
                                            2015020797

A catalogue record for this book is available from the British Library.

Wiley also publishes its books in a variety of electronic formats. Some content that appears in print may not be available in electronic books.

Cover image: iStock_000014424928/**copyright - teekid**

Set in 9/11pt MinionPro-Regular by Thomson Digital, Noida, India

Printed in Singapore by Markono Print Media Pte Ltd

1 2016

Contents

Contributors

Olujimi Ajijola
UCLA Cardiac Arrhythmia Center, Ronald Reagan UCLA
Health System, David Geffen School of Medicine at UCLA,
Los Angeles, CA, USA

Jason G. Andrade
Electrophysiology Service, Montreal Heart Institute,
Montreal, Canada and Department of Medicine,
Université de Montréal, Montreal, Canada
Department of Medicine, The University of British
Columbia,r, Vancouver, Canada

Jeffrey S. Arkles
Cardiology Division, Hospital of the University of
Pennsylvania, Philadelphia, PA, USA

Rong Bai
Texas Cardiac Arrhythmia Institute, St. David's Medical
Center, Austin, TX, USA

Chirag Barbhaiya
Shapiro Cardiovascular Center, Brigham and Women's
Hospital, Boston, MA, USA

Conor Barrett
Al-Sabah Arrhythmia Institute (AI) at St. Luke's Hospital,
New York, NY, USA

Kazim Baser
Division of Cardiovascular Medicine, University of
Michigan, Ann Arbor, MI, USA

Benjamin Berte
CHU de Bordeaux, Hopital Cardiologique Haut Leveque,
Pessac, France
Université de Bordeaux, IHU LIRYC, Bordeaux, France

Deepak Bhakta
Krannert Institute of Cardiology, Department of Medicine,
Indiana University School of Medicine, Indianapolis,
IN, USA

Eric Buch
UCLA Cardiac Arrhythmia Center, Ronald Reagan UCLA
Health System, David Geffen School of Medicine at UCLA,
Los Angeles, CA, USA

Scott W. Burke
Arrhythmia Institute, Newtown, PA, USA

John David Burkhardt
Texas Cardiac Arrhythmia Institute, St. David's Medical
Center, Austin, TX, USA

Hugh Calkins
Division of Cardiology, Department of Medicine, Johns
Hopkins University School of Medicine, Baltimore, MD,
USA

David J. Callans
Cardiology Division, Hospital of the University of
Pennsylvania, Philadelphia, PA, USA

Riccardo Cappato
Arrhythmia and Electrophysiology Center, University of
Milan, I.R.C.C.S. Policlinico San Donato, Milan, Italy

Farooq A. Chaudhry
Mount Sinai School of Medicine, New York, NY, USA

Matthew Daly
CHU de Bordeaux, Hopital Cardiologique Haut Leveque,
Pessac, France
Université de Bordeaux, IHU LIRYC, Bordeaux, France

Stephan Danik
Al-Sabah Arrhythmia Institute (AI), St. Luke's Hospital, New
York, NY, USA

Mithilesh K. Das
Krannert Institute of Cardiology, Department of Medicine,
Indiana University School of Medicine, Indianapolis,
IN, USA

D. Wyn Davies
Department of General Medicine, St. Mary's Hospital,
London, UK

Isabel Deisenhofer
German Heart Center Munich, Department for
Electrophysiology, TechnischeUniversitätMünchen,
München, Germany

Arnaud Denis
CHU de Bordeaux, Hopital Cardiologique Haut Leveque,
Pessac, France
Université de Bordeaux, IHU LIRYC, Bordeaux, France
INSERM U1045 – L'Institut de Rythmologie et Modeling
Cardiaque, Bordeaux, France

Nicolas Derval
CHU de Bordeaux, Hopital Cardiologique Haut Leveque,
Pessac, France
Université de Bordeaux, IHU LIRYC, Bordeaux, France
INSERM U1045 – L'Institut de Rythmologie et Modeling
Cardiaque, Bordeaux, France

Luigi Di Biase
Texas Cardiac Arrhythmia Institute, St. David's Medical
Center, Austin, TX, USA
Department of Biomedical Engineering, University of Texas,
Austin, TX , USA
Department of Cardiology, University of Foggia, Foggia,
Italy

Mark A. Dixon
Indiana University Health La Porte Hospital,
La Porte, IN, USA

Hatice Duygu Bas
Division of Cardiovascular Medicine, University of
Michigan, Ann Arbor, MI, USA

Charlotte Eitel
Department of Electrophysiology, University of Leipzig
Heart Center, Leipzig, Germany

Kenneth A. Ellenbogen
Department of Medicine and Division of Cardiology,
Virginia Commonwealth University Medical Center and
McGuire VA Medical Center, Richmond, VA, USA

Gregory K. Feld
Department of Medicine, Division of Cardiology,
Electrophysiology Program at the University of California
and the Sulpizio Family Cardiovascular Center, La Jolla, CA,
USA

Anand N. Ganesan
Centre for Heart Rhythm Disorders (CHRD), South
Australian Health and Medical Research Institute
(SAHMRI), University of Adelaide and Royal Adelaide
Hospital, Adelaide, SA, Australia

Michel Haïssaguerre
CHU de Bordeaux, Hopital Cardiologique Haut Leveque,
Pessac, France
Université de Bordeaux, IHU LIRYC, Bordeaux, France
INSERM U1045 – L'Institut de Rythmologie et Modeling
Cardiaque, Bordeaux, France

Henry Halperin
Heart and Vascular Institute, Johns Hopkins University,
Baltimore, MD, USA

Gerard Hindricks
Department of Electrophysiology, University of Leipzig
Heart Center, Leipzig, Germany

Mélèze Hocini
CHU de Bordeaux, Hopital Cardiologique Haut Leveque,
Pessac, France
Université de Bordeaux, IHU LIRYC, Bordeaux, France
INSERM U1045 – L'Institut de Rythmologie et Modeling
Cardiaque, Bordeaux, France

Darren Hooks
CHU de Bordeaux, Hopital Cardiologique Haut Leveque,
Pessac, France
Université de Bordeaux, IHU LIRYC, Bordeaux, France
INSERM U1045 – L'Institut de Rythmologie et Modeling
Cardiaque, Bordeaux, France

Rodney Horton
Texas Cardiac Arrhythmia Institute, St. David's Medical
Center, Austin, TX, USA

Jose F. Huizar
Department of Medicine and Division of Cardiology,
Virginia Commonwealth University Medical Center and
McGuire VA Medical Center, Richmond, VA, USA

John D. Hummel
Division of Cardiovascular Medicine, The Ohio State
University, Columbus, OH, USA

Rahul Jain
Krannert Institute of Cardiology, Department of Medicine,
Indiana University School of Medicine, Indianapolis,
IN, USA

Pierre Jaïs
CHU de Bordeaux, Hopital Cardiologique Haut Leveque,
Pessac, France
Université de Bordeaux, IHU LIRYC, Bordeaux, France

German Kamalov
Division of Cardiovascular Medicine, The Ohio State
University, Columbus, OH, USA

Simon Kircher
Department of Electrophysiology, University of Leipzig
Heart Center, Leipzig, Germany

Karoly Kaszala
Department of Medicine and Division of Cardiology,
Virginia Commonwealth University Medical
Center and McGuire VA Medical Center, Richmond,
VA, USA

Pipin Kojodjojo
Department of General Medicine, St. Mary's Hospital,
London, UK

Aravindan Kolandaivelu
Heart and Vascular Institute, Johns Hopkins University,
Baltimore, MD, USA

Yuki Komatsu
CHU de Bordeaux, Hopital Cardiologique Haut Leveque,
Pessac,
France Université de Bordeaux, IHU LIRYC, Bordeaux,
France

Jayanthi N. Koneru
Virginia Commonwealth University, Richmond, VA, USA

David E. Krummen
Division of Cardiovascular Medicine, Department of
Medicine, University of California at San Diego,
San Diego, CA, USA

Karl-Heinz Kuck
Department of Cardiology, AsklepiosKlinik St. Georg,
Hamburg, Germany

Dennis H. Lau
Centre for Heart Rhythm Disorders (CHRD), South
Australian Health and Medical Research Institute
(SAHMRI), University of Adelaide and Royal Adelaide
Hospital, Adelaide, SA, Australia

Han S. Lim
HôpitalCardologique du Haut-Lévêque and the Université
Victor Segalen Bordeaux II, Bordeaux, France

Carlos Macias
UCLA Cardiac Arrhythmia Center, Ronald Reagan UCLA
Health System, David Geffen School of Medicine at UCLA,
Los Angeles, CA, USA

Laurent Macle
Electrophysiology Service, Montreal Heart Institute, Canada
and Department of Medicine, Université de Montréal,
Montreal, Canada

Saagar Mahida
CHU de Bordeaux, Hopital Cardiologique Haut Leveque,
Pessac, France
Université de Bordeaux, IHU LIRYC, Bordeaux, France

Francis E. Marchlinski
Cardiovascular Division, Hospital of the University of
Pennsylvania, Philadelphia, PA, USA

Nassir F. Marrouche
Comprehensive Arrhythmia Research and Management
Center (CARMA), University of Utah School of Medicine,
Salt Lake City, UT, USA

Andreas Metzner
Department of Cardiology, AsklepiosKlinik St. Georg,
Hamburg, Germany

Gregory F. Michaud
Shapiro Cardiovascular Center, Brigham and Women's
Hospital, Boston, MA, USA

John M. Miller
Krannert Institute of Cardiology, Department of Medicine,
Indiana University School of Medicine, Indianapolis,
IN, USA

Suneet Mittal
Arrhythmia Institute, the Valley Hospital Health System,
Ridgewood, NJ, USA

Sanghamitra Mohanty
Texas Cardiac Arrhythmia Institute, St. David's Medical
Center, Austin, TX, USA

Siva K. Mulpuru
Division of Cardiovascular Diseases, Mayo Clinic, Rochester,
MN, USA

Dan L. Musat
Valley Health System, New York, NY, USA

Koonlawee Nademanee
Pacific Rim Electrophysiology Research Institute, Los
Angeles, CA, USA

Mehdi Namdar
Service de Cardiologie, Hôpitaux Universitaires de Genève,
Geneva, Switzerland

Sanjiv M. Narayan
Cardiovascular Medicine, Stanford University, Stanford,
CA, USA

Andrea Natale
Texas Cardiac Arrhythmia Institute, St. David's Medical
Center, Austin, TX, USA
Department of Biomedical Engineering, University of Texas,
Austin, TX, USA
EP Services, California Pacific Medical Center, San Francisco,
California, USA
Dell Medical School, Austin, Texas, USA

Leenhapong Navaravong
Comprehensive Arrhythmia Research and Management
Center (CARMA), University of Utah School of Medicine,
Salt Lake City, UT, USA

Justin Ng
Shapiro Cardiovascular Center, Brigham and Women's
Hospital, Boston, MA, USA

Naoya Oketani
Department of Cardiovascular Medicine and Hypertension, Graduate School of Medical and Dental Sciences, Kagoshima University, Kagoshima, Japan

Hakan Oral
Division of Cardiovascular Medicine, University of Michigan, Ann Arbor, MI, USA

Feifan Ouyang
Department of Cardiology, AsklepiosKlinik St. Georg, Hamburg, Germany

Alessandro Paoletti Perini
Texas Cardiac Arrhythmia Institute, St. David's Medical Center, Austin, TX
Department of Heart and Vessel, University of Florence, Florence, Italy

Evgeny Pokushalov
State Research Institute of Circulation Pathology, Novosibirsk, Russia

Riccardo Proietti
University of Milan, Ospedale Sacco, Milan, Italy
McGill University Health Centre, Montreal, Canada

Frédéric Sacher
CHU de Bordeaux, Hopital Cardiologique Haut Leveque, Pessac, France
Université de Bordeaux, IHU LIRYC, Bordeaux, France
INSERM U1045 – L'Institut de Rythmologie et Modeling Cardiaque, Bordeaux, France

Javier E. Sanchez
Texas Cardiac Arrhythmia Institute, St. David's Medical Center, Austin, TX, USA

Prashanthan Sanders
Centre for Heart Rhythm Disorders (CHRD), South Australian Health and Medical Research Institute (SAHMRI), University of Adelaide and Royal Adelaide Hospital, Adelaide, SA, Australia

Pasquale Santangeli
Texas Cardiac Arrhythmia Institute, St. David's Medical Center, Austin, TX, USA
Department of Cardiology, University of Foggia, Foggia, Italy
University of Pennsylvania, Philadelphia, USA

Francesco Santoro
Texas Cardiac Arrhythmia Institute, St. David's Medical Center, Austin, TX, USA
Department of Cardiology, University of Foggia, Foggia, Italy

Kazuhiro Satomi
Department of Cardiology, AsklepiosKlinik St. Georg, Hamburg, Germany

Dipen Shah
Service de Cardiologie, HôpitauxUniversitaires de Genève, Geneva, Switzerland

Ashok J. Shah
CHU de Bordeaux, Hopital Cardiologique Haut Leveque, Pessac, France
Université de Bordeaux, IHU LIRYC, Bordeaux, France

Kalyanam Shivkumar
UCLA Cardiac Arrhythmia Center, Ronald Reagan UCLA Health System, David Geffen School of Medicine at UCLA, Los Angeles, CA, USA

David J. Slotwiner
Department of Medicine and School of Health Policy and Research, Weill Cornell Medical College, New York, NY

Antonio Sorgente
Heart & Vascular Institute, Cleveland Clinic Abu Dhabi, Abu Dhabi, UAE, Milan, Italy

David Spragg
Division of Cardiology, Department of Medicine, Johns Hopkins University School of Medicine, Baltimore, MD, USA

Jonathan S. Steinberg
Arrhythmia Institute, The Valley Health System, University of Rochester School of Medicine & Dentistry, New York, NY and Ridgewood, NJ, USA

Chintan Trivedi
Texas Cardiac Arrhythmia Institute, St. David's Medical Center, Austin, TX, USA

Seigo Yamashita
CHU de Bordeaux, Hopital Cardiologique Haut Leveque, Pessac, France
Université de Bordeaux, IHU LIRYC, Bordeaux, France

Junaid A. B. Zaman
Cardiovascular Medicine, Stanford University, Stanford, CA, USA

Stephan Zellerhoff
CHU de Bordeaux, Hopital Cardiologique Haut Leveque, Pessac, France
Université de Bordeaux, IHU LIRYC, Bordeaux, France

CHAPTER 1

Indications for catheter and surgical ablation of atrial fibrillation

Hugh Calkins

Division of Cardiology, Department of Medicine, Johns Hopkins University School of Medicine, Professor of Medicine, Baltimore, MD, USA

Introduction

The indications for catheter ablation of atrial fibrillation have been defined by three major documents. The first is the 2012 HRS Consensus Document on Catheter and Surgical Ablation of Atrial Fibrillation [1], the second is the European Society of Cardiology 2010 Guidelines for the Management of Atrial Fibrillation [2,3], and the third are the ACC/AHA/HRS Guideline for the Management of the Patients with Atrial Fibrillation [4]. In this chapter, we will review, compare, and contrast the indications for AF ablation, as defined in each of these three documents. We will also discuss areas of controversy.

The 2012 HRS/EHRA/ECAS consensus document on Catheter ablation of atrial fibrillation

The 2012 HRS/EHRA/ESC Expert Consensus Document on Catheter and Surgical Ablation of Atrial Fibrillation was an update on the original Expert Consensus Document that was published in 2007. The recommendations concerning the indications for catheter and surgical ablation of atrial fibrillation as defined by the 2012 HRS/EHRA/ECAS Consensus Document are as follows:

Symptomatic AF refractory of intolerant to at least one class 1 or 3 antiarrhythmic medication

---

Practical Guide to Catheter Ablation of Atrial Fibrillation, Second Edition. Edited by Jonathan S. Steinberg, Pierre Jaïs and Hugh Calkins.

Paroxysmal AF: Catheter ablation is recommended. Class 1, LOE A.

Persistent AF: Catheter ablation is reasonable. Class 2A, LOE B.

Long-standing Persistent AF: Catheter ablation may be considered class 2B, LOE B.

Symptomatic AF prior to initiation of antiarrhythmic drug therapy with a class 1 or 3 antiarrhythmic agent

Paroxysmal: Catheter ablation is reasonable. Class 2A, LOE B.

Persistent: Catheter ablation may be considered. Class 2A, LOE C.

Long-standing persistent: Catheter ablation may be considered. Class 2A, LOE C.

Concomitant surgical ablation of atrial fibrillation

Symptomatic AF refractory of intolerant to at least one class 1 or 3 antiarrhythmic medication.

Paroxysmal AF: Concomitant surgical ablation is recommended. Class 2A, LOE C.

Persistent AF: Concomitant surgical ablation is reasonable. Class 2A, LOE C.

Long-standing Persistent AF: Concomitant surgical ablation may be considered class 2A, LOE C.

Symptomatic AF prior to initiation of antiarrhythmic drug therapy with a class 1 or 3 antiarrhythmic agent

Paroxysmal: Concomitant surgical ablation is reasonable. Class 2A, LOE C.

Persistent: Concomitant surgical ablation may be considered. Class 2A, LOE C.

Long-standing persistent: Concomitant surgical ablation may be considered. Class 2B, LOE C.

Stand-alone surgical ablation of atrial fibrillation

Symptomatic AF refractory of intolerant to at least one class 1 or 3 antiarrhythmic medication.

Paroxysmal AF: Stand-alone surgical ablation is recommended. Class 2A, LOE C.

Persistent AF: Stand-alone surgical ablation is reasonable. Class 2A, LOE C.

Long-standing Persistent AF: Stand-alone surgical ablation may be considered class 2A, LOE C.

Symptomatic AF prior to initiation of antiarrhythmic drug therapy with a class 1 or 3 antiarrhythmic agent

Paroxysmal: Stand-alone surgical ablation is reasonable. Class 2A, LOE C.

Persistent: Stand-alone surgical ablation may be considered. Class 2A, LOE C.

Long-standing persistent: Stand-alone surgical ablation may be considered. Class 2B, LOE C.

Indications for catheter ablation of atrial fibrillation as defined by the 2010 European Society of Cardiology guidelines for atrial fibrillation management

The most recent document on AF management put forth by the European Society of Cardiology was published in 2012 [3]. This document is an update of the 2010 European Society of Cardiology AF Guidelines [2].

The updated 2012 indications are as follows:

1 Catheter ablation of symptomatic paroxysmal AF is recommended in patients who have symptomatic recurrences of AF on antiarrhythmic drug therapy and who prefer further rhythm control therapy, when performed by an electrophysiologist who has received appropriate training and is performing the procedure in an experienced center. Class 1, LOE A.

2 Catheter ablation of AF should be considered as first-line therapy in selected patients with symptomatic paroxysmal AF as an alternative to antiarrhythmic drug therapy, considering patient choice, benefit, and risk. Class 2A, LOE B.

The indications that remain unchanged from the 2010 document are as follows:

3 Ablation of persistent symptomatic AF that is refractory to antiarrhythmic therapy should be considered as a treatment option. Class 2a, LOE B.

4 Catheter ablation of AF in patients with heart failure may be considered when antiarrhythmic medication, including amiodarone, fails to control symptoms. Class 2b, LOE B.

5 Catheter ablation of AF may be considered in patients with symptomatic long-standing persistent AF refractory to antiarrhythmic drugs. Class 2b, LOE C. Indications for catheter ablation of atrial fibrillation as defined by the 2014 ACC/EHRA/ECAS AF Management Guidelines.

In 2014, the ACC/AHA/and HRS published a guidelines document focused on atrial fibrillation management [4]. The recommendations put forth in this document concerning the indications for catheter ablation of atrial fibrillation are as follows:

Class I

1 AF ablation is useful for symptomatic paroxysmal AF refractory or intolerant to at least one class 1 or 3 antiarrhythmic medication when a rhythm control strategy is desired *(Level of Evidence: A)*

2 Prior to consideration of ablation of AF, careful assessment of the procedural risks and outcomes relevant to the individual patient is recommended. *(Level of Evidence: C)*

Class IIa

1 AF ablation is reasonable for selected patients with symptomatic persistent AF refractory or intolerant to at least one class 1 or 3 antiarrhythmic medication. *(Level of Evidence: A)*

2 In selected patients with recurrent symptomatic paroxysmal AF, AF ablation is a reasonable initial rhythm control strategy prior to therapeutic trials of antiarrhythmic drug therapy, after carefully weighing risks and outcomes of drug and ablation therapy. *(Level of Evidence: B)*

Class IIb

1 AF ablation may be considered for symptomatic long-standing persistent AF refractory or intolerant to at least one class 1 or 3 antiarrhythmic medication when a rhythm control strategy is desired. *(Level of Evidence: B)*

2 In patients with recurrent symptomatic paroxysmal AF, it is a reasonable initial rhythm control strategy prior to therapeutic trials of antiarrhythmic drug therapy, after weighing the risks and outcomes of drug and ablation therapy (LOE B).

Class III: Harm

1 AF ablation should not be performed in patients who cannot be treated with anticoagulant therapy during and following the procedure. *(Level of Evidence: C)*

2 AF ablation of AF to restore sinus rhythm should not be performed with the sole intent of obviating need for anticoagulation. *(Level of Evidence: C)*

Considerations on the published guidelines for AF ablation

These indications are categorized into class I, class IIa, class IIb, and class III indications. The evidence supporting these indications is graded as level A through C. In making these recommendations, the writing groups considered the body of literature published that has defined the safety and efficacy of catheter and surgical ablation of AF. Both the number of clinical trials and the quality of these trials were considered. Catheter and surgical ablation of AF are highly complex procedures, and a careful assessment of benefit and risk must be considered for each patient.

As demonstrated in a large number of published studies, the primary clinical benefit from catheter ablation of AF is an improvement in quality of life resulting from elimination of arrhythmia-related symptoms such as palpitations, fatigue, or effort intolerance (see section on Outcomes and Efficacy of Catheter Ablation of AF). Thus, the primary selection criterion for catheter ablation should be the presence of symptomatic AF. As noted above, there are many considerations in patient selection other than type of AF alone. In clinical practice, many patients with AF may be asymptomatic but seek catheter ablation as an alternative to long-term anticoagulation with warfarin or other drugs with similar efficacy. One of the important features of the indications for AF ablation described in these documents is that the guidelines viewed collectively tell us that a desire to stop anticoagulation is not an appropriate indication for AF ablation. This is stated most clearly in the 2014 ACC/AHA/HRS AF guidelines that provide a class 3 indication "harm" for performing AF ablation because of a desire to stop anticoagulation. Although retrospective studies have demonstrated that discontinuation of warfarin therapy after catheter ablation may be safe over medium-term follow-up in some subsets of patients, this has never been confirmed by a large prospective randomized clinical trial and therefore remains unproven. Furthermore, it is well recognized that symptomatic and/or asymptomatic AF may recur during long-term follow-up after an AF ablation procedure. It is for these reasons that Heart Rhythm Society Consensus Document recommends that discontinuation of warfarin or equivalent therapies post-ablation is not recommended in patients who have a high stroke risk as determined by the $CHADS_2$ or CHA_2DS_2VASc score. Either aspirin or warfarin is appropriate for patients who do not have a high stroke risk. If anticoagulation withdrawal is being considered, additional ECG monitoring may be required, and a detailed discussion of risk versus benefit should be entertained. A patient's desire to eliminate the need for long-term anticoagulation by itself should not be considered an appropriate selection criterion. In arriving at this recommendation, the Task Force recognizes that patients who have undergone catheter ablation of AF represent a new and previously unstudied population of patients. Clinical trials, therefore, are needed to define the stroke risk of this patient population and to determine whether the risk factors identified in the $CHADS_2$ or CHA_2DS_2VASc or other scoring systems apply to these patients.

A review of the above guidelines reveals that there is a remarkable consistency among the three published guidelines. This is not surprising given that the same worldwide body of evidence was reviewed in order to create these guidelines. These guidelines, taken as a whole, remind us that the outcomes of catheter ablation are superior in patients with paroxysmal atrial fibrillation compared to persistent or particularly long-standing persistent AF. They also remind us of the importance of patient preference. In my experience, patients fall into two main groups. For some patients, the notion of an AF ablation procedure, that is a lengthy procedure performed usually under general anesthesia with measureable risks, is an unattractive option unless all attempts at pharmacologic therapy have failed. Other patients view this decision from a very different stand point and would gladly undergo an invasive procedure to avoid anti-arrhythmic drug therapy. These guidelines also reflect the body of literature that informs us of the outcomes and safety of AF ablation. In the case of paroxysmal AF, more than eight prospective randomized trials have been performed. In contrast, remarkably little literature is available to inform us of the safety and efficacy of AF ablation in patients with long-standing persistent AF. This is particularly the case for patients who have been in continuous AF for many years.

A reader of this chapter cannot help but wonder that there is no mention in any of the three guideline documents on what the role of AF ablation is in the truly asymptomatic patient. Although none of these documents provides a clear indication for ablation in this patient group, one of these documents states that catheter ablation is inappropriate. This silence on the part of the experts reflects a number of subtle issues concerning the field of AF ablation. The first issue concerns how symptoms are defined. In my experience, many patients with AF when asked if they have symptoms will reply that they are symptom free. And yet, if the effort is made to restore the sinus rhythm in a particular patient, the patient will recognize that they feel much better with improved sinus rhythm. It is for this reason that it is becoming an increasingly common practice for cardiologists and electrophysiologists to give a patient a "trial of sinus rhythm" before declaring they have permanent AF and abandoning all attempts at rhythm control. This is particularly the case for young individuals. The next issue concerns how a truly asymptomatic young patient with AF should be handled. We all recognize that there are the "proven" and also the "unproven" benefits of restoration of sinus rhythm. The proven benefits of a rhythm control strategy are the improvement in quality of life and reduction of symptoms. But there are also many "unproven" and "theoretical" benefits of a rhythm control strategy. AF has been shown to increase mortality, increase the risk of heart failure, and increase the risk of dementia. And there is some data suggesting that stroke risk is higher in AF patients persistent AF than those with paroxysmal AF. Although studies have not been completed to prove that the elimination of AF reduces these risks, this may be the case. Some might argue that the AFFIRM study resolved this issue in demonstrating that "rate" and "rhythm" control did not differ in terms of stroke risk and mortality, this is really not the case. Not only was antiarrhythmic therapy ineffective in maintaining rhythm control in many patients and many patients in the rate control arm were in sinus rhythm but also the duration of follow-up was less than 5 years. So, can we really apply these findings when having a detailed discussion with a 50-year-old man recently diagnosed with persistent AF on a routine physical examination? I do not believe this is the case. We also need to be aware of the important issue of atrial remodeling. It is well established that the longer a patient is in atrial fibrillation, the harder it is to restore and maintain sinus rhythm. Because of this when one chooses to pursue a rate control strategy in a 50-year-old with persistent AF, the opportunity to change direction and pursue a rhythm control strategy 5 years later, perhaps when new data proves that rhythm control lowers stroke risk, will be lost.

Considerations on discussions of the risks and benefits of AF ablation with patients

A physician plays an important role in a patient's decision whether to proceed with catheter ablation or pursue further attempts at antiarrhythmic drug therapy. In my experience, many physicians "oversell" AF ablation, informing patients that the "success of AF ablation is approximately 90%, with up to 50% of patients needing a second procedure." What such physicians mean to explain to the patient is that the single procedure success rate of AF ablation, defined as being AF free of antiarrhythmic drug therapy12 months postablation, is 50 to 60%. And among patients doing well 12 months postablation, AF recurs in about one in four after 5 years postablation. In my experience, it is a mistake to oversell the procedure. I always explain to the patients that AF ablation continues to evolve, and if we can control

their AF with an antiarrhythmic medication the AF ablation procedure they will get in the future will have higher safety and efficacy than the AF ablation they undergo now. Some patients feel an urgency to have their AF ablation procedure sooner than later because they are getting "older." My response to this concern is that they are getting older more slowly that the procedure is getting better. In my opinion, the only situation where it is a mistake not to proceed with AF ablation now is when a patient is in continuous AF despite drug therapy on an antiarrhythmic medication. The importance of continuous AF as a major determinant of poor outcomes of AF ablation is so powerful that the concept of deferring the procedure in a patient in continuous AF never pays off, especially when viewed in the long term.

Conclusions

In conclusion, the indications for AF ablation have been spelled out in three major documents. These documents, although different in some minor respects, are remarkably similar and consistent. Although it is important for electrophysiologists to be aware of these documents and their indications, the final decision will always rest with the patient. It is important to take the time and effort to fully inform the patient so that an informed and thoughtful decision can be made. In most situations, the patient faces the question "should I undergo AF ablation now or should I wait and defer this decision to a later point?" Many well-informed patients will defer the procedure only to decide to proceed months or years later.

References

1 Calkins H, Kuck KH, Cappato R, Brugada J, Camm AJ, Chen SA, Crijns HJ, Damiano RJ Jr, Davies DW, DiMarco J, Edgerton J, Ellenbogen K, Ezekowitz MD, Haines DE, Haissaguerre M, Hindricks G, Iesaka Y, Jackman W, Jalife J, Jais P, Kalman J, Keane D, Kim YH, Kirchhof P, Klein G, Kottkamp H, Kumagai K, Lindsay BD, Mansour M, Marchlinski FE, McCarthy PM, Mont JL, Morady F, Nademanee K, Nakagawa H, Natale A, Nattel S, Packer DL, Pappone C, Prystowsky E, Raviele A, Reddy V, Ruskin JN, Shemin RJ, Tsao HM, Wilber D. HRS/EHRA/ ECAS Expert Consensus Statement on Catheter and Surgical Ablation of Atrial Fibrillation: recommendations for patient selection, procedural techniques, patient management and follow-up, definitions, endpoints, and research trial design. Europace. 2012;14(4):528–606.
2 European Heart Rhythm Association and European Association for Cardio-Thoracic Surgery, Camm AJ, Kirchhof P, Lip GY, Schotten U, Savelieva I, Ernst S, Van Gelder IC, Al-Attar N, Hindricks G, Prendergast B, Heidbuchel H, Alfieri O, Angelini A, Atar D, Colonna P, De Caterina R,

De Sutter J, Goette A, Gorenek B, Heldal M, Hohloser SH, Kolh P, Le Heuzey JY, Ponikowski P, Rutten FH. ESC Committee for Practice Guidelines. Guidelines for the management of atrial fibrillation: the Task Force for the Management of Atrial Fibrillation of the European Society of Cardiology (ESC). Eur Heart J. 2010;31(19):2369–429.

3 Camm AJ, Lip GY, De Caterina R, Savelieva I, Atar D, Hohnloser SH, Hindricks G, Kirchhof P. ESC Committee for Practice Guidelines-CPG and Document Reviewers. 2012 focused update of the ESC Guidelines for the management of atrial fibrillation: an update of the 2010 ESC Guidelines for the management of atrial fibrillation. Developed with the special contribution of the European Heart Rhythm Association. Europace. 2012;14(10):1385–413.

4 January CT, Wann LS, Alpert JS, Calkins H, Cleveland JC Jr, Cigarroa JE, Conti JB, Ellinor PT, Ezekowitz MD, Field ME, Murray KT, Sacco RL, Stevenson WG, Tchou PJ, Tracy CM, Yancy CW. AHA/ACC/HRS Guideline for the Management of Patients with Atrial Fibrillation: a Report of the American College of Cardiology/American Heart Association Task Force on Practice Guidelines and the Heart Rhythm Society. J Am Coll Cardiol. 2014 Mar 28.

CHAPTER 2

Catheter ablation for atrial fibrillation: past, present, and future

David Spragg & Hugh Calkins

Division of Cardiology, Department of Medicine, Johns Hopkins University School of Medicine, Baltimore, MD, USA

Introduction

Atrial fibrillation (AF) is the most common sustained tachyarrhythmia encountered by physicians. The prevalence of AF in patients over the age of 65 is approximately 6% and approaches 10% in patients over the age of 85 [1]. As the median age of the population in the United States becomes older, the epidemiologic burden of AF in this country is likely to increase. At present, over 2.2 million people in the United States have AF [1]. AF, while typically not a life-threatening arrhythmia per se, is associated with increased risk of stroke [2], heart failure, and increased mortality. The stroke risk in patients with AF, for instance, is increased between five- and sevenfold compared to similar patients without AF [3,4].

Therapy for AF can be divided into two major paradigms – rate control and rhythm control. Rate control, as the name implies, focuses exclusively on preventing an uncontrolled, rapid ventricular response rate in the setting of AF. Strategies to achieve rate control typically include either pharmacological agents to slow conduction through the atrioventricular (AV) node (i.e., beta-blockers or calcium-channel blockers) or ablation of the AV junction and implantation of a permanent pacemaker. Large prospective randomized trials have validated rate control as a reasonable option in patients with AF,

particularly in terms of overall mortality [5,6]. However, such a strategy does nothing to reduce the stroke risk and loss of AV synchrony seen in patients with AF, and as such, it represents a suboptimal strategy in many patients.

The second paradigm, rhythm control, has historically involved the use of antiarrhythmic medications and/or DC cardioversion from AF into sinus rhythm. Antiarrhythmic medications used for the maintenance of sinus rhythm include class I and class III agents. Randomized prospective data has demonstrated that amiodarone, compared to other class III and to class I medications, is the most effective antiarrhythmic drug to prevent AF [7,8]. Long-term therapy with amiodarone is imperfect, however, both due to limited efficacy and due to attendant end-organ toxicities. Recurrence rates in patients treated with amiodarone are approximately 35% [7]. As importantly, amiodarone has dose-dependent effects on thyroid, liver, and pulmonary function. In patients treated with DC cardioversion alone (i.e., without the suppressive effects of antiarrhythmic medications), AF recurrence is predictably high, with nearly 66% of cardioverted patients developing recurrent AF within 15 months [9]. In part because of the limitations of effective and safe pharmacological therapy for AF suppression, clinicians have sought nonpharmacological interventions to achieve rhythm control. Over the past 20 years, techniques for catheter-based ablation of atrial fibrillation have evolved and now provide a widely accepted therapeutic option for the treatment and potential cure of AF. This chapter reviews that evolution, summarizes current trends

Practical Guide to Catheter Ablation of Atrial Fibrillation, Second Edition. Edited by Jonathan S. Steinberg, Pierre Jaïs and Hugh Calkins.

in practice, and speculates on the future directions of AF ablation.

Catheter-based treatment for atrial fibrillation

In 1959, Moe hypothesized that AF was due to multiple randomly propagating reentrant waves in the atrium, suggesting that functional reentry was the mechanism underlying fibrillation [10–12]. In subsequent work by Allessie and coworkers [13–15], Moe's hypothesis was confirmed. AF was demonstrated to require at least six to eight circulating reentrant wave fronts. Maintenance of AF depended both on a critical atrial mass and on conduction velocity and refractory periods in the atrial tissue to support functional reentry. This paradigm has been challenged recently by investigators who have described stable rotors, rather than wandering, unstable wave fronts, responsible for the maintenance of persistent AF (see section on the future, below).

Catheter ablation for atrial tachyarrhythmias is a relatively recent phenomenon [16–20]. The propagation of electrical activation from atria to ventricles over myocardial fibers was originally described in 1883 [21]. Nearly a century later, Scheinman and colleagues described the first catheter-based ablation procedure – His bundle interruption for the control of ventricular response rates to refractory supraventricular tachycardias [22]. Over the past 25 years, catheter ablation techniques have become standard curative therapy for AVNRT [17], accessory pathway ablation [18,20], and ablation of macro-reentrant atrial flutter [19]. While ablation of the AV junction has long been accepted as a palliative treatment for AF, curative catheter-based therapy has evolved rapidly since the early 1990s. Initial work focused on linear and MAZE-like lesions sets in the right [23,24], right and left [25], and left atria [26]. More recently, the importance of AF triggers (particularly those located in the PVs) has been recognized and targeted [27].

The past

Initial ablation attempts to cure atrial fibrillation focused on linear lesions confined to the right atrium. Between 1994 and 1996, Haissaguerre and colleagues investigated the effects of linear lesion sets in patients with symptomatic, drug-refractory AF [25]. Forty-five initial patients were studied and followed over the long term. Patients initially underwent right atrial ablation only, with either a single ablation line from SVC to IVC over the atrial septum or multiple ablation lines (longitudinal and transverse) to compartmentalize the right atrium. The procedure led to stable

sinus rhythm in 18 of 45 patients (40%) during the procedure. Sustained AF was inducible in 40 of 45 patients, however, and 19 patients underwent repeat ablation of left- or right-sided atrial flutter or focal atrial tachycardia. After a follow-up period of 11 ± 4 months, only six patients were free of AF off antiarrhythmic drugs, with another nine patients free of AF on a previously ineffective medication (overall success of 33%). Nine of forty-five patients had significant improvement of their symptom burden with the aid of an antiarrhythmic medication, while the remaining twenty-one of forty-five patients had no appreciable effect from RA-only ablation. After 26 ± 5 months of follow-up [24], there was a further reduction in therapeutic benefit, with seven previous respondents (either cured or with significant reduction in AF burden) reverting to frequent AF. Successful results with RA-only lesions were seen in only 17 of 45 patients.

Other investigators have prospectively attempted curative lesion sets confined to the right atrium. Natale et al. studied 18 patients with symptomatic, drug-refractory AF [28]. While the lesion sets varied somewhat among the patients (seven with two intercaval lesions, ablation of the cavotricuspid isthmus, and an anterior RA line and eleven with a single intercaval line, a septal line, and cavo-tricuspid isthmus ablation), the results were generally poor. After a follow-up period of 22 ± 11 months, only 5 of 18 patients remained free from atrial arrhythmia recurrence. Most of the 13 recurrences occurred within 2 months of the procedure. The particular lesion set did not predict procedural efficacy. Thus, while linear ablation confined to the right atrium to cure AF is attractive from a technical and safety standpoint, multiple trials with intermediate- and long-term follow-up have shown it to be a largely ineffective procedure [24,29].

Recognizing the limited efficacy of RA-only ablation for AF, several groups began prospective investigations of biatrial and left-atrial linear ablation. Haissaguerre performed left atrial ablation in 10 of 45 patients described above [25]. Linear ablation in this group terminated AF during the procedure in 8 of 10 patients. In 5 of 10 patients, sustained AF could not be induced after the procedure. Intermediate follow-up demonstrated success in 6 of 10 patients (with 2 patients requiring ongoing antiarrhythmic medications).

Between 1996 and 1998, the same group systematically studied biatrial linear ablation to cure AF [26]. Forty-four patients were enrolled prospectively, the majority of whom suffered from paroxysmal, drug-refractory AF ($n = 40$). Four patients had persistent AF. All patients underwent a similar ablative procedure.

In the right atrium, an intercaval septal line and ablation of the cavotricuspid isthmus were made. In the left atrium, linear lesions were applied from the superior PVs to the posterior MV annulus, including the inferior PV ostia. A roof line connecting the two superior PVs was performed in all patients. A septal left-sided line from the right superior PV to the fossa ovalis was performed in 23 of 44 patients.

This complex lesion set was technically difficult, requiring multiple procedures (2.7 ± 1.3) and prolonged fluoroscopy (171 ± 94 min) [26]. After a follow-up period of 19 ± 7 months, 25 of the 44 patients were successfully treated, 12 patients showed significant improvement, and 7 reported no improvement. Success rates increased to 37 of 44 patients with the use of antiarrhythmic medications. However, there were clearly important caveats to the study. Only seven of the patients were treated with a single procedure, while the rest were treated with multiple procedures for AF recurrence, ablation of AF triggers, and/or the ablation of iatrogenic left atrial flutters. Perhaps most importantly, triggers of AF arising from the PVs were identified and ablated in 26 of the 44 patients studied. Given the clear importance of trigger elimination in catheter-based cures of AF (discussed below), these results undoubtedly confounded an analysis of left atrial linear lesions alone as a curative approach to AF. Indeed, ablation of triggering foci and the creation of at least one successful line of block were the two sole predictors of success in the 37 patients with a favorable outcome.

Other linear left atrial lesion sets have been investigated. Schwartz and colleagues pursued a catheter-based recreation of the Cox MAZE lesion set. Technical difficulty and complication rates limited the widespread application of the procedure, however [30]. A much simpler left atrial lesion pattern was investigated prospectively by Pappone et al. [31]. Twenty-five patients with highly symptomatic, drug-refractory, paroxysmal AF underwent biatrial lesion application using a novel (at the time) mapping system. Fourteen patients underwent biatrial ablation, with three linear lesions in the RA (posterior intercaval, cavotricuspid isthmus, and septal) and a single, long linear lesion surrounding the PV ostia and connecting to the MV annulus in the left atrium. The left atrial lesion alone was performed in isolation in five patients, while only the RA lesion set was performed in eight patients. The success and complication rates reported by Pappone et al. were relatively good, with 16 of 27 patients entirely asymptomatic from AF (4 on antiarrhythmic medications), and another 4 with markedly reduced symptoms. No acute complications were reported. Success appeared to be predicted by biatrial ablation (85% success versus 50–60% with single-chamber ablation).

The present

In part because of the limited efficacy of linear ablation alone for AF and in part because of critically important observations by Haissaguerre of the triggered nature of AF (discussed below), linear ablation alone for AF is not widely performed. However, observations made by the groups that pursued linear ablation – unmasked triggering foci in patients undergoing linear ablation and the development of simple lesion sets around the PV ostia, in particular – continue to inform current catheter-based ablation strategies for AF.

A seminal event in the catheter-based treatment of AF was the observation by Haissaguerre and colleagues that fibrillation could be triggered by rapidly firing ectopic atrial foci [27,32,33]. In a series of publications in the mid- and late-1990s, Haissaguerre's group reported the successful ablation of AF through radiofrequency ablation of focal trigger points. In 1994, they described three patients with atrial tachyarrhythmias [32]. In the first patient, a focal, rapidly firing atrial tachycardia mimicked AF on ECG and was successfully ablated. The second patient had AT-induced AF, again with successful ablative therapy targeting the ectopic trigger. In the third patient of the series, a focal right atrial septal trigger was found and ablated, with marked diminution of AF burden. These initial results were expanded upon by a larger series of patients ($n = 9$), in whom paroxysmal AF was found to be triggered from ectopic atrial foci [33]. In three patients, these foci were located in the RA; in the other six patients, triggers were at the ostium of the right ($n = 5$) or left ($n = 1$) PVs. All patients underwent successful ablation, with a mean of 4 ± 4 RF applications. One patient suffered an early recurrence of AF and underwent reablation. After 10 ± 10 months of follow-up, there were no observed recurrences of AT or AF.

In a larger landmark study of 45 patients with symptomatic, drug-refractory paroxysmal AF, Haissaguerre et al. reported that all 45 had demonstrable focal atrial triggers [27]. Most patients ($n = 29$) had a single triggering site, although as many as four triggering sites were observed. A total of 69 triggering foci were found, the majority of which (31/69) were located in the left superior PV (LSPV). Other frequent sites included the right superior PV (RSPV; 17/69), left inferior PV (LIPV; 11/69), and right inferior PV (RIPV; 6/69). Three ectopic foci were located in the RA. AF induction was spontaneously observed in 36 patients, and was characterized by short bursts of two or more repetitive focal firings (40/45 patients). Ablation of ectopic foci was successfully achieved in 38/45 patients. Short-term recurrence of AF was seen in 2 of the 38 ablated patients. After 8 ± 6 months, 28 of the 45 patients remained free of AF (62%), without the use of antiarrhythmic medications; 17 patients, including the early failures, had recurrence of AF.

The observation that AF is frequently triggered by ectopic, rapidly firing atrial foci amounted to a paradigm shift in ablative treatment. Surgical and catheter-based strategies to date had focused principally on substrate modification, in an effort to disrupt the maintenance of AF. Many of these strategies involved surgical or ablative isolation of the PV ostia from the body of the left atrium, which may in part explain their effectiveness. Current ablation strategies are focused more on the elimination and/or isolation of AF triggers, although many strategies combine both trigger isolation and substrate modification. Ablation of PV-located triggers has evolved rapidly, from focal to segmental and ultimately to linear ablation lesions.

With the initial observation that AF triggers are predominantly located in the PVs, focal trigger ablation within the veins became more widespread [27,33–40]. Quickly, though, the limitations and dangers of this strategy were discovered. The recurrence rates of AF in patients undergoing focal PV trigger ablation was high, primarily either due to other PV triggers unrecognized at the time of initial ablation or due to recovery of identified and ablated PV triggers. As importantly, ablation within the PVs led to an unacceptably high rate of PV stenosis [41,42]. This complication has serious downstream sequellae, including pulmonary hypertension, hemoptysis, dyspnea, and (rarely) death [43]. Accordingly, strategies to isolate the PVs, either through segmental or through circumferential lesion sets, were developed in an effort to avoid injury to the PVs themselves.

Segmental PV isolation refers to the application of lesion arcs immediately outside the ostia of the PVs and is based on the observation that discrete strands of myocardial tissue are found in PV ostia and represent attractive ablation targets. Segmental isolation is typically guided by a lasso catheter inserted into the PV, allowing for identification of the earliest activated region. A second ablation catheter is then used for lesion application. Ablation is performed at the region of earliest activation, with lesions placed outside the PV ostium.

Segmental ablation has been carefully studied in a number of prospective clinical trials (see Table 1 [44]) and remains a preferred method of some operators. Oral et al. investigated the efficacy of segmental ablation for patients with paroxysmal ($n = 58$) or

persistent ($n = 12$) AF [45]. In all patients, at least three PVs were targeted (with variable inclusion of the RIPV), with 94% success in acute isolation. Patients were followed for 150 ± 85 days. There was a 70% cure rate (freedom from AF) and 83% clinical improvement rate (freedom from or marked reduction of symptomatic AF) in patients with paroxysmal AF. Those patients with persistent AF had markedly worse results, with only 22% of patients getting cured of AF. Subsequent data from this group demonstrated inferiority of their segmental approach to circumferential PV isolation (discussed below). A review of the compiled data evaluating segmental PV isolation demonstrates a combined efficacy that reflects the disparities in success rates seen between patients with paroxysmal and persistent AF described by Oral et al. [45]. Intermediate-term success with segmental ablation was seen in 196 of 280 patients (70%) with paroxysmal AF, contrasted with 21 of 70 patients (30%) with persistent or permanent AF. PV stenosis remained a significant complication in these collected studies (incidence of 4.3%). Long-term data on this group is limited.

Pappone et al. have championed an alternative strategy for PV isolation, in which large circumferential lesions are placed around the ostia of the PVs [31,46–48]. Several variations of the procedure are practiced: a single long lesion encompassing the ostia of all four PVs, twin lesions around the left and right PV ostia, or four lesions, each targeting a single PV. In each case, lesions are made empirically, rather than targeting particular regions of early PV activation. Success rates using wide, circumferential lesions have been favorable, typically ranging between 56 and 95% [44].

Pappone et al. studied 251 patients consecutively between 1998 and 2000 [49], employing the circumferential approach. The majority of their patients had symptomatic, drug-refractory paroxysmal AF ($n = 179$), though some patients had permanent AF ($n = 72$). In most cases, each PV was isolated individually, with circumferential lesions applied > 5 mm outside the PV ostium. Some patients with closely paired or common PV ostia had larger lesions incorporating both ipsilateral PVs. The study reported follow-up data after 10 ± 4.5 months. In 179 patients with paroxysmal AF, 85% were free of AF; in 49 patients with persistent or permanent AF, 68% were free of AF. Importantly, the procedure appeared to markedly reduce the incidence of PV stenosis (none), and was generally well tolerated (tamponade in two patients).

Oral et al. have directly compared the segmental and circumferential approaches in a randomized,

Table 1 Summary of clinical studies of segmental PV ablation.

Study	Year	Success				Complications			
		Follow up (mo)	Overall	Paroxysmal AF	Persistent or permanent AF	PV stenosis (>50%)	Stroke	Cardiac tamponade	Mitral valve injury
Haissaguerre et al.	2000	4 ± 5	51/70 (73)	51/70 (73)	–	0	0	0	0
Oral et al.	2002	5 ± 3	44/70 (63)	41/58 (71)	3/12 (25)	0	1 (1.4)	0	0
Deisenhofer et al.[a]	2003	8 ± 4	38/75 (51)	N/A	NA	6 (8)	0	4 (53)	0
Marrouche et al.[b]	2003	14 ± 5	271/315 (86)	N/A	NA	22 (7)	2 (0.6)	0	0
Arentz et al.	2003	12	34/55 (62)	26/37 (70)	8/18 (44)	1 (1.8)	0	1 (1.8)	0
Oral et al.	2003	6	27/40 (67)	27/40 (67)	–	0	0	0	3
Mansour et al.	2004	21 ± 5	22/40 (55)	19/33 (58)	3/7 (43)	0	0	2 (5)	0
Vasamreddy et al.	2004	11 ± 8	39/75 (52)	32/42 (76)	7/33 (21)	3 (4)	2 (2.6)	2 (2.6)	1 (1.3)
Overall	–	–	526/740 (71)	196/280 (70)	21/70 (30)	32 (4.3)	5 (0.7)	9 (1.2)	1 (0.1)

Values are given as n (%); success was defined as tree of AF recurrence without antiarrhythmic drugs.
Source: Marine et al., 2005 [44]. Reproduced with permission of Elsevier.
[a] Seven-day Holter monitoring was used to screen AF recurrence.
[b] Intracardiac echocardiography was used to monitor ablation in 259 patients.

prospective trial [50]. Eighty patients, all with symptomatic paroxysmal AF, were evenly assigned to segmental or circumferential ablation. Ipsilateral veins were isolated in a single lesion with the circumferential technique. Procedure and fluoroscopy times did not vary significantly between the two groups. Success after 6 months, however, favored the circumferential (88% freedom from symptomatic AF) over the segmental approach (67% freedom from symptomatic AF). Complications did not vary meaningfully between the two groups, and were minimal (single iatrogenic LA flutter).

A recent review summarized the recent clinical trials investigating circumferential PV isolation efficacy (Table 2 [44]). Long-term success was seen in 290 of 393 patients (74%) with paroxysmal AF. In patients with persistent or permanent AF, success rates were predictably lower (73 of 149 patients – 49%). Also predictably, the incidence of PV stenosis was markedly reduced compared to focal or segmental ablation (0.4%). Other complications, including tamponade, stroke, and death, were all under 1%. Based in large part on these trials, and on the aforementioned limitations of focal and segmental PV isolation, circumferential ablation around the PVs remains a commonly used technique, either alone or in conjunction with alternative approaches, in the catheter-based treatment of AF.

The present – Johns Hopkins Hospital

At Johns Hopkins Hospital, we have prospectively investigated both segmental and circumferential techniques for AF ablation, publishing both intermediate- and long-term results [51–55]. We have chosen a stringent definition for success following AF ablation, defined as freedom from AF off all antiarrhythmic drugs. An important consideration in evaluating clinical trials describing success rates in AF ablation is the often protean and changing definition of success (ranging from reduction of symptoms to elimination of the rhythm per se). Using the segmental approach to ablation in a series [51] of 75 patients with paroxysmal (n = 42), persistent (n = 21), or permanent (n = 12) AF, acute isolation of electrically active PVs was achieved in 100% of cases. Forty-two of seventy-five patients required isolation of all four PVs. After 10.5 ± 7.5 months following a single (n = 75) or second (n = 11) procedure, 39 of the 75 patients were free from AF, 10 of 75 patients were markedly improved, and 26 reported no benefit from the procedure(s).

We prospectively investigated the circumferential approach in a series of 64 consecutive patients with

Table 2 Summary of clinical studies of CPVA.

Study	Year	Success				Complications			
		Follow-up (mo)	Overall	Paroxysmal AF	Persistent or permanent AF	PV stenosis (>50%)	Cardiac tamponade	Stroke	Left atrial flutter
Pappone et al.	2001	10 ± 5	188/251 (75)	148/179 (83)	40/72 (56)	0	2 (0.8)	0	0
Oral et al.	2003	6	35/40 (88)	35/40 (88)	–	0	0	0	1 (2.5)
Mansour et al.	2004	11 ± 3	25/40 (63)	21/32 (66)	4/8 (50)	0	1 (2.5)	1 (2.5)	0
Kottkamp et al.[a]	2004	12	37/100 (37)	34/80 (43)	3/20 (15)	0	0	0	4 (5)
Ouyang et al.[b]	2004	6 ± 1	39/41 (95)	39/41 (95)	–	0	0	0	0
Vasamreddy et al.	2004	6 ± 3	39/70 (56)	13/21 (62)	26/49 (53)	2 (2.8)	1 (1.4)	1 (1.4)	0
Overall	–	–	363/542 (67)	290/393 (74)	73/149 (49)	2 (0.4)	4 (0.7)	2 (0.4)	5 (0.9)

Values are given as *n* (%); success was defined as free of AF recurrence without antiarrhythmic drugs.
Source: Marine et al., 2005 [44]. Reproduced with permission of Elsevier.
[a] Seven-day Holter monitoring was used to screen AF recurrence.
[b] Two Lasso catheters were used to guide ablation to achieve PV isolation.

paroxysmal ($n = 29$) or persistent/permanent ($n = 35$) AF. Patients were followed for a mean of 13 ± 1 months [52]. After a single procedure, long-term success (freedom from AF) was found in 45% of patients. Nineteen patients with initial procedure failure elected to undergo a second procedure. The results including patients undergoing two procedures improved to an overall cure rate of 62%, with an additional 9% of patients significantly improved.

Based in part on these imperfect results, AF ablation techniques have continued to evolve at Johns Hopkins. At present, we perform a hybrid procedure that combines wide, circumferential ablation and limited segmental PV isolation. During this procedure, a double transseptal puncture is performed. PV electrical activity is monitored by lasso catheter. The right and left PVs are initially isolated in twin circumferential lesions. Following circumferential ablation, each vein is electrically isolated using a segmental approach, with care taken to avoid ablation in the PV itself. Long-term results from this procedure are forthcoming and appear to be promising.

Finally, it is important to note that other centers have investigated extra-PV foci as targets for ablation and have reported encouraging results. Nademanee, for instance, has described ablation of atrial foci in which high-frequency atrial electrograms are recorded [56]. He found that these sites are typically located in nine regions of the atria. Ablation during spontaneous or induced AF resulted in termination of fibrillation in 91% of cases, with a single-procedure success rate (freedom from AF off antiarrhythmic medications) after 12 month follow-up of 70%. Success increased to 83% after a redo procedure.

The future
The field of AF ablation is rapidly evolving. How the field is evolving can be broken down, for the purposes of discussion, into incremental developments and disruptive approaches.

Incremental developments
There are a number of ongoing incremental developments, principally in the area of technological approaches to delivery of PVI lesion sets, which are ongoing. Some of these novel techniques are mature and in widespread use. Cryoballoon ablation to achieve PVI, for instance, is now an established approach using second-generation technology (i.e., the Arctic Front Advance balloon now in common use). Other techniques, still designed to achieve PV isolation as the mainstay of therapy, are more experimental. These technologies include balloon-based ablation systems with laser or microwave energy systems, multipolar ablation catheters capable of delivering linear lesion sets, and also include novel mapping systems that allow for more detailed assessment of atrial conduction patterns.

It is clear that electrophysiologists are striving to find an ablation system or strategy that will deliver the best outcomes for their patients. At present, all of the futuristic ablation systems described above are no more than promising possibilities. In order for these new ablation systems to gain widespread acceptance, clinical trials will need to be performed that demonstrate increased efficacy, improved safety, and hopefully both shorter procedure times and reduced cost. Even if the first three are achieved, at an increased overall cost, this ablation system/approach will likely gain widespread acceptance.

Disruptive approaches

In parallel to the incremental steps toward achieving safe, rapid, and effective PV isolation described above, there are entirely novel approaches to rhythm control of AF that are being investigated that may play a significant role in shaping how we treat patients with symptomatic AF in the future. One of these potentially revolutionary approaches is a change in AF ablation targets from triggers to substrate. There is a growing appreciation that at least in select patients, AF is maintained by a pattern of stable reentry and that targeting reentrant rotors for ablation (either in addition to triggering sites or alone) may be a more effective and durable means of AF elimination [57]. To date there are only a limited number of centers performing rotor-based AF ablation, and it will certainly be interesting to see if AF ablation changes from a largely anatomic to a more electrophysiologically targeted procedure.

Second, there is the ongoing CABANA investigation, looking at whether drug therapy or first-line ablation therapy for AF is most beneficial. The data from this and other large clinical trials may impact who we send for AF ablation and what the relationship is between antiarrhythmic and ablative therapy in the hierarchy of rhythm-controlling strategies for AF ablation [58].

Conclusions

Catheter-based therapies for AF have evolved rapidly over the last 15 years. One of the striking aspects of that evolutionary process has been the discovery of fundamental mechanisms underlying AF, often revealed during the course of clinical investigation. Triggering of AF from ectopic foci, atrial electrophysiological properties permitting arrhythmia maintenance, and the physical and electrophysiological remodeling that occurs in the setting of AF all have been elucidated, in large part, through clinical investigations.

As importantly, the efficacy and risk-to-benefit ratio of nonpharmacological interventions for AF continues to improve. New modalities of ablation, including ultrasound, laser, microwave, and cryoablation are all subjects of ongoing investigation. Given the rate of progress in AF therapy over the past quarter century, safer and more effective techniques seem certain to emerge over the next 25 years. Given the aging of the US population, and the likely attendant flood of patients with AF at our doorstep, such advances are certainly worthy of aggressive pursuit.

References

1 Feinberg WM, Blackshear JL, Laupacis A, Kronmal R, Hart RG. Prevalence, age distribution, and gender of patients with atrial fibrillation. Analysis and implications. Arch Intern Med. 1995;155:469–473.

2 Singer DE. Overview of the randomized trials to prevent stroke in atrial fibrillation. Ann Epidemiol. 1993;3:563–567.

3 Singer DE. Anticoagulation for atrial fibrillation: epidemiology informing a difficult clinical decision. Proc Assoc Am Physicians. 1996;108:29–36.

4 Stroke Prevention in Atrial Fibrillation Study. Final results. Circulation. 1991;84:527–539.

5 Wyse DG, Waldo AL, DiMarco JP, Domanski MJ, Rosenberg Y, Schron EB, Kellen JC, Greene HL, Mickel MC, Dalquist JE, Corley SD. Atrial Fibrillation Follow-up Investigation of Rhythm Management (AFFIRM) Investigators: a comparison of rate control and rhythm control in patients with atrial fibrillation. N Engl J Med. 2002;347:1825–1833.

6 Van Gelder IC, Hagens VE, Bosker HA, Kingma JH, Kamp O, Kingma T, Said SA, Darmanata JI, Timmermans AJ, Tijssen JG, Crijns HJ, Rate Control versus Electrical Cardioversion for Persistent Atrial Fibrillation Study Group: a comparison of rate control and rhythm control in patients with recurrent persistent atrial fibrillation. N Engl J Med. 2002;347:1834–1840.

7 Roy D, Talajic M, Dorian P, Connolly S, Eisenberg MJ, Green M, Kus T, Lambert J, Dubuc M, Gagne P, Nattel S, Thibault B. Amiodarone to prevent recurrence of atrial fibrillation. Canadian Trial of Atrial Fibrillation Investigators. N Engl J Med. 2000;342:913–920.

8 Singh BN, Singh SN, Reda DJ, Tang XC, Lopez B, Harris CL, Fletcher RD, Sharma SC, Atwood JE, Jacobson AK, Lewis HD, Raisch DW, Jr, Ezekowitz MD. Sotalol Amiodarone Atrial Fibrillation Efficacy Trial (SAFE-T) Investigators. Amiodarone versus sotalol for atrial fibrillation. N Engl J Med. 2005;352:1861–1872.

9 Dogan A, Ergene O, Nazli C, Kinay O, Altinbas A, Ucarci Y, Ergene U, Ozaydin M, Gedikli O. Efficacy of propafenone for maintaining sinus rhythm in patients with recent onset or persistent atrial fibrillation after conversion: a randomized, placebo–controlled study. Acta Cardiol. 2004;59:255–261.

10 Moe GK, Abildskov JA. Atrial fibrillation as a self-sustaining arrhythmia independent of focal discharge. Am Heart J. 1959;58:59–70.

11 Moe GK, Rheinboldt WC, Abildskov JA. A Computer Model of Atrial Fibrillation. Am Heart J. 1964; 67:200–220.

12 Moe GK. A conceptual model of atrial fibrillation. J Electrocardiol. 1968;1:145–146.

13 Wijffels MC, Kirchhof CJ, Dorland R, Allessie MA. Atrial fibrillation begets atrial fibrillation: a study in awake chronically instrumented goats. Circulation. 1995; 92:1954–1968.

14 Allessie MA, Konings K, Kirchhof CJ, Wijffels M. Electrophysiologic mechanisms of perpetuation of atrial fibrillation. Am J Cardiol. 1996;77:10A–23A.

15 Allessie MA, Kirchhof CJ, Konings KT. Unravelling the electrical mysteries of atrial fibrillation. Eur Heart J. 1996;17 Suppl C: 2–9.

16 Bhandari A, Morady F, Shen EN, Schwartz AB, Botvinick E, Scheinman MM. Catheter-induced His bundle ablation in a patient with reentrant tachycardia associated with a nodoventricular tract. J Am Coll Cardiol. 1984;4:611–616.

17 Lee MA, Morady F, Kadish A, Schamp DJ, Chin MC, Scheinman MM, Griffin JC, Lesh MD, Pederson D, Goldberger J. Catheter modification of the atrioventricular junction with radiofrequency energy for control of atrioventricular nodal reentry tachycardia. Circulation. 1991; 83:827–835.

18 Calkins H, Sousa J, el-Atassi R, Rosenheck S, de Buitleir M, Kou WH, Kadish AH, Langberg JJ, Morady F. Diagnosis and cure of the Wolff–Parkinson–White syndrome or paroxysmal supraventricular tachycardias during a single electrophysiologic test. N Engl J Med. 1991; 324:1612–1618.

19 Calkins H, Leon AR, Deam AG, Kalbfleisch SJ, Langberg JJ, Morady F. Catheter ablation of atrial flutter using radiofrequency energy. Am J Cardiol. 1994;73:353–356.

20 Jackman WM, Wang XZ, Friday KJ, Roman CA, Moulton KP, Beckman KJ, McClelland JH, Twidale N, Hazlitt HA, Prior MI. Catheter ablation of accessory atrioventricular pathways (Wolff–Parkinson–White syndrome) by radiofrequency current. N Engl J Med. 1991;324:1605–1611.

21 Gaskell WH. On the innervation of the heart, with especial reference to the heart of the tortoise. J Physiol. 1883;4:43–230. 14.

22 Scheinman MM, Morady F, Hess DS, Gonzalez R. Catheter-induced ablation of the atrioventricular junction to control refractory supraventricular arrhythmias. JAMA. 1982;248:851–855.

23 Haissaguerre M, Gencel L, Fischer B, Le Metayer P, Poquet F, Marcus FI, Clementy J. Successful catheter ablation of atrial fibrillation. J Cardiovasc Electrophysiol. 1994;5:1045–1052.

24 Jais P, Shah DC, Takahashi A, Hocini M, Haissaguerre M, Clementy J. Long-term follow-up after right atrial radiofrequency catheter treatment of paroxysmal atrial fibrillation. Pacing Clin Electrophysiol. 1998; 21:2533–2538.

25 Haissaguerre M, Jais P, Shah DC, Gencel L, Pradeau V, Garrigues S, Chouairi S, Hocini M, Le Metayer P, Roudaut R, Clementy J. Right and left atrial radiofrequency catheter therapy of paroxysmal atrial fibrillation. J Cardiovasc Electrophysiol. 1996;7:1132–1144.

26 Jais P, Shah DC, Haissaguerre M, Takahashi A, Lavergne T, Hocini M, Garrigue S, Barold SS, Le Metayer P, Clementy J. Efficacy and safety of septal and left-atrial linear ablation for atrial fibrillation. Am J Cardiol. 1999;84:139R–146R.

27 Haissaguerre M, Jais P, Shah DC, Takahashi A, Hocini M, Quiniou G, Garrigue S, Le Mouroux A, Le Metayer P, Clementy J. Spontaneous initiation of atrial fibrillation by ectopic beats originating in the pulmonary veins. N Engl J Med. 1998;339:659–666.

28 Natale A, Leonelli F, Beheiry S, Newby K, Pisano E, Potenza D, Rajkovich K, Wides B, Cromwell L, Tomassoni G. Catheter ablation approach on the right side only for paroxysmal atrial fibrillation therapy: long-term results. Pacing Clin Electrophysiol. 2000;23:224–233.

29 Gaita F, Riccardi R, Calo L, Scaglione M, Garberoglio L, Antolini R, Kirchner M, Lamberti F, Richiardi E. Atrial mapping and radiofrequency catheter ablation in patients with idiopathic atrial fibrillation: electrophysiological findings and ablation results. Circulation. 1998; 97:2136–2145.

30 Cox JL. Cardiac surgery for arrhythmias. J Cardiovasc Electrophysiol. 2004;15:250–262.

31 Pappone C, Oreto G, Lamberti F, Vicedomini G, Loricchio ML, Shpun S, Rillo M, Calabro MP, Conversano A, Ben-Haim SA, Cappato R, Chierchia S. Catheter ablation of paroxysmal atrial fibrillation using a 3D mapping system. Circulation. 1999;100:1203–1208.

32 Haissaguerre M, Marcus FI, Fischer B, Clementy J. Radiofrequency catheter ablation in unusual mechanisms of atrial fibrillation: report of three cases. J Cardiovasc Electrophysiol. 1994;5:743–751.

33 Jais P, Haissaguerre M, Shah DC, Chouairi S, Gencel L, Hocini M, Clementy J. A focal source of atrial fibrillation treated by discrete radiofrequency ablation. Circulation. 1997;95:572–576.

34 Lau CP, Tse HF, Ayers GM. Defibrillation-guided radiofrequency ablation of atrial fibrillation secondary to an atrial focus. J Am Coll Cardiol. 1999;33:1217–1226.

35 Tsai CF, Chen SA, Tai CT, Chiou CW, Prakash VS, Yu WC, Hsieh MH, Ding YA, Chang MS. Bezold-Jarisch-like reflex during radiofrequency ablation of the pulmonary vein tissues in patients with paroxysmal focal atrial fibrillation. J Cardiovasc Electrophysiol. 1999;10:27–35.

36 Chen SA, Hsieh MH, Tai CT, Tsai CF, Prakash VS, Yu WC, Hsu TL, Ding YA, Chang MS. Initiation of atrial fibrillation by ectopic beats originating from the pulmonary veins: electrophysiological characteristics, pharmacological responses, and effects of radiofrequency ablation. Circulation. 1999;100:1879–1886.

37 Lin WS, Prakash VS, Tai CT, Hsieh MH, Tsai CF, Yu WC, Lin YK, Ding YA, Chang MS, Chen SA. Pulmonary vein morphology in patients with paroxysmal atrial fibrillation initiated by ectopic beats originating from the pulmonary

veins: implications for catheter ablation. Circulation. 2000;101:1274–1281.

38 Haissaguerre M, Shah DC, Jais P, Hocini M, Yamane T, Deisenhofer I, Garrigue S, Clementy J. Mapping-guided ablation of pulmonary veins to cure atrial fibrillation. Am J Cardiol. 2000;86:9K–19K.

39 Haissaguerre M, Jais P, Shah DC, Garrigue S, Takahashi A, Lavergne T, Hocini M, Peng JT, Roudaut R, Clementy J. Electrophysiological end point for catheter ablation of atrial fibrillation initiated from multiple pulmonary venous foci. Circulation. 2000;101:1409–1417.

40 Haissaguerre M, Jais P, Shah DC, Arentz T, Kalusche D, Takahashi A, Garrigue S, Hocini M, Peng JT, Clementy J. Catheter ablation of chronic atrial fibrillation targeting the reinitiating triggers. J Cardiovasc Electrophysiol. 2000;11:2–10.

41 Saad EB, Marrouche NF, Saad CP, Ha E, Bash D, White RD, Rhodes J, Prieto L, Martin DO, Saliba WI, Schweikert RA, Natale A. Pulmonary vein stenosis after catheter ablation of atrial fibrillation: emergence of a new clinical syndrome. Ann Intern Med. 2003;138:634–638.

42 Saad EB, Rossillo A, Saad CP, Martin DO, Bhargava M, Erciyes D, Bash D, Williams-Andrews M, Beheiry S, Marrouche NF, Adams J, Pisano E, Fanelli R, Potenza D, Raviele A, Bonso A, Themistoclakis S, Brachmann J, Saliba WI, Schweikert RA, Natale A. Pulmonary vein stenosis after radiofrequency ablation of atrial fibrillation: functional characterization, evolution, and influence of the ablation strategy. Circulation. 2003;108:3102–3107.

43 Nilsson B, Chen X, Pehrson S, Jensen HL, Sondergaard L, Helvind M, Andersen LW, Svendsen JH. Acute fatal pulmonary vein occlusion after catheter ablation of atrial fibrillation. J Interv Card Electrophysiol. 2004; 11:127–130.

44 Marine JE, Dong J, Calkins H. Catheter ablation therapy for atrial fibrillation. Prog Cardiovasc Dis. 2005; 48:178–192.

45 Oral H, Knight BP, Tada H, Ozaydin M, Chugh A, Hassan S, Scharf C, Lai SW, Greenstein R, Pelosi F, Strickberger SA, Jr, Morady F. Pulmonary vein isolation for paroxysmal and persistent atrial fibrillation. Circulation. 2002;105:1077–1081.

46 Pappone C, Rosanio S, Oreto G, Tocchi M, Gugliotta F, Vicedomini G, Salvati A, Dicandia C, Mazzone P, Santinelli V, Gulletta S, Chierchia S. Circumferential radiofrequency ablation of pulmonary vein ostia: a new anatomic approach for curing atrial fibrillation. Circulation. 2000;102:2619–2628.

47 Pappone C, Rosanio S, Oreto G, Tocchi M, Gugliotta F, Salvati A, Dicandia C, Mazzone P, Santinelli V, Gulletta S, Vicedomini G. Prospects of the treatment of atrial fibrillation: circumferential radiofrequency ablation of pulmonary vein ostia. Recenti Prog Med. 2001;92:508–512.

48 Pappone C, Rosanio S, Augello G, Gallus G, Vicedomini G, Mazzone P, Gulletta S, Gugliotta F, Pappone A, Santinelli V, Tortoriello V, Sala S, Zangrillo A, Crescenzi

G, Benussi S, Alfieri O. Mortality, morbidity, and quality of life after circumferential pulmonary vein ablation for atrial fibrillation: outcomes from a controlled non-randomized long-term study. J Am Coll Cardiol. 2003; 42:185–197.

49 Pappone C, Oreto G, Rosanio S, Vicedomini G, Tocchi M, Gugliotta F, Salvati A, Dicandia C, Calabro MP, Mazzone P, Ficarra E, Di Gioia C, Gulletta S, Nardi S, Santinelli V, Benussi S, Alfieri O. Atrial electroanatomic remodeling after circumferential radiofrequency pulmonary vein ablation: efficacy of an anatomic approach in a large cohort of patients with atrial fibrillation. Circulation. 2001;104:2539–2544.

50 Oral H, Scharf C, Chugh A, Hall B, Cheung P, Good E, Veerareddy S, Pelosi F, Jr, Morady F. Catheter ablation for paroxysmal atrial fibrillation: segmental pulmonary vein ostial ablation versus left atrial ablation. Circulation. 2003;108:2355–2360.

51 Vasamreddy CR, Lickfett L, Jayam VK, Nasir K, Bradley DJ, Eldadah Z, Dickfeld T, Berger R, Calkins H. Predictors of recurrence following catheter ablation of atrial fibrillation using an irrigated-tip ablation catheter. J Cardiovasc Electrophysiol. 2004;15:692–697.

52 Vasamreddy CR, Dalal D, Eldadah Z, Dickfeld T, Jayam VK, Henrikson C, Meininger G, Dong J, Lickfett L, Berger R, Calkins H. Safety and efficacy of circumferential pulmonary vein catheter ablation of atrial fibrillation. Heart Rhythm. 2005;2:42–48.

53 Vasamreddy CR, Dalal D, Dong J, Cheng A, Spragg D, Lamiy SZ, Meininger G, Henrikson CA, Marine JE, Berger R, Calkins H. Symptomatic and asymptomatic atrial fibrillation in patients undergoing radiofrequency catheter ablation. J Cardiovasc Electrophysiol. 2006; 17:134–139.

54 Cheema A, Vasamreddy CR, Dalal D, Marine JE, Dong J, Henrikson CA, Spragg D, Cheng A, Nazarian S, Sinha S, Halperin H, Berger R, Calkins H. Long-term single procedure efficacy of catheter ablation of atrial fibrillation. J Interv Card Electrophysiol. 2006;15:145–155.

55 Cheema A, Dong J, Dalal D, Vasamreddy CR, Marine JE, Henrikson CA, Spragg D, Cheng A, Nazarian S, Sinha S, Halperin H, Berger R, Calkins H. Long-term safety and efficacy of circumferential ablation with pulmonary vein isolation. J Cardiovasc Electrophysiol. 2006;17:1080–1085.

56 Nademanee K, McKenzie J, Kosar E, Schwab M, Sunsaneewitayakul B, Vasavakul T, Khunnawat C, Ngarmukos T. A new approach for catheter ablation of atrial fibrillation: mapping of the electrophysiologic substrate. J Am Coll Cardiol. 2004;43:2044–2053.

57 Narayan SM, Krummen DE, Shivkumar K, Clopton P, Rappel WJ, Miller JM. Treatment of atrial fibrillation by the ablation of localized sources: CONFIRM (Conventional Ablation for Atrial Fibrillation With or Without Focal Impulse and Rotor Modulation) trial. J Am Coll Cardiol. 2012;60:628–36.

58 Packer D. CABANA Investigator Meeting, 2009.

CHAPTER 3

Staffing, training, and ongoing volume requirements

Mehdi Namdar & Dipen Shah

Service de Cardiologie, Hôpitaux Universitaires de Genève, Geneva, Switzerland

Catheter ablation of atrial fibrillation (AF) has undergone substantial development over the past 15 years. Advances in catheter technology and the plethora of scientific observations have contributed to our understanding of underlying mechanisms and reasonable, evidence-based, therapeutic strategies have been developed leading to the adoption of wide area circumferential ablation and substrate modification by an increasing number of electrophysiologists. A recent survey of practicing electrophysiologists revealed that 30% performed AF ablations [1]. Nevertheless, the currently used techniques are still evolving and the long-term risk–benefit ratio remains to be determined. It needs to be emphasized that AF ablation is a technically challenging procedure and has a higher periprocedural risk than the ablation of any other arrhythmia (see Chapter 26). This is certainly why this procedure should be performed only in appropriately equipped electrophysiology laboratories staffed by experienced and well-trained operators and support personnel. These considerations should play an important role in the decision whether or not to offer an AF ablation program and a respective training program.

Staffing

The extent of an electrophysiologic laboratory staff and its skill level varies with the complexity of the procedures but should, however, always guarantee patient safety and positive outcomes. Generally, the entire personnel may include staff physicians (EP lab medical director, teaching attending physicians, EP lab attending), secondary operators and/or EP fellows, and anesthesia service and nonphysician members such as nurses/certified EP technicians, nurse anesthetists, patient preparation and recovery staff, radiological and IT technologists/biomedical engineers, scheduling coordinators, purchasing, inventory and supply personnel, and housekeeping. Finally, some mapping, recording, and/or ablation systems may be assisted by industry representatives according to the laboratory's policies [2]. Naturally, minimum permanent and temporary staffing recommendations for EP procedures are based on the type of procedure. While a basic EP study might require an independent electrophysiologist, one nurse, and one EP technician as permanent staff, more extended permanent and temporary staff recommendations may be applied for AF ablation procedures (Table 1).

Training

Accomplishing as well as maintaining the cognitive and technical skills, which are necessary for the adequate performance of any particular cardiovascular procedure generally implicate the awareness of details on indications and patient selection, potential procedural risks and benefits, basic theoretical and anatomical knowledge, technical competence, management of complications, and meaningful follow-up strategies. Such basic points should be an inherent part of continued education not only for electrophysiology trainees but also for nurses and technical staff since achieving greater knowledge and understanding of any procedure guarantees a highly effective team work in order to achieve a reasonable therapeutic goal for the patient. Naturally, AF ablation procedures

Practical Guide to Catheter Ablation of Atrial Fibrillation, Second Edition. Edited by Jonathan S. Steinberg, Pierre Jaïs and Hugh Calkins.
© 2016 John Wiley & Sons, Ltd. Published 2016 by John Wiley & Sons, Ltd.

Table 1 Permanent and temporary staffing recommendations.

Type of procedure	Permanent staff	Temporary staff
EP study	1 Electrophysiologist 1 Nurse (patient care) 1 EP technician	No specific requirements
AF ablation	1 Electrophysiologist 1 Nurse (patient care) 1 EP technician	1 Secondary operator (MD) 1 Nurse (anesthesia/sedation) 1 Nurse helps with catheters/fluoroscopy 1 Industry representative (3D-mapping system) 1 Industry representative (ICE, Cryo-Console, robotic navigation systems)

comprise further distinctive features such as the interpretation of pulmonary vein electrograms, related pacing maneuvers, the use of three-dimensional mapping systems and other imaging modalities (registration of preacquired images, intracardiac echo. etc.), and left atrial access by transseptal puncture.

Indications, patient selection, and procedural issues

Electrophysiologists involved in catheter ablation of AF should be updated on current clinical guidelines and recommendations with regard to indications/contraindications and patient selection (see Chapter 1). To that effect, preprocedural examinations (physical examination, TTE/TEE, and Holter-ECG), drug regimen (antiarrhythmic agents, generally to be stopped five half-lives prior to the procedure/anticoagulation) and basic laboratory results (electrolytes, blood urea nitrogen, creatinine, GFR, complete blood count, and INR) should be reviewed systematically for every patient. Furthermore, individual potential risks and benefits of the procedure should be evaluated carefully and explained to the patient optimally in the outpatient setting prior to the EP procedure. Accordingly, comorbidities and factors adversely impacting procedural outcome and anesthesia management (allergies, previous complications, and obstructive sleep apnea) have to be identified. Finally, formal informed consent has to be obtained before the procedure and should include full disclosure of risks.

Basic theoretical and anatomical knowledge

A comprehensive and detailed knowledge of the basic electrophysiological principles including the correct recognition of intracavitary electrograms, arrhythmia mechanisms, and pacing maneuvers is essential before starting catheter ablation of AF. This should include a detailed knowledge of diagnostic electrophysiology, the differential diagnosis of SVTs and their

appropriate, effective and safe ablation by catheter. The next prerequisite step in training is a similar detailed knowledge of typical flutter and understanding of entrainment and activation mapping as well as effective ablation with special emphasis on the techniques of creating and recognizing linear conduction block. Correspondingly, identification of PV potentials both at baseline and during different pacing maneuvers and when PV isolation is achieved remains crucial. Different ablation strategies and specific targets for paroxysmal and persistent AF (e.g., complex fractionated atrial electrograms, linear ablation in the left atrium) should be recognized. The electrophysiologist must also be proficient in peripheral vascular, cardiac, particularly left atrial anatomy, and adjacent structures both actual and fluoroscopic.

Furthermore, a relatively advanced level of interventional skills is certainly desirable in order to minimize the risk of procedure-related complications when performing technical steps such as transseptal puncture, cannulation of pulmonary veins, navigation and ablation in the left atrium with different types of catheters (see below).

Technical skills

Every procedure comes along with the use of many different occasionally sophisticated technical modalities. It is, therefore, mandatory to get familiar with the functionality, correct preparation, and adequate manipulation of the latter. Hereby, applying a systematic, algorithmic approach is strongly advised. Generally required technical skills for trainees before being involved in AF ablation are as follows:
• Correct manipulation of fluoroscopic system and projections/landmarks
• Proper preparation of materials used including flushing of sheaths, guidewires
• Vascular access, cannulation, and hemostasis
• Catheter/guidewire manipulation and correct positioning

• Technique of recording intracardiac pressures and their interpretation
• Left-sided catheter and sheath management
• Intraprocedural anticoagulation monitoring and use
• Preparation and comprehension of EP and 3D electroanatomical systems
• Preparation and understanding of materials – in the form of prepared ready-to-use kits – to be used in case of complications

Owing to both the rapid technological progress and the rising concerns on radiation exposure over the past so many years, three-dimensional electroanatomical mapping systems have become an integral part of many electrophysiologic laboratories and procedures. Here again, electrophysiologists involved in AF ablation should have knowledge not only of the technical aspects of the respective system, its handling, and interpretation of acquired maps but also its limitations. Although indications and the integration of an electroanatomical mapping into different procedures strongly depends on the philosophy of each laboratory, trainees should be familiar with activation mapping (for atrial macro-reentrant tachycardia) and voltage mapping (for substrate-guided ablation).

Transseptal puncture

An in-depth knowledge of the anatomy of both atria and adjacent structures and transseptal puncture materials and techniques is crucial for interventional cardiologists involved in any left-sided procedure. Initially introduced for left-sided pressure measurements, it is nowadays integrated into a variety of procedures. Finally, despite the broad establishment of AF ablation procedures, transseptal catheterization remains a technically demanding procedure requiring a certain level of experience in order to avoid eventually life-threatening complications. Accordingly, the trainee must be fully aware of advantages and limitations of available options in the transseptal puncture approach, of signs, which are suggestive of successful access in the left atrium, recognize high-risk cases for transseptal puncture or contraindications [3]. Generally, it needs to be emphasized on the one hand that the more experienced the operator, the quicker she or he will learn new techniques and on the other hand that experience remains the main determinant for procedural safety.

Follow-up

Postinterventional observational and follow-up principles of rhythm monitoring define the rates of acute, mid-, and long-term success. Thus, every physician encountering patients, who have undergone AF

ablation, must be aware of these principles. Furthermore, indications/contraindications including risk–benefit considerations for cardioversion, concomitant use of drugs (antiarrhythmic regimen and anticoagulation), and timing of a repeat procedure have to be recognized [4,5].

Volume requirements

Basic training

Many factors determine successful training, and it is a difficult undertaking to set requirements for a number of procedures to gain proficiency. This is especially true of a multistep, multifaceted complex procedure such as catheter ablation of AF. Individual differences in interventional cardiology background and familiarity with LA anatomy also play a large role in generating differences in aptitude. Thus, there are no strict norms or rules. Yet, expert committees have been trying to formulate recommendations and establish precise criteria specifically addressing this matter (Table 2) [6–8]. Generally, the beginning of an electrophysiology training should be envisaged after the completion of a 3-year formation in cardiovascular medicine with proficiency in acute management of potential complications [6,9]. Nevertheless, backup of an experienced physician with skills in emergency needle pericardiocentesis is highly recommended and training in pericardiocentesis, whenever possible, advised [8].

Both the European Heart Rhythm Association and Heart Rhythm Society (EHRA and HRS) generally agree that a minimum of 12 months of basic training in conventional electrophysiology procedures including simpler (mostly right-sided) ablations is needed to

Table 2 Minimum recommended numbers for trainees involved in AF ablation.

Procedure	Training	Recredentialing
Transseptal punctures	10–20	20
Diagnostic EP studies	150	50
SVT studies and maneuvers	75	25
Catheter ablations Including AVNRT, typical AFL, accessory pathways (15 with retrograde aortic approach), VT	100–150 30–50 as primary operator	50
Atrial fibrillation	30–50	20
Complex flutter ablations	15–25	15

acquire the cognitive and technical skills before being involved in AF ablation procedures [6,10]. Consequently, the second year of the fellowship should provide training in more complex, including left-sided, procedures. While such recommendations strongly depend on the skills of the trainee and the "size" of the laboratory and whether experience with a diverse patient population manifesting a broad variety of arrhythmias can be offered, most of the scientific organizations still agree that an acceptable basic training in most frequently encountered arrhythmias and most important aspects of electrophysiology, including ablation, is expected to take up to 24 months [11]. Until here, the electrophysiology trainee should have been directly involved in 100–150 ablation procedures, whereof at least 30–35 as the primary operator, that is, level of competence III as defined by the HRS and EHRA [8,11–13]. These numbers include the ablation of a mix of arrhythmias, namely, AV nodal reentrant tachycardia, typical atrial flutter, AV junction ablation, accessory pathways (explicitly 15 ablations required with a retrograde aortic approach), and ventricular tachycardia [6,14].

When it comes to AF ablation, the establishment of such numeric guidelines and criteria remains justifiably difficult. This may be due to the higher degree of procedural complexity, concomitant life-threatening complications, and the variety of different ablation strategies and lesion sets to treat AF. A common denominator, however, is the access to the left atrium, achieved via transseptal puncture. The American College of Cardiology recommends 10 transseptal punctures to be performed in order to be considered trained for this task [6]. Others suggest the performance of 20 supervised transseptal punctures as a reasonable amount of competence [15]. Furthermore, the 2012 HRS/EHRA/ECAS Expert Consensus Statement on Catheter and Surgical Ablation of Atrial Fibrillation recommends for physicians' training in AF ablation and complex atrial tachycardias to perform at least 25 cases of each as primary operator, mentored by an experienced electrophysiologist [16]. Thus, it is strongly advisable that electrophysiologists, who have accomplished their fellowship training, are proficient in performing conventional ablation procedures and wish to undergo further training in AF ablation, should observe colleagues with a high degree of expertise [4]. This is in line with the former published update of the clinical competence statement on invasive electrophysiology studies, catheter ablation, and cardioversion by the American College of Cardiology/American Heart Association and the Canadian Guidelines, proposing for trainees to perform a minimum of 30–50 AF ablation procedures and 15–20 complex flutter

ablations [11,16,17]. Furthermore, electrophysiologists should perform several AF ablation procedures per month if they wish to remain active in this field along with tracking the outcomes of their ablations [4]. Most of the experts agree that it may be inappropriate to perform AF ablations without any training in electrophysiology since the patient population as well as frequently encountered arrhythmias such as atypical atrial flutters and other atrial tachycardias require training that is unique to electrophysiology fellowships [4,18]. In any case, exact numerical requirements remain difficult and a delicate matter, as technical skills vary on an individual basis and develop at different rates. Nevertheless, it has to be emphasized that complication and recurrence rates as well as fluoroscopy times are lower and general outcomes better at experienced centers exhibiting more than 100 AF ablation procedures/year [19–21]. Moreover, joint efforts have been made in recent years by different national heart rhythm associations for the assessment of established training programs in order to promote continuous improvement of the latter [10,11]. These assessment methods imply new strategies such as the use of reports by the training program supervisor, a logbook of procedures performed by the trainee, self-assessment programs, and competence examinations in electrocardiography and written theoretical exams aiming to develop not only a certification but also a recertification or recredentialing system [11,13]. For the time being, required numbers of ablations for recredentialing have been set as summarized in Table 2. However, these numbers may need to be adapted periodically according to revised clinical competence statements and requirements.

Training strategies: New technologies

In the context of training strategies, various high-fidelity simulator and/or virtual reality training systems have been developed in the past decades in order to improve procedural skills. In fact, superior post-training performance and reduction in radiation exposure were shown to be linked with mentored simulation training despite a shorter simulator training time compared to conventional training [22–25]. It seems further that the less proficient the operator is, the greater the benefit from the mentored simulator-based training, avoiding patient exposure to the early phase of the operator's learning curve – a less safe period in terms of complications such as tamponade [23,26]. However, such systems do not and cannot represent a fully comprehensive stand-alone training modality and should be understood as sophisticated (and eventually expensive – US$ 6000 to $250'000) complementary tools. Thus, mentoring by proficient and experienced operators stays instrumental in teaching the procedural steps.

In the course of recent developments, novel ablation modalities ("single-shot" devices with a purely anatomical approach, different energy sources, and remote robotic navigation systems) have been introduced focusing on optimization of AF ablation procedures both for patients and for operators. Of note, the new tools were also drafted to make AF ablation "simple, fast, and safe" and to be used by operators with little prior experience. Many of them stood the test of feasibility and clinical applicability and showed initial promising results with regard to outcomes compared to established techniques, however, in *experienced* hands. Hence, the main question remains as to which extent such new modalities and their positive effects might be reproducible in less-experienced centers, which, nonetheless, would want to offer these new technologies. In this regard, data (mainly analyzing procedural/fluoroscopy time and safety as crucial stages of the learning curve) are scarce and rather conflicting, yet come to one and the same conclusion: whatever technology may be applied, the more experienced the operator, the shorter the learning curve [27–29].

Finally, where available, mentored simulator-based training may certainly also help to acquire skills required to make use of such new technologies and transfer these skills readily to actual procedures. Otherwise, international proctorships may be of great benefit, as has been experienced in many other purely interventional/operative medical domains, representing a modern form of an old apprenticeship model, which after all proved valuable in passing skills and expertise from one generation to the next: see one, do one, teach one.

References

1 Mickelsen S, Dudley B, Treat E, Barela J, Omdahl J, Kusumoto F. Survey of physician experience, trends and outcomes with atrial fibrillation ablation. J Interv Card Electrophysiol. 2005;12(3):213–220.

2 Haines DE. 2013. HRS Expert Consensus Statement on Electrophysiology (EP) Lab Standards: Ergonomics, Equipment, Personnel, Policy and Safety. Unpublished data.

3 Tzeis S, Andrikopoulos G, Deisenhofer I, Ho SY, Theodorakis G. Transseptal catheterization: considerations and caveats. Pacing Clin Electrophysiol. 2010;33(2):231–242.

4 Calkins H, Brugada J, Packer DL, Cappato R, Chen SA, Crijns HJ, et al. HRS/EHRA/ECAS expert consensus statement on catheter and surgical ablation of atrial fibrillation: recommendations for personnel, policy, procedures and follow-up. A report of the Heart Rhythm Society (HRS) Task Force on catheter and surgical ablation of atrial fibrillation. Heart Rhythm. 2007;4(6):816–861.

5 Kirchhof P, Auricchio A, Bax J, Crijns H, Camm J, Diener HC, et al. Outcome parameters for trials in atrial fibrillation: recommendations from a consensus conference organized by the German Atrial Fibrillation Competence NETwork and the European Heart Rhythm Association. Europace. 2007;9(11):1006–1023.

6 Tracy CM, Akhtar M, DiMarco JP, Packer DL, Weitz HH, Creager MA, et al. American College of Cardiology/American Heart Association 2006 update of the clinical competence statement on invasive electrophysiologystudies, catheterablation, andcardioversion: a report of the American College of Cardiology/American Heart Association/American College of Physicians Task Force on Clinical Competence and Training developed in collaboration with the Heart Rhythm Society. J Am Coll Cardiol. 2006;48(7):1503–1517.

7 Naccarelli GV, Conti JB, DiMarco JP, Tracy CM. Task Force 6: training in specialized electrophysiology, cardiac pacing, and arrhythmia management: endorsed by the Heart Rhythm Society. J Am Coll Cardiol. 2006;47(4):904–910.

8 Natale A, Raviele A, Arentz T, Calkins H, Chen SA, Haissaguerre M, et al. Venice Chart International Consensus Document on Atrial Fibrillation Ablation. J Cardiovasc Electrophysiol. 2007;18(5):560–580.

9 Mitchell LB, Dorian P, Gillis A, Kerr C, Klein G, Talajic M. Standards for training in adult clinical cardiac electrophysiology. Canadian Cardiovascular Society Committee. Can J Cardiol. 1996;12(5):476–480.

10 Merino JL, Arribas F, Botto GL, Huikuri H, Kraemer LI, Linde C, et al. Core curriculum for the heart rhythm specialist. Europace. 2009;11Suppl 3:iii1–26.

11 Naccarelli GV, Conti JB, DiMarco JP, Tracy CM. Task force 6: training in specialized electrophysiology, cardiac pacing, and arrhythmia management endorsed by the Heart Rhythm Society. J Am Coll Cardiol. 2008;51(3):374–380.

12 Scheinman MM. Catheter ablation for cardiac arrhythmias, personnel, and facilities. North American Society of Pacing and Electrophysiology Ad Hoc Committee on Catheter Ablation. Pacing Clin Electrophysiol. 1992;15(5):715–721.

13 Merino JL, Arribas F, Botto GL, Huikuri H, Kraemer LI, Linde C, et al. Core curriculum for the heart rhythm specialist: executive summary. Europace. 2009;11(10):1381–1386.

14 Josephson ME, Maloney JD, Barold SS, Flowers NC, Goldschlager NF, Hayes DL, et al. Guidelines for training in adult cardiovascular medicine. Core Cardiology Training Symposium (COCATS). Task Force 6: training in specialized electrophysiology, cardiac pacing and arrhythmia management. J Am Coll Cardiol. 1995;25(1):23–26.

15 Linker NJ, Fitzpatrick AP. The transseptal approach for ablation of cardiac arrhythmias: experience of 104 procedures. Heart. 1998;79(4):379 382.

16 Calkins H, Kuck KH, Cappato R, Brugada J, Camm AJ, Chen SA, et al. HRS/EHRA/ECAS Expert Consensus Statement on Catheter and Surgical Ablation of Atrial Fibrillation: recommendations for patient selection,

procedural techniques, patient management and follow-up, definitions, endpoints, and research trial design. Europace. 2012;14(4):528–606.

17 Green MS, Guerra PG, Krahn AD. Canadian Cardiovascular Society/Canadian Heart Rhythm Society Training Standards and Maintenance of Competency in Adult Clinical Cardiac Electrophysiology. Can J Cardiol. 2010;27(6):859–861.

18 Scheinman M, Calkins H, Gillette P, Klein R, Lerman BB, Morady F, et al. NASPE policy statement on catheter ablation: personnel, policy, procedures, and therapeutic recommendations. Pacing Clin Electrophysiol. 2003;26 (3):789–799.

19 Cappato R, Calkins H, Chen SA, Davies W, Iesaka Y, Kalman J, et al. Updated worldwide survey on the methods, efficacy, and safety of catheter ablation for human atrial fibrillation. Circ Arrhythm Electrophysiol. 2005;3 (1):32–38.

20 Calkins H, el-Atassi R, Kalbfleisch SJ, Langberg JJ, Morady F. Effect of operator experience on outcome of radiofrequency catheter ablation of accessory pathways. Am J Cardiol. 1993; 71(12):1104–1105.

21 Rosenheck S, Rose M, Sharon Z, Weiss TA, Gotsman MS. The ongoing influence of staff training on the performance of radiofrequency catheter ablation. Pacing Clin Electrophysiol. 1997;20(5 Pt 1):1312–1317.

22 De Ponti R, Marazzi R, Ghiringhelli S, Salerno-Uriarte JA, Calkins H, Cheng A. Superiority of simulator-based training compared with conventional training methodologies in the performance of transseptal catheterization. J Am Coll Cardiol. 2011;58(4):359–363.

23 De Ponti R, Marazzi R, Doni LA, Tamborini C, Ghiringhelli S, Salerno-Uriarte JA. Simulator training reduces radiation exposure and improves trainees' performance in placing electrophysiologic catheters during patient-based procedures. Heart Rhythm. 2012;9 (8):1280–1285.

24 De Ponti R. Transseptal catheterization: a matter of technology, training, or both? Europace. 2012;14 (5):615–616.

25 Bagai A, O'Brien S, Al Lawati H, Goyal P, Ball W, Grantcharov T, et al. Mentored simulation training improves procedural skills in cardiac catheterization: a randomized, controlled pilot study. Circ Cardiovasc Interv. 2012;5(5):672–679.

26 Sairaku A, Nakano Y, Oda N, Makita Y, Kajihara K, Tokuyama T, et al. Learning curve for ablation of atrial fibrillation in medium-volume centers. J Cardiol. 2011;57 (3):263–268.

27 Maagh P, Butz T, Plehn G, Christoph A, Meissner A. Pulmonary vein isolation in 2012: is it necessary to perform a time consuming electrophysical mapping or should we focus on rapid and safe therapies? A retrospective analysis of different ablation tools. Int J Med Sci. 2012;10(1):24–33.

28 Rillig A, Meyerfeldt U, Birkemeyer R, Treusch F, Kunze M, Miljak T, et al. Remote robotic catheter ablation for atrial fibrillation: how fast is it learned and what benefits can be earned? J Interv Card Electrophysiol. 2010;29 (2):109–117.

29 Schmidt B, Tilz RR, Neven K, Julian Chun KR, Furnkranz A, Ouyang F. Remote robotic navigation and electroanatomical mapping for ablation of atrial fibrillation: considerations for navigation and impact on procedural outcome. Circ Arrhythm Electrophysiol. 2009;2(2): 120–128.

CHAPTER 4

Equipment options for the ablation of atrial fibrillation

German Kamalov & John D. Hummel

Division of Cardiovascular Medicine, The Ohio State University, Columbus, OH, USA

In this chapter, we will discuss the following equipment options for ablation of atrial fibrillation:

1 Sedation: general anesthesia and conscious sedation
2 X-ray equipment and shielding
3 EP recording and pacing systems
4 Equipment for transseptal puncture
5 Echocardiography options
6 Catheters, ablation generators and electroanatomic mapping

Sedation

AF ablation procedures are complex and can last for several hours, during which the patients can feel significant discomfort and restlessness. Patient respiration and motion can affect catheter stability and can impact both efficacy and safety of the AF ablation. Either general anesthesia or conscious sedation is used in electrophysiology laboratories performing catheter ablation of AF. The choice of sedation or general anesthesia is generally determined by physician preference, patient characteristics, and hospital resources, and this choice carries implications for equipment options that need to be available.

Both *moderate* and *deep* sedation can be employed for AF ablation. Typically, *moderate* sedation is achieved by administering a benzodiazepine combined with analgesia using a short-acting narcotic. Patients are sedated to the point of sleeping, but remain easily arousable. No interventions are required

to maintain a patent airway as spontaneous ventilation is adequate. The EP staff performing the procedure must be trained in procedural sedation techniques and airway management. According to the guidelines of American Society of Anesthesiology, blood pressure, heart rate, oxygen saturation, and EKG monitoring should be available and provided during both sedation and general anesthesia [3]. Adhesive defibrillation patches are placed on the patient's chest and attached to an external defibrillator to allow prompt resuscitation if needed. The lab should be equipped with resuscitation equipment including the external pacemaker/defibrillator, Ambu bags and masks for ventilation, a crash cart for emergent intubation, and a full selection of medications required for resuscitation. Moderate sedation is a safe approach; however, the long procedure time, the large number of painful radiofrequency (RF) energy applications, and the need for motionless supine posture on the operating table may limit the ease of the procedure for the operator and patient. Deep sedation is an alternative to general anesthesia. Deep sedation can utilize many different agents, but the best described approach employs benzodiazapines and narcotics followed by an intravenous propofol bolus with maintenance of sedation via continuous intravenous administration of propofol [4]. This approach does compromise the airway and generally requires that an anesthesiologist be present in the hospital on call at all times.

General anesthesia

Intermittent positive pressure ventilation is commonly employed, though the successful use of high-frequency jet ventilation has also been reported to limit respiratory motion during the procedure [5].

Practical Guide to Catheter Ablation of Atrial Fibrillation, Second Edition. Edited by Jonathan S. Steinberg, Pierre Jaïs and Hugh Calkins.
© 2016 John Wiley & Sons, Ltd. Published 2016 by John Wiley & Sons, Ltd.

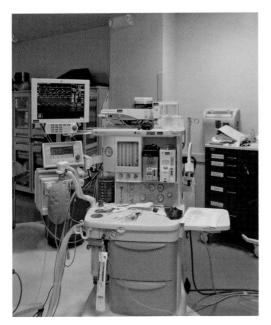

Figure 1 Typical anesthesia cart used during AF ablation.

General anesthesia requires the presence of anesthesia staff throughout the duration of the case, as well as anesthesia cart(s) (Figure 1). Advantages of general anesthesia include optimal airway management, pain control, and prevention of a patient's movement during catheter manipulation as well as enhanced tolerance of esophageal temperature probes. Thus, a randomized study showed both a higher cure rate and a reduction in pulmonary vein (PV) reconnection compared to the conscious sedation [6]. Disadvantages of anesthesia include the risk of trauma during intubation, the need for anesthesia staff, anesthesia equipment (cart(s)), and increased cost of procedure. Moreover, the use of general anesthesia is associated with the increased risk of esophageal damage as detected by capsule endoscopy [7]. Ultimately, without general anesthesia support and equipment availability, patients with high-risk airways, significant sleep apnea, and significant pulmonary disease may not be able to undergo ablation of atrial fibrillation.

Anticoagulation

Anticoagulation with IV heparin to maintain activated clotting time (ACT) > 350 ms significantly reduces the incidence of left atrial clot formation during AF ablation. ACT monitoring throughout the procedure requires a dedicated ACT machine.

Esophageal probe

The esophagus lies close to the posterior left atrial wall and to the PV ostia. RF ablation in these areas carries the risk of injury to the esophagus due to local heat transfer. This can lead to esophageal lesions including mucosal changes, necrotic ulcers, or, in extreme cases, to atrio-esophageal fistula. Two main approaches are typically used to minimize the risk of esophageal injury: imaging methods to define esophagus position in relation to the posterior LA wall (fluoroscopy, electroanatomic mapping, ultrasound, and barium paste) and luminal esophageal temperature monitoring using esophageal temperature probes. Data from a luminal probe can provide information about esophageal heating and has been reported to help guide RF energy titration to minimize thermal injury to the esophagus during catheter ablation [8,9]. It is important to recognize the possibility for a significant underestimation of RF-induced esophageal heating using luminal esophageal temperature monitoring [10,11]. Esophageal temperature probes are available from many companies and can have single or multiple thermocouple sensors (three–five poles).

X-ray equipment and shielding

Fluoroscopy

Fluoroscopy continues to serve an important imaging role during AF ablation in spite of the advances in 3D navigation systems. Most laboratories employ single C-arm or biplane fluoroscopic systems (Figure 2). Current fluoroscopy systems fall into two distinct categories: image intensifier and flat-panel detector (FPD) systems. The more conventional and older design is the image intensifier system, which is coupled with a television camera and displays. FPD fluoroscopy systems represent more modern solid-state detector arrays used as the image receptor. FDP systems do not require a television camera to convert the X-ray intensity distribution into an electronic signal, as the electronic signal automatically emerges from the image receptor. FDP receptors have a number of advantages over image intensifier fluoroscopy systems including better stability, lower patient radiation doses, and wider dynamic ranges. However, image intensifier systems are widely used, especially for mobile C-arms and have a smaller physical footprint over the patient, which can enhance dual use both for device implantation and for AF ablation.

Modern fluoroscopy systems with digital image acquisition allow high resolution real-time X-ray imaging with lower radiation rates. Pulse fluoroscopy reduces radiation levels to the patient and image degradation caused by motion blur. Copper filtration

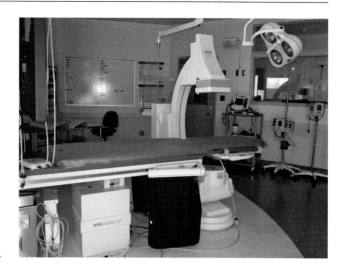

Figure 2 Typical C-arm fluoroscopy system (flat-panel detector) and fluoroscopic table.

is used to preferentially remove the lower energy X-rays that do not effectively penetrate the patient's tissues. New automatic dose rate control (ADRC) systems modulate milliampere, kilovolt peak, pulse width, and filtration in a manner aimed at minimizing patient dose rates while maintaining good image quality [12].

Radiation protection

The fluoroscopic exposure to the patient and lab personnel follows the ALARA standard: as low as reasonably acceptable. Scatter (or secondary) radiation is the primary exposure source of radiation for the physician. It occurs when the primary radiation beam comes in contact with the patient, scatters, and emanates out from the patient in all directions. The closer the physician is positioned to the primary beam, the greater the exposure to the scatter radiation.

The following steps are recommended to minimize personnel exposure in the electrophysiology laboratory.
1 Customization of the X-ray system: Pulsed fluoroscopy, lowering the frame rate to seven per second, reducing the dose per frame, strict beam collimation, reducing tube voltage and milliamperage [13,14].
2 Workflow adaptations: Position image intensifier close to the patient to reduce scatter, avoidance of cine imaging (use of recording fluoroscopy instead), avoiding left anterior oblique imaging if possible [15].
3 Personal protection: Radiation protection badges to monitor X-ray exposure; lead apron, eye glasses, and thyroid shield – 0.35 mm lead-equivalent apron reduces effective dose by a factor of 10, while a 0.5 mm thyroid collar provides a further 1.5-fold decrease [14].

External protective equipment including hanging shields, table skirts, radiation drapes, and rolling shields are all helpful. Overhead, suspended lead aprons in front of the operator, instead of lead apparel is available through systems such as the Zero Gravity™ radiation protection system.

EP recording and pacing systems

Recording systems consist of amplifiers, junction boxes, pulse generators, and monitors that are coupled to stimulators. The junction boxes receive the pin electrodes from the ablation catheters in the heart and carry these signals to the amplifiers. The recording system allows the operator to adjust the amplitude and filters of the signal for display and most systems allow up to 64 channels to be displayed. The recording system is married to a stimulator that allows the operator to deliver timed electrical stimulation to the heart via a pulse generator connected to the mapping and ablation catheters (Figure 3). Various manufacturers of EP recording systems include Prucka, EPMed, Bard, and others.

Equipment for transseptal puncture

Successful transseptal puncture is a crucial step in AF ablation and can be safely performed under fluoroscopy with or without intracardiac echocardiographic guidance. It requires the use of special transseptal sheaths and a needle. Sheaths for transseptal puncture can be steerable or fixed. The shape and curve of the sheath are designed to provide support for the transseptal needle during transseptal puncture and give stability for the mapping or ablation catheter inside

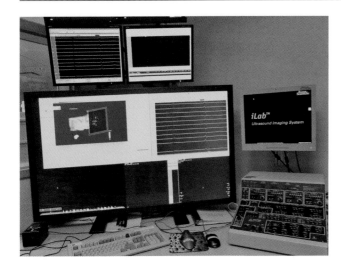

Figure 3 A large and small flat screen displaying 12 surface leads from an EP recording system with a stimulator to the right with multiple channels to stimulate from.

the left atrium. Fixed sheaths generally are 59–63 cm in length and include a side port with a hemostatic valve. They come with dilators that fit within the lumen of the sheath and extend beyond the sheath tip. These dilators add structural support both during transseptal puncture and during cannulation of the vein used for access. Multiple transseptal sheaths have been developed to provide improved catheter delivery to the various portions of the left atrium. Steerable sheaths provides uni- or bidirectional deflection that can be controlled from the handle and come in various diameter curves. These steerable sheaths are generally longer than fixed curve sheaths and require a longer transseptal needle (Figure 4). Fixed curve sheaths are also available with curves of 45°–150° and are produced by various manufacturers (Figure 5). Guide-wires are required for safe advancement of sheaths and dilators through the vascular anatomy to allow positioning for transseptal puncture. Most sheaths come with standard J-tipped wires of maximum diameter of 0.032 inch.

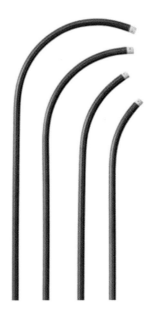

Figure 5 St Jude Swartz braided fixed curve transseptal sheaths with different distal curves. *Source*: St Jude Medical. Reproduced with permission.

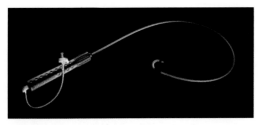

Figure 4 Agilis Nxt™ steerable sheath. *Source*: St Jude Medical. Reproduced with permission.

Brockenbrough needle

The transseptal needle is a long, curved, stainless steel needle that is designed to be introduced via the right femoral vein. Varying curvatures of the Brockenbrough needle have been developed to accommodate variations in right atrial anatomy. The needle has an arrow-shaped handle that indicates the direction of the needle tip and allows the operator to control the direction of the needle tip (Figure 6). The needles are

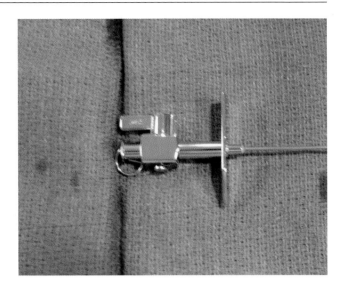

Figure 6 Arrow-shaped handle of transseptal needle that indicates the direction of the needle tip.

18-gauge and taper to a size of 21-gauge at the tip. Most transseptal procedures are accomplished with a BRK-shaped Brockenbrough needle with the shaft to the needle tip angle of 19°. Adult patients with marked right atrial enlargement may require the enhanced curvature of the BRK-1 Brockenbrough needle to reach the interatrial septum (approximately 55°) and thus this equipment should be available if needed. The majority of transseptal sheaths accommodate a standard-length needle of 71 cm, whereas longer sheaths such as the steerable sheaths may require a longer needle of 98 cm. The NRG® RF Transseptal Needle is designed to assist in gaining access to the left atrium by using RF energy as opposed to mechanical force (Baylis Medical, Montreal, QC).

Smaller diameter guidewires (0.014 inch diameter) that fit through the hub of the transseptal needle are available and can be advanced through the needle tip to confirm a left atrial entry. If using the guidewire to confirm successful transseptal puncture, a durable preferably metal wire should be used to prevent the tip of the needle from easily cutting the wire loose in the left atrium. Other techniques for confirmation of the left atrial position would include contrast injection and/or checking the oxygen concentration of blood aspirated from the transseptal needle.

Echocardiography

Echocardiography is frequently used during atrial fibrillation ablation as a complementary tool to fluoroscopy to guide safe transseptal access. Intracardiac echocardiography (ICE) allows the operator to visualize the position of the needle when tenting of the septum is observed, significantly reducing fluoroscopy time and the incidence of complications [16,17]. Additionally, ICE may be used to monitor procedural complications such as intracardiac thrombus formation, pericardial effusion or tamponade, and pulmonary vein stenosis. It can be utilized to define pulmonary vein (PV) anatomy and guide accurate positioning of the lasso catheter at the PV ostium. The development of CartoSound (Biosense Webster, Diamond Bar, CA) allows three-dimensional (3D) reconstruction of the images obtained by ICE and integration with an electroanatomic mapping (EAM) system for better visualization of anatomic landmarks throughout the procedure [17].

ICE systems consist of radial ultrasound or phased array transducers mounted on the tip of 8 or 9 F catheters and are supplied as sterile, disposable, single-use only devices [17,18].

The radial intracardiac ultrasound (Boston Scientific UltraICE™) uses a mechanical radial 9 MHz single element transducer mounted on the tip of an 8 F catheter that has an insertable length of 110 cm. It can be used only with a proprietary platform to allow visualization of the images. The catheter has a flexible drive shaft that connects to a motor drive unit, but it is not steerable. A piezoelectric crystal rotates at 1800 revolutions per minute generating a 360° image perpendicular to the catheter, with the tip as a central reference point. The imaging depth is 4–8 cm. This allows the user to visualize structures directly adjacent to the catheter tip and still see a detailed cross section of the entire septum. Axial and lateral resolution is 0.27 mm and 0.26 mm, respectively. Phased array intracardiac echo probes employ a 64-element phased array multiple-frequency transducer (5–10 MHz) incorporated into an 8 F steerable catheter (four directions), which provides 90° sector images with depth control and Doppler ultrasound. The phased array ICE catheter provides high-resolution 2D images with a penetration ranging from 2 mm to 12 cm. This allows imaging of the entire heart. The phased array ultrasound creates sector (pie shaped) images comparable to those obtained by TEE, as opposed to the 360° view of the rotating ICE catheter. The catheter offers lockable steering in four directions – anterior, posterior, left, and right. Imaging planes can be fixed with the locking tensioning wheel. Phased array ultrasound catheters can be used with standard ultrasound machines and connect to the compatible ultrasound systems with a reusable universal connector.

Thus, the rotational ultrasound catheter offers radial two-dimensional imaging with excellent near-field spatial resolution but limited depth of penetration. Phased array ultrasound offers increased depth of penetration, steering capabilities for additional imaging planes, and full Doppler capabilities. The rotational system is much less expensive and may be adequate if ICE is used to guide only transseptal access. Additional cost of phased array ultrasound is justified if ICE is used for guiding pulmonary vein isolation.

Transesophageal echocardiography (TEE) is most commonly used prior to the AF ablation procedure to rule out left atrial thrombus in patients prior to left atrial instrumentation. In some labs, TEE is utilized to facilitate transseptal catheterization. TEE can readily image the fossa ovalis and needle assembly, but it requires another operator other than the electrophysiologist and greater degrees of sedation than intracardiac echocardiography to allow adequate imaging. If the case is performed under general anesthesia, a trained cardiac anesthesiologist can function as the other operator and use TEE to guide the transseptal puncture and to monitor complications such as pericardial tamponade or thrombus.

Transthoracic echocardiography plays a limited role in AF ablation. It is mostly used for quick assessment for pericardial tamponade and to exclude or confirm the need for immediate pericardiocenthesis.

Catheters, ablation generators, and electroanatomic mapping

The cornerstone of AF ablation is isolation of conduction from the PVs. Circular mapping catheters are positioned at the ostium of PV during ablation to ensure isolation of the PV antrum. These catheters have been shown to improve the success of

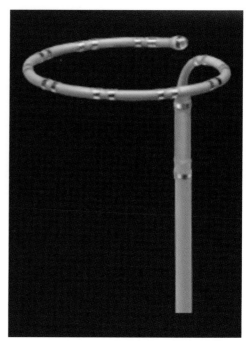

Figure 7 Lasso® NAV mapping catheter (Biosense Webster). Electrode positions can be readily visualized on Carto® 3 System. *Source*: Biosense Webster, Inc. Reproduced with permission.

circumferential pulmonary vein isolation compared to the use of an ablation catheter alone [19]. Lasso (Biosense Webster, USA) and Inquiry™ AFocus™ II EB (St Jude) are examples of such catheters (Figure 7).

Standard electrophysiology catheters used for mapping and pacing in AF ablation include both steerable multipolar catheters to ease placement at the His bundle and within the coronary sinus and fixed curve catheters for the right atrium and ventricle from various manufacturers. At times a 64-pole basket catheter is deployed for mapping within the PV or to map conduction patterns and rotor patterns from the right and left atria. All of these catheters may be required and the use will depend upon the operator's preferences. Electroanatomic mapping systems allow the operator to record intracardiac points reflecting electrical activation time and voltage amplitude in relation to anatomic position in space, thus creating a three-dimensional cardiac chamber using interpolation between acquired points on the endocardial surface (Figure 8). This technology allows one to accurately target locations of arrhythmia origin, delineate areas of anatomic interest, and allow catheter manipulation and positioning without fluoroscopic guidance. The use of EAM to facilitate pulmonary vein isolation for treatment for AF ablation has been

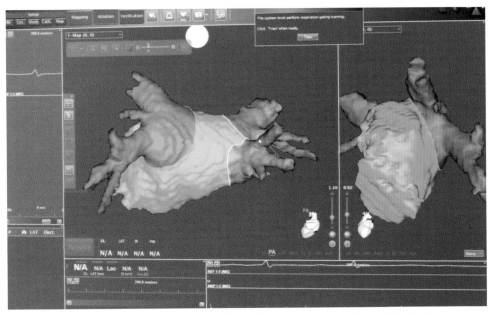

Figure 8 Carto® 3 mapping system displaying imported three-dimensional reconstruction of a CT of the heart.

shown to reduce fluoroscopy time, radiation dose, and procedure time [20]. Most AF ablation programs employ EAM unless they depend entirely on phased RF or Cryoablation for AF ablation.

Stereotaxis Niobe™ is a magnetic navigation system designed to allow a complete, remote RF catheter ablation. The system consists of two permanent large magnets positioned on either side of the single-plane fluoroscopy table. The positions of these magnets are computer-controlled. In the "navigate" mode, the magnets create a uniform spherical magnetic navigation field inside the patient's chest. The mapping and ablation catheter is very flexible distally and is equipped with three small permanent magnets positioned at the distal shaft. By changing the orientation of the outer magnets relative to each other, the orientation of the magnetic field changes, thereby leading to deflection of the catheter. The Hansen Robotic™ system allows the use of multiple types of standard ablation catheters that are mounted and then remotely maneuvered by an operator via robotic controls.

Radiofrequency ablation catheters and generators

Standard RF generators used for catheter ablation monitor the temperature at the tip of the catheter, the power required to achieve that temperature, the impedance measured by the system, and the duration of energy delivery. Irrigated catheters are the most frequently used type of catheter for AF ablation. Irrigated catheters produce deeper lesions than solid tip catheters, at the same time reducing the risk for char formation at the catheter tip [21]. The Boston Scientific Chilli catheter employs a closed, internally irrigated catheter tip. Its development was followed by the open-irrigated tip of the Biosense Webster Thermocool® and Thermocool® SF catheters that have a magnetic sensor at the tip and are designed to be used only with CARTO mapping system. The Thermocool™ SF catheter achieves the same power as conventional Thermocool® catheter at half the flow rate, thus reducing fluid load to the patient. Ablation with irrigated tip catheters is performed via a generator that interacts with irrigation pumps. It delivers power with the irrigation flow adjusted from 10 to 60 mL/min to keep the temperature below 45 °C at the desired power. Other examples of open-irrigated catheters include Boston Scientific Open Irrigated™, St Jude CoolPath™, St Jude CoolPath Duo™, St Jude Cool Flex™ catheters. These catheters can be used with NavX St Jude mapping system that has an open platform. Regardless of the specific system used, the catheters used will require both an RF generator and an irrigation pump that can work together.

ThermoCool® SmartTouch™ (Biosense Webster) is an ablation catheter that measures the catheter tip contact force in real time. This should allow more efficient energy delivery during ablation. The nMARQ™ catheter (Biosense Webster) is an open-irrigated circular 10-electrode ablation catheter that combines the ability to map and multiablate simultaneously. It requires a special nMARQ™ generator. The catheter is being evaluated in a clinical trial in the United States.

Nonirrigated solid-tip catheters have also been used for AF ablation. Eight-mm solid-tip catheters such as the Blazer series (Boston Scientific) have been used for AF ablation with RF energy up to 50–70 W and target temperatures of 50–55 °C. Char has been noted with the use of these catheters leading to the development of irrigated catheters and nonirrigated catheters with less risk of char formation.

Duty-cycled phased RF allows for phased delivery of uni- and bipolar RF energy via mutielectrode ablation catheters. Unipolar energy delivery modulates the depth of the desired lesion, while bipolar energy fills the space between electrodes. Phased RF Ablation is delivered via the pulmonary vein ablation catheter (PVAC™), multiarray septal catheter (MASC™), multiarray ablation catheter (MAAC™), and tip versatile ablation catheter (TVAC™). A multichannel RF ablation generator (GENius™ Multi-Channel RF Generator) directs RF energy independently to each of the catheter's electrodes. Duty-cycling is used to cool the electrode during off-phases to prevent overheating and char formation. RF energy can be simultaneously applied to 12 electrodes. RF energy is usually applied for a fixed 60 s to achieve a target temperature of 60 °C using a maximum of 10-W energy (temperature controlled, power limited) [22].

Non-RF systems

PV isolation cryoablation is achieved using Arctic Front™ balloon catheters (Medtronic AF Solutions) designed to achieve isolation with a single energy application after seating the balloon in the PV over a wire or the circular mapping wire (Achieve™). Complete occlusion of the PV by the balloon is confirmed before ablation by PV angiography distal to the balloon or by color Doppler using ICE. Arctic Front does not require 3D mapping, thus reducing procedure time and complexity. However, it requires a large 12 F introducer sheath and carries a higher risk of phrenic nerve paralysis. The STOP AF trial demonstrated that cryoballoon ablation is safe for the treatment of patients with symptomatic paroxysmal AF with risks within accepted standards for ablation therapy. At 12 months, treatment success of cryoablation was 69.9%. Eleven percent of the patients in the trial developed phrenic nerve palsy, while

in eighty-six percent patients palsy resolved by 12 months [23]. Finally, a visually guided laser ablation (VGLA) catheter has been designed to facilitate PV isolation. VGLA employs a laser that is positioned via an insertable balloon at the antrum of the pulmonary vein. This system is undergoing clinical evaluations in the United States [24].

Conclusions

One could argue that the equipment requirements for AF ablation are as complex and challenging to orchestrate as the ablation itself. The options continue to evolve and the operators' preferences evolve as our understanding of the safest and most effective means to cure AF move forward. Continued reassessment of new and old technologies is required to stay abreast of the field and provide the best care to the patient.

References

1 Haissaguerre M, Jais P, Shah DC, et al. Spontaneous initiation of atrial fibrillation by ectopic beats originating in the pulmonary veins. N Engl J Med 1998;339:659–666.
2 Chen SA, Hsieh MH, Tai CT, et al. Initiation of atrial fibrillation by ectopic beats originating from the pulmonary veins: electrophysiological characteristics, pharmacological responses, and effects of radiofrequency ablation. Circulation 1999;100:1879–1886.
3 Practice Guidelines for Sedation and Analgesia by Non-Anesthesiologists (An Updated Report by the American Society of Anesthesiologists Task Force on Sedation and Analgesia by Non-Anesthesiologists). Anesthesiology 2002;96:1004–1017.
4 Kottkamp H, Hindricks G, Eitel C, et al. Deep sedation for catheter ablation of atrial fibrillation. J Cardiovasc Electrophysiol 2011;22(12):1339–1343.
5 Elkassabany N, Garcia F, Tschabrunn C, et al. Anesthetic management of patients undergoing pulmonary vein isolation for treatment of atrial fibrillation using high-frequency jet ventilation. J Cardiothorac Vasc Anesth. 2012;26(3):433–438.
6 Di Biase L, Conti S, Mohanty P, et al. General anesthesia reduces the prevalence of pulmonary vein reconnection during repeat ablation when compared with conscious sedation: results from a randomized study. Heart Rhythm. 2011;8(3):368–372.
7 Di Biase L, Saenz LC, Burkhardt DJ, et al. Esophageal capsule endoscopy after radiofrequency catheter ablation for atrial fibrillation: documented higher risk of luminal esophageal damage with general anesthesia as compared with conscious sedation. Circ Arrhythm Electrophysiol. 2009;2(2):108–112.
8 Singh SM, d'Avila A, Doshi SK, et al. Esophageal injury and temperature monitoring during atrial fibrillation ablation. Circ Arrhythmia Electrophysiol. 2008;1:162–168.
9 Sause A, Tutdibi O, Pomsel K, et al. Limiting esophageal temperature in radiofrequency ablation of left atrial

tachyarrhythmias results in low incidence of thermal esophageal lesions. BMC Cardiovasc. Disord. 2010;10:52.

10 Perzanowski C, Teplitsky L, Hranitzky PM, et al. Real-time monitoring of luminal esophageal temperature during left atrial radiofrequency catheter ablation for atrial fibrillation: observations about esophageal heating during ablation at the pulmonary vein ostia and posterior left atrium. J Cardiovasc Electrophysiol. 2006;17:166–170.

11 Cummings JE, Seil O, Kilicaslan F, Salida WI, et al. Esophageal luminal temperature measurement significantly underestimates esophageal tissue temperature during radiofrequency ablation within the left atrium, in an experimental model. Circulation 2005;112: II-393.

12 Nickoloff EL. AAPM/RSNA Physics Tutorial for Residents: physics of flat-panel fluoroscopy systems. RadioGraphics 2011;31:591–602.

13 Kuon E, Schmitt M, Dahm JB. Significant reduction of radiation exposure to operator and staff during cardiac interventions by analysis of radiation leakage and improved lead shielding. Am J Cardiol. 2002;89(1):44–49.

14 Theocharopoulos N, Damilakis J, Perisinakis K. Occupational exposure in the electrophysiology laboratory: quantifying and minimizing radiation burden. Br J Radiol. 2006;79:644–651.

15 Kuon E, Dahm JB, Empen K, Robinson DM, Reuter G, Wucherer M. Identification of less-irradiating tube angulations in invasive cardiology. J Am Coll Cardiol. 2004;44:1420–1428.

16 Dravid SG, Hope B, McKinnie JJ. Intracardiac echocardiography in electrophysiology: a review of current applications in practice. Echocardiography. 2008;25 (10):1172–1175.

17 Biermann J, Bode C, Asbach S. Intracardiac echocardiography during catheter-based ablation of atrial fibrillation. Cardiol Res Pract. 2012;2012:921746.

18 Silvestry F. Intracardiac echocardiography: currently available ICE systems. In: Silvestry F, Wiegers S (eds), Intracardiac Echocardiography, (1st edn). Informa, 2006; 19–29.

19 Tamborero D, Mont L, Berruezo A, et al. Circumferential pulmonary vein ablation: does use of a circular mapping catheter improve results? A prospective randomized study. Heart Rhythm. 2010;7(5):612–618.

20 Reddy VY, Morales G, Ahmed H, et al. Catheter ablation of atrial fibrillation without the use of fluoroscopy. Heart Rhythm. 2010;11:1644–1653.

21 Houmsse M, Daoud EG. Biophysics and clinical utility of irrigated-tip radiofrequency catheter ablation. Expert Rev Med Devices. 2012;9(1):59–70.

22 Boersma L, Wijffels M, Oral H, et al. Pulmonary vein isolation by duty-cycled bipolar and unipolar radiofrequency energy with a multielectrode ablation catheter. Heart Rhythm. 2008;5:1635–1642.

23 Packer DL, Kowal RC, Wheelan KR, et al. STOP AF Cryoablation Investigators. Cryoballoon ablation of pulmonary veins for paroxysmal atrial fibrillation: first results of the North American Arctic Front (STOP AF) pivotal trial. J Am Coll Cardiol. 2013;61(16):1713–1723.

24 Dukkipati SR, Kuck KH, Neuzil P, et al. Pulmonary vein isolation using a visually guided laser balloon catheter: the first 200-patient multicenter clinical experience. Circ Arrhythm Electrophysiol. 2013;6(3):467–472.

CHAPTER 5

Preprocedure preparation for catheter-based ablation of atrial fibrillation

José F. Huizar, Karoly Kaszala & Kenneth A. Ellenbogen
Department of Medicine and Division of Cardiology, Virginia Commonwealth University
Medical Center and McGuire VA Medical Center, Richmond, VA, USA

Introduction

In preparation for catheter-based ablation of atrial fibrillation (AF), a significant amount of pertinent information should be collected to perform this procedure as safely as possible. Two facts should always be kept in mind: (1) atrial fibrillation is most commonly a relatively benign disease with the primary indication for ablation at this time being amelioration of symptoms and the reversal of tachycardia-induced cardiomyopathy in selected patients [1] and (2) catheter ablation is almost always an elective procedure. As such, AF ablation should be performed in an ideal setting under optimal conditions. In this chapter, we will discuss all the pertinent data that should be considered and obtained prior to catheter ablation for AF.

Due to the potential risks of AF ablation, we typically evaluate all patients in the outpatient setting in order to discuss alternative approaches and therapies. At this time, all relevant details of the medical history should be explored, from type and duration of AF (paroxysmal, persistent, or permanent) to prior ablation(s), prior surgeries, medical conditions, medications, and allergies [1,2]. Some of these factors may increase the risk of the procedure (Table 1) or increase the likelihood of AF recurrence after ablation

(Table 2). For example, the presence of rods in the spine from scoliosis surgery could increase morbidity due to difficult visualization of the left atrium (LA), whereas incomplete left atrial ablation lines from prior procedures predispose the patient to occurrence of left atrial macroreentry [3]. A complete evaluation should be performed similar to any patient with new onset AF, including evaluation for reversible causes of AF. Recent laboratory data should be reviewed to exclude abnormalities that could complicate procedure or recovery such as significant anemia, thrombocytopenia or coagulopathy, infection, renal insufficiency, and electrolyte disturbance.

A resting 12-lead electrocardiogram (ECG), a rhythm strip, and a 24-h Holter or 30-day event monitor should be obtained to document atrial fibrillation and measure the burden of atrial fibrillation. A cardiac ultrasound, typically a transthoracic or if indicated a transesophageal echocardiogram, should be obtained to document cardiac anatomy and function, such as LA size, left ventricular (LV) function and dimensions, valvular function, interatrial septal anatomy, and exclusion of possible anomalies or appendage thrombus. Other imaging studies can also provide further detailed information about cardiac anatomy and function, such as cardiac computed tomography (CT) or magnetic resonance (MRI) scan (see below). However, these studies are considered optional and may be used in selected patients dictated by clinical evaluation, institutional protocol, financial resources, procedural complexity, and specific ablation approach.

Practical Guide to Catheter Ablation of Atrial Fibrillation,
Second Edition. Edited by Jonathan S. Steinberg, Pierre Jaïs and Hugh Calkins.
© 2016 John Wiley & Sons, Ltd. Published 2016 by John Wiley & Sons, Ltd.

Table 1 Factors probably associated with increased morbidity of AF ablation.

Age
Body mass index/obesity
Prior ablations and complications
Prior cardiac surgeries
   Valvular repair/replacement
Cardiac diseases
   LV dysfunction/heart failure/end-stage cardiomyopathy
   Severe valvular heart disease
IVC filters/DVT
Prior spine surgery (e.g., Harrington rods)
Anticoagulation (contraindications, adverse events, or complications)
Allergies (including IV contrast adverse effects)
Sedation history (complications and medical conditions)
Relative contraindications to transseptal access
   PFO or ASD closure device
   Complex congenital heart disease

Table 2 Factors probably associated with increased risk of recurrent AF.

Age [42]
LA size > 55–60 mm/LA scar [1,13,32,43]
Type and duration of atrial fibrillation [42]
Body mass index/obesity [44]
Prior ablations and complications [3]
Prior cardiac surgeries
   Valvular repair/replacement [45]
   MAZE procedure
   Elevated biomarkers
   B-type natriuretic peptide [46]
   C-reactive protein >0.5 mg/dL [47]
Cardiac diseases
   Hypertrophic cardiomyopathy [14]
   LV dysfunction/heart failure/end-stage cardiomyopathy [48]
   Severe valvular heart disease [49]
Pulmonary diseases
   Emphysema/asthma [50]
   Sleep apnea [51]
Anxiety and Depression [52]

A thorough evaluation of patients includes a discussion of alternative therapies, including rate control and anticoagulation strategy, a pace and ablate strategy, and surgical procedures.

ECG and ambulatory ECG recordings

A resting 12-lead electrocardiogram (ECG) and rhythm strip should be performed to document AF.

In the absence of AF, a 12-lead ECG will both provide important information, such as baseline sinus rate, QT interval, and possible triggers of AF, and exclude ongoing or active ischemia that would defer or postpone AF ablation.

The baseline sinus rate and QT interval are important to better select appropriate antiarrhythmic therapy if required during and/or immediately after the ablation. For example, propafenone, sotalol, and beta-blockers should be used cautiously in patients with significant bradycardia or tachycardia–bradycardia syndrome due to their significant negative chronotropic effect. Sotalol, dofetilide, ibutilide (class III antiarrhythmics) will significantly prolong QT interval, which can result in polymorphic ventricular tachycardia in susceptible patients.

Triggers of atrial fibrillation have been well described. Tachycardia-induced tachycardia was described several decades ago and refers to one tachycardia that can degenerate or trigger a second tachycardia. Examples of tachycardias that may precipitate atrial fibrillation include atrial tachycardia, atrioventricular (AV), nodal reentrant tachycardia (AVNRT), AV reentrant tachycardia (AV accessory pathway), and premature atrial contractions [4]. These triggers may be potentially recognizable with a 12-lead ECG (Figure 1) or ambulatory ECG recordings (24-h Holter or 30-day event monitor, Figure 2). Atrial ectopy that triggers AF has been most frequently documented to originate from the pulmonary veins (PVs), left atria (LA), vein of Marshall, crista terminalis, superior vena cava (SVC), and coronary sinus (CS) [5,6]. The frequency of triggers and the site of triggers may be higher in younger patients. For example, a study in adolescents with documented AF and structurally normal hearts was found to have more underlying supraventricular arrhythmias [5]. The P-wave axis and morphology in a 12-lead ECG can more precisely identify the source of atrial ectopy and focal tachycardia. Several studies have described the ECG P-wave morphology that helps localize the source of atrial ectopy and/or tachycardia (Figure 3) [7–9]. Yamane et al. described an algorithm based on P-wave morphology to identify the PV origin of atrial ectopic beats with an accuracy of 79% (Figure 4) [9].

An attempt to control and treat such triggers should be made in order to better prevent recurrences of atrial fibrillation and allow the electrophysiologists to focus on an area that may require further attention. In some centers, eliciting triggers during electrophysiological study in patients referred for AF ablation is a critical component of the procedure. Sauer et al. demonstrated that slow-pathway ablation alone (without

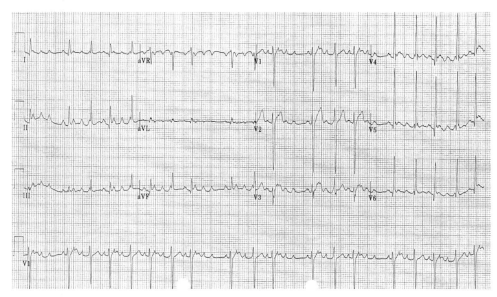

Figure 1 Right superior pulmonary vein tachycardia recorded from an 18-year-old male with atrial fibrillation.

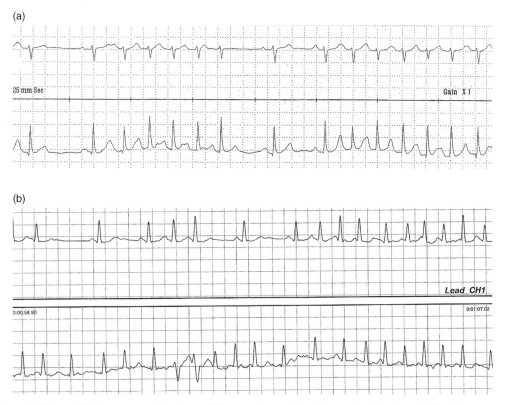

Figure 2 Holter and 30-day event monitor in two different patients with atrial ectopy/atrial tachycardia that degenerates to atrial fibrillation.

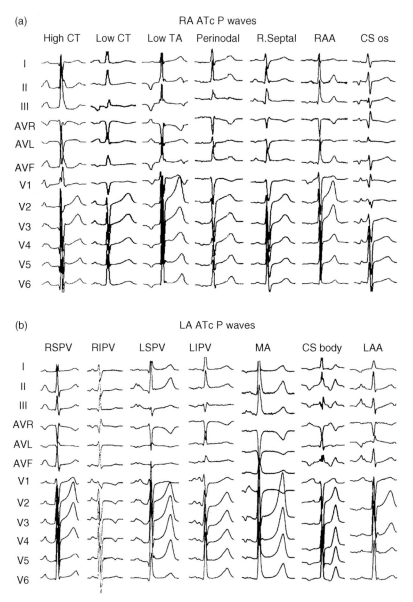

Figure 3 Representative examples of tachycardia P-wave morphology of tachycardia from right atrial sites (a) and from left atrial sites (b). CT, crista terminalis; TA, tricuspid annulus; RAA, right atrial appendage; CS, coronary sinus; PV, pulmonary vein; RS, right superior; RI, right inferior; LS, left superior; LI, left inferior; MA, mitral annulus; LAA, left atrial appendage. *Source:* Kistler et al., 2006 [7]. Reproduced with permission of Elsevier.

pulmonary vein isolation) in patients referred for AF ablation with inducible AVNRT during electrophysiological study had a very low rate of AF recurrence without antiarrhythmic drugs after 21 months [4]. Similarly, Haissaguerre et.al. and other groups have shown that successful catheter ablation of accessory pathways prevents further recurrence of AF in 91% of patients [10].

In patients with intermittent symptoms, a Holter or event monitor and 12-lead ECG during symptoms accurately diagnose AF and avoid misdiagnosis of other arrhythmias, which would require a different procedure or therapy. Dixit et al. demonstrated that AF could be erroneously diagnosed in patients with dual AV nodal pathways manifesting with a double response and/or AVNRT [11]. In another study,

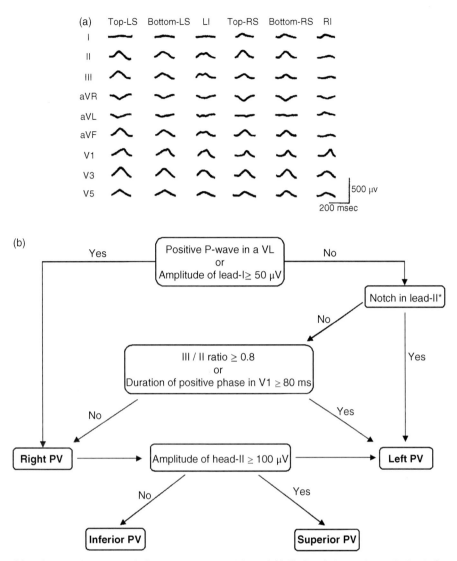

Figure 4 (a) Surface ECG P-wave morphology in one patient with atrial fibrillation during pacing at six sites in four pulmonary veins, (b) algorithm to determine PV origin. For abbreviations refer to Figure 3. *Source:* Yamne et al., 2001 [7]. Reproduced with permission of Elsevier.

almost 10% of ECGs interpreted as showing AF were incorrectly classified [12]. In addition, ambulatory ECG recordings will correlate symptoms with paroxysms and burden of atrial fibrillation. Ambulatory ECG recordings in patients with chronic AF are useful both to assess ventricular rate and response to medical therapy and to correlate symptoms associated with rapid ventricular response.

Finally, it is important to identify other coexistent conditions such as typical or atypical atrial flutter and other supraventricular arrhythmias, which would necessitate additional ablation and therefore will increase the complexity and time of the procedure.

Transthoracic and transesophageal echocardiogram

Transthoracic echocardiography (TTE) is paramount in the preprocedure evaluation of AF ablation. Detailed data on the cardiac function, anatomy, and possible anomalies will both maximize the safety of the procedure and provide information that can predict the response or failure of AF ablation.

The most important data pertinent to AF ablation include (1) LA size; (2) LV dimension, thickness, and ejection fraction; (3) valvular function; (4) pulmonary artery pressure; (5) interatrial septal anatomy;

(6) pericardial space and effusion; and (7) cardiac anomalies, if any exist.

The LA size can predict the response to AF ablation or direct the operator to perform more extensive LA substrate ablation. Studies have documented a higher AF recurrence rate after ablation in patients with larger LA size prior to the procedure [13]. Hypertrophic cardiomyopathy may also have a higher AF recurrence rate after catheter-based ablation [14]. Severe LV dilatation and depressed systolic function could facilitate volume overload and precipitate congestive heart failure during the ablation, particularly if an open-irrigated catheter is used. Additionally, knowledge of LV systolic function will guide appropriate antiarrhythmic drug selection in the pre- and postablation phase.

Special attention should be paid to evaluate the right atrium and ventricle (e.g., abnormal insertion of the tricuspid valve may suggest Ebstein's anomaly that is associated with the presence of accessory pathways and trigger of AF. Moreover, pulmonary hypertension, congenital heart disease with significant shunts, and severe valvular heart disease are associated with a higher incidence of AF and likely associated with a higher recurrence rate of AF after catheter ablation (Table 2). The transthoracic echocardiogram will also provide a baseline evaluation of the pericardial space prior to ablation, to accurately diagnose any suspected acute complications during the ablation procedure, such as pericardial effusion and cardiac tamponade.

The integrity and possible anomalies of the interatrial septum should be assessed in order to safely perform the transseptal puncture. In the presence of a patent foramen ovale or interatrial septal defect, the septum may be probed to obtain transseptal access and introduce catheters into the LA without the need for transseptal puncture. The transseptal puncture can be more difficult in patients with an interatrial septal aneurysm, due to significant bowing of the septum. In such cases, a radiofrequency transseptal needle maybe particularly useful as its use maybe associated with a shorter instrumentation time and lower incidence of tamponade [15]. Any prior detailed history of patent foramen closure (including type of device and indication) is important to ascertain prior to the procedure.

Prior to AF ablation, an LA appendage clot should be excluded if appropriate anticoagulation has not been adequate for the past 3–4 weeks. Its presence should lead to additional anticoagulation and likely repetition of the transesophageal echocardiogram (TEE) because of a higher risk of stroke during or after the procedure [1]. Unfortunately, TTE has a very limited role for the assessment of left atrial thrombus

due to its relative inability to adequately visualize the LA appendage. Therefore, most AF ablation centers rely on a TEE within 12–24 h before the ablation procedure. Nevertheless, TEE is not necessary in patients who are in sinus rhythm at the time of and prior to AF ablation or patients who have been in AF for less than 48 h prior to AF ablation or those with lone AF and appropriate preprocedure anticoagulation [2]. The 2012 HRS/EHRA/ECAS guidelines of AF ablation recommend to consider TEE in patients with long-standing persistent AF with high thromboembolic risk (CHADS$_2$ score > 2) and large LA even if full anticoagulation (INR >2) has been present for 4 weeks or more prior to AF ablation [2]. It is important to understand that intracardiac echocardiogram (ICE) has significant limitations visualizing the LA appendage and thus, it should not replace screening TEE [2]. The ICE-CHIP study [16] demonstrated that while ICE is an acceptable modality to assess LA and interatrial septum anatomy, ICE does not have a good concordance with TEE for the detection of LA and LA appendage thrombus and spontaneous echo contrast (concordance 66 and 60%, respectively). Thus, ICE imaging during AF ablation should be considered complimentary and should not replace preprocedure TEE due to the limited sensitivity of ICE to detect LA appendage thrombus [2,16].

TEE can also assist in documenting baseline PV flow prior to ablation if ICE is not used during the ablation procedure. TEE has a few limitations in the preprocedure evaluation of AF ablation, including restricted visualization of the PV size and number [17]. Recent data has shown multiplane TEE had a 95% concordance with MRI for evaluation of PV anatomy and its variants [18].

Cardiac CT and MRI

More sophisticated cardiac imaging, such as cardiac computed tomography (CT) or magnetic resonance (MRI), has been routinely performed as part of the preprocedure evaluation in most high-volume AF ablation centers.

Cardiac CT and MRI can now provide detailed anatomical and functional information of cardiac valves and chambers. Due to the many anatomic variations in PV number and position, the evaluation of the LA and PV anatomy can be invaluable in preparing a safe and complete ablation strategy. Cardiac CT and MRI have a clear advantage in delineating LA anatomy including size, number, location, and possible anomalies of PVs [17]. MRI has helped to identify variant anatomy of the PV in about 38% of cases (Figure 5) [19]. Similarly, cardiac CT found

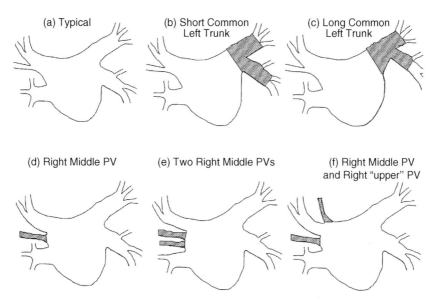

Figure 5 Branching pattern of pulmonary vein (PV) anatomy in controls and patients with atrial fibrillation. Shaded portions indicate different parts from typical anatomy. (a) Typical branching pattern. (b) Short common left trunk. (c) Long common left trunk. (d) Right middle PV. (e) Two middle PVs. (f) Right middle PV and right upper PV. *Source:* Kato et al., 2003 [19]. Reproduced with permission of Lippencott, Williams & Wilkins.

three or five right-sided pulmonary veins in 28%, a single right-sided PV ostium in 2%, and a single left PV ostium in 14% of the patients without AF (Figures 6 and 7) [20]. Unusual PV anomalies that have been described include a common ostium of the right and left PVs and a PV arising from the LA roof [21]. The left PV with a common ostium has been implicated as a common source of arrhythmogenic ectopy in patients with AF [22].

MRI has shown that the PV orifices are not fixed in size or position. Dynamic analysis of the PVs have revealed changes in the orifice size with cardiac cycle (a decrease of 32.5% during atrial systole) and location changes in the range of up to 7.2 mm [23]. MRI and

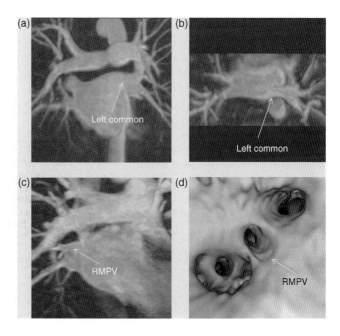

Figure 6 Examples of unusual PV anatomy. MRI demonstrating a long left common trunk ((a), AP view; (b) axial view) and right middle PV with discrete ostium ((c), AP view; (d), virtual endoscopic imaging). *Source:* Kato et al., 2003 [19]. Reproduced with permission of Lippencott, Williams & Wilkins.

(a)

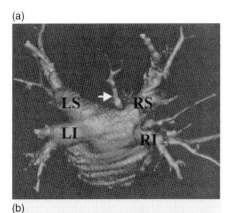

(b)

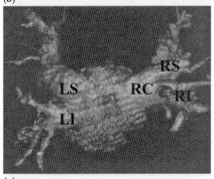

(c)

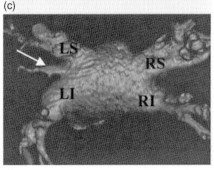

Figure 7 Atrial CT images from three patients with atrial fibrillation. (a) Anomalous insertion of right superior PV into LA body (arrow), (b) right common (RC) PV, and (c) independent insertion of the lingula branch of the left PV into LA. For abbreviations refer to Figure 3. *Source:* Schwartzman et al., 2003 [20]. Reproduced with permission of Lippencott, Williams & Wilkins.

CT scan can also recognize and characterize LA roof pouches (15%), septal ridges (32%) and the width of the ridges separating the left PV from the LA appendage (29%), and the right middle PV from the right superior and inferior PV (Figures 8 and 9). These LA variants appear to challenge the AF ablation procedure due to difficulty of obtaining a stable catheter position [24,25]. Moreover, these noninvasive imaging techniques may

identify the presence of an LA appendage clot, even though the sensitivity and specificity of MRI visualization of the LA appendage is a controversial subject [26]. Having preprocedure information about LA anatomy and esophageal location can help better plan the procedure.

In addition, cardiac CT or MRI can provide detailed position and relationship of the esophagus with the LA and CS, as well as esophageal abnormalities that could increase the risk of thermal injury (Figure 10). CT imaging has shown (1) large area of contact between esophagus and LA (mean length of contact: 58 mm), (2) direct esophageal contact with the mid to distal CS in up to 57% of patients (mean length of contact 6.1 ± 3.4 mm) (Figure 11), (3) a variable course of the esophagus along the posterior LA (parallel to the left-sided PV in 56% and an oblique course from left superior to right inferior PV in 36% of cases) (Figure 12), and (4) a thin posterior LA and esophageal walls (mean: 2.2 and 3.6 mm, respectively) (Figure 13) [27–29]. Therefore, imaging of the esophagus may aid ablation by avoiding delivery of radiofrequency ablation in sites adjacent to the esophagus [30]. However, the esophagus appears to be a dynamic structure that may change its diameter and position during the procedure.

These imaging techniques have been extensively used early in the AF ablation experience to monitor for the presence and severity of PV stenosis, when the incidence of this complication was seen in up to 10–12% of patients undergoing a more focal procedure (Figure 14a). Now, that the incidence of PV stenosis has decreased dramatically due to a number of factors, but primarily as a realization that ablation should be proximal to the pulmonary vein ostium or in the venous antrum, the need for these imaging techniques are much lower. CT or MRI of the LA is still performed prior to ablation at many centers, in order to perform image integration with electroanatomical mapping systems such as CARTO^{TM} Merge (Biosense Webster, Irwindale, CA, USA), which can facilitate the mapping and ablation procedures and lead to decrease in radiation exposure. Confirmation and comparison of the LA and PV size and structure are also important in the 15–20% of patients who may require a second or third repeat intervention.

It is important to have an appreciation of normal PV anatomy when analyzing CT or MRI scans. Recent CT analysis of the PV diameter demonstrated a gradual increase of the caliber of the right and left superior, as well as the right inferior PV, as they enter the LA. On the contrary, the diameter of the left inferior PV decreases as it enters the LA (Figure 14b) [31]. Therefore, careful

(a)

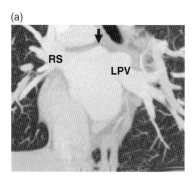

(b)

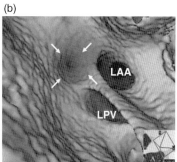

Figure 8 CT images from (a) coronal and (b) virtual endoscopic view of a pouch located in the anterior roof of the LA (arrows). For abbreviations refer to Figure 3. *Source:* Wongcharoen et al., 2006 [25]. Reproduced with permission of Wiley.

(a)

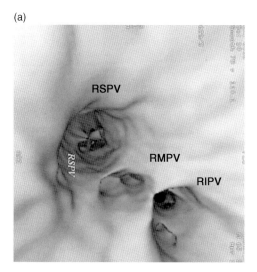

(b)

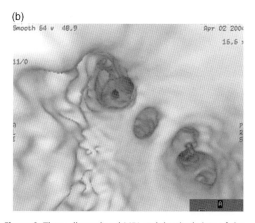

Figure 9 Three-dimensional MRI endoluminal view of the LA showing interpatient variability in the width of ridges between the right superior PV, the right middle (RM), and the right inferior PV. (a) Patient with thin ridges and (b) patient with thicker ridges. For abbreviations refer to Figure 3. *Source:* Mansour et al., 2006 [24]. Reproduced with permission of Wiley.

assessment should be performed when the left inferior PV is evaluated for stenosis.

Finally, the DECAAF trial recently demonstrated that atrial scar burden using a delayed enhancement MRI may be an independent predictor of response to RFA [32].

Cardiac CT and MRI are not considered mandatory in the preprocedure evaluation. CT and MRI have a number of limitations: (1) anatomical information provided by images (obtained a day prior to AF ablation) may differ from normal status since patient may have a different volume status, images are obtained during inspiration with inferior displacement of PV ostia, (2) increased administrative and financial burden, (3) higher radiation exposure associated with cardiac CT, and (4) potential nephrotoxicity of CT/MRI contrast media [33].

Many centers obtain complementary information from careful ICE imaging with the ICE probe either in the right or in the left atrium. A combination of ICE imaging plus contrast injection of the PV and LA or contrast-enhanced rotational X-ray angiography of LA and PVs can provide similar information and eliminate the need for preprocedural imaging. Kriatselis et al. demonstrated that rotational LA and PV angiography during adenosine-induced asystole has excellent correlation with CT imaging (correlation coefficient > 0.90 for all PVs) [33]. We believe that detailed knowledge of the cardiac anatomy and more specifically the LA, PV, and relationship with the esophagus may likely decrease the complications related to AF ablation, such as PV stenosis, LA perforation, phrenic nerve palsy, esophageal damage, and decrease radiation exposure [1]. In patients undergoing a repeat procedure, imaging of the veins is critical to make sure there is no preprocedure stenosis or other anatomic changes following the initial ablation. In the future, periprocedure *in vivo*

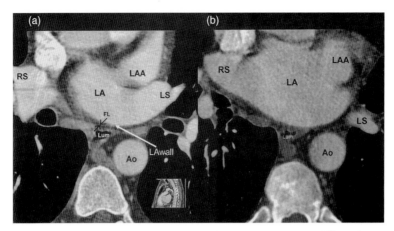

Figure 10 CT images of the esophagus and posterior LA at level of superior PVs. (a) Three different layers are visible, including the LA wall, thin layer of adipose tissue, and anterior esophageal wall. (b) No fat layer visible between LA and esophagus. Ao, Aorta; for abbreviations refer to Figure 3. *Source:* Lemola et al., 2004 [27]. Reproduced with permission of Lippencott, Williams & Wilkins.

or online/live CT and MRI may increase the safety and accuracy of the procedure.

Drug therapy

In preparation for the ablation procedure, medical therapy should be addressed in detail several weeks prior to ablation in order to optimize procedural safety.

All antiarrhythmic agents should be discontinued at least five half-lives prior to AF ablation. This will unmask potential triggers, such as atrial tachycardia, which need to be ablated in addition to LA ablation. This may also provide more accurate evaluation of complex fractionated electrograms (CFAEs) and areas of slow conduction to perform substrate modification procedure if indicated. Some centers will have the patient placed on amiodarone for one or more months at a low dose prior to AF ablation for chronic AF, while in most centers all antiarrhythmic drugs are stopped prior to ablation. In the case of amiodarone, we typically discontinue it at least 3 weeks prior to AF ablation and even longer if possible.

Expert consensus has always recommended that patients should be fully anticoagulated (e.g., INR 2.0–3.0) for at least 3–4 weeks prior to AF ablation. Any deviation from this standard, such as a single INR below 2.0 or unknown anticoagulation status in the

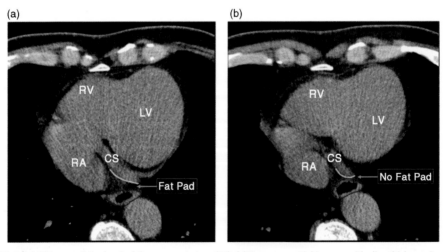

Figure 11 Axial CT image at the level of the coronary sinus (CS). (a) Two sequential images with slice thickness 3 mm showed direct contact between the anterior esophageal wall (red line) and the posterior aspect of the CS (yellow line). (b) No adipose tissue could be identified between structures. LV, left ventricle; RV, right ventricle; CS, coronary sinus; RA, right atrium. *Source:* Tsao et al., 2006 [29]. Reproduced with permission of Wiley.)

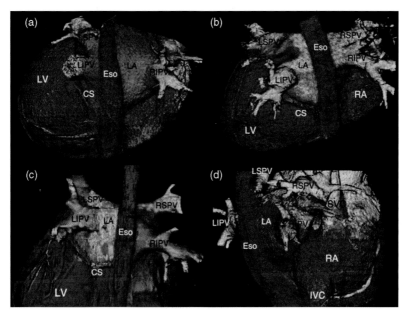

Figure 12 Relationship of esophagus to posterior wall: 3-dimensional CT images. Esophagus (Eso) may be positioned very close to the left-sided PVs ostia (a), may have an oblique course from left to right as it travels caudal (b), or may be closer to right-sided PVs than left-sided PVs (c). In sagittal projection, esophagus wraps around posterior left atrium (LA) along its entire length (d). SVC, superior vena cava; IVC, inferior vena cava; RA, right atrium. For abbreviations refer to Figure 3. *Source:* Lemola et al., 2004 [27]. Reproduced with permission of Lippencott, Williams & Wilkins.

weeks prior to AF ablation, should lead us to perform a TEE to exclude LA appendage clot.

For the past few years, a new strategy of continuous warfarin during AF ablation has been adopted widely. Recent clinical data has shown that AF ablation can be performed safely with therapeutic levels of warfarin [34,35]. Overall, these studies demonstrated a lower risk of thromboembolic events (odds ratio, OR, 0.10) and minor bleeding (OR 0.38) without significant increase in complications such as major bleeding or tamponade [34]. Thus, current 2012 HRS/

EHRA/ECAS guidelines for AF ablation [2] recommend to continue warfarin in preparation of AF ablation, avoiding bridging with low molecular weight heparin. Kim et al. [36] showed that complications were less prevalent with INR range of 2.0–3.0, with an optimal INR between 2.1 and 2.5, while an INR <2.0 and >3.0 had a twofold increase in complications with a sharp increase if INR was above 3.5. However, clopidogrel should be discontinued if possible prior to the procedure due to an increase in bleeding [36] while we generally continue aspirin.

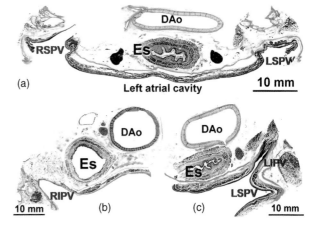

Figure 13 Transverse histological sections (Masson's trichrome stain) showing the proximity of the esophagus to middle of the posterior wall of the LA (a), the right inferior PV (b), and the left PV (c). DAo, descending aorta; Es, esophagus; LIPV, left inferior cava vein; LSPV, left superior PV; RIPV, right inferior PV. *Source:* Sanchez-Quintana et al., 2005 [28]. Reproduced with permission of Lippencott, Williams & Wilkins.

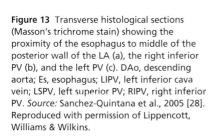

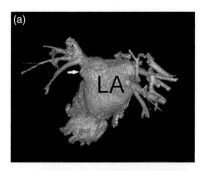

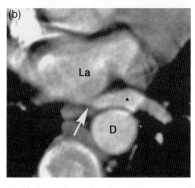

Figure 14 (a), CT angiography with a 3D-reconstruction of LA (posterior view) demonstrates complete occlusion of the left inferior PV at the ostium (arrow). (b) Transverse CT scan of the left inferior PV in a young woman shows normal tapering (arrow) of the left inferior pulmonary vein (*) as it enters the left atrium (LA). *Source:* Part (b), Kim et al., 2005 [31]. Reproduced with permission of Radiological Society of North America.

The safety of new oral anticoagulants (such as dabigatran, rivaroxaban, and apixaban) during AF ablation remains unclear at present. Observational studies and meta-analysis have addressed the periprocedural safety of dabigatran during AF ablation [37–41], with only one showing an increased risk of bleeding and thromboembolic events [37]. Due to the lack of large randomized trials with these newer anticoagulants, many electrophysiologists do not perform AF ablation while the patient is on dabigatran, rivaroxaban or apixiban and will require patients to hold these anticoagulants for at least 24 h prior to AF ablation. Some electrophysiologists feel uncomfortable using these newer agents until a tested antidote is available. Furthermore, the optimal time for stopping the newer agents during AF ablation is also unknown. An acceptable strategy for those patients is to switch to warfarin 3–4 weeks before the ablation, to continue warfarin during the ablation and to switch back to the new oral anticoagulants either immediately or shortly after the ablation.

Other interventions to consider before ablation are to optimize hydration to avoid or minimize risks of contrast-induced nephropathy. In diabetic patients, metformin should be held 3 days prior to the procedure and resumed 2–3 days after ablation, in an attempt to prevent lactic acidosis and acute renal failure associated with coadministration of IV contrast.

Patients with significant sleep apnea are encouraged to bring their CPAP machine on the day of the procedure. This is particularly important in laboratories where the AF ablation is performed with conscious sedation. Some other laboratories perform AF ablation under general anesthesia. In this situation, prior consultation with an anesthesiologist or nurse anesthetist is generally performed to evaluate the airway and risks for general anesthesia.

Finally, prior to catheter ablation of AF, the patient and relatives should be informed and educated about all aspects associated with this procedure. These include benefits, expectations, duration, limitations, safety, and risks of AF ablation. Furthermore, details of the recovery phase including return to work and activities should be discussed. The indications for the procedure are discussed in Chapter 1.

In summary, AF ablation is an elective procedure and a series of actions and studies should be performed in advance. These should include complete physical examination, complete and updated laboratory data, 12-lead ECG, 24-h Holter or 30-day event monitor, cardiac imaging studies, and adjustment of medical therapy. The duty of any physician performing AF catheter ablation is to be aware of all required patient information and studies that would help improve the outcome and safety of the procedure (Table 3). A careful review of all anatomic studies

Table 3 Checklist prior to atrial fibrillation ablation.

- Electrocardiographic documentation of AF
- Exclude reversible causes of AF (e.g., hyperthyroidism)
- Exclude and/or treat AF triggers (e.g., AP, AVNRT, and AT)
- Assess comorbidities and allergies (e.g., sleep apnea, IVC filter, etc.)
- Discuss risks, benefits, and alternatives of ablation
- Anticoagulation for at least 3 weeks unless TEE performed (documentation INR: 2–3)
- Assess left ventricular systolic function
- Assess anatomy, variants, and anomalies of LA, PV, and esophagus (MRI or CT preprocedure imaging)
- TEE to exclude intracardiac thrombus, if indicated
- Discontinuation of antiarrhythmic drugs for at least five half-lives in most cases
- Evaluate laboratory data prior to ablation
- Optimize hydration status prior to IV contrast load

is critical prior to bringing the patient to the electrophysiology laboratory.

References

1 Oral H, Morady F. How to select patients for atrial fibrillation ablation. Heart Rhythm. 2006;3(5):615–618.

2 Calkins H, Kuck KH, Cappato R, Brugada J, Camm AJ, Chen SA, et al. 2012 HRS/EHRA/ECAS expert consensus statement on catheter and surgical ablation of atrial fibrillation: recommendations for patient selection, procedural techniques, patient management and follow-up, definitions, endpoints, and research trial design: a report of the Heart Rhythm Society (HRS) Task Force on Catheter and Surgical Ablation of Atrial Fibrillation. Developed in partnership with the European Heart Rhythm Association (EHRA), a registered branch of the European Society of Cardiology (ESC) and the European Cardiac Arrhythmia Society (ECAS); and in collaboration with the American College of Cardiology (ACC), American Heart Association (AHA), the Asia Pacific Heart Rhythm Society (APHRS), and the Society of Thoracic Surgeons (STS). Endorsed by the governing bodies of the American College of Cardiology Foundation, the American Heart Association, the European Cardiac Arrhythmia Society, the European Heart Rhythm Association, the Society of Thoracic Surgeons, the Asia Pacific Heart Rhythm Society, and the Heart Rhythm Society. Heart Rhythm. 2012;9(4):632–696, e21.

3 Jais P, Shah DC, Haissaguerre M, Hocini M, Peng JT, Takahashi A, et al. Mapping and ablation of left atrial flutters. Circulation 2000;101(25):2928–2934.

4 Sauer WH, Alonso C, Zado E, Cooper JM, Lin D, Dixit S, et al. Atrioventricular nodal reentrant tachycardia in patients referred for atrial fibrillation ablation: response to ablation that incorporates slow-pathway modification. Circulation 2006;114(3):191–195.

5 Nanthakumar K, Lau YR, Plumb VJ, Epstein AE, Kay GN. Electrophysiological findings in adolescents with atrial fibrillation who have structurally normal hearts. Circulation 2004;110(2):117–123.

6 Yamada T, Murakami Y, Plumb VJ, Kay GN. Focal atrial fibrillation originating from the coronary sinus musculature. Heart Rhythm. 2006;3(9):1088–1091.

7 Kistler PM, Roberts-Thomson KC, Haqqani HM, Fynn SP, Singarayar S, Vohra JK, et al. P-wave morphology in focal atrial tachycardia: development of an algorithm to predict the anatomic site of origin. J Am Coll Cardiol. 2006;48(5):1010–1017.

8 Rajawat YS, Gerstenfeld EP, Patel VV, Dixit S, Callans DJ, Marchlinski FE. ECG criteria for localizing the pulmonary vein origin of spontaneous atrial premature complexes: validation using intracardiac recordings. Pacing Clin Electrophysiol. 2004;27(2):182–188.

9 Yamane T, Shah DC, Peng JT, Jais P, Hocini M, Deisenhofer I, et al. Morphological characteristics of P waves during selective pulmonary vein pacing. J Am Coll Cardiol. 2001;38(5):1505–1510.

10 Haissaguerre M, Fischer B, Labbe T, Lemetayer P, Montserrat P, d'Ivernois C, et al. Frequency of recurrent atrial fibrillation after catheter ablation of overt accessory pathways. Am J Cardiol. 1992;69(5):493–497.

11 Dixit S, Callans DJ, Gerstenfeld EP, Marchlinski FE. Reentrant and nonreentrant forms of atrio-ventricular nodal tachycardia mimicking atrial fibrillation. J Cardiovasc Electrophysiol. 2006;17(3):312–316.

12 Bogun F, Anh D, Kalahasty G, Wissner E, Bou Serhal C, Bazzi R, et al. Misdiagnosis of atrial fibrillation and its clinical consequences. Am J Med. 2004;117(9): 636–642.

13 Zhuang J, Wang Y, Tang K, Li X, Peng W, Liang C, et al. Association between left atrial size and atrial fibrillation recurrence after single circumferential pulmonary vein isolation: a systematic review and meta-analysis of observational studies. Europace. 2012;14(5):638–645.

14 Kilicaslan F, Verma A, Saad E, Themistoclakis S, Bonso A, Raviele A, et al. Efficacy of catheter ablation of atrial fibrillation in patients with hypertrophic obstructive cardiomyopathy. Heart Rhythm. 2006;3(3):275–280.

15 Winkle RA, Mead RH, Engel G, Patrawala RA. The use of a radiofrequency needle improves the safety and efficacy of transseptal puncture for atrial fibrillation ablation. Heart Rhythm. 2011;8(9):1411–1415.

16 Saksena S, Sra J, Jordaens L, Kusumoto F, Knight B, Natale A, et al. A prospective comparison of cardiac imaging using intracardiac echocardiography with transesophageal echocardiography in patients with atrial fibrillation: the intracardiac echocardiography guided cardioversion helps interventional procedures study. Circ Arrhythm Electrophysiol. 2010;3(6):571–577.

17 Wood MA, Wittkamp M, Henry D, Martin R, Nixon JV, Shepard RK, et al. A comparison of pulmonary vein ostial anatomy by computerized tomography, echocardiography, and venography in patients with atrial fibrillation having radiofrequency catheter ablation. Am J Cardiol. 2004;93 (1):49–53.

18 Toffanin G, Scarabeo V, Verlato R, De Conti F, Zampiero AA, Piovesana P. Transoesophageal echocardiographic evaluation of pulmonary vein anatomy in patients undergoing ostial radiofrequency catheter ablation for atrial fibrillation: a comparison with magnetic resonance angiography. J Cardiovasc Med (Hagerstown). 2006;7(10): 748–752.

19 Kato R, Lickfett L, Meininger G, Dickfeld T, Wu R, Juang G, et al. Pulmonary vein anatomy in patients undergoing catheter ablation of atrial fibrillation: lessons learned by use of magnetic resonance imaging. Circulation. 2003;107 (15):2004–2010.

20 Schwartzman D, Lacomis J, Wigginton WG. Characterization of left atrium and distal pulmonary vein morphology using multidimensional computed tomography. J Am Coll Cardiol. 2003;41(8):1349–1357.

21 Shapiro M, Dodd JD, Brady TJ, Abbara S. Common pulmonary venous ostium of the right and left inferior pulmonary veins: an unusual pulmonary vein anomaly depicted with 64-slice cardiac computed tomography. J Cardiovasc Electrophysiol. 2007;18(1):110.

22 Schwartzman D, Bazaz R, Nosbisch J. Common left pulmonary vein: a consistent source of arrhythmogenic atrial ectopy. J Cardiovasc Electrophysiol. 2004;15(5): 560–566.

23 Lickfett L, Dickfeld T, Kato R, Tandri H, Vasamreddy CR, Berger R, et al. Changes of pulmonary vein orifice size and location throughout the cardiac cycle: dynamic analysis using magnetic resonance cine imaging. J Cardiovasc Electrophysiol. 2005;16(6):582–588.

24 Mansour M, Refaat M, Heist EK, Mela T, Cury R, Holmvang G, et al. Three-dimensional anatomy of the left atrium by magnetic resonance angiography: implications for catheter ablation for atrial fibrillation. J Cardiovasc Electrophysiol. 2006;17(7):719–723.

25 Wongcharoen W, Tsao HM, Wu MH, Tai CT, Chang SL, Lin YJ, et al. Morphologic characteristics of the left atrial appendage, roof, and septum: implications for the ablation of atrial fibrillation. J Cardiovasc Electrophysiol. 2006;17(9):951–956.

26 Ohyama H, Hosomi N, Takahashi T, Mizushige K, Osaka K, Kohno M, et al. Comparison of magnetic resonance imaging and transesophageal echocardiography in detection of thrombus in the left atrial appendage. Stroke. 2003;34(10):2436–2439.

27 Lemola K, Sneider M, Desjardins B, Case I, Han J, Good E, et al. Computed tomographic analysis of the anatomy of the left atrium and the esophagus: implications for left atrial catheter ablation. Circulation. 2004;110(24): 3655–3660.

28 Sanchez-Quintana D, Cabrera JA, Climent V, Farre J, Mendonca MC, Ho SY. Anatomic relations between the esophagus and left atrium and relevance for ablation of atrial fibrillation. Circulation. 2005;112(10):1400–1405.

29 Tsao HM, Wu MH, Chern MS, Tai CT, Lin YJ, Chang SL, et al. Anatomic proximity of the esophagus to the coronary sinus: implication for catheter ablation within the coronary sinus. J Cardiovasc Electrophysiol. 2006;17(3): 266–269.

30 Kenigsberg DN, Lee BP, Grizzard JD, Ellenbogen KA, Wood MA. Accuracy of intracardiac echocardiography for assessing the esophageal course along the posterior left atrium: a comparison to magnetic resonance imaging. J Cardiovasc Electrophysiol. 2007;18(2):169–173.

31 Kim YH, Marom EM, Herndon JE 2nd, McAdams HP. Pulmonary vein diameter, cross-sectional area, and shape: CT analysis. Radiology. 2005;235(1):43–49; discussion 9–50.

32 Marrouche N. Delayed enhancement MRI determinant of successful catheter ablation for atrial fibrillation (decaaf): a doubleblinded, multi-center, prospective trial (Abstract LB 01–04). Heart Rhythm. 2013;10(5).

33 Kriatselis C, Tang M, Roser M, Fleck E, Gerds-Li H. A new approach for contrast-enhanced X-ray imaging of the left atrium and pulmonary veins for atrial fibrillation ablation: rotational angiography during adenosine-induced asystole. Europace. 2009;11(1):35–41.

34 Santangeli P, Di Biase L, Horton R, Burkhardt JD, Sanchez J, Al-Ahmad A, et al. Ablation of atrial fibrillation under therapeutic warfarin reduces periprocedural complications: evidence from a meta-analysis. Circ Arrhythm Electrophysiol. 2012;5(2):302–311.

35 Di Biase L, Burkhardt JD, Mohanty P, Sanchez J, Horton R, Gallinghouse GJ, et al. Periprocedural stroke and management of major bleeding complications in patients undergoing catheter ablation of atrial fibrillation: the impact of periprocedural therapeutic international normalized ratio. Circulation. 2010;121(23):2550–2556.

36 Kim JS, Jongnarangsin K, Latchamsetty R, Chugh A, Ghanbari H, Crawford T, et al. The optimal range of international normalized ratio for radiofrequency catheter ablation of atrial fibrillation during therapeutic anticoagulation with warfarin. Circ Arrhythm Electrophysiol. 2013;6(2):302–309.

37 Lakkireddy D, Reddy YM, Di Biase L, Vanga SR, Santangeli P, Swarup V, et al. Feasibility and safety of dabigatran versus warfarin for periprocedural anticoagulation in patients undergoing radiofrequency ablation for atrial fibrillation: results from a multicenter prospective registry. J Am Coll Cardiol. 2012;59(13):1168–1174.

38 Kim JS, She F, Jongnarangsin K, Chugh A, Latchamsetty R, Ghanbari H, et al. Dabigatran vs warfarin for radiofrequency catheter ablation of atrial fibrillation. Heart Rhythm. 2013;10(4):483–489.

39 Bassiouny M, Saliba W, Rickard J, Shao M, Sey A, Diab M, et al. Use of Dabigatran for peri-procedural anticoagulation in patients undergoing catheter ablation for atrial fibrillation. Circ Arrhythm Electrophysiol. 2013;6(3):460–466.

40 Bin Abdulhak AA, Khan AR, Tleyjeh IM, Spertus JA, Sanders SU, Steigerwalt KE, et al. Safety and efficacy of interrupted dabigatran for peri-procedural anticoagulation in catheter ablation of atrial fibrillation: a systematic review and meta-analysis. Europace. 2013; doi: 10.1093/europace/eut239 (First published online: August 16, 2013).

41 Hohnloser S, Camm AJ. Safety and efficacy of dabigatran etexilate during catheter ablation of atrial fibrillation: a meta-analysis of the literature. Europace 2013; doi: 10.1093/europace/eut241 (First published online: August 16, 2013).

42 Gerstenfeld EP, Sauer W, Callans DJ, Dixit S, Lin D, Russo AM, et al. Predictors of success after selective pulmonary vein isolation of arrhythmogenic pulmonary veins for treatment of atrial fibrillation. Heart Rhythm. 2006;3(2):165–170.

43 Chang SL, Tsao HM, Lin YJ, Lo LW, Hu YF, Tuan TC, et al. Characteristics and significance of very early recurrence of atrial fibrillation after catheter ablation. J Cardiovasc Electrophysiol. 2011;22(11):1193–1198.

44 Cai L, Yin Y, Ling Z, Su L, Liu Z, Wu J, et al. Predictors of late recurrence of atrial fibrillation after catheter ablation. Int J Cardiol. 2013;164(1):82–87.

45 Santangeli P, Di Biase L, Bai R, Horton R, Burkhardt JD, Sanchez J, et al. Advances in catheter ablation: atrial fibrillation ablation in patients with mitral mechanical prosthetic valve. Curr Cardiol Rev. 2012;8(4):362–367.

46 Hussein AA, Saliba WI, Martin DO, Shadman M, Kanj M, Bhargava M, et al. Plasma B-type natriuretic peptide levels and recurrent arrhythmia after successful ablation

of lone atrial fibrillation. Circulation. 2011;123(19): 2077–2082.

47 Sotomi Y, Inoue K, Ito N, Kimura R, Toyoshima Y, Masuda M, et al. Incidence and risk factors for very late recurrence of atrial fibrillation after radiofrequency catheter ablation. Europace. 2013;15(11):1581–1586.

48 Cha YM, Wokhlu A, Asirvatham SJ, Shen WK, Friedman PA, Munger TM, et al. Success of ablation for atrial fibrillation in isolated left ventricular diastolic dysfunction: a comparison to systolic dysfunction and normal ventricular function. Circ Arrhythm Electrophysiol. 2011;4(5):724–732.

49 Nair M, Shah P, Batra R, Kumar M, Mohan J, Kaul U, et al. Chronic atrial fibrillation in patients with rheumatic heart disease: mapping and radiofrequency ablation of flutter circuits seen at initiation after cardioversion. Circulation. 2001;104(7):802–809.

50 Gu J, Liu X, Tan H, Zhou L, Jiang W, Wang Y, et al. Impact of chronic obstructive pulmonary disease on procedural outcomes and quality of life in patients with atrial fibrillation undergoing catheter ablation. J Cardiovasc Electrophysiol. 2013;24(2):148–154.

51 Naruse Y, Tada H, Satoh M, Yanagihara M, Tsuneoka H, Hirata Y, et al. Concomitant obstructive sleep apnea increases the recurrence of atrial fibrillation following radiofrequency catheter ablation of atrial fibrillation: clinical impact of continuous positive airway pressure therapy. Heart Rhythm. 2013;10(3):331–337.

52 Yu S, Zhao Q, Wu P, Qin M, Huang H, Cui H, et al. Effect of anxiety and depression on the recurrence of paroxysmal atrial fibrillation after circumferential pulmonary vein ablation. J Cardiovasc Electrophysiol. 2012;23 (Suppl 1):S17–S 23.

6 CHAPTER 6

Intracardiac ultrasound

Dan L. Musat,[1] Jayanthi N. Koneru,[2] Scott W. Burke,[3] Farooq A. Chaudhry,[4] & Jonathan S. Steinberg[5]

[1]Valley Health System, New York, NY, USA
[2]Virginia Commonwealth University, Richmond, VA, USA
[3]Arrhythmia Institute, Newtown, PA, USA
[4]Mount Sinai School of Medicine, New York, NY, USA
[5]Arrhythmia Institute, The Valley Health System University of Rochester School of Medicine & Dentistry New York, NY and Ridgewood, NJ, USA

Percutaneous ablation procedures require the accurate placement of catheters at target tissues to deliver ablative energy to interrupt arrhythmia circuits, create lines of block or destroy triggering foci. Traditionally, the only tools used for guiding catheters into proper target zones have been electrical recordings and fluoroscopic imaging, the latter providing at best only indirect information, as judged by catheter position in relationship to the imaged cardiac silhouette, based on known anatomic relationships. Besides the less than optimal location guidance, it carries the risk of ionizing radiation exposure for the patients, operator, and support staff.

Intracardiac ultrasound (ICUS) is a valuable EP imaging modality, which allows real-time continuous, safe, and direct ultrasonic visualization of natural cardiac structures and intravascular catheters, and online instantaneous monitoring for unwanted complications. These characteristics offer the potential to enhance the success and safety of technically complex catheter ablation procedures, like those for atrial fibrillation (AF).

ICUS uses a catheter-based ultrasound probe that allows visualization of the heart from within the cardiac chambers or the great vessels. The catheter is positioned in the right atrium (RA) during the entire procedure with excellent patient tolerance [1–4]. The current longitudinal phased array, with variable ultrasound frequency, ICUS can provide comparable images to transesophageal echocardiography especially of the left heart, the interatrial septum, the valves, and the pulmonary veins (PVs).

In this chapter, we will describe the uses and advantages of ICUS.

Technical requirements: imaging equipment and transducer

Historical perspective

Over the years, ICUS catheters have become more miniaturized with improved maneuverability and dramatic image quality enhancement from single-element transducers to the current phased array electric crystal technology.

Technology has evolved from the late 1970s real-time M-mode intracardiac echocardiography [5,6] to the 1990s high-frequency transducers (10–20 MHz) with better resolution but limited tissue penetration [7,8], then the 9 MHz catheter (Boston Scientific Company, Watertown, MA) improving ultrasound penetration even further [9–13], to current electronic longitudinal phased array-based ultrasound catheter (8–10 F, 90 cm length) with a wide dynamic frequency range (5.5–10 MHz), with both pulse and continuous wave spectral Doppler and color flow imaging (AcuNav, Siemens Medical Solutions, Inc., Mountainview, CA) (Figure 1). The AcuNav utilizes single-plane imaging, with a single-use probe that can be connected to standard ultrasound imaging system. The variable frequency, steerability, and flexibility of the probe provide both higher resolution and deeper penetration and ability to image most of the

Practical Guide to Catheter Ablation of Atrial Fibrillation, Second Edition. Edited by Jonathan S. Steinberg, Pierre Jaïs and Hugh Calkins.

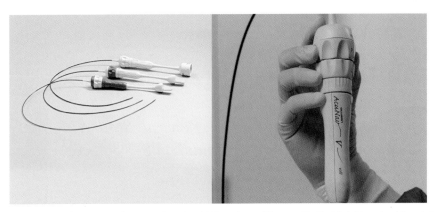

Figure 1 The bidirectional AcuNav catheters and AcuNav V 3D catheter (Siemens Medical Solutions, Inc, Mountainview, CA). The top knob rotates the catheter either anteriorly or posteriorly. The bottom knob is used to direct the catheter in a right–left orientation, while the last white knob locks the catheter in position. *Source:* Siemens Medical Solutions, Inc, Mountainview, CA. Reproduced with permission.

cardiac structures from the RA, right ventricle (RV), or inferior vena cava positions.

Real-time volume mode is the latest advance in ICE, allowing cardiac electrophysiologists to perform ablation in three-dimensional mode. It became commercially available as the ACUSON AcuNav V ultrasound catheter and comes with an imaging platform (SC2000 imaging platform, Siemens Healthcare, Mountain View, CA). Imaging can be performed in real-time volume mode using a 90-cm, 10-F phased array catheter capable of articulating 160° in four directions at 8-MHz frequency [14] (Figure 1).

Ultrasound principles and techniques

Ultrasound, as the name suggests, consists of sound waves with frequencies far above the upper limits of normal range for human hearing (20 Hz–20 KHz). Image resolution and penetration of the ultrasound

beam is based on the frequency of the transducer. As the frequency of the transducer increases, the resolution of the image improves but at the expense of decreased penetration (Figure 2a). Resolution of the image is based on the ultrasound speed (a constant) divided by the frequency of the transducer (Figure 2b). Thus, for transthoracic (surface) echocardiography, a lower frequency probe is used compared to transesophageal or ICUS, where the required penetration is lower as the probe is positioned right behind the heart or within the cardiac chambers. Understanding these basic concepts is important for any physician involved with ultrasound imaging.

Technique for visualization of critical anatomic structures

Placement and manipulation: The ultrasound catheter is introduced through a sheath inserted in a femoral

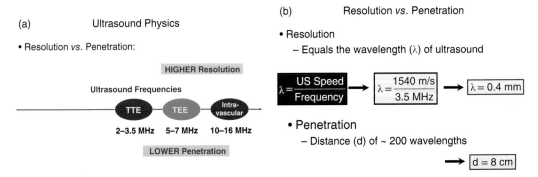

Figure 2 (a) Basic principles of ultrasound physics dictate that as you increase the ultrasound frequency of the imaging probe, the tissue penetration decreases. Thus, for optimal imaging, the image resolution has to be counterbalanced with the penetration of the ultrasound beam. (b) The resolution at a specific frequency is determined by dividing the wavelength of the ultrasound beam (1540 m/s) by the frequency of the imaging probe. In this example, using a 3.5 MHz probe the resolution is 0.4 mm. Conversely, the penetration is 8 cm, approximately 200 times the wavelength of the ultrasound.

vein and advanced to the RA using fluoroscopy or direct ultrasound visualization of the vessels to guide accurate placement, as the probe does not accommodate a guidewire system. Upon entry in the RA, the probe is usually positioned in the mid-RA in a *neutral position*: 1–2 cm above the IVC/RA junction, with visualization of the tricuspid valve and right ventricle. This position (Figure 3a) will be a common starting point for many of the anatomical destinations used in the electrophysiology laboratory including the tricuspid valve and the right ventricle, the mitral valve and the left ventricle, the short axis of the aortic valve, the interatrial septum, and the left atrium (LA), LA appendage (LAA), and the PVs. An imaging frequency of 7.5 MHz is optimal, and the position marker should be placed at the level of the

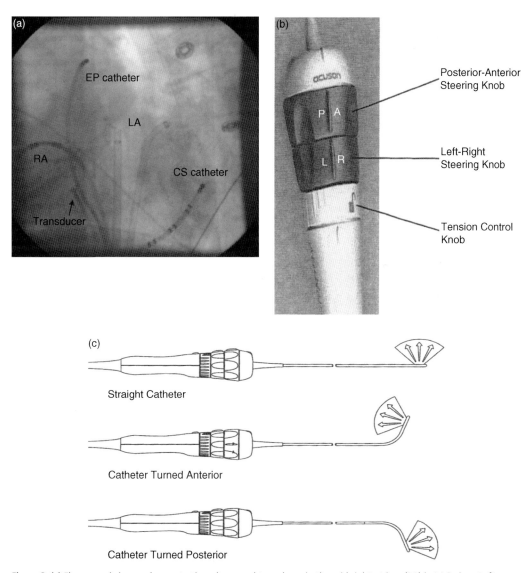

Figure 3 (a) Fluoroscopic image demonstrating ultrasound transducer in the mid-right atrium (RA) in LAO view. Left atrium (LA) and coronary sinus (CS) sheaths and catheters are also shown. (b) The AcuNav catheter has two steerable knobs: a posterior–anterior knob (P&A) and a left–right knob (L&R). Steerable knobs allow you to bend the tip of the catheter during imaging for acquisition of different imaging planes. (c) The imaging face of the AcuNav catheter faces anteriorly and the scanning plane is longitudinal. The catheter can be steered anteriorly/posteriorly or left to right maneuvering the respective knobs. *Source:* Part (b) and (c), Siemens Medical Solutions, Inc, Mountainview, CA. Reproduced with permission.

deepest cardiac structure imaged and depth should be adjusted to see the esophagus and the aorta.

The ICUS probe can then be manipulated to acquire different views by advancing, withdrawing, and rotation, similar to monoplane transesophageal imaging. Furthermore, the tip of the probe can be flexed or tilted using dials at the base of the probe to further optimize the imaging planes (Figure 3b–d). In all the views, 2D measurements as well as pulse and continuous wave spectral Doppler and color Doppler measurements can be obtained.

The probe can be further advanced into the RV to view the outflow tract (RVOT) and the pulmonary artery as well as the left ventricle for assessment of wall motion and presence of pericardial effusion, or RVOT and pulmonary artery to better visualize the LAA. If the probe is pulled further back to the inferior vena cava (IVC), the Eustachian valve and abdominal aorta can be readily visualized.

Manipulation of the probe to visualize specific structures: From the neutral position, a clockwise rotation (toward posterior) of the catheter permits imaging of all the left-sided structures helpful for AF ablation. The first structure to appear is the aortic valve in transversal plane with the three leaflets well visualized.

Left atrial appendage: Because the presence of LAA thrombus is a contraindication for LA ablation, detection of thrombus in at-risk patients is critical. Both TEE and ICUS can be used with excellent sensitivity to image the LAA and search for thrombus. With slight clockwise rotation of the probe from the neutral position, the LAA is the first structure visualized anteriorly in the LA, after passing the trileaflet view of the aortic valve, in the same plane as mitral valve, and can be inspected for thrombus. On the screen, LAA is the most lateral structure and has a typical pouch-like triangular or half-crescent appearance, with the tip pointing inferiorly, and has prominent trabeculae, to distinguish it from the PVs (Figure 4a). Infrequently, due to atypical cardiac anatomy, the LAA cannot be seen easily and additional adjustments of echo probe is necessary either by advancing or withdrawing while applying posterior or anterior

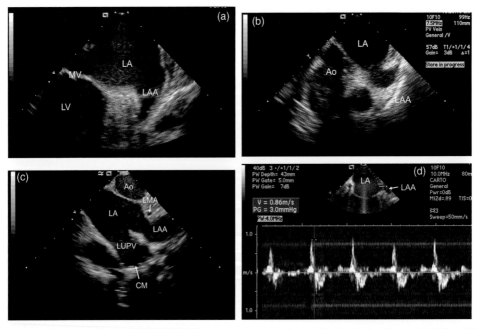

Figure 4 (a) Left atrial appendage the most lateral structure, triangular shape with tip pointing down. LAA, left atrial appendage; LA, left atrium; MV, mitral valve; LV, left ventricle. (b) The intracardiac echocardiographic image of the left atrial appendage (LAA) and left atrium (LA) from the coronary sinus. Ao, aorta. (c) The intracardiac echocardiographic image of the left atrial appendage (LAA) and left atrium (LA) from the right ventricular outflow tract (RVOT). LMA, left main artery; Ao, aorta; LUPV, left upper pulmonary vein; CM, circular mapping catheter. (d) Pulse Doppler velocities recorded at the entrance of left atrial appendage (LAA), sharp, with very high acceleration and deceleration of short duration, characteristic of LAA, depicting the blood flow ejected fast from the appendage.

flexion of the catheter to the cross-sectional image of the aortic valve or by placing the probe in the coronary sinus, RVOT, or pulmonary artery. (Figure 4b,c). Pulsed wave Doppler with the characteristic short-lived emptying and filling wave pattern of the LAA (Figure 4d) should always be obtained to verify that the imaged structure is LAA rather than the neighboring left upper PV. Lower LAA emptying velocity has been associated with a higher recurrence rate after AF ablation [15] and values below 20 cm/s are associated with higher risk of stroke.

Fossa ovalis: At about the same plane of LAA visualization, the interatrial septum can be seen in the near-field and can be spanned with clockwise/counterclockwise rotation. Some posterior deflection or slight withdrawal of the echo probe may be required. The septum has a thicker area (limbus) and a thinner area in the middle, the fossa ovalis, the identification of which is paramount for transseptal sheath placement (described below).

Pulmonary veins: If the catheter continues to be rotated clockwise slightly, the left PVs are visualized. From this position, the left common PV can be differentiated from two separate PVs (upper and lower) (Figure 5a). If the junction between the upper and the lower PVs joins the plane of the LA wall, two separate left PVs are defined and if the junction falls short of the plane of the LA wall, a common trunk is defined (Figure 5b). This differentiation is very important since some ablation strategies will be based on this information. While imaging the left PVs, pulsed wave Doppler and color flow can be obtained to confirm venous structures from LAA. Subtle clockwise/counterclockwise rotation may be necessary to obtain images of each PV and the LAA. The left PVs can usually be seen in their long axis. Applying more clockwise rotation, the right PVs are identified in sagittal view. They may look like "owl's eyes" in the near field of the image (Figure 5c). With slight movements, the veins could be seen in longitudinal axis as well; however these views might be difficult (Figure 5c). The right superior PV being located more anteriorly and closer to the septum can be more challenging; therefore, advancing the catheter to the junction of superior vena cava and anterior flexion of the catheter can help visualize this structure.

The diameter of each PV can be measured at the LA–PV junction from leading edge to edge. Color and pulsed wave Doppler information can be recorded by obtaining a sample volume 1–2 cm into the mouth of the PV to qualify venous flow. The typical tracing in sinus rhythm has three components: the forward flow components represent systole (S) and diastole (D), while a retrograde flow represents atrial contraction (AR) (Figure 5d).

Esophagus: Atrio-esophageal fistula is a rare but very severe complication of ablation for AF. The esophagus is in close proximity to the posterior wall of the LA and renders it susceptible to convection thermal injury with RF delivery, especially at the posterior wall. Good et al. have reported significant (≥2 cm) excursion of the esophagus during RF ablation performed under conscious sedation [16]. Thus, real-time knowledge of the location of the esophagus in relation to key LA landmarks is not only desirable but also vital in reducing the potentially fatal complication of atrio-esophageal fistula. The ability of ICUS to accurately identify the location of the esophagus is comparable to that of MRI [17], and Ren et al. [18] could identify the longitudinal extent of the posterior LA and the esophageal wall with the help of ICUS in all 152 patients studied. They also noted that monitoring the posterior LA thickness and reduction of power and titration of duration of RF delivery limited the risk of esophageal involvement [18]. The esophagus could be visualized in long axis at the level of left inferior PV, with fine clockwise movement of the probe, after passing the longitudinal view of the descending aorta. It is the deepest structure visible, beyond the cardiac structures and is identified by the railway track appearance with narrow, irregular lumen. If placed, the esophageal probe is readily seen in the lumen (Figure 6a). In rare difficult identification cases, a useful maneuver is oral administration of a carbonated beverage that provides echogenic contrast in the esophageal lumen facilitating the visualization (Figure 6b) [17].

As with other methods of esophageal visualization, like barium swallow, electro anatomical 3D tagging, and the use of an indwelling temperature probe, the ICUS delineate the lumen of the esophagus better than the outer wall. Therefore, when ablation is performed along the posterior LA wall or the PVs near the esophagus, a buffer zone is desirable. The optimal buffer zone has not been determined as yet; however, results from our studies indicate that a minimum of 24 mm is optimal [19] and greatly limits the likelihood of esophageal heating.

Other visualized structures: When the ICUS probe is at the junction of RA/IVC, the RA, tricuspid valve,

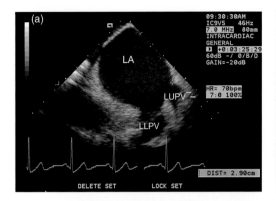
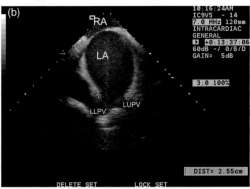
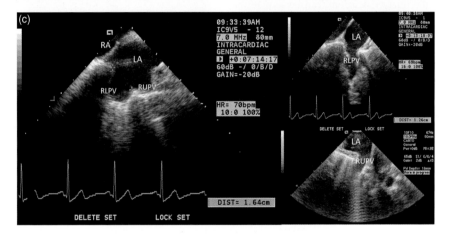
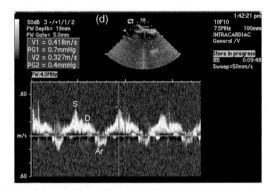

Figure 5 (a) Independent left lower (LLPV) and left upper (LUPV) veins emptying into left atrium (LA). (b) Image recorded with the probe near fossa ovalis in right atrium (RA), showing left atrium (LA) with a common left-sided pulmonary vein (orifice delineated by "+" signs) with left lower pulmonary vein (LLPV) and left upper pulmonary vein (LUPV). (c) Image recorded with the probe in high right atrium (RA), showing right upper (RUPV) and right lower (RLPV) pulmonary veins simultaneously and adjacently left atrium (LA) with long axis of RLPV and RUPV. (d) Pulsed Doppler velocity signals recorded with transducer in right atrium with sampling volume in ostium of the RLPV prior to ablation, showing peak flow velocity during systole (S) as well as flow during diastole (D) and atrial reversal (Ar).

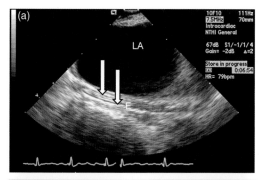

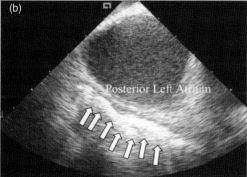

Figure 6 (a) Esophagus is the most posterior structure seen with appearance of "railway tracks" (arrows). (b) Image of the esophagus (arrows) after the administration of carbonated beverage as contrast. *Source:* Part (b), Kenigsberg, 2007 [17]. Reproduced with permission of Wiley.

and RV are visualized. Counterclockwise rotation of the probe from this position can bring the crista terminalis into view. By upward movement of the probe and clockwise rotation, the Eustachian ridge and cavo-tricuspid isthmus can be seen. The catheter in mid-RA allows imaging of the aortic valve and the RVOT. More clockwise rotation of the catheter makes imaging of the cross section of the coronary sinus and the aorta possible. By flexing the catheter into the RV and clockwise rotation to position it in RVOT, a cross section of the LV as well as papillary muscles and mitral valve leaflets can be visualized.

Transseptal catheterization

With the constantly increasing complexity of left-sided catheter-based ablative procedures, it has become mandatory that electrophysiologists be experts in the technique of transseptal catheterization. ICUS is an invaluable tool in performing transseptal catheterization safely and in a location-specific manner (anterior versus posterior and superior versus

inferior) depending on the nature of the intervention. Transseptal catheterization is performed to access the LA from the RA by crossing the fossa ovalis. In approximately, 10–15% of patients this maneuver is performed via a probe-patent foramen ovale [20]. In the remainder, mechanical puncture of this area with a needle and catheter combination is required. Transseptal puncture is safe, but an inherent danger of this procedure is the potential of the catheter or the needle to puncture adjacent structures: posterior wall of the RA or LA, the coronary sinus, or the aortic root. Inadvertent puncture of any of these structures is a dreaded and potentially deadly complication especially during anticoagulant therapy. Other complications of transseptal puncture include systemic arterial embolism and perforation of the inferior caval vein. Herein lies the importance of utmost accuracy in identifying the regional anatomy of the atrial septum. This regional anatomy may be variable depending on the underlying structural disease in an individual patient.

The advent of ICUS has vastly enhanced the safety and success of transseptal access during electrophysiological procedures and can supplant other traditional imaging modalities like fluoroscopy. Several prior studies of ICUS-guided transseptal catheterization have shown that successful puncture site was visualized in 100% of patients [21]. In a study by Daoud et al., 53 patients underwent transseptal puncture guided by ICUS and the success rate of the first attempt was 96% [22]. In our own experience, in thousands of patients, the transseptal access rate with ICUS guidance is virtually 100% with no significant adverse events.

Because ICUS is a direct method of imaging, the fossa can be visualized with a high degree of confidence. Occasionally, we have been convinced that despite the presence of all characteristic fluoroscopic signs, the sheath has not engaged the fossa, as judged by ICUS. In these patients, using direct imaging by ICUS, transseptal catheterization in a misleading location was avoided.

Transseptal technique

The current phased array ultrasound catheters provide a 90° sector image with tissue penetration of up to 15 cms, making imaging of the LA from an RA position feasible. Two planes of bidirectional steering (anterior–posterior and left–right, each to an extent of 160°) are possible.

The classic approach for transseptal catheterization is from the right femoral vein, although left femoral vein and transjugular approaches have been described. We typically monitor the position of the sheath in two

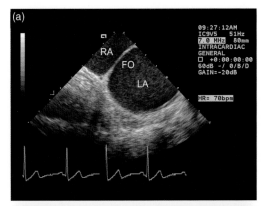

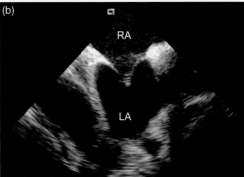

Figure 7 (a) The fossa ovalis (FO) is easily identified between right atrium (RA) and left atrium (LA) as thin walled membrane. (b) ICUS image of 'tenting' caused by the transseptal sheath in the right atrium (RA) pressing on the fossa ovalis and pushing it toward cavity of left atrium (LA).

fluoroscopy planes, antero-posterior and left anterior oblique. The ICUS catheter is positioned in the mid-RA, providing a clear view of the interatrial septum (see above). The ICUS catheter is moved slightly to gain a full view of the fossa in the center (Figure 7a). Some deflections of the ICUS catheter might be required. The fossa ovalis is clearly delineated, and its size, length, and proximity to the posterior and lateral LA walls are noted. Interatrial septal aneurysm can be visualized, if present.

The entire transseptal sheath is withdrawn from the SVC to the RA with the sheath via the transseptal needle rotated in a posterior direction. A characteristic downward "jump" of the sheath, detected by fluoroscopy, is an indirect radiological sign of the position of the fossa; the sheath appears directly in the view of the ICUS [21]. The sheath is then gently advanced toward the fossa. Once the transseptal sheath is in position, the operator surveys above and below the point of contact, as well as the point of entry, in order to visually verify appropriate angulation and prevent

the possibility of penetrating into an undesirable structure. If the dilator tip is too proximal to the LA wall, it can be rotated anteriorly or posteriorly until there is sufficient atrial space on the left side of the fossa ovalis for a safe needle puncture. We typically perform transseptal puncture when the ICUS images display tenting of the atrial septum and the left PVs in the same view (Figure 7b), thus confirming appropriate angulation for AF ablation.

The transseptal needle is then advanced from the dilator through the fossa ovalis, with the operator monitoring the ICUS images for any change in tenting. When a decrease in fossa ovalis tenting and microbubbles in the LA are observed, the dilator and sheath can be advanced safely into the LA and flushing the sheath with heparinized saline results in echogenic microbubbles within the LA, easily visible on the ICUS screen, providing additional confirmation.

Methodological variations

In patients who have had prior ablations and in those with lipomatous hypertrophy, the septum is thickened and/or a distinct fossa ovalis is not detectable on ICE. Additionally, aneurysmal atrial septum is particularly problematic because the process of tenting might result in apposition of the atrial septum to the posterior wall. There is a risk of posterior LA wall puncture in these scenarios. Electrocautery energy applied to the tip of the transseptal needle can aid the operator in achieving transseptal access without using undue force in some instances. Occasionally, transseptal puncture might have to be performed in patients with atrial septal defect closure devices. ICUS is invaluable in these instances, because the puncture has to be performed with pinpoint accuracy [23].

The visualization of the fossa ovalis and "catheter tenting" becomes particularly advantageous if transseptal access is required when the patient is already anticoagulated and some operators perform transseptal catheterization after the patient has been fully heparinized. Also in case of inadvertent proximal displacement of mapping catheter/sheath into RA during the procedure, reaccess of the LA can then be safely and confidently anticipated with ICUS guidance.

Pulmonary vein anatomy

Successful isolation of the PVs is widely considered to be the cornerstone of long-term clinical procedural response. This can be accomplished by segmental electrophysiologically guided delivery of RF ablation lesions at the LA–PV junction, contiguous RF lesion set designed to encircle one or both ipsilateral PVs just outside of the PV orifice or in a wider region, or ostial cryo energy delivery using a cryoballoon (Artic Front® Medtronic, Inc., Minneapolis, MN). All tactics depend clearly on the accurate identification of the PV orifice, both to successfully achieve the desired ablation results and to avoid specific complications. RF or cryo delivery within the PVs has been associated with a greater risk of PV stenosis, hence the evolution away from intra-PV lesion creation to ostial or extra-ostial sites.

There are a number of different ways to carefully identify the PV and its anatomical configuration. A preprocedure CT or MRI will beautifully render the atrial and PV anatomic relationships. This could be imported into the 3D electroanatomic mapping systems and merged with intraprocedural 3D schematic anatomy, but still requires time-consuming registration to align the images. Fluoroscopy is used throughout all ablation procedures but exposes patient and operator to radiation and does not image specific anatomic structures, only silhouettes and catheter positions relative to one another or estimated critical structure locations. Contrast imaging can help; LA or PV angiography will indeed be informative and accurate about the visualized anatomic structures. However, the image is recorded before the ablation catheter begins its tour of lesion sites and can be used only as a reference image for comparison with the live fluoroscopic image, incapable of online and continuous visual feedback of catheter location vis-a vis the structure of interest and lacking spatial resolution as well.

Hence, we and others [3,24] have resorted to the regular performance of ICUS for, among other uses, the accurate positioning of ablation and mapping catheters throughout the AF ablation procedure. The sheaths, ablation, and mapping catheters all can be visualized with ICUS in their real-time position relative to imaged anatomic sites (Figure 8a). Indeed their movement to and from positions can be monitored online on the ICUS. An enhancement for ICUS usage as monitoring tool during ablation is the CartoSound® module (Biosense Webster Inc., Diamond Bar, CA), which has the capability of integrating the real-time ICUS images into the 3D CARTO 3 mapping system with ability of online ablation catheter tip position identification (Figure 11)

We typically perform a full interrogation of all PVs (see above for specific advice regarding ICUS protocol) at the beginning of the procedure to:

1 determine the number of major and minor PV openings and their relative positions, ascertain the presence of common ostia (created by the confluence of the two major ipsilateral branches – a particularly common phenomenon on the left, seen in up to 50% of patients) [25]. Identification of a common PV is critical and its targeting during the ablation procedure very important for the long-term elimination of all potential PV trigger sites. These large antra are particularly difficult to ablate and require greater technical skill, effort, and perseverance to stabilize mapping and ablation catheters/cryoballoon.

2 assess the anatomic relationship of the LAA and the left upper PV, often very close to one another as well as the ridge between them, a common trigger site

3 measure the diameter of the PV orifice to help in choosing appropriately sized circumferential mapping catheter or cryoballoon to assure a good consistent contact at all PV ostial sites. PV diameters on ICUS appear to be larger in AF patients than controls and this observation is consistent with the hypothesis that stretch plays a role in PV arrhythmogenesis [25]. PV diameter increases as LA size increases. The PV size measured on ICUS is accurate and correlates well with other imaging modalities, such as CT and angiography [25].

4 determine if there is very proximal branching of the main PV vessel – the presence of proximal branching indicates that there should be no effort at moving the mapping system deeper into the PV and care exercised in establishing a rail for cryoballoon; energy delivery too close to the branches should be avoided.

5 quantify the systolic and diastolic flow velocity of each PV prior to ablation. If the ablation procedure is not the initial procedure, the presence of elevated PV flow velocity on the Doppler tracing is an indication of PV stenosis and the entire ablation tactical plan will need to be reviewed and possibly altered. PV Doppler results obtained by ICUS correlate very well with those simultaneously from TEE, with correlation coefficients exceeding 0.90 [26].

At the conclusion of the procedure, the PVs can be reimaged and the flow velocity requantified. We typically observe a slight increase in flow velocity, probably due to some edema at the LA–PV ostium, but not at levels indicative of stenosis. PV diameters also might shrink slightly. Although postablation observation of increased PV flow does not seem to predict subsequent PV stenosis [27], we do become concerned if PV flow velocity exceeds 100 cm/s especially if there has been a major change from baseline and sometimes institute short-term corticosteroid therapy in addition to the usual postprocedure measures.

Catheter vizualization, contact, and lesion-formation monitoring

Mapping catheter: After successful transseptal procedure, a circumferential mapping catheter is typically

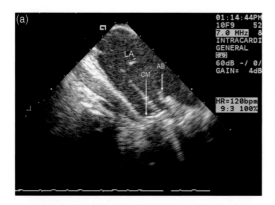
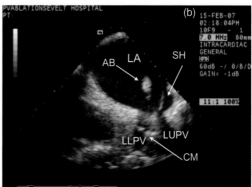
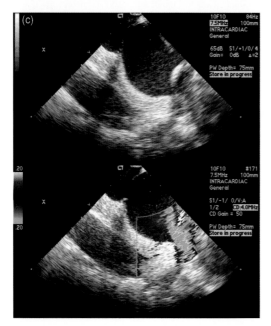
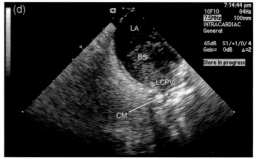

Figure 8 (a) An ablation catheter (AB) is positioned just at the ostium of the left lower pulmonary vein, guided by a circumferential mapping (CM) placed just inside the vein. The ablation catheter is making nice contact at the left atrial–pulmonary vein junction. (b) View of left atrial chamber and posterior wall with left lower (LLPV) and left upper (LUPV) pulmonary veins. Circumferential mapping (CM) catheter is positioned at the opening of LLPV, with its sheath (SH) crossing over the LUPV. The echodense ablation catheter (AB) and sheath sit near the opening of the LLPV. (c) Imaging of the cryo balloon (CB) with incomplete occlusion of the left pulmonary vein (LPV), demonstrated by color Doppler flow (cDf) coming out of the vein. (d) With good occlusion several seconds after balloon deflation, there is a "bubble shower" (BS) rushing out from the occluded vein. LCPV, left common pulmonary vein; CM, circular mapping catheter.

deployed at or near the ostium of the targeted PV, used for mapping, remapping, and as guidance for ablation. This catheter's characteristic structure is easily visualized (Figure 8a,b) and its relationship to the ostium of the PVs could be continuously assessed by ICUS. Moreover, the movement of the catheter from one to the other ispilateral vein could be done safely under only ICUS guidance.

Radiofrequency ablation: The ablation catheter's precise location and movement around the target

zone can be assessed and adjusted easily as needed on ICUS, especially if using the tip visualization with CartoSound module, whether the goal is ostial or extraostial positioning. Catheter drift from the desired position, either into the LA or deeper into the PV, can be detected immediately and corrected by continuous ICUS monitoring during the procedure. This advantage can become quite relevant when there are smaller PVs (e.g., right middle) where energy delivery is to be avoided.

Successful ablation depends on firm and stable contact between the RF catheter electrode and the target tissue, which results in local resistive and deeper tissue heating by conductive heat transfer. Poor contact results in loss of heat by convective transfer to circulating blood and inadequate tissue heating, resulting in a failed ablation attempt or nonpermanent loss of electrical function/lesion. Studies using ICUS have suggested that the conventional radiographic approach leaves much to be desired [28,29], and catheter contact was better detected and maintained by direct ICUS visualization than by fluoroscopy [29] as confirmed by indices of tissue heating and lesion size at pathologic examination. Nowadays, better ICUS quality and CartoSound integration makes possible to identify real-time minor catheter movements, such as sliding of the tip from the target zone (Figure 11).

Radiofrequency lesion formation monitoring: Certainly, the ability to verify lesion creation and quantify lesion size and contiguity would be advantageous during catheter ablation, especially when attempting to connect sites in a linear fashion. ICUS may be of value, but demonstration of clinical utility has been challenging. In carefully performed experimental studies, echocardiographic evolution of ablative lesion was observed as pitting on the ICUS image and offline measurement correlated very well with pathologic lesion volume [30]. Echocardiographic evidence of lesion formation includes tissue swelling or increased tissue thickness, pitting or dimpling of the endocardial surface, and increased echogenicity of the deeper tissue indicating tissue necrosis.

Because lesion size and depth can be accurately predicted *in vitro* by ICUS characterization of the target atrial tissue, there is the theoretical possibility that ICUS can alert the operator of nontransmural or noncontiguous lesions that may necessitate additional or more aggressive RF delivery or alternative ablation strategies. In practice, however, this type of strategy has proven quite challenging as clinical echocardiographic assessment of lesions is difficult, time-consuming, and likely not sufficiently accurate to guide clinical ablation.

During RF delivery, fine scattered microbubbles may be observed, suggestive of tissue heating and lesion creation. A rapid escape of a dense array of coarse bubbles may herald (within seconds) excessive tissue or blood heating and be associated with coagulum formation with impedance rise; thus some consider this an online indication to discontinue RF delivery [3]. Microbubbles are a sign of adequate catheter–tissue contact and likely lesion formation, whereas rapid release of coarse bubbles is an early warning to lower power output or halt ablation. Routine use of ICUS for continuous detection of microbubble formation to guide power settings during RF delivery in PV isolation procedures during the era of nonirrigated tip catheters was associated with better short-term success and few recurrences than ablation not using this approach [3] and has been advocated as a means to titrate energy delivery. However, at present most labs use open irrigated tip catheters, thus making it impossible to accurately differentiate the microbubble formation due to tissue heating from the echogenic bubbles produced by the irrigated solution.

Cryo-energy ablation: ICUS has provided helpful insight with the new cryoballoon ablation technique, which targets a circumferential scar at the ostium of PVs by freezing the tissue using liquid nitrogen delivered into a balloon. The balloon has to provide occlusion of the vein in order to reach temperatures low enough for transmural lesions, but care has to be taken for the balloon to be outside the vein. The occlusion and balloon position is usually evaluated by pulmonary venograms. ICUS could provide accurate information about good occlusion by the absence of the microbubbles in the left atrium during saline injection into the occluded vein. Another method to assess for occlusion is color Doppler evaluation at the ostium of the vein: if a leak is present one could see jets around the balloon. Also ICUS gives precise visualization of the balloon and the PV ostium, thus preventing cryo-energy delivery inside the vein [31,32]. An assessment of good occlusion after the freeze is a long thaw followed by a "bubble shower" that rushes out form the vein either immediately after balloon deflation or some seconds later after the occlusive intravenous ice melts (Figure 8c,d).

Early detection and treatment of complications

Pericardial effusion

Perhaps, the most frequent serious complication encountered during LA ablation procedures for AF is the development of pericardial effusion and progression to pericardial tamponade. In a large cohorts of patients undergoing AF ablation, asymptomatic pericardial effusion not requiring intervention was reported in 2.5% cases, while pericardial tamponade requiring intervention was reported in 0.29–1.3% of all cases [33–35]. During an AF ablation, if the patient becomes hypotensive, it is imperative to rule out pericardial effusion and tamponade.

In our labs, we immediately maneuver the ICUS catheter through the tricuspid valve, into the RV inflow tract and rotate the probe clockwise to look for the presence of pericardial effusion if a patient develops acute hypotension (Figure 9a). The absence of pericardial fluid essentially excludes the presence of tamponade (except in rare instances of loculated effusions) and other causes of hypotension need to be sought. Conversely, when a new significant effusion is found, with the accompanying physical signs, one can be confident that tamponade is present and begin preparations for emergent pericardiocentesis.

Ideally, detection of pericardial effusion prior to progression to tamponade can allow interruption of the procedure without the potentially deleterious consequences of tamponade and its treatment. ICUS is ideally suited to allow periodic and quick assessment of the pericardial effusion and any progressive changes in quantity.

Intra-atrial thrombus

One of the serious complications of LA procedures is thromboembolism, particularly cerebral thromboembolism. Transseptal procedures have long been known to have this risk, and all left-sided procedures require therapeutic parenteral anticoagulation. Although cerebrovascular accident can be caused by air embolism, spontaneous hemorrhage, or dislodgement of preexisting clot, the most likely cause is thrombus generated by the presence of left-sided intracardiac catheters, and may occur despite adequate anticoagulation. The risk of stroke is variable, but has been reported to be as high as 2–5%. Thrombus or char can also form at the tissue interface with the ablation catheter if overheating occurs. ICUS is very useful to identify intracardiac thrombus. When attached to catheters, thrombus will appear as an adherent mobile and serpiginous echodensity of varying size (Figure 9b).

Our consecutive series of 90 patients studied for the presence of thrombus formation detected by phased array ICUS during left-sided ablation procedures sheds some light on the most likely mechanisms [36]. We identified thrombus in 9% of patients, most commonly early in the procedure, within minutes of transseptal passage, and typically on the transseptal sheath. The space between the dilator and the sheath was thought to encourage blood stasis and a nidus for clot that propagates when exposed in the LA. A virtually identical incidence of thrombus, 10%, was observed in another series of AF ablation patients [37]. Similarly, this series found the majority of thrombus detected was not related to RF delivery and was observed on the sheaths and the mapping catheter. Neither study found thrombus at the endocardial site of RF delivery. Both series report that the thrombus formed despite adequate heparinization. In order to

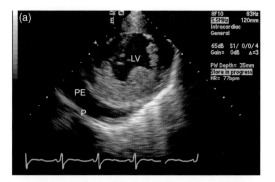

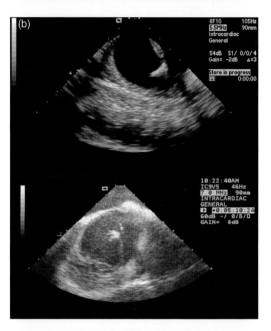

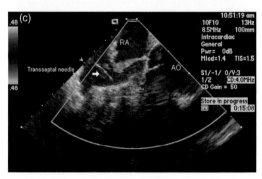

Figure 9 (a) View of left ventricle (LV) from RVOT used to demonstrate the presence of large pericardial effusion (PE); P, pericardium. (b) Large thrombus (white arrow) on sheath positioned in mid-left atrium. (c) Flow jet coming from the aorta into the right atrium after inadvertent puncture of the aortic sinus of Valsalva.

combat the development of embolization, it is crucial to prevent thrombus formation on sheaths, mapping catheters, and ablation catheters, and a variety of techniques are employed. Some have suggested the presence of spontaneous echo contrast is a predisposing factor [37]. Thus, vigilance is called upon for the entire procedure and during all procedures. We strongly believe that detection of thrombus before it embolizes is crucial to keeping the stroke rate as low as possible. ICUS is indispensable in this effort. When thrombus is detected on the sheath, the most typical location, we can aspirate the thrombus, and confirm its disappearance by ICUS [36]. The procedure can then be continued to completion. Adherent thrombus to catheter or sheath has also been successfully withdrawn to the RA without cardioembolic sequelae [37].

ICUS can also identify acute wall motion abnormalities that can occur after air embolism through the sheaths.

Pulmonary vein stenosis

PV stenosis is now much less common. It is usually neither an acute complication nor is it observable during the ablation procedure, but develops in the weeks and months later. Certainly, Doppler interrogation of the PVs will detect markedly increased flow velocity (>120 cm/s) with turbulent flow, or even no flow, if severe stenosis was present. Thus the hemodynamic detection of stenosis by ICUS would likely be encountered only at a repeat procedure. Of course, this can be confirmed by ICUS observation of a narrowed lumen with similar findings on CT/MRI and direct contrast angiography.

The best approach to prevent this complication is to perform ablation away from the PV ostium and as antral as possible.

Inadvertent puncture of aorta during transseptal catheterization

Inadvertent puncture of the aorta can happen when the transseptal apparatus "rides" up the septum and needle perforates the aorta or if the initial "drop" of the transeptal apparatus is mistaken for engaging the fossa ovalis. This usually happens when the aortic knob is prominent and ICUS is not used for confirmation of "tenting." Immediate recognition of this complication with the help of ICUS should alert the operator not to advance the sheath over the needle (Figure 9c).

Other preventative measures

The careful screening of the LAA and the LA for *in situ* thrombus by ICUS prior to LA access is almost certainly beneficial to prevent dislodgement of thrombus. Proper catheter positioning as guided by ICUS and avoidance of tissue or catheter overheating also likely prevents complications. Avoiding RF delivery near the ICUS-imaged esophagus is also advantageous.

Catheter ablation of atrial fibrillation without fluoroscopy

With the increase in the use of ablative therapies for cardiac arrhythmias came the increased exposure of patients and operators alike to fluoroscopy, presenting a significant risk. The advance of ICUS and 3D mapping technologies over the last several years affords the opportunity to alter this risk. Many laboratories have adopted an aggressive fluoroscopy reduction program, even eliminating the need for fluoroscopy in some cases.

These efforts rely heavily on 3D mapping technologies and their integration with ICUS. This allows for live catheter and electrode visualization, significantly reducing the need for fluoroscopy to navigate, while offering better intracardiac detail and visualization of the entire catheter to assist with maneuverability.

One of us (SB) has developed and safely employed in large numbers of patients a virtually radiation-free ablation procedure. After femoral vein access, venous structures are navigated with the ICUS probe by advancing the catheter toward the echolucent zone, representing the vein body (Figure 10a). If resistance is met, the catheter is withdrawn and redirected. As the probe is advanced, the liver is identified. At this level, the long guidewires for the transseptal sheaths can be seen.

The ICUS catheter is advanced to the junction of the RA and the SVC to confirm the location of the two long guidewires. The long sheaths are then safely delivered to the SVC under ultrasound guidance in preparation for transseptal puncture.

Next, the entire LA is surveyed using ICUS as described above. Transseptal catheterization is then performed using the standard technique with ICUS visualization of fossa tenting and microbubble spray once the needle crosses the septum (Figure 10b–d).

When placing the reference coronary sinus (CS) catheter, nonfluoroscopic access is possible utilizing one of the two techniques. The first approach is to take the processed ultrasound CS images and develop them in a biplane view in the 3D mapping system and then advance a decapolar catheter with electrode and shaft visualization via the femoral vein gently to the RA. The tip of the electrode is then positioned into the CS os and advanced into the CS with standard technique (Figure 11a–d). If this is unsuccessful, electroanatomic

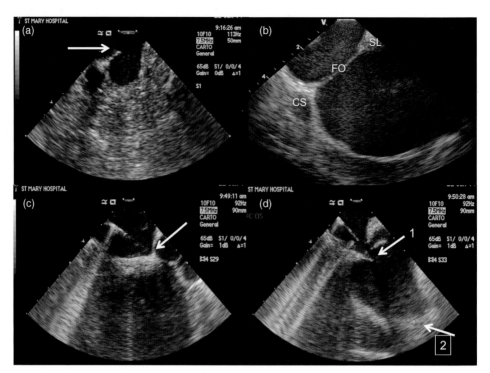

Figure 10 (a) Confluence of the femoral veins during ICE introduction (arrow). (b) Detailed view of the interatrial septum with the superior limbus (SL), fossa ovalis (FO), and coronary sinus (CS). (c) Transseptal dilator during descent from SVC toward FO arriving in the superior RA septum with the aortic root just beyond the needle (arrow). (d) Transseptal dilator arriving in the FO upon further descent (arrow 1). Note the needle was directed toward the 5 o'clock position and the assembly was followed within the vasculature by ICE only. Also note the ICE notation of the LPV carina as a 'target' (arrow 2).

data from the RA is acquired and the zone of the CS os is detailed, typically showing the course of the CS and allowing access without fluoroscopy.

All imaging data are then used to design the complete PV antral lesion set until complete PVI is demonstrated. After PVI, entrance and exit block along the linear lesion sets is confirmed.

Future directions

From time of publication of the previous edition of this book to now, several of the possible advances have indeed occurred. Namely, we now routinely place anatomic and ablation lesions directly on the US map and interface for live use during the procedure. Also, the catheters have been made in smaller caliber. Transponders now allow live ablation catheter visualization. We can expect several more advances in the ICUS realm in the near future.

1 Further miniaturization will allow incorporation of more elements into the phased array catheters that will add more flexibility in tissue penetration and tissue characterization. Therapeutic elements such as radiofrequency current delivery may be incorporated.

2 While 3D ICUS exists, its incorporation into the ablation workflow has yet to occur. The current workflow includes a basic 3D reconstruction of US. However, it is anticipated that an automated 3D reconstruction will occur, improving the speed of this modality and its application to a live ablation procedure.

3 4D ICUS will be the next stage, with a live rendering of 3D ultrasound images. Incorporation of live catheter positions and allowing labeling of critical structures will offer significant advantage. It is likely that 3D goggles will be utilized by operators to achieve a true 3D/4D experience.

4 Characterizing the ablation lesion will be a major step forward. Being able to identify areas of incompletely ablated tissue with higher resolution US will potentially improve the success rates of the ablative procedures. Adding labels from the live electroanatomic map of pressure and impedance values may give further advantage.

5 Automation of echocardiographic settings will allow for live rapid refinement of images that will improve speed and safety of these procedures.

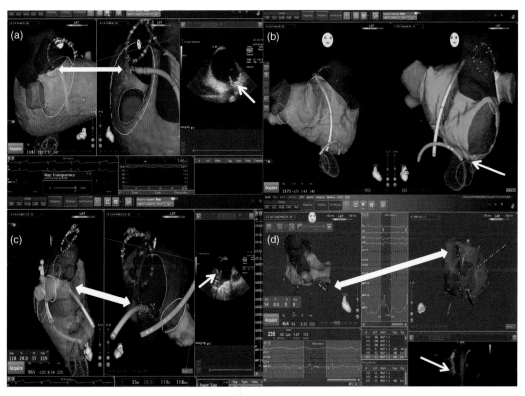

Figure 11 (a) Nonfluoroscopic positioning of the reference catheter just prior to CS access (arrow); (b) ICUS confirmation of ablation catheter on the carina between the left PV's (arrows) (c) ICUS confirmation of ablation catheter on the anterior carina between the right PV's (arrows); (d) ICUS confirmation of the ablation catheter on the distal CTI during ablation of typical atrial flutter (arrows).

6 Incorporating live or virtual electroanatomic elements into the 4D maps of the future will reverse the current process of using the electroanatomic map first, allowing one to use live ICUS to 'visualize' electrical activity and more rapidly design ablation strategy.

References

1 Packer DL, Stevens CL, Curley MG, et al. Intracardiac phased-array imaging: methods and initial clinical experience with high resolution, under blood visualization: initial experience with intracardiac phased-array ultrasound. J Am Coll Cardiol. 2002;39(3):509–516.

2 Cooper JM, Epstein LM. Use of intracardiac echocardiography to guide ablation of atrial fibrillation. Circulation 2001;104(25):3010–3013.

3 Marrouche NF, Martin DO, Wazni O, et al. Phased-array intracardiac echocardiography monitoring during pulmonary vein isolation in patients with atrial fibrillation: impact on outcome and complications. Circulation 2003;107(21):2710–2716.

4 Ren JF, Marchlinski FE, Callans DJ, Herrmann HC. Clinical use of AcuNav diagnostic ultrasound catheter imaging during left heart radiofrequency ablation and transcatheter closure procedures. J Am Soc Echocardiogr. 2002;15(10 Pt 2):1301–1308.

5 Conetta DA, Christie LG Jr., Pepine CJ, Nichols WW, Conti CR. Intracardiac M-mode echocardiography for continuous left ventricular monitoring: method and potential application. Catheter Cardiovasc Diagn. 1979;5(2):135–143.

6 Glassman E, Kronzon I. Transvenous intracardiac echocardiography. Am J Cardiol. 1981;47(6):1255–1259.

7 Pandian NG, Kumar R, Katz SE, et al. Real-time, intracardiac, two-dimensional echocardiography: enhanced depth of field with a low-frequency (12.5 MHz) ultrasound catheter. Echocardiography 1991;8(4):407–422.

8 Schwartz SL, Gillam LD, Weintraub AR, et al. Intracardiac echocardiography in humans using a small-sized (6F), low frequency (12.5 MHz) ultrasound catheter. Methods, imaging planes and clinical experience. J Am Coll Cardiol. 1993;21(1):189–198.

9 Callans DJ, Ren JF, Schwartzman D, Gottlieb CD, Chaudhry FA, Marchlinski FE. Narrowing of the superior vena cava–right atrium junction during radiofrequency catheter ablation for inappropriate sinus tachycardia: analysis with intracardiac echocardiography. J Am Coll Cardiol. 1999;33(6):1667–1670.

10 Kalman JM, Olgin JE, Karch MR, Lesh MD. Use of intracardiac echocardiography in interventional

electrophysiology. Pacing Clin Electrophysiol. 1997; 20(9 Pt 1):2248–2262.

11 Ren JF, Schwartzman D, Callans DJ, Marchlinski FE, Zhang LP, Chaudhry FA. Intracardiac echocardiographic imaging in guiding and monitoring radiofrequency catheter ablation at the tricuspid annulus. Echocardiography 1998;15(7):661–664.

12 Ren JF, Schwartzman D, Chaudhry FA. Intracardiac echocardiographic imaging of right atrial appendage: mass vs. pectinate muscle. J Interv Card Electrophysiol. 1998;2(3):247–248.

13 Ren JF, Schwartzman D, Michele JJ, et al. Lower frequency (5 MHZ) intracardiac echocardiography in a large swine model: imaging views and research applications. Ultrasound Med Biol. 1997;23(6):871–877.

14 Brysiewicz N, Mitiku T, Haleem K, et al. 3D Real-time intracardiac echocardiographic visualization of atrial structures relevant to atrial fibrillation ablation. JACC. Cardiovascular Imaging 2014;7(1):97–100.

15 Verma A, Marrouche NF, Yamada H, et al. Usefulness of intracardiac Doppler assessment of left atrial function immediately post-pulmonary vein antrum isolation to predict short-term recurrence of atrial fibrillation. Am J Cardiol. 2004;94(7):951–954.

16 Good E, Oral H, Lemola K, et al. Movement of the esophagus during left atrial catheter ablation for atrial fibrillation. J Am Coll Cardiol. 2005;46(11):2107–2110.

17 Kenigsberg DN, Lee BP, Grizzard JD, Ellenbogen KA, Wood MA. Accuracy of intracardiac echocardiography for assessing the esophageal course along the posterior left atrium: a comparison to magnetic resonance imaging. J Cardiovasc Electrophysiol. 2007;18(2):169–173.

18 Ren JF, Lin D, Marchlinski FE, Callans DJ, Patel V. Esophageal imaging and strategies for avoiding injury during left atrial ablation for atrial fibrillation. Heart Rhythm 2006;3(10):1156–1161.

19 Musat D, Aziz EF, Koneru J, et al. Computational method to predict esophageal temperature elevations during pulmonary vein isolation. Pacing Clin Electrophysiol. 2010;33(10):1239–1248.

20 Baim DS, Simon DI. Percutaneous approach, including trans-septal and apical puncture. Grossman's Cardiac Catheterization, Angiography, and Intervention, 7th ed. Lippincott Williams & Wilkins, 2005.

21 Szili-Torok T KG, Theuns D, Res J, Roelandt JR, Jordaens LJ. Transseptal left heart catheterization guided by intracardiac echocardiography. Heart 2001;86: E11.

22 Daoud EG, Kalbfleisch SJ, Hummel JD. Intracardiac echocardiography to guide transseptal left heart catheterization for radiofrequency catheter ablation. J Cardiovasc Electrophysiol. 1999;10(3):358–363.

23 Santangeli P, Di Biase L, Burkhardt JD, et al. Transseptal access and atrial fibrillation ablation guided by intracardiac echocardiography in patients with atrial septal closure devices. Heart Rhythm 2011;8(11):1669–1675.

24 Herweg B, Sichrovsky T, Polosajian L, Vloka M, Rozenshtein A, Steinberg JS. Anatomic substrate, procedural results, and clinical outcome of ultrasound-guided left atrial-pulmonary vein disconnection for treatment of atrial fibrillation. Am J Cardiol. 2005;95(7):871–875.

25 Herweg B, Sichrovsky T, Polosajian L, Rozenshtein A, Steinberg JS. Hypertension and hypertensive heart disease are associated with increased ostial pulmonary vein diameter. J Cardiovasc Electrophysiol. 2005;16(1):2–5.

26 Morton JB, Sanders P, Sparks PB, Morgan J, Kalman JM. Usefulness of phased-array intracardiac echocardiography for the assessment of left atrial mechanical "stunning" in atrial flutter and comparison with multiplane transesophageal echocardiography(*). Am J Cardiol. 2002;90(7):741–746.

27 Saad EB, Cole CR, Marrouche NF, et al. Use of intracardiac echocardiography for prediction of chronic pulmonary vein stenosis after ablation of atrial fibrillation. J Cardiovasc Electrophysiol. 2002;13(10):986–989.

28 Chu E, Fitzpatrick AP, Chin MC, Sudhir K, Yock PG, Lesh MD. Radiofrequency catheter ablation guided by intracardiac echocardiography. Circulation 1994;89(3): 1301–1305.

29 Kalman JM, Fitzpatrick AP, Olgin JE, et al. Biophysical characteristics of radiofrequency lesion formation *in vivo*: dynamics of catheter tip–tissue contact evaluated by intracardiac echocardiography. Am Heart J. 1997;133(1): 8–18.

30 Kalman JM, Jue J, Sudhir K, Fitzgerald P, Yock P, Lesh MD. *In vitro* quantification of radiofrequency ablation lesion size using intracardiac echocardiography in dogs. Am J Cardiol. 1996;77(2):217–219.

31 Catanzariti D, Maines M, Angheben C, Centonze M, Cemin C, Vergara G. Usefulness of contrast intracardiac echocardiography in performing pulmonary vein balloon occlusion during Cryo-ablation for atrial fibrillation. Indian Pacing Electrophysiol J. 2012;12(6):237–249.

32 Nolker G, Heintze J, Gutleben KJ, et al. Cryoballoon pulmonary vein isolation supported by intracardiac echocardiography: integration of a nonfluoroscopic imaging technique in atrial fibrillation ablation. J Cardiovasc Electrophysiol. 2010;21(12):1325–1330.

33 Cappato R, Calkins H, Chen SA, et al. Updated worldwide survey on the methods, efficacy, and safety of catheter ablation for human atrial fibrillation. Circ Arrhythm Electrophysiol. 2010;3(1):32–38.

34 Hammerstingl C, Tripp C, Schmidt H, von der Recke G, Omran H. Periprocedural bridging therapy with low-molecular-weight heparin in chronically anticoagulated patients with prosthetic mechanical heart valves: experience in 116 patients from the prospective BRAVE registry. J Heart Valve Dis. 2007;16(3):285–292.

35 Santangeli P, Di Biase L, Horton R, et al. Ablation of atrial fibrillation under therapeutic warfarin reduces periprocedural complications: evidence from a meta-analysis. Circ Arrhythm Electrophysiol. 2012;5(2):302–311.

36 Maleki K, Mohammadi R, Hart D, Cotiga D, Farhat N, Steinberg JS. Intracardiac ultrasound detection of thrombus on transseptal sheath: incidence, treatment, and prevention. J Cardiovasc Electrophysiol. 2005;16(6): 561–565.

37 Ren JF, Marchlinski FE, Callans DJ. Left atrial thrombus associated with ablation for atrial fibrillation: identification with intracardiac echocardiography. J Am Coll Cardiol. 2004;43(10):1861–1867.

CHAPTER 7

Electroanatomic mapping systems

Carlos Macias, Olujimi Ajijola,
Kalyanam Shivkumar, & Eric Buch

UCLA Cardiac Arrhythmia Center, Ronald Reagan UCLA Health System,
David Geffen School of Medicine at UCLA, Los Angeles, CA, USA

Introduction to electroanatomic mapping systems

Safe and effective catheter ablation of atrial fibrillation (AF) depends on a comprehensive understanding of cardiac anatomy, including the left atrium (LA), pulmonary veins (PV), and neighboring structures. Although fluoroscopy can show catheter location in a two-dimensional plane, it requires ionizing radiation that carries risk for both patients and the electrophysiology lab staff. Electroanatomic mapping (EAM) systems can provide real-time three-dimensional anatomic information to guide radiofrequency (RF) catheter ablation of AF without radiation exposure, and have become routine in many electrophysiology laboratories. Their role in cryoballoon ablation is less well established; other modalities such as intracardiac echocardiography may complement fluoroscopy sufficiently so that EAM is not needed.

Among the benefits of EAM for AF ablation are the ability to map the LA and its relationship to sites of interest such as the PV ostia, left atrial appendage (LAA), mitral annulus, coronary sinus, and others. With EAM, the operator can track the location of intracardiac catheters without fluoroscopy and record the signals obtained at each site for later review in order to delineate scar or abnormal electrograms (Figure 1). In addition, structures to avoid during ablation, such as the bundle of His, phrenic nerve, and LA sites near the esophagus, can be tagged on the map to prevent collateral damage. EAM systems also permit mapping other arrhythmias that may be encountered during AF ablation, such as focal atrial tachycardia and macroreentrant atrial flutter. Finally, preprocedure imaging with computerized tomography (CT) scan or cardiac magnetic resonance imaging (cMRI) can be imported into the EAM system, reducing time required for mapping and further reducing radiation exposure.

EAM systems are broadly divided into two main groups based on the technology employed for determining catheter location. Localization based on magnetic field (magnetic EAM) is used by the CARTO system (Biosense-Webster, Inc, Diamond Bar, CA). Impedance-based systems, such as EnSite NaVX (St Jude Medical, St Paul, MN), record changes in electrical impedance from each catheter as low-level current is applied across skin reference patches. More recently, a hybrid model for catheter location, combining magnetic and impedance technology, has been employed by the Rhythmia Medical system (Boston Scientific, Inc, Natick, MA, USA).

Regardless of the technology used for catheter localization, currently available EAM systems have been shown to be accurate and precise. Bourier et al. compared spatial and point localization accuracy between the CARTO and the EnSite systems, finding them to be similar, with a discrepancy generally less than 3 mm between systems [1].

CARTO system

The CARTO mapping system (Biosense, Diamond Bar, CA, USA) utilizes a low-level magnetic field (5×10^{-6} to 5×10^{-5} Tesla) delivered from three separate coils in a locator pad beneath the patient and two reference patches placed in anterior and

Practical Guide to Catheter Ablation of Atrial Fibrillation, Second Edition. Edited by Jonathan S. Steinberg, Pierre Jaïs and Hugh Calkins.

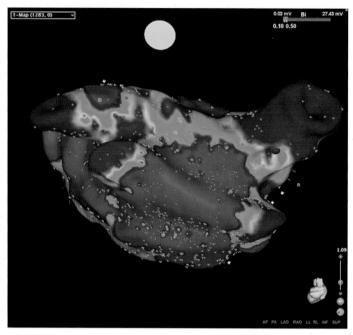

Figure 1 LA postero-anterior (PA) view using CARTO 3 for voltage mapping. Regions of normal voltage are marked with purple and in this case involved the majority of the posterior wall. Border zone and low voltage are identified as green and red localized to the LA roof the PV ostia, respectably.

posterior positions along the patient's chest wall, over the region of interest. The magnetic field strength of each coil is detected by a location sensor proximal to the tip of a proprietary mapping and ablation catheter (NaviSTAR, Biosense-Webster, Inc, Diamond Bar, Ca), available in solid-tip and open-irrigation versions. The catheter tip location and orientation is calculated and displayed to six degrees of freedom (x, y, z, roll, pitch, yaw). The strength of each coil's magnetic field as measured by the location sensor is inversely proportional to the distance between sensor and coil. The location of the catheter within a cardiac chamber is obtained by integrating each coil's field strength and converting the measurement into distance [2,3].

CARTO-guided ablation in atrial fibrillation

Since ablation of AF is primarily based on anatomical approaches such as circumferential PV isolation, the CARTO mapping system is useful in creating an accurate three-dimensional model of the LA and surrounding structures. Accurate LA and PV geometry is important both for efficacy and safety during the ablation procedure. Software-mediated respiratory compensation (AccuResp, Carto 3, Biosense Webster)

corrects for respiratory movement of the heart, resulting in more accurate representation of the PV ostia and LA geometry [4], and decreased fluoroscopy and ablation times [5]. Image integration has been associated with reduced fluoroscopy time and arrhythmia recurrence, as well as increased restoration of sinus rhythm [6–8].

Geometry acquisition can be performed using point-by-point mapping with the ablation catheter or more rapidly with a multipolar catheter equipped with a magnetic location sensor (LassoNav, Biosense Webster). Preprocedure imaging with CT or cMRI can be integrated with the EA map (Cartomerge, Biosense Webster) to yield greater detail with less fluoroscopy exposure (Figure 2). Special attention should be given to accurately define the LA roof, mitral annulus, anterior and posterior wall, along with the PVs and LAA. Additionally, a quadripolar catheter may be delivered into the esophagus to determine its location relative to the LA posterior wall.

CartoSound Image Integration Software (Biosense Webster, Inc.) integrates real-time catheter location acquired from the NaviSTAR mapping and ablation catheter in combination with images obtained from the Soundstar intracardiac echocardiogram (ICE) resulting in the creation of accurate 3D images of the LA and its adjacent structures (Figure 3). The

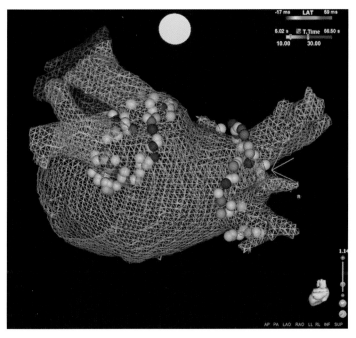

Figure 2 LA PA projection with circumferential ablation of all four PVs using Cartomerge. The EAM was made with the LassoNav catheter and was then registered to the CT using anatomical landmarks. During ablation the lesions are projected to the CT surface.

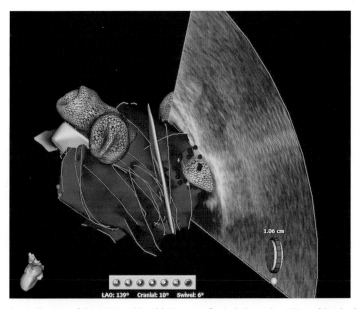

Figure 3 CartoSound. Localization of the RIPV and its ablation tags for isolation using ICE resulting in the creation of accurate 3D images of the LA and its adjacent structures. The created 3D volumetric structures are a result of cardiac cycle gated image acquisition without chamber deformity, which is a limitation of the contact mapping systems.

Soundstar catheter tip location can be visualized in three dimensions on the CARTO system due to a sensor in the tip of the specialized ICE catheter [9,10]. The CartoSound images can then be merged with a preprocedure CT or MRI; mismatches related to changes in volume status and patient position can be identified and corrected [10].

EnSite NaVX

The EnSite NaVX System (St Jude Medical, St Paul, MN) is an impedance-based EAM system utilizing orthogonally placed surface patches to detect real-time catheter position and motion. Three pairs of patches, placed on the patient's body surface in the antero-posterior, left–right, and superoinferior positions, generate X–Y–Z axes (coordinates). A low-current, high-frequency (5.6 kHz) electrical field is created between each pair of patches, and the impedance drop created by the catheter tip's position between patches effectively localizes the catheter position in three dimensions. Multiple catheters, including nonproprietary mapping and ablation catheters, can be simultaneously triangulated, facilitating simultaneous mapping and ablation.

Movement of a uni- or multipolar mapping catheter to contact the endothelial surface of the cardiac chambers or vessel wall allows creation of 3D chamber or vessel geometry. As shown in Figure 4, the posterior view of left atrial (LA) geometry with corresponding left and right pulmonary venous (PV) anatomy (left image). The image on the right demonstrates a reconstructed computed tomography (CT) image. The left atrial appendage in both images is colored green. The high degree of similarity between the two imaging modalities can be readily appreciated. Since RF energy is not delivered inside the PVs, the definition of secondary and tertiary branches of the main pulmonary veins offers little additional benefit for atrial fibrillation ablation. Simultaneous measurement of recorded electrogram amplitude allows characterization of the atrial myocardial substrate, to delineate regions of normal voltage from those with low voltage, suggestive of fibrosis or scar.

EnSite NaVX-guided ablation of atrial fibrillation

The comprehensive evaluation of the chamber geometry, pulmonary vein (PV) anatomy, catheter position, and substrate characterization achieved with EnSite NaVX can be helpful for catheter ablation of AF. Figure 5 shows three commonly used ablation strategies for PVI. A right posterior oblique (RPO) image of the left atrium and pulmonary veins (PVs) is shown in Figure 5a, where PVI has been achieved by circular ablation lesion sets delivered around each individual PV. In Figure 5b, an RPO cranial view of the LA and PVs is depicted with a wide area circumferential ablation performed around the left PVs, while the right-sided veins were isolated individually. Figure 5c shows the addition of an LA roof line, a set of ablation lesions created between the two superior pulmonary veins. Left atrial voltage mapping with EnSite NavX can also be helpful in identifying and characterizing abnormal atrial substrate. Scarred regions with abnormally low voltage tissue can be identified by electroanatomic mapping (EAM), and may guide atrial fibrillation

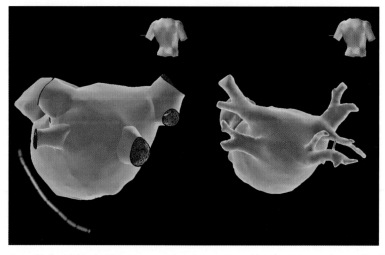

Figure 4 Comparison of left atrial and pulmonary venous geometry created by electroanatomic mapping (EnSite NavX) and reconstructed computed tomography.

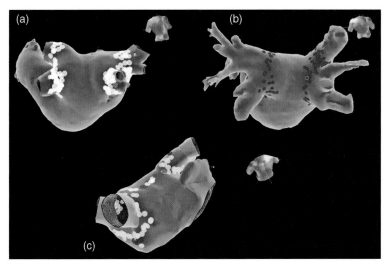

Figure 5 Pulmonary vein isolation (PVI) strategies guided by electroanatomic mapping with EnSite NavX.

ablation (Figure 6a–b). A voltage map of the LA in the left anterior oblique view, with a mesh structure of the right atrium is shown in Figure 6a. In Figure 6b, a right posterior oblique projection of the LA shows extensive areas of low voltage and scar. In patients who present for a second pulmonary vein isolation or patients with persistent atrial fibrillation, voltage mapping may identify regions of PV reconnection or LA fibrosis, which can serve as targets for ablation.

The use of NavX has been associated with reduced fluoroscopic exposure and total procedure time [11,12]. A novel approach using MediGuide technology (MGT, St Jude Medical Inc, St. Paul, MN) has recently been developed to work synergistically with NAVX [13].

Figure 6 Left atrial voltage mapping with EnSite NavX. Regions corresponding to scar or electrically silent tissue and abnormal low-voltage tissue can be identified by electroanatomic mapping. Voltage map color scheme: Purple, normal tissue; gray, scar tissue; and other colors, abnormal low-voltage tissue.

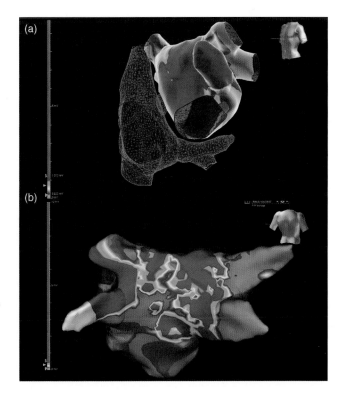

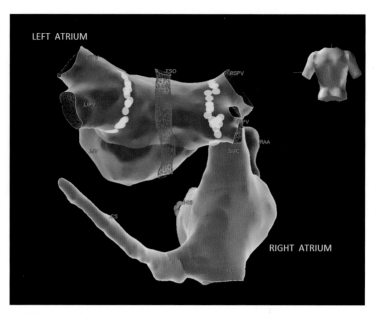

Figure 7 Definition of The atria and esophagus using electroanatomic mapping. The location of the esophagus (ESO), coronary sinus (CS), and His bundle (HIS) has been identified anatomically. LSPV/LIPV, left superior/inferior pulmonary vein; RSPV/RIPV, right superior/inferior pulmonary vein; SVC/IVC, superior/inferior vena cava; RAA, right atrial appendage.

This approach involves collecting a series of cinematic fluoroscopic loops, to which the electromagnetic sensors used for EAM are then aligned, minimizing the need for fluoroscopy.

Catheter ablation of atrial fibrillation with zero fluoroscopy, guided by NAVX and intracardiac echocardiography (ICE), has been described [14]. In this study, an ICE catheter was advanced into the SVC, and a quadripolar catheter advanced to the noncoronary cusp via femoral arterial access and used as a reference. This allowed creation of right atrial and coronary sinus geometry using electrode catheters guided by NAVX into the respective chambers. Transeptal access was achieved using ICE. Geometry of the left atrium and pulmonary veins was then created, guided by ICE.

Anatomic mapping using NaVX alone is limited to anatomic locations reached by the catheter. As a result, regions of significant interest, for example, a fifth pulmonary vein or a small PV ostium, may be missed if not encountered by the catheter, especially without preprocedural cardiac imaging.

This limitation can be mitigated by NaVX Fusion, which merges preprocedural MRI or CT with intraprocedural anatomic mapping. This has the added advantage of guiding ablation with an anatomically accurate shell. Mapping and ablation using NaVX Fusion is accurate and reduces fluoroscopy time relative to procedural duration [12]. Although both CT

and MRI can be fused to real-time anatomical mapping obtained during EAM, CT may provide better LA reconstruction, especially in patients with AF at the time of imaging [15]. Outside of atrial anatomical delineation, NaVX fusion with CT may also be useful in esophageal localization (Figure 7), in order to prevent atrio-esophageal fistula, a rare but often fatal complication of AF ablation [16].

Rhythmia medical system

Compared to the previously discussed EAM systems that employ either magnetic or impedance-based navigation and acquisition platforms, Rhythmia Medical (Boston Scientific, Inc, Natick, MA, USA) utilizes both magnetic and impedance technology with automated processing of intracardiac recordings from a bidirectional 64-electrode basket catheter (IntellaMap Orion, Boston Scientific, Inc, Natick, MA, USA) while maintaining an open architecture to visualize nonproprietary diagnostic and ablation catheters. The system uses predetermined operator parameters to allow automated point annotation during continuous mapping, resulting in greater efficiency and map density with reduced need for manual EGM annotation.

Animal studies with canine and swine models have shown promising results in atrial and ventricular mapping of focal and reentrant arrhythmias [17,18]. In 2013, the Rhythmia Medical mapping system and its 64-electrode IntellaMap Orion high-resolution mapping catheter received FDA 510(k) approval.

Noncontact mapping

One method of cardiac electrical mapping without myocardial contact involves a balloon-mounted 64-electrode array catheter (Ensite, St Jude Medical, St. Paul, MN, USA). Once advanced into the cardiac chamber of choice, the balloon is inflated with saline and/or contrast solution to produce a global multi-electrode array (MEA), from which multiple areas of endocardial activation can be recorded simultaneously [19], such that an activation map of the entire chamber can be obtained from one beat. Similar to other forms of EAM, the anatomic delineation of the cardiac chamber can also be obtained by contact of the catheter with the vessel wall, although the shape of the MEA in certain cardiac chambers may significantly limit this. Plotting and reconstruction of the resulting point cloud yields chamber geometry, with similar accuracy to uni- or multipolar mapping catheters [19,20]. Overall accuracy of the noncontact mapping system is much better at distances less than 50 mm from the electrode plane [19].

The use of the noncontact system to guide ablation of AF is perhaps most applicable to identify focal triggers of atrial fibrillation, especially when they occur infrequently [21,22]. Noncontact mapping may also provide additional value in defining the fidelity of box lesions made to isolate the PVs and to identify sites of conduction gaps [23].

Real-time position management (RPM) system

This system utilizes ultrasonic ranging to localize catheter positions. Specially built catheters (reference, mapping, or ablation) contain ultrasonic transducers within the catheter shaft, which receive continuously emitted ultrasonic waves at 558.5 kHz from a separate emitting device. The distance and position of the catheter is calculated based on the time it takes emitted ultrasound waves to reach the transducer. The RPM system (Cardiac Pathways, Sunnyvale, CA, USA) utilizes two reference catheters placed in fiducial locations such as the coronary sinus or right atrium. Although not as widely used as CARTO and EnSite NAVX, the system has been validated in human atrial and ventricular catheter ablation. As detailed by Bhakta et al [3], RPM offers a distinct advantage, the ability to visualize catheter deflection, in addition to noted advantages of EAM systems in general, such as ability to display multiple catheters, lesion tagging, and construction of chamber geometry. Disadvantages include requirement for specialized ultrasound transducer-equipped catheters, which may interfere with other ultrasound-based systems used in the EP lab such as transesophageal or intracardiac echocardiography.

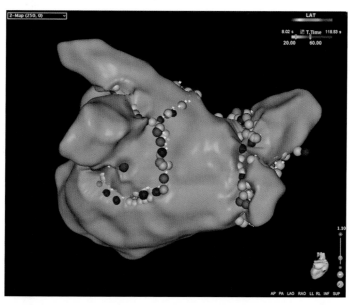

Figure 8 LA PA projection with circumferential ablation of all four PVs using Visitag™. Visitag™ visually confirms lesion location and formation by color based on operator-defined ablation parameters.

Contact force-guided radiofrequency ablation

Lesion formation during RF ablation is directly proportional to tissue contact. In the absence of adequate contact, the result of RF delivery will be intracavitary blood heating with insufficient myocardial energy delivery to cause necrosis of targeted tissue.

Catheters that measure and report real-time contact force are now available and include the TactiCath Quartz contact force ablation Catheter (Ensite, St Jude Medical, St. Paul, MN, USA) and SmartTouch (Biosense Webster Inc., MA, US) (Figure 8). Using either fine optical cables or a magnetic spring coil that deform in response to force at the tip, these systems display both contact pressure and catheter angle. Information about contact force can be integrated with maps from the EAM system. Preclinical studies showed that average contact force, as quantified by the force–time integral, correlates with tissue temperature and lesion volume at a given power setting [24,25].

The benefits of contact force monitoring include decreased risk of cardiac perforation and other complications of ablation associated with excessive contact force [25,26]. In cases of recurrence of atrial fibrillation following catheter ablation, incomplete PV isolation is often related to low force–time integral [27,28]. Contact force-guided PV isolation ablation might improve procedure success while decreasing procedural time and complication rate [29].

Conclusions

EAM systems are invaluable in radiofrequency catheter ablation of atrial fibrillation. While they vary in the technology used to collect data, each aims to provide a highly accurate anatomical model, real-time data on areas targeted for ablation, integration of imaging data, and decreased use of radiation. When used effectively, they can decrease procedure time and increase the safety and effectiveness of AF ablation.

References

1 Bourier F, Fahrig R, Wang P, et al. Accuracy assessment of catheter guidance technology in electrophysiology procedures: a comparison of a new 3D-based fluoroscopy navigation system to current electroanatomic mapping systems. J Cardiovasc Electrophysiol 2014;25(1):74–83.

2 Gepstein L, Hayam G, Ben-Haim SA. A novel method for nonfluoroscopic catheter-based electroanatomical mapping of the heart. *In vitro* and *in vivo* accuracy results. Circulation 1997;95(6):1611–1622.

3 Bhakta D, Miller JM. Principles of electroanatomic mapping. Indian Pacing Electrophysiol J. 2008;8(1):32–50.

4 Beinart R, Kabra R, Heist KE, et al. Respiratory compensation improves the accuracy of electroanatomic mapping of the left atrium and pulmonary veins during atrial fibrillation ablation. J Interv Card Electrophysiol. 2011; 32(2):105–110.

5 Ozcan EE, Szeplaki G, Tahin T, et al. Impact of respiration gating on image integration guided atrial fibrillation ablation. Clinical Res Cardiol. 2014.

6 Kistler PM, Earley MJ, Harris S, et al. Validation of three-dimensional cardiac image integration: use of integrated CT image into electroanatomic mapping system to perform catheter ablation of atrial fibrillation. J Cardiovasc Electrophysiol. 2006;17(4):341–348.

7 Kistler PM, Rajappan K, Jahngir M, et al. The impact of CT image integration into an electroanatomic mapping system on clinical outcomes of catheter ablation of atrial fibrillation. J Cardiovasc Electrophysiol. 2006;17 (10):1093–1101.

8 Dong J, Dickfeld T, Dalal D, et al. Initial experience in the use of integrated electroanatomic mapping with three-dimensional MR/CT images to guide catheter ablation of atrial fibrillation. J Cardiovasc Electrophysiol. 2006;17 (5):459–466.

9 Kabra R, Singh J. Recent trends in imaging for atrial fibrillation ablation. Indian Pacing Electrophysiol J. 2010;10(5):215–227.

10 Banchs JE, Patel P, Naccarelli GV, et al. Intracardiac echocardiography in complex cardiac catheter ablation procedures. J Interv Card Electrophysiol. 2010;28 (3):167–184.

11 Estner HL, Deisenhofer I, Luik A, et al. Electrical isolation of pulmonary veins in patients with atrial fibrillation: reduction of fluoroscopy exposure and procedure duration by the use of a non-fluoroscopic navigation system (NavX). Europace 2006;8(8):583–587.

12 Brooks AG, Wilson L, Kuklik P, et al. Image integration using NavX Fusion: initial experience and validation. Heart Rhythm. 2008;5(4):526–535.

13 Rolf S, John S, Gaspar T, et al. Catheter ablation of atrial fibrillation supported by novel nonfluoroscopic 4D navigation technology. Heart Rhythm. 2013;10(9): 1293–1300.

14 Reddy VY, Morales G, Ahmed H, et al. Catheter ablation of atrial fibrillation without the use of fluoroscopy. Heart Rhythm. 2010;7(11):1644–1653.

15 Kettering K, Greil GF, Fenchel M, et al. Catheter ablation of atrial fibrillation using the Navx-/Ensite-system and a CT-/MRI-guided approach. Clinical Res Cardiol. 2009;98 (5):285–296.

16 Scazzuso FA, Rivera SH, Albina G, et al. Three-dimensional esophagus reconstruction and monitoring during ablation of atrial fibrillation: combination of two imaging techniques. Int J Cardiol. 2013;168(3):2364–2368.

17 Ptaszek LM, Chalhoub F, Perna F, et al. Rapid acquisition of high-resolution electroanatomical maps using a novel multielectrode mapping system. J Interv Card Electrophysiol. 2013;36(3):233–242.

18 Nakagawa H, Ikeda A, Sharma T, et al. Rapid high resolution electroanatomical mapping: evaluation of a new system in a canine atrial linear lesion model. Circ Arrhythm Electrophysiol. 2012;5(2):417–424.

19 Gornick CC, Adler SW, Pederson B, et al. Validation of a new noncontact catheter system for electroanatomic mapping of left ventricular endocardium. Circulation 1999;99(6):829–835.

20 Schilling RJ, Peters NS, Davies DW. Simultaneous endocardial mapping in the human left ventricle using a noncontact catheter: comparison of contact and reconstructed electrograms during sinus rhythm. Circulation 1998;98(9):887–898.

21 Hindricks G, Kottkamp H. Simultaneous noncontact mapping of left atrium in patients with paroxysmal atrial fibrillation. Circulation 2001;104(3):297–303.

22 Schneider MA, Ndrepepa G, Zrenner B, et al. Noncontact mapping-guided catheter ablation of atrial fibrillation associated with left atrial ectopy. J Cardiovasc Electrophysiol. 2000;11(4):475–479.

23 Kumagai K, Nakashima H. Noncontact mapping-guided catheter ablation of atrial fibrillation. Circulation J. 2009;73(2):233–241.

24 Shah DC, Lambert H, Nakagawa H, et al. Area under the real-time contact force curve (force–time integral) predicts radiofrequency lesion size in an *in vitro* contractile model. J Cardiovasc Electrophysiol. 2010;21(9):1038–1043.

25 Nakagawa H, Kautzner J, Natale A, et al. Locations of high contact force during left atrial mapping in atrial fibrillation patients: electrogram amplitude and impedance are poor predictors of electrode–tissue contact force for ablation of atrial fibrillation. Circ Arrhythm Electrophysiol. 2013;6(4):746–753.

26 Perna F, Heist EK, Danik SB, et al. Assessment of catheter tip contact force resulting in cardiac perforation in swine atria using force sensing technology. Circ Arrhythm Electrophysiol. 2011;4(2):218–224.

27 Neuzil P, Reddy VY, Kautzner J, et al. Electrical reconnection after pulmonary vein isolation is contingent on contact force during initial treatment: results from the EFFICAS I study. Circ Arrhythm Electrophysiol. 2013; 6(2):327–333.

28 Reddy VY, Shah D, Kautzner J, et al. The relationship between contact force and clinical outcome during radiofrequency catheter ablation of atrial fibrillation in the TOCCATA study. Heart Rhythm. 2012;9(11):1789–1795.

29 Wutzler A, Huemer M, Parwani AS, et al. Contact force mapping during catheter ablation for atrial fibrillation: procedural data and one-year follow-up. Arch Med Sci. 2014;10(2):266–272.

CHAPTER 8

Magnetic and robotic catheter navigation

John M. Miller,[1] Mark A. Dixon,[2] Deepak Bhakta,[1] Rahul Jain,[1] & Mithilesh K. Das[1]

[1]Krannert Institute of Cardiology, Department of Medicine, [†]Indiana University School of Medicine, Indianapolis, IN, USA
[2]Indiana University Health La Porte Hospital, La Porte, IN, USA

Introduction

Catheter ablation for treatment of atrial fibrillation and associated arrhythmias (right atrial (RA) cavotricuspid isthmus-dependent atrial flutter and macroreentrant atrial tachycardias) has become a very common procedure in the electrophysiology laboratory. Pulmonary vein (PV) isolation, consisting of a series of contiguous applications of radiofrequency (RF) energy on the left atrial (LA) aspect of PV antrum in order to effect entrance block into and exit block out of the PV, continues to form the basis of most strategies for treatment of atrial fibrillation. Standard manual catheter manipulation, with the operator standing at the patient's side and physically moving the electrode at the catheter tip to desired mapping and ablation locations using controls on the catheter handle as well as advancing or withdrawing the catheter, has several shortcomings. Getting the catheter to all desired locations may be challenging, and although the operator has some sense of "feedback" from the catheter when its tip is against a wall, his or her sense of whether the tip has optimal tissue contact (enough for effective mapping and ablation, but not enough for perforation) is poor. In addition, the operator accumulates a certain amount of fluoroscopic exposure, has back strain from wearing lead, and in most cases cannot control the stimulator,

Practical Guide to Catheter Ablation of Atrial Fibrillation, Second Edition. Edited by Jonathan S. Steinberg, Pierre Jaïs and Hugh Calkins.

recording, and mapping systems while at the bedside. Long, manually deflectable sheaths and use of intracardiac echocardiography have aided in achieving and improving some degree of contact in all desired locations, and reduction in fluoroscopic exposure, but do not address all of these shortcomings. Remote catheter manipulation, using either magnetic navigation of the electrode tip or robotic manipulation of deflectable sheaths, has been developed to further improve procedures for atrial fibrillation ablation.

Remote magnetic catheter navigation

Remote magnetic navigation (RMN) of catheters uses operator-designated changes in magnetic fields centered on the patient's torso to deflect and maintain the position of an electrode at the end of a mapping/ablation catheter. The clinically available system manufactured by Stereotaxis, Inc. (St Louis, MO) uses fixed magnets composed of rare earth elements housed in large pods, situated to the right and left of the patient's torso during the procedure, to deflect the tip electrode with an embedded magnet (Figure 1). Additional magnets on the shaft up to 3 cm proximal to the tip enable deflection and shaping of the end of the catheter (not just tip electrode) in any direction desired. Forward and backward motion of the electrode is accomplished by a motor drive attached to the catheter shaft just outside its sheath in the groin, operated in the control room via joystick. With this system, an electrode at the end of a very soft and flexible catheter shaft (Figure 2) can be directed with

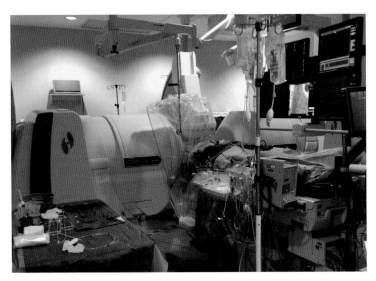

Figure 1 RMN laboratory. The patient is beneath standard blue drapes, with a single plane fluoroscopy unit above the chest. The large beige cylinders to the patient's sides house the magnets, the movement of which within the housing controls deflection of the electrode at the catheter tip.

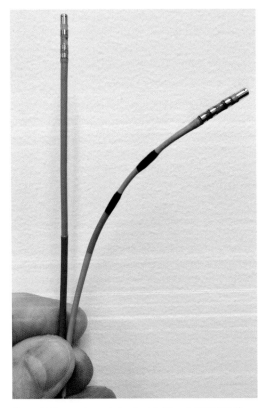

Figure 2 Comparison of standard (left) and RMN (right) catheters, held upright by their shafts. The standard catheter is relatively stiff compared to the "floppy" RMN catheter. Large dark lobes on the RMN catheter are magnets that help in deflecting the distal electrode, which also contains a magnet.

great precision to any location in the atria by an operator who is sitting in the control room (Figure 3); in principle, with proper logistics, the operator can be in a different building or even a different continent.

Setup of the system requires only a few minutes; standard catheters are positioned and LA access obtained as usual. When used with the CARTO system (Biosense Webster, Diamond Bar, CA), the patient and patch locations are fluoroscopically registered to be within the operating range of each system. The magnet pods are then rotated into position astride the patient's torso and catheter manipulation using the RMN system can begin. The operator uses a mouse on the control screen to direct a vector for the catheter tip destination that is followed by automatically reconfiguring the orientation of the large fixed magnets to match the programmed vector. The desired location is achieved in 1–2 s and precision of movement is 1 mm. The field strength (maximum 0.1T) is far less than used in magnetic resonance imaging. The ability to precisely move the catheter tip remotely results in dramatic reduction in fluoroscopic exposure for the operator, who is not physically in the room with the patient during catheter manipulation; however, experience has shown a marked reduction in fluoroscopic exposure for patients and nursing and other personnel in the procedure room since the electrode can be safely manipulated to all atrial sites with adequate contact pressure for ablation, without concern for perforation. In addition, the system has

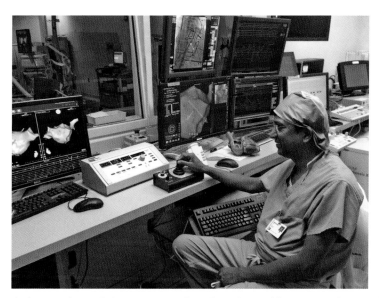

Figure 3 Operator in the control room during a RMN procedure. The patient and fluoroscopy unit are on the other side of the glass wall. The operator, comfortably seated and without lead, uses a joystick and mouse to move the mapping electrode in all degrees of freedom. The RMN system is integrated with the electroanatomic mapping system (at left) such that it can be controlled almost entirely from the mapping system keyboard and mouse.

preprogrammed vectors that, when activated, automatically direct the catheter to specific locations; sites of interest can be designated during mapping and the system can direct the electrode back to the same site later in the study. An "AutoMap" feature systematically moves the electrode to sample the entire chamber in a matter of minutes.

Originally, the decrease in operator fluoroscopic exposure and attendant time wearing lead was offset somewhat by his or her still having to move other catheters, such as ring catheters to monitor PV conduction. However, a new addition to the system, Vdrive™, allows the operator to use a joystick mechanism to remotely manipulate the ring catheter in all its axes of motion (forward/backward, torque in either direction, deflection, and increase/decrease in diameter of the ring) [1]. This is accomplished by fixing the catheter handle in a cradle with mechanisms that remotely move each control on the handle as would be done manually. A similar mechanism is available for intracardiac echocardiography catheters (V-Sono™). Experience has shown these to be very effective, such that after situating catheters in the left atrium and making the proper mechanical connections, the entire procedure may be completed without the operator having to leave his or her seat in the control room.

The initial commercial release of the RMN system used a 4 mm, nonirrigated tip electrode with two magnets in the catheter shaft. While this configuration

sufficed for simple supraventricular tachycardia ablation, it was suboptimal for treatment of AF. Char formation was relatively common and acute efficacy was inferior to that of manual catheters, which by that time were 8 mm or irrigated tip in some cases. An 8 mm catheter was later introduced and while this was initially thought to have less flexibility than the 4 mm tip, it was actually more flexible (the 4 mm catheter had an approximately 9 mm stiff segment at the tip). Outcomes were improved, but were still not as good as contemporaneous manual catheters (largely irrigated tip at the time). A 3.5 mm irrigated tip electrode was introduced in 2009 and improved by 2010 and has resulted in comparable acute and long-term efficacy rates to those of manual catheters. Handling characteristics are superior to prior iterations of RMN catheters, with three shaft magnets and a short (4 mm) stiff segment at the catheter tip.

Contact force (CF), or the amount of consistent pressure on tissue during delivery of RF energy, has been shown to correlate with both lesion depth and steam pops (rupture of tissue either inward or externally as a result of steam generation below the endocardial surface) [2]. CF of 20 gm is a good target; amounts less than 10 gm are unlikely to produce transmural atrial damage, whereas CF >40 gm may result in steam pops and CF >60 may result in perforation. Since atrial tissue thickness varies greatly, these numbers represent generalization rather than absolute cutoff values. Achievable CF is generally less with RMN (15–20 gm) than with other methods due to the inherent highly flexible nature of the catheter tip; however, to a degree, this shortcoming is mitigated in part or completely by the greater consistency of contact at a specific site over the course of the time of RF application. With either manual or robotic catheter manipulation, the catheter tip contact with tissue may vary greatly as the atrial walls move during cardiac and respiratory cycles, but due to the flexibility of the RMN-guided catheter tip, its contact can be more constant during usual cardiac motion. On the other hand, perforation resulting in cardiac tamponade and steam pops (each a function at least in part of excessive CF) are almost nonexistent with the RMN catheter.

Performance

An early publication, using a 4 mm nonirrigated ablation electrode, showed less efficacy in achieving PV isolation with the RMN system as opposed to manual catheter manipulation (Table 1) [3]. Subsequent generations of electrodes have markedly improved PV isolation rates and 6–12-month freedom from recurrent AF (currently equivalent to manual catheter

ablation). Procedure times are generally somewhat longer (up to an hour more so) and fluoroscopic times significantly shorter (1/3 or less) than with manual catheter movement [4–8]. One study showed a comparatively longer fluoroscopic time, but this was during the "learning curve" phase for the facility [7].

Safety

As noted, two of the most significant advantages of the RMN system and catheter are the very low likelihood of perforation and resultant cardiac tamponade with the catheter (almost physically impossible), and rarity of steam pops. In addition, marked decreases in fluoroscopic exposure have been observed for all individuals involved in the procedure. In the authors' experience, RMN fluoroscopic times versus those for contemporaneous manual catheter ablation are dramatically reduced (by 60%); in many cases, after situating catheters in the LA, no additional fluoroscopy is necessary for the remainder of the procedure. Esophageal injury including ulceration has been reported with the system; it does not appear to be significantly different from that with manual catheter movement [9]. Other complications (thromboembolic events, phrenic nerve damage, those related to femoral

Table 1 Comparison of remote versus manual catheter manipulation clinical parameters.

Study	Tool	Cases	Procedure duration (minutes)	Fluoroscopic time (minutes)	Acute success	Freedom from AF at 6 or 12 mo	Complications
Katsiyiannis [4]	Magnetic	20 RMN versus 20 MAN	209 ± 56 versus 279 ± 60^{a}	19.5 ± 9.8 versus 58.6 ± 21^{a}	100% versus 100%	75% versus 80%	<1% versus 2.4%
Miyazaki [7]	Magnetic	30 RMN versus 44 MAN	246 ± 50 versus 153 ± 51^{a}	58 ± 24 versus 40 ± 14^{a}	97% versus 100%	69% versus 61.8%	0% versus 0.5%
Arya [6]	Magnetic	70 RMN versus 286 MAN	223 ± 44 versus 166 ± 52^{a}	13.7 ± 7.8 versus 34.5 ± 15^{a}	87.6% versus 99.6%^{a}	57.8% versus 66.4%^{b}	<1% versus 2.4%
Luthje [5]	Magnetic	107 RMN versus 54 MAN	226 ± 55 versus 166 ± 52^{a}	12 ± 4 versus 37 ± 7^{a}	90% vs 87%	53.5% versus 55.5%	4.3% versus 0%
Di Biase [15]	Robotic	193 ROB versus 197 MAN	186 ± 66 versus 186 ± 54	49 ± 25 versus 58 ± 20^{a}	100% vs 100%	85% versus 81%	1.3% versus 1%
Steven [18]	Robotic	30 ROB versus 30 MAN	156 ± 44 versus 134 ± 12	9.0 ± 3.4 versus 22 ± 6.5^{a}	100% versus 100%	73% versus 77%^{b}	0% versus 0%
Thomas [19]	Robotic	25 ROB versus 61 MAN	NA	40 ± 12 versus 54 ± 17^{a}	92% versus 92%	NA	4.0% versus 4.9%

Abbreviations: RMN, remote magnetic navigation; MAN, manual; ROB, robotic mechanical navigation; NA, not available from paper
$^{a}P < 0.05$
^{b} = 6 month follow-up

access site, etc.) are not significantly different from that with manual catheter manipulation.

Other considerations

Although the magnetic field strength even at the patient's torso is quite weak, patients and medical personnel in the room (nursing, physicians) must remove magnetically sensitive items from their person (credit cards, etc.) due to possible damage from the magnets. Implanted cardiac devices such as pacemakers and defibrillators are generally not adversely affected; the magnetic field does not displace devices or leads [10]. Occasional fixed rate (VOO) pacing or power-on-reset behavior has been reported, which is always reprogrammable at the end of the procedure [11–13]. Component damage has not been reported. Anesthetic and monitoring equipment near the patient's head must be composed of materials unaffected by magnetic fields; instrument tables, chairs, etc. have been attracted to the ends of the magnetic housing pods and can be difficult to remove.

Advantages and disadvantages

The major advantages of the RMN system are in the area of safety (very low likelihood of perforation or steam pop and a marked decrease in fluoroscopic exposure to operator and personnel in the procedure room, including the patient) and precision of electrode movement. Disadvantages include need for the magnetic system and thus lack of portability from room to room, proprietary mapping/ablation catheters, difficulty regaining LA access if the catheter falls back into the RA, and in some cases, difficulty isolating the right PVs (particularly right inferior), requiring exchanging the catheter for a manual system. This seems to be mitigated if the LA access used for the RMN catheter is relatively anterior on the septum, allowing better access to more posteromedial LA sites.

Another still-experimental system uses electromagnets rather than fixed rare earth magnets. The Catheter Guidance Control and Imaging (CGCI) system, manufactured by Magnetecs Corporation (Inglewood, CA) uses large electromagnets around the patient's torso to deflect a magnetic element in the tip electrode of a mapping/ablation catheter [14]. Clinical experience with this system is very limited thus far. Potential advantages, compared to the Stereotaxis system, include more rapid motion response of the electrode to operator-directed position changes (due to a stronger magnetic field, up to 0.15T) and perhaps greater stability with reactive changes in field strength, while disadvantages include lack of portability of the system and high power and cooling requirements for the electromagnets.

Robotic catheter manipulation

Catheters can also be maneuvered by nonmagnetic, robotic manipulation of the catheter tip. The Sensei® X system (Hansen Medical, Mountain View, CA), at present the only clinically available unit, uses a robotic arm to direct the catheter tip within universally deflectable sheaths; the catheter tip can be further manipulated independently, but most of the movement derives from sheath deflection. The catheter is advanced or withdrawn remotely as well. Controls are concentrated at a workstation, where the operating physician directs catheter positioning while seated in the control room, away from fluoroscopic exposure. The sheath can be smoothly deflected to 260° and rotated in all directions, allowing positioning with great precision (1–2 mm).

Setup is relatively simple. After standard catheters are positioned and LA access has been obtained, the transseptal sheath is exchanged for the deflectable sheath (Artisan® Extend); this sheath has an outer 14F and a coaxial, inner 10.5F sheath. Alternatively, transseptal access can be obtained using the robotic controls. The mapping/ablation catheter is placed into this sheath, which extends the length of the catheter shaft; the catheter's control handle is affixed to the robotic arm, which is in turn attached to the operating table (Figure 4). Remote catheter manipulation with the system can then begin using a handle mechanism to mechanically deflect the sheath (activating combinations of six internal pull-wires) and move the catheter forward and backward within it (Figure 5). With this, all areas of each atrium are fully accessible for mapping and ablation. Initial experience with the system showed that perforation with resultant cardiac tamponade could occur in the absence of tactile or other feedback regarding electrode–tissue contact. Subsequently, a feature has been added (IntelliSense®) that gives the operator an indicator of CF that is useful for both safety (avoidance of perforation) and efficacy (accuracy of mapping data, producing dense ablation lesions). CF information is displayed graphically as well as with a tactile vibration in the handle of the robotic control system to alert the operator that CF exceeds predetermined limits (usually 30 gm). The system integrates with either the CARTO™ or EnSite™/EnSite Velocity™ (St. Jude Medical, Minneapolis, MN) mapping systems; the display includes mapping system and IntelliSense® graphics for monitoring catheter position and CF.

Performance

As with the RMN system (Table 1), several studies have demonstrated robotic ablation's ability to isolate

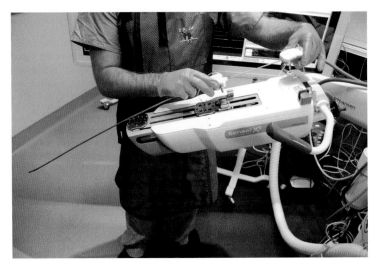

Figure 4 Robotic catheter manipulation arm (white apparatus) with remotely activated, mechanically deflected sheath system (in operator's hands). The latter is attached to the robotic arm that is positioned above the patient's thigh during the procedure.

PVs in nearly 100% of cases, with very infrequent need for manual catheter "touch-up." The number of procedures needed for an operator to become facile is significant (roughly 50–75 cases [15,16]) but achievable. In the relatively small number of studies comparing robotic with manual catheter movement, procedure times were very similar as were 6- or 12-month freedom from recurrent AF; fluoroscopy times tend to be roughly 25% lower with robotic manipulation (far lower for the operator seated in the control room) [15,17–19]. A randomized "Man and Machine"

trial [20] is underway to assess efficacy and safety of robotic ablation compared to manual ablation.

Safety

Instantaneous contact force monitoring has largely allayed initial concerns about perforation risk; however, it is still possible to exert excessive pressure sufficient to perforate the atrial wall (i.e., the mechanical system is capable of delivering excessive CF; the monitoring system notifies the operator but does not prevent this). Esophageal injury is possible with the

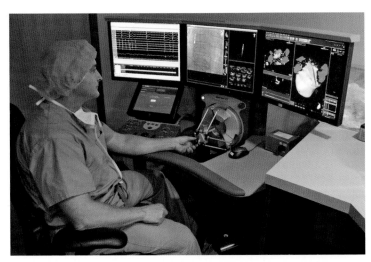

Figure 5 Operator in the control room during a robotic procedure. The operator, comfortably seated and without lead, uses a horizontal handle to move the catheter tip with mapping electrode in all degrees of freedom.

system but in general does not appear to be more likely than with manual catheter movement; of note, in one study, only patients with body mass index <26 had esophageal lesions [21]. As noted, fluoroscopic exposure to the operator is greatly reduced since he or she can operate the device from a separate control room; exposure to patient and staff in the procedure room is also slightly less than with manually manipulated catheter mapping and ablation. The operator is still subject to additional fluoroscopic exposure and has to use protective lead when moving other catheters, such PV ring catheters, during the procedure.

Advantages and disadvantages

The system is portable from one procedure room to another and integrates with both major mapping systems. Remote catheter manipulation decreases operator fluoroscopic exposure and fatigue, but these advantages do not benefit the patient and staff in the procedure room. The sheath is larger than standard (14 F outer dimension), with the potential for more problems with hemostasis and a larger residual atrial septal hole. Such

iatrogenic atrial septal defects (>3 mm) have been reported to occur in up to 95% of cases, but tend to close in up to 79% within 6 months [22].

Another mechanical remote catheter manipulation system (Amigo™, Catheter Robotics, Inc., Mt. Olive, NJ) uses a standard mapping/ablation catheter affixed to a mounting arm similar to the Sensei® X system, but remote activation is via a handheld emulation of the control handle of a catheter; advancement and withdrawal of the catheter as well as rotation and deflection are accomplished much as an operator would with the actual catheter handle in hand, but can be done from several feet away (thus avoiding fluoroscopic exposure and fatigue related to standing/wearing protective lead). Clinical experience with this system is limited. It has the advantages of simplicity, lower cost than other systems, portability from one procedure room to another, ability to use a variety of catheters, and, as noted, less operator fluoroscopic exposure and fatigue.

A comparison of commercially available systems' features is presented in Table 2.

Table 2 Comparison of technologies for catheter manipulation during mapping and ablation of atrial arrhythmias.

	Standard manual	Robotic (Hansen Medical)	Magnetic (Stereotaxis)
Means of electrode movement	Bedside manual control using catheter handle	Remote control by mechanical sheath movement	Remote control by magnetic deflection
Fluoroscopic exposure			
Operator	Moderate	Far less than manual	Far less than manual
Patient/nursing	Moderate	Same as manual	Far less than manual
Procedure time	Moderate	Same as manual	Same as manual
Efficacy			
Contact force	10–60 gm; manual feedback	10–80 gm; electronic and tactile feedback	15–20 gm; electronic feedback
Acute outcomes			
PV isolation	Excellent	Same as manual	Same as manual
Bidirectional CTI block	Excellent	Same as manual	Same as manual
Elimination of MRAT	Excellent	Same as manual	Same as manual
Safety			
Perforation	Low	Same as/more than manual	Less than manual
Steam pop	Low	Same as manual	Less than manual
Other aspects			
Portability from lab to lab	Good	Good	Not feasible
Catheter choice	Any	Any	Proprietary
Sheath size	8–12 Fr[a]	14 Fr	8–8.5 Fr
Regaining LA access[b]	Moderately easy	Same as manual	Harder than manual
Mapping system integration	Any can be used	Any can be used	Best with CARTO
Per-case cost	Moderate	More than manual	More than manual

Abbreviations: gm, gram; PV, pulmonary vein; CTI, right atrial cavotricuspid isthmus; MRAT, macroreentrant atrial tachycardia; LA, left atrium; Fr, French size
[a] Up to 12 Fr if one of a several deflectable sheaths is used.
[b] If the catheter in the left atrium slips back into the right atrium, how difficult is it to regain access to the left atrium?

Summary

Catheter ablation of atrial fibrillation continues to be a challenging procedure, requiring skill and patience. Historically, long procedure durations and significant fluoroscopic exposure to patients, staff, and operator have been major problems; outcomes (both efficacy and safety) have been suboptimal. Moving the operator away from the bedside to a control room, where the ablation catheter can be manipulated remotely either mechanically or using magnetic deflection of the catheter tip, has greatly decreased not only operator fluoroscopic exposure but also that to patient and staff as well without sacrificing efficacy either short or long term. Procedure duration appears to be somewhat longer with magnetic as opposed to manual catheter movement, with tradeoff benefits of more precise electrode movement, more consistent electrode–tissue contact, and almost nonexistent perforation or steam pop risk. Procedure times for mechanical robotic and manual catheter manipulation are similar; the risk of perforation with the former appears to have been significantly reduced with contact force-sensing technology that provides the operator with instantaneous feedback. Newer technologies for remote catheter manipulation may further improve procedure times and outcomes and lower fluoroscopic exposure while improving efficiency.

References

1 Nolker G, Gutleben KJ, Muntean B, Vogt J, Horstkotte D, Dabiri Abkenari L, et al. Novel robotic catheter manipulation system integrated with remote magnetic navigation for fully remote ablation of atrial tachyarrhythmias: a two-centre evaluation. Europace 2012;14(12):1715–1718. PubMed PMID: 22719063.

2 Yokoyama K, Nakagawa H, Shah DC, Lambert H, Leo G, Aeby N, et al. Novel contact force sensor incorporated in irrigated radiofrequency ablation catheter predicts lesion size and incidence of steam pop and thrombus. Circ Arrhythm Electrophysiol. 2008;1(5):354–362. PubMed PMID: 19808430.

3 Di Biase L, Fahmy TS, Patel D, Bai R, Civello K, Wazni OM, et al. Remote magnetic navigation: human experience in pulmonary vein ablation. J Am Coll Cardiol. 2007;50(9):868–874. PubMed PMID: 17719473.

4 Katsiyiannis WT, Melby DP, Matelski JL, Ervin VL, Laverence KL, Gornick CC. Feasibility and safety of remote-controlled magnetic navigation for ablation of atrial fibrillation. Am J Cardiol. 2008;102(12):1674–1676. PubMed PMID: 19064022.

5 Luthje L, Vollmann D, Seegers J, Dorenkamp M, Sohns C, Hasenfuss G, et al. Remote magnetic versus manual catheter navigation for circumferential pulmonary vein ablation in patients with atrial fibrillation. Clin Res Cardiol. 2011;100(11):1003–1011. PubMed PMID: 21706198. Pubmed Central PMCID: 3203998.

6 Arya A, Zaker-Shahrak R, Sommer P, Bollmann A, Wetzel U, Gaspar T, et al. Catheter ablation of atrial fibrillation using remote magnetic catheter navigation: a case–control study. Europace 2011;13(1):45–50. PubMed PMID: 21149511.

7 Miyazaki S, Shah AJ, Xhaet O, Derval N, Matsuo S, Wright M, et al. Remote magnetic navigation with irrigated tip catheter for ablation of paroxysmal atrial fibrillation. Circ Arrhythm Electrophysiol. 2010;3(6):585–589. PubMed PMID: 20937723.

8 Proietti R, Pecoraro V, Di Biase L, Natale A, Santangeli P, Viecca M, et al. Remote magnetic with open-irrigated catheter vs. manual navigation for ablation of atrial fibrillation: a systematic review and meta-analysis. Europace 2013. PubMed PMID: 23585253.

9 Konstantinidou M, Wissner E, Chun JK, Koektuerk B, Metzner A, Tilz RR, et al. Luminal esophageal temperature rise and esophageal lesion formation following remote-controlled magnetic pulmonary vein isolation. Heart Rhythm. 2011;8(12):1875–1880. PubMed PMID: 21802392.

10 Jilek C, Lennerz C, Stracke B, Badran H, Semmler V, Reents T, et al. Forces on cardiac implantable electronic devices during remote magnetic navigation. Clin Res Cardiol. 2013;102(3):185–192. PubMed PMID: 23052333.

11 Eitel C, Hindricks G, Sommer P, Wetzel U, Bollmann A, Gaspar T, et al. Safety of remote magnetic navigation in patients with pacemakers and implanted cardioverter defibrillators. J Cardiovasc Electrophysiol. 2010;21(10):1130–1135. PubMed PMID: 20455985.

12 Jilek C, Tzeis S, Reents T, Estner HL, Fichtner S, Ammar S, et al. Safety of implantable pacemakers and cardioverter defibrillators in the magnetic field of a novel remote magnetic navigation system. J Cardiovasc Electrophysiol. 2010;21(10):1136–1141. PubMed PMID: 20522155.

13 Luthje L, Vollmann D, Seegers J, Sohns C, Hasenfuss G, Zabel M. Interference of remote magnetic catheter navigation and ablation with implanted devices for pacing and defibrillation. Europace 2010;12(11):1574–1580. PubMed PMID: 20810533.

14 Filgueiras-Rama D, Estrada A, Shachar J, Castrejon S, Doiny D, Ortega M, et al. Remote magnetic navigation for accurate, real-time catheter positioning and ablation in cardiac electrophysiology procedures. J Vis Exp. 2013 (74). PubMed PMID: 23628883. Pubmed Central PMCID: 3665328.

15 Di Biase L, Wang Y, Horton R, Gallinghouse GJ, Mohanty P, Sanchez J, et al. Ablation of atrial fibrillation utilizing robotic catheter navigation in comparison to manual navigation and ablation: single-center experience. J Cardiovasc Electrophysiol. 2009;20(12):1328–1335. PubMed PMID: 19656244.

16 Rillig A, Meyerfeldt U, Birkemeyer R, Treusch F, Kunze M, Miljak T, et al. Remote robotic catheter ablation for atrial fibrillation: how fast is it learned and what benefits can be earned? J Interv Card Electrophysiol. 2010;29 (2):109–117. PubMed PMID: 20878222.

17 Bai R, DIB L, Valderrabano M, Lorgat F, Mlcochova H, Tilz R, et al. Worldwide experience with the robotic

navigation system in catheter ablation of atrial fibrillation: methodology, efficacy and safety. J Cardiovasc Electrophysiol. 2012;23(8):820–826. PubMed PMID: 22509886.

18 Steven D, Servatius H, Rostock T, Hoffmann B, Drewitz I, Mullerleile K, et al. Reduced fluoroscopy during atrial fibrillation ablation: benefits of robotic guided navigation. J Cardiovasc Electrophysiol. 2010;21(1):6–12. PubMed PMID: 19793149.

19 Thomas D, Scholz EP, Schweizer PA, Katus HA, Becker R. Initial experience with robotic navigation for catheter ablation of paroxysmal and persistent atrial fibrillation. J Electrocardiol. 2012;45(2):95–101. PubMed PMID: 21714971.

20 Rillig A, Schmidt B, Steven D, Meyerfeldt U, Di Biase L, Wissner E, et al. Study design of the man and machine trial: a prospective international controlled noninferiority trial comparing manual with robotic catheter ablation for treatment of atrial fibrillation. J Cardiovasc Electrophysiol. 2013;24(1):40–46. PubMed PMID: 23131063.

21 Rillig A, Meyerfeldt U, Birkemeyer R, Wiest S, Sauer BM, Staritz M, et al. Oesophageal temperature monitoring and incidence of oesophageal lesions after pulmonary vein isolation using a remote robotic navigation system. Europace 2010;12(5):655–661. PubMed PMID: 20233761.

22 Rillig A, Meyerfeldt U, Kunze M, Birkemeyer R, Miljak T, Jackle S, et al. Persistent iatrogenic atrial septal defect after a single-puncture, double-transseptal approach for pulmonary vein isolation using a remote robotic navigation system: results from a prospective study. Europace 2010;12(3):331–336. PubMed PMID: 20080903.

CHAPTER 9

MRI-guided procedures

Henry Halperin & Aravindan Kolandaivelu
Heart and Vascular Institute, Johns Hopkins University, Baltimore, MD, USA

Catheter ablation is successful at curing a number of arrhythmias [1]. However, ablation has been less successful at managing arrhythmias with more complex and variable arrhythmogenic substrate, such as atrial fibrillation (AF). Improving the management of complex arrhythmias has motivated the development of more sophisticated tools for guiding ablation procedures.

Modern imaging techniques such as magnetic resonance imaging (MRI), intracardiac ultrasound (ICE), and X-ray computed tomography (CT) are increasingly used to approach the shortcomings of current mapping and ablation systems. MRI is a particularly flexible imaging modality with excellent soft tissue contrast. Of particular relevance to EP procedures guidance is that MRI can provide 3D imaging of complex cardiovascular anatomy, visualization of myocardial scar and ablation lesions, and real-time imaging along arbitrary imaging planes. This chapter will survey applications of preprocedure MRI for guidance of AF ablation and provide an update on the progress toward full MRI guidance of electrophysiology procedures.

Preprocedure MRI for EP procedure guidance

3D angiography

MRI angiography provides a 3D perspective of the left atrium and surrounding anatomy without need for ionizing radiation. Pulmonary vein (PV) variants are common [2] and are relevant for planning ablation strategy. Triggering foci for AF can originate from variant PVs requiring their isolation [3]. Ablating

near small or early branching PVs increases the risk of pulmonary vein stenosis [4,5]. Atrial size and variant anatomy can also affect procedure outcomes and could play a role when selecting geometry-sensitive ablation modalities such as cryo-balloon ablation [6–8].

For such reasons, MRI or CT angiography is considered an appropriate pre-AF ablation study [9,10].

Preprocedure 3D angiography is now commonly imported into standard electroanatomic mapping systems (EAM) to provide a real-time sense of catheter position in relation to a patient's specific LA and PV anatomy [11,12]. Application of this technique requires careful attention to accurate registration between the EAM space and the preprocedure 3D angiogram. This registration is subject to potential errors including changes in volume status, respiratory phase, and cardiac rhythm that may occur after image acquisition. Accepting these limitations, angiogram integration can be helpful for tailoring ablation to variant PV anatomy and to guide lesion placement in areas where stable catheter positioning is more difficult, such as along the tissue ridge separating the left atrial appendage from the left pulmonary veins [4,13] (Figure 1 left). An increased confidence in catheter manipulation has been reflected in randomized trial evidence that fluoroscopy use can decrease when image integration is used [14–17]. However, the consensus of these trials is that angiogram integration does not reduce AF recurrence suggesting that outcomes are limited by other procedural factors.

Ablation lesion imaging

Recovery of PV conduction is a typical finding in patients who undergo repeat AF ablation despite electrical isolation after previous procedures [18–21]. This is likely due to resolution of transient factors that acutely affect conduction but can resolve anywhere from minutes to weeks following ablation [22,23].

Practical Guide to Catheter Ablation of Atrial Fibrillation, Second Edition. Edited by Jonathan S. Steinberg, Pierre Jaïs and Hugh Calkins.
© 2016 John Wiley & Sons, Ltd. Published 2016 by John Wiley & Sons, Ltd.

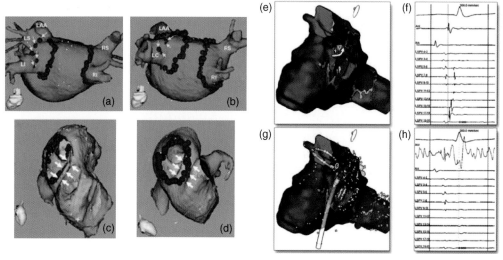

Figure 1 MRI integration with electroanatomic (EAM) mapping. (a-d) 3D angiogram integration with EAM. (a) Illustrates circumferential ablation performed followed by segmental ablation, marked by yellow arrows, to achieve pulmonary vein isolation. (c) Shows that ablation was guided to the PV side of a narrow left atrial appendage ridge, marked by white arrows. (b) Illustrates a patient with a left common PV and (d) in this case ablation could be directed onto a wider left atrial appendage ridge. (e–h) DEMRI ablation lesion integration with EAM. Ablation maps in (e) and (g) were obtained by processing 3D DEMRI images acquired prior to repeat ablation. (e) The white arrow highlights a DEMRI lesion gap that corresponded to early PV activation by lasso catheter (f). (g) Shows that positioning ablation catheter at this gap and delivering ablation resulted in isolation of the PV (h). *Sources:* (a)–(d), Dong et al., 2006 [13]. Reproduced with permission of Wiley; (e)–(h), Bisbal et al., 2014 [13]. Reproduced with permission of Elsevier.

The ability to reliably target additional ablation to "gaps" in regions of incomplete ablation would address an important limitation of current ablation procedures.

There has been steady progress toward using MRI lesion imaging to guide ablation gap completion following AF ablation. Dickfeld et al. performed early work to characterize gadolinium contrast and non-contrast MRI ablation lesion imaging methods [24,25]. Of these, delayed gadolinium enhancement MRI (DEMRI) has been the most clinically applied method thus far. DEMRI is based on the preferential distribution of IV gadolinium into regions with increased extracellular space and slowed washout kinetics. This results in enhancement of scarred myocardium relative to normal tissue on T1 weighted MRI [26]. In 2007, Peters et.al. first described a method for visualizing ablation lesions in the thin-walled atrium following AF ablation using high-resolution 3D DEMRI [27]. Using this technique, Taclas et.al. found that 20% of lesions they marked with CARTO did not have associated DEMRI enhancement [28]. This study also associated more DEMRI ablation gaps with greater AF recurrence postablation. Conversely, Badger et al. found that more veins with circumferential ablation by DEMRI predicted increasing

freedom from AF at one year [29]. Their study, however, showed only a modest correlation between specific low-voltage locations by EAM and lesion location by DEMRI ($R^2 = 0.57$). Spragg et al. were subsequently able to find an association between reduced local bipolar voltage by EAM and DEMRI lesion location ($-0.72 +/- 0.09$ mV, $P < 0.001$) [30]. However, they did not find an association between specific DEMRI gap locations and the sites of earliest electrical activation within the PV by lasso catheter. Most recently, Bisbal et al. were able to find a correlation between DEMRI and electrical gap location [31]. They were also able to achieve reisolation of 95% of PVs and conduction block across all roof lines by targeting ablation to DEMRI lesion gaps (Figure 1 right). However, though DEMRI had a 93–100% sensitivity for identifying sites of electrical reconnection, specificity was low with wide confidence intervals (19–90%) in this small 15 patient study [32]. Still, these encouraging results will motivate future work into the best methods and utility of ablation lesion imaging to guide AF ablation.

One caveat to the DEMRI studies above is that lesion imaging was performed after the resolution of transient tissue injury, weeks after ablation. Lesion imaging acutely after ablation, in order to guide the initial procedure, is an area of active investigation. This topic will be discussed further in the intraprocedure lesion imaging section below.

Atrial substrate imaging

There may be additional benefit to using atrial tissue characteristics to guide ablation. Oakes et al. first reported the use of DEMRI prior to ablation to assess atrial fibrosis [33]. They found that more atrial fibrosis by MRI was associated with progressively more AF recurrence following ablation, a finding corroborated in a recent multicenter study [34]. Akoum et al. suggested that atrial fibrosis MRI might have additional use for guiding ablation strategy [35]. They found that while complete circumferential ablation by MRI was predictive of ablation success in those with less atrial fibrosis, only more extensive atrial ablation was associated with ablation success in those with more fibrosis. More specific relationships between atrial fibrosis distribution and atrial fibrillation propagation are now being investigated that may more directly contribute to procedure guidance [36,37]. One challenge of atrial fibrosis imaging has been reliable image acquisition and postprocessing. Efforts to standardize this technique are underway [34,38]. MRI can also visualize atrial epicardial fat pads, which harbor ganglionic plexi and may be targets for ablation [39].

Fully MRI-guided EP procedures

Performing EP procedures entirely within the MRI scanner offers a number of potential advantages. First, real-time MRI (rtMRI) does not utilize ionizing radiation and provides good soft tissue visualization, unlike X-ray fluoroscopy. rtMRI can also image along arbitrary image planes, unlike ICE. Second, MRI offers a number of methods for evaluating tissue injury following ablation that could be useful for targeting gaps in ablation during the procedure. Third, because rtMRI uses the same coordinate system as 3D imaging, the error-prone registration process required for conventional EAM can be avoided. This simplifies guiding EP catheters to specific image-based targets, such as lesion gaps, and may improve procedure efficacy and risk. Over the last 15 years, the basic techniques for fully MRI-guided EP procedures have been described.

Studies using real-time MRI guidance

Lardo et al. introduced the potential of using rtMRI for guiding EP procedures in 2000 [40]. Continuous MR imaging of dogs was used to guide a low-magnetic susceptibility EP catheter (Figure 2a,b) from the internal jugular vein to selected locations in the right atrium (RA) and right ventricle (RV). RV ablation was performed after assessing catheter–tissue contact

Figure 2 Illustrates the importance of specific EP tools for use in the MRI scanner. (a) Stainless steel braiding and electrodes in a standard EP catheters results in significant image artifact that obscures the catheter position and surrounding anatomy, yellow arrow. (b) Making catheters from low magnetic susceptibility materials dramatically reduces this artifact such that the tip contact with the myocardium can now be seen. (c) Noise almost completely obscures this MRI image during delivery of RF ablation. (d) Image quality can be significantly restored by appropriately filtering the ablation source. *Source:* Lardo et al., 2000 [40]. Reproduced with permission of Lippincott Williams & Wilkins.

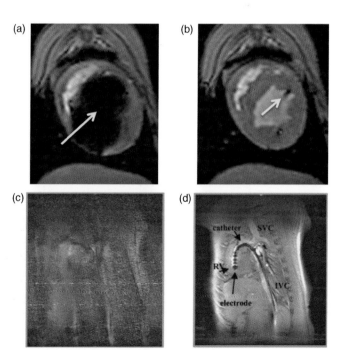

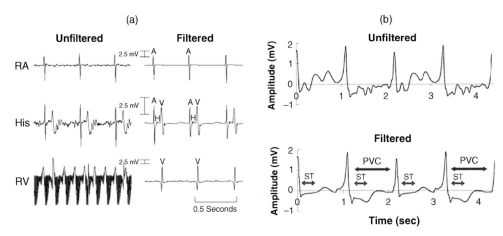

Figure 3 Illustrates cardiac electrogram recording in the MRI environment. (a) Shows intracardiac electrograms (icEGM) from a three catheter EP study during MRI scanning. Scanning-induced noise varies based on the catheter and image location, but in this case completely obscures the RV icEGM. (a) Shows that proper filtering and catheter design can significantly suppress icEGM noise during MRI scanning. (b) Top row illustrates surface ECG distortion in the MRI scanner even without MRI scanning due to the magnetohydrodynamic effect. (b) Bottom row shows this distortion can be suppressed through the use of adaptive filtering. *Sources:* Part (a), Nazarian et al., 2008 [41]. Reproduced with permission of Lippincott Williams & Wilkins; Part (b), Tse et al., 2013 [80]. Reproduced with permission of Wiley.

by MRI. Delivery of RF ablation energy during imaging can cause significant image degradation, but this noise was dramatically suppressed by low-pass filtering of the ablation source (Figure 2c,d). Postablation MRI showed that ablation lesion position and extent could be visualized by both T2 weighted and gadolinium enhanced DEMRI. Nazarian et al. subsequently demonstrated that electrogram recording and pacing could also be performed under rtMRI guidance [41]. Using continuous MR imaging in dogs, catheters were guided from femoral venous access sites to the high RA, His bundle, and RV apex. Interpretable electrogram recording could be performed at these sites during MRI scanning through the use of filtering (Figure 3a). Atrial and ventricular pacing was also demonstrated during MRI scanning without unintentional myocardial stimulation. More recently, Hoffman et al. used rtMRI to guide linear ablation of the cavo-tricuspid isthmus (CTI) in pigs [42]. Ganesan et al. similarly performed CTI ablation and also performed pacing maneuvers to demonstrate CTI block using rtMRI guidance [43]. In a nice integration of currently available techniques, Ranjan et al. demonstrated fusion of rtMRI, 3D MR angiogram, and 3D DEMRI lesion imaging to direct a catheter to a gap between atrial ablation lesions, perform additional ablation to fill in the gap, and demonstrate completion of the ablation line by repeat DEMRI [44] (Figure 7c). Accurate gap completion was achieved without the need for image registration because rtMRI and 3D imaging was performed in the same MRI system.

These studies have paved the way for basic real-time MRI-guided EP studies in patients. Nazarian et al. took the first step by obtaining FDA IDE approval for a steerable nonferromagnetic catheter [41]. rtMRI was used to guide this catheter and record intracardiac electrograms in two patients. A commercial MRI-compatible EP system has since been used to perform multicatheter EP recording and pacing in six patients [45,46]. Grothoff et al. recently applied this system to perform irrigated ablation of the CTI under real-time MRI guidance in 10 patients [47]. Though successful isthmus block was achieved only in two patients within the 90 min allotted study time, this study provided important support to the premise that the MRI heating safety concerns of an RF ablation capable catheter can be addressed. The important topic of interventional device heating during MRI will be discussed further in the MRI safety section below.

Studies using MRI electroanatomic mapping guidance

EAM is an important adjunct for guiding complex EP procedures and can also be performed in the MRI scanner. Dumoulin et al. first described using 1D MR imaging along the x, y, and z directions to identify the 3D position of a small receiver coil located in the catheter tip [48]. Dukkipati et al. used this technique to guide a five-receiver coil EP catheter around the LV of infarcted dogs to generate endocardial voltage

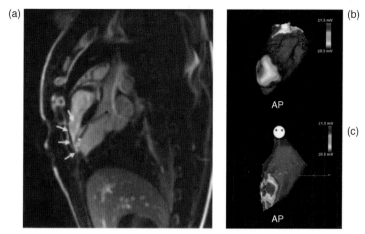

Figure 4 MRI-based electroanatomic mapping. (a) Illustrates MRI guidance of a catheter, in magenta, to a region of anteroseptal infarct, yellow arrows, seen on preacquired DEMRI roadmap images. The marked points along the catheter are the locations of the MRI tracking coils that are used to determine catheter position relative to the roadmap. (b) Illustrates this system can generate voltage substrate maps that are comparable to (c) the maps acquired by a conventional EAM system. *Source:* Dukkipati et al., 2008 [49]. Reproduced with permission of Lippincott Williams & Wilkins.

maps [49]. They found that the maps generated by MRI EAM were at least equivalent to those obtained using the CARTO EAM system in a conventional fluoroscopy suite. However, because MRI EAM was superimposed on 3D DEMRI infarct imaging, more detailed voltage maps could be created because dense mapping could be guided to the imaged infarct border. Also, unlike conventional EAM, registration of MRI EAM position to the MRI scar images was not needed because both used the same MRI coordinate system. Schmidt et al. subsequently utilized this system to perform MRI EAM guided ablation of the PV ostium and AV node in pigs [50]. Though their modest ablation outcomes could be attributed to inadequate catheter maneuverability and limited electrophysiologic mapping, they felt the tracking features of this system performed similar to conventional EAM (Figure 4). Recently, the feasibility of MRI EAM activation mapping was also shown [51]. MRI EAM has not yet been demonstrated in patients because of concerns about the heating safety of tracking coils. However, a technique for suppressing this heating has been described as discussed in the MRI safety section below [52,53].

Ongoing work toward fully MRI-guided clinical procedures

Current work focuses on taking MRI-guided EP from feasibility to safe and effective practice in patients. This includes (1) developing reliable techniques for acute ablation lesion imaging, (2) optimizing device

visualization and navigation, (3) integrated visualization of rtMRI with 3D anatomy and electrograms, (4) developing full featured, MRI-compatible electrogram recording and pacing systems, and (5) constructing clinical-grade MRI safe EP devices.

Intraprocedure ablation lesion imaging

Perhaps, the most significant advantage of MRI-guided ablation therapy is the potential to visualize incomplete regions of ablation, and direct additional treatment in order to ensure a complete, durable result during the initial procedure. Ablation lesions can be visualized because MRI is able to detect changes in proton precession and relaxation properties resulting from many factors including ablation-induced temperature changes, perfusion changes, interstitial edema, protein conformational changes, membrane disruption, and tissue coagulation [24,25,40,54–58]. Work is currently underway to determine the most reliable MRI techniques for determining the region permanent tissue destruction following ablation.

As discussed earlier, gadolinium contrast DEMRI has been increasingly used for ablation lesion assessment following AF ablation. However, this technique may have limitations for lesion imaging acutely after ablation. Badger et al. observed that the extent of DEMRI enhancement within 24 h of AF ablation was significantly greater than the enhancement seen at 3 and 6 months after ablation [59]. This suggests that early postablation gadolinium also accumulates in areas of transient injury that do not correlate well with eventual atrial scarring. McGann et al. subsequently noted that hypoenhancement of acutely ablated areas was more specific than hyperenhancement for identifying lesions that persisted 3 months following ablation [60] (Figure 5a). However, they also found that 40% of lesion persisting at 3 months arose from hyperenhancing or nonenhancing tissue. Also, restrictions on total gadolinium dose limit the number of time DEMRI can be performed during an EP study.

The limitations of DEMRI have renewed investigation of noncontrast enhanced MRI methods for assessing acute ablation lesions. There is growing evidence that noncontrast T1 weighted MRI is a more specific indicator of acute postablation tissue necrosis (Figure 5b) [61]. By comparison, T2 weighted MRI is sensitive to transient edema and provides poorer delineation of permanent tissue damage [42,61]. More quantitative proton density, T1, and T2 mapping techniques show promise for better distinguishing permanent from transient tissue injury acutely following ablation [61,62] (Figure 5c).

Methods for monitoring ablation lesion formation during energy delivery are also being investigated. Vergara et al. applied T2 weighted imaging to assess atrial tissue injury during RF energy delivery [63]. MR thermography may be able to more reliably determine the extent of permanent tissue damage by visualizing the extent of necrosis inducing tissue temperatures [54,55]. Its ability to assess RF ablation in the beating heart has been demonstrated and work is underway to assess its feasibility in the thin-walled atrium [64,65] (Figure 5d).

Device visualization and navigation

While fluoroscopy provides projection images where the entire catheter body and tip are easily visualized, 2D MR images typically depict a slice through the body that is around 5–10 mm thick. Curved devices such as catheters may pass in and out of the MR imaging plane leading to misinterpretation of the device tip position. Poor delineation of the tip position during catheter manipulation can result in tissue trauma [41]. Most real-time imaging studies to date have required manual image plane adjustment to properly locate the device tip. For procedures where the device is mostly constrained to a coplanar region, such CTI ablation, this is acceptable since only minor image translations are needed to visualize the device tip and relevant anatomy. For navigation in cardiac chambers where the device tip location is less

constrained, such as the left atrium, the frequent need for manual image repositioning necessitates a skilled operator and can distract from efficient procedure workflow. Fortunately, a number of methods are available to improve MRI catheter visualization and guidance that will see increased use in future studies.

Catheter visibility is significantly improved using "active" visualization techniques (Figure 6a,b). Using a similar method to the MRI EAM studies discussed above, active visualization utilizes localized imaging coils embedded within the device to generate regions of high signal around points or segments of the device. Because the MRI signals from each coil can be wired separately to the MRI system, different portions of the device can be clearly distinguished from one another and from the rest of the image [66] (Figure 6b). This localized region of high signal can be identified even on very thick imaging planes to producing an effect similar to the full-body thickness projection imaging provided by X-ray fluoroscopy [67]. Unlike thin-slice rtMRI, the device tip can be readily visualized on these "projection" images (Figure 6c.1, c.2). The major concern with using active visualization in patients, however, is the risk of unintentional heating of the active catheter coils during MRI scanning. The cause of this heating and progress toward mitigating this risk is discussed in the MRI safety section below.

Unambiguous catheter tip detection can also be performed using MRI EAM. MRI EAM can be interleaved with real-time MRI, in a manner analogous to conventional EAM and ICE. Also, because real-time MRI permits arbitrary image plane positioning, the imaged slice can be automatically moved to the catheter tip location, reducing the need for cumbersome manual image repositioning [68,69]. To delineate the curve and orientation of catheter sections that fall outside the real-time MRI slice, it is desirable to have multiple tracking points per catheter. However, making catheters with multiple tracking coils can be challenging given the space constraints of catheter lumens, particularly after MRI heating safety elements are incorporated. Multicoil designs and tracking algorithms have been developed to reduce the need for separate tuning circuits within the catheter [70,71]. Other MRI catheter tracking techniques can also be used that may have simpler heating mitigation solutions. One magnetic field-based tracking method is referenced to the MRI scanner coordinate system so that registration of catheter position to MR images is not needed [72]. Commercial electric field based EAM systems have also been adapted for use in the MRI that could permit any device with electrodes to be tracked in the MRI without the need for specific tracking components [73].

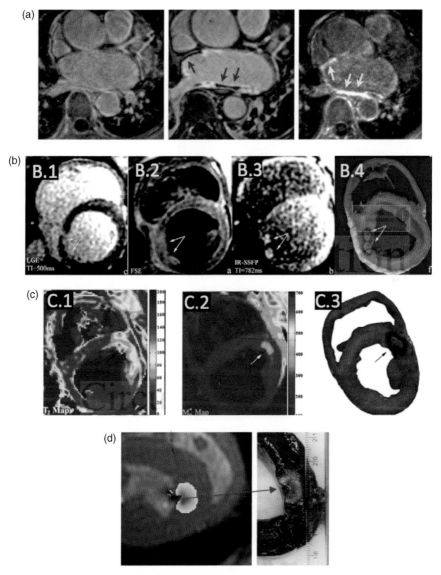

Figure 5 Acute ablation lesion imaging using MRI. (a) Illustrates acute and chronic ablation lesions on the equivalent slice of 3D atrial DEMRI images. (a) Left figure illustrates the atrial appearance prior to ablation. (a) Middle figure shows that within 24 h of ablation both hyperenhancement and hypoenhancement, red arrows, are seen. (a) Right figure shows weeks after ablation hyperenhancement can be seen in some regions that initially appeared to have hypoenhancement. Some regions that enhanced within 24 h, white arrow, no longer enhance suggesting transient injury. (b) Compares acute ablation lesion features of (b.1) DEMRI, (b.2) T2 weighted MRI, and (b.3) T1 weighted MRI with (b.4) pathology. Two discrete adjacent lesion are noted on T1 weighted MRI and pathology, supporting that T1 MRI may be more specific for identifying ablation lesion necrosis. (c) Illustrates ablation lesion imaging by quantitative MRI parameter mapping. In this case, (c.1) T2 mapping and (c.3) M0 proton density mapping are compared with (c.3) pathology. Quantitative mapping could better distinguish signal changes due to tissue properties from signal variation due to other factors such as proximity to MRI receiver coils. (d) Illustrates the potential of MRI for lesion monitoring during delivery of ablation energy. The left figure shows MRI thermography performed during RF energy delivery. The yellow lesion border indicating tissue heating to 50 °C. The right figure shows the necrotic lesion by TTC stained pathology corresponded well with the expected lesion extent based on thermography. *Sources:* Part (a), McGann et al., 2011 [60]. Reproduced with permission of Elsevier; Part (b) and (c), Celik et al., 2014 [61]. Reproduced with permission of Lippincott Williams & Wilkins; Part (d), Kolandaivelu et al., 2010 [64]. Reproduced with permission of Lippincott Williams & Wilkins.

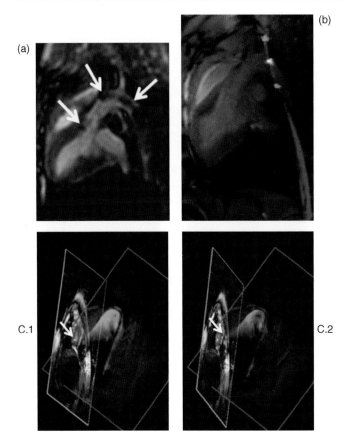

Figure 6 Device visualization by real-time MRI (rtMRI). (a) Illustrates rtMRI guidance of an MRI-safe guidewire, marked by white arrows, from the aortic root to cross the aortic valve. (b) Shows visualization can be much improved by the use of "active" imaging coils located within the device. In this case, focal coils mark points along the distal portion of the device and a longer antenna is used to delineate the shaft in blue. Because each coil is connected separately to the MRI system, they can be easily distinguished by coloring each differently. (c) Illustrates the use of thick slice "projection" rtMRI. In this case, the projection image is interleaved with a standard anatomic rtMRI slice. The tip of the device in red, marked by a white arrow for clarity, can be visualized on the "projection" image whether (c.1) the tip is in the rtMRI slice, or (c.2) the tip is pulled back out of that slice. *Sources:* Part (a), Tzifa et al., 2010 [108]. Reproduced with permission of LWW; Part (b), Kocaturk et al., 2009 [66]. Reproduced with permission of Wiley; Part (c), Guttman et al., 2007 [67]. Reproduced with permission of Wiley.

Ongoing developments in MRI acceleration will alleviate additional limitations of current rtMRI guidance. While cardiac gating can be used to generate MR images with excellent spatial resolution by splitting data collection over multiple heartbeats, rtMRI requires a more deliberate trade-off between temporal and spatial resolution. To reasonably visualize catheters, MRI-guided EP procedures require an in-plane spatial resolution of around $2\,\text{mm}^2$. The target temporal resolution has been seven frames per second (fps), similar to X-ray fluoroscopy frame rates for clinical EP procedures. rtMRI has advanced from re 1 fps imaging used to guide the first MRI-guided EP procedure to around 7 fps in recent studies [40,47]. However, higher spatial and temporal resolutions are desirable for confidently assessing detailed features such as catheter/tissue contact [42]. This can be done by switching to gated imaging when needed, but ideally would be possible while guiding catheter manipulation with real-time imaging. In addition, while current real-time MRI is acceptable for single-plane imaging, ideal visualization of multiple devices, target anatomy, and surrounding reference anatomy may require multiple real-time 2D image planes. Advances in more efficient image sampling, reconstruction, and parallel computing hardware now permit rtMRI that approaches the spatial and temporal resolution of gated cine MRI and could be applied to more rapid multislice rtMRI [74–76].

Integrated visualization of real-time imaging, 3D anatomy, electrograms

The ability to generate real-time images in any orientation in addition to anatomically detailed 3D images with flexible tissue contrast makes MRI well suited for navigating complex arrhythmia anatomy and delineating complex ablation patterns. Appropriate displays and user-interfaces tailored to the workflow of an EP procedure are needed to manage this flexibility. Because thin-slice real-time imaging can intersect anatomy in unfamiliar ways, 3D visualizations that plot real-time images oriented relative to reference images are helpful (Figure 7a). A basic imaging interface for MR-guided EP procedures would also provide

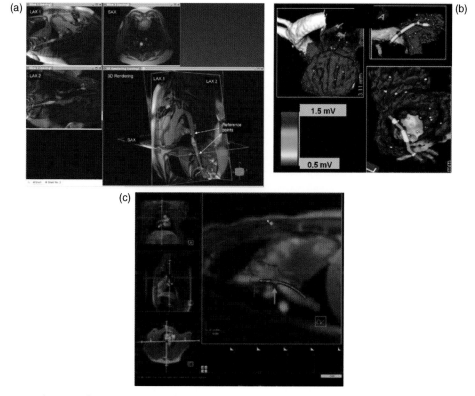

Figure 7 Development of integrated systems for MRI-guided procedures. (a) Shows a system displaying multiple rtMRI slices with different orientations to clarify device position, in green, relative to the surrounding anatomy. (b) Shows an example of MRI-based EAM mapping of the atrium that integrates catheter position, 3D angiogram surface anatomy, voltage mapping information, and ablation lesion locations. (c) Shows integration of rtMRI together with an MRI-tracked catheter, segmented MRI angiogram of the atrium, and segmented DEMRI ablation lesion images, marked by arrows. *Sources:* Part (a), Guttman et al., 2007 [67]. Reproduced with permission of Wiley; Part (b), Schmidt et al., 2009 [50]. Adapted with permission of Lippencott, Williams & Wilkins; Part (c), Ranjan et al., 2012 [44]. Reproduced with permission of Lippencott, Williams & Wilkins.

a convenient way to "bookmark" and access reference cardiac views, switch between real-time and lesion visualization sequences during the procedure, and appropriately present lesion images for ablation continuity assessment. Similar to current EAM systems, the MRI guided procedure interface should also display the relationship of catheter tracking positions to image information and intracardiac electrogram characteristics. Though still a work in progress, interventional MRI systems are steadily incorporating larger subsets of these features [44,49,53,67,77] (Figure 7).

Full-featured electrogram recording and pacing systems

In order to perform clinical EP studies, MRI compatible multichannel electrogram recording and pacing systems are needed. These systems must integrate appropriate filtering to suppress MRI image noise

introduced by the EP systems (Figure 2c,d) and electrogram noise created by the MRI environment (Figure 3). To minimize the risks of shock and cardiac stimulation, attention must also be paid to suppress current loops between filters and ground [78] and between different catheter channels. A commercial MRI EP system that acknowledges these issues has recently been demonstrated in patients [46,47].

As efforts turn to clinical application, acquiring accurate electrograms in the MRI environment becomes more important. Electromagnetic interference created by the MRI gradient magnetic field system overlaps the frequencies of interest in intracardiac electrograms (icEGM) and the surface ECG. Reasonable suppression of icEGM noise during MRI scanning has been demonstrated using conventional filter settings and closely spacing catheter electrodes and wiring to minimize the loop area available for noise induction [41]. However, noise can increase to noticeable levels depending on catheter and image plane position. One solution is to avoid active MR imaging during detailed electrogram interpretation. Adaptive filtering techniques and active blocking of electrogram sampling during MRI gradient activity can also be used to improve the fidelity of electrogram signals during imaging [79,80]. Another source of electrical interference, which is present even without MRI scanning, is the "magnetohydrodynamic effect" (MHD). MHD is caused by blood flowing perpendicular to the strong static magnetic field of the MRI scanner. This flow induces a voltage that distorts QRS and P waves and prevents ST segment interpretation. Adaptive filtering techniques that are calibrated using ECG characteristics outside and inside the MRI scanner have been developed to improve ECG interpretation in the MRI scanner [80] (Figure 3b).

MRI safety

Safety is a primary consideration for any new diagnostic or therapeutic approach.

A number of studies have been performed to determine the safety of conventional MRI with regard to electromagnetic energy exposure and tissue heating [81,82]. Interventional MRI procedures raise additional safety concerns [83–87]. The most straightforward aspect of MRI safety is the avoidance of ferromagnetic materials that could experience significant forces when brought close to the scanner. Although unsafe objects, such as ferromagnetic scissors and needle drivers, may be used during the preparatory phase of a procedure a system must be in place to methodically track and remove such objects before approaching the scanner. Similar attention is needed to address the ferromagnetic properties of other equipment associated with electrophysiology procedures including physiology monitoring equipment, ablation and pacing sources, and anesthesia apparatus. Clear marking of high field areas and secure placement of objects that may experience magnetic forces is mandatory so that appropriate pieces of equipment are kept at a safe distance from the MRI scanner [87–89].

The other major safety concern is the significant heating that can result from MRI RF transmission-induced current in extended metallic objects such as guidewires and wired electrodes [84,85]. This induction is more pronounced when portions of the device are located close to the MRI RF transmit coil housed within the edge of the scanner bore. The simplest way to avoid RF induction heating is to construct devices from nonmetallic components when possible.

Polymer materials and composites such as glass fiber-reinforced plastics have been used for catheter braiding and guidewires to reduce the heating risk introduced by catheter structural elements while maintaining device functional characteristics such as torquability, stiffness, and tensile strength [40,90,91]. Several approaches have also been developed to suppress induction heating in structures that require conductivity. Wires made from high-resistance alloys can adequately suppress inductive heating and can be used for electrogram recording and pacing electrodes [53,92]. For tasks where more efficient power transfer is required, such as RF ablation, high-frequency RF filters can allow passage of signals lower than a few MHz while blocking unwanted MR transmit frequency currents [92–94]. The fluid flow used for irrigated ablation may also be effective for suppressing heating of the ablation electrode [95]. Transformer transmission lines are a promising heating suppression technique for active visualization and position tracking coils, which need to pass differential mode signals at the same frequencies as unwanted common mode induced currents [52,96,97]. A number of other strategies for induction heating mitigation have also been developed that may have utility in some situations [92,93,98–103].

With a number of heating mitigation strategies now available, the current focus is to develop the interventional tools needed to conduct EP studies in patients. A commercial nonferromagnetic and heating mitigated ablation catheter was recently used in an early clinical CTI ablation study in Europe [47]. A heating mitigated active visualization and tracking system has also been developed but awaits integration into clinical-grade diagnostic and ablation devices [53]. In order to perform access procedures under MRI guidance, compatible guide sheaths, transseptal needles, and guidewires are also needed [104–107]. Though clinical-grade forms of these tools are becoming available [108], "actively visualized" devices would be preferable [104,105] (Figure 6). Development of a heating safe active guidewire is a remaining challenge with potential solutions under investigation [109–112]. In the mean time, vascular access procedures may be performed with fluoroscopy or ultrasound guidance before transfer to the MRI scanner area [89].

Conclusions

The flexibility of preprocedure MRI for visualizing complex 3D cardiovascular anatomy and more detailed atrial tissue characteristics such as ablated tissue provides a number of ways MRI may contribute to guidance of current AF ablation procedures. Performing procedures under full real-time MRI guidance could address additional limitations of current ablation procedures including avoidance of ionizing radiation and more accurate targeting of detailed anatomic features such as gaps in ablation lines. Availability of clinical-grade nonferromagnetic and MRI heating safe interventional EP tools is a rate-limiting step for application of full MRI guidance to EP procedures in patients. However, the technologies to enable these devices are largely available and suitable MRI-compatible EP devices are under active development and testing.

References

1 Calkins H, Yong P, Miller JM, et al. Catheter ablation of accessory pathways, atrioventricular nodal reentrant tachycardia, and the atrioventricular junction: final results of a prospective, multicenter clinical trial. The Atakr Multicenter Investigators Group. Circulation 1999;99(2):262–270.

2 Kato R, Lickfett L, Meininger G, et al. Pulmonary vein anatomy in patients undergoing catheter ablation of atrial fibrillation: lessons learned by use of magnetic resonance imaging. Circulation 2003;107(15):2004–2010.

3 Tsao HM, Wu MH, Yu WC, et al. Role of right middle pulmonary vein in patients with paroxysmal atrial fibrillation. J Cardiovasc Electrophysiol. 2001;12(12):1353–1357.

4 Mansour M, Refaat M, Heist EK, et al. Three-dimensional anatomy of the left atrium by magnetic resonance angiography: implications for catheter ablation for atrial fibrillation. J Cardiovasc Electrophysiol. 2006;17(7):719–723.

5 Scharf C, Sneider M, Case I, et al. Anatomy of the pulmonary veins in patients with atrial fibrillation and effects of segmental ostial ablation analyzed by computed tomography. J Cardiovasc Electrophysiol. 2003;14(2):150–155.

6 Hunter RJ, Ginks M, Ang R, et al. Impact of variant pulmonary vein anatomy and image integration on long-term outcome after catheter ablation for atrial fibrillation. Europace. 2010;12(12):1691–1697.

7 Kubala M, Hermida JS, Nadji G, Quenum S, Traulle S, Jarry G. Normal pulmonary veins anatomy is associated with better AF-free survival after cryoablation as compared to atypical anatomy with common left pulmonary vein. Pacing Clin Electrophysiol. 2011;34 (7):837–843.

8 McLellan AJ, Ling LH, Ruggiero D, et al. Pulmonary vein isolation: the impact of pulmonary venous anatomy on long-term outcome of catheter ablation for paroxysmal atrial fibrillation. Heart Rhythm. 2014;11(4):549–556.

9 Hendel RC, Patel MR, Kramer CM, et al. ACCF/ACR/SCCT/SCMR/ASNC/NASCI/SCAI/SIR 2006 appropriateness criteria for cardiac computed tomography and cardiac magnetic resonance imaging: a report of the American College of Cardiology Foundation Quality Strategic Directions Committee Appropriateness Criteria Working Group, American College of Radiology, Society of Cardiovascular Computed Tomography, Society for Cardiovascular Magnetic Resonance, American Society of Nuclear Cardiology, North American Society for Cardiac Imaging, Society for Cardiovascular Angiography and Interventions, and Society of Interventional Radiology. J Am Coll Cardiol. 2006;48(7):1475–1497.

10 Calkins H, Brugada J, Packer DL, et al. HRS/EHRA/ECAS Expert Consensus Statement on Catheter and Surgical Alation of Atrial Fibrillation: recommendations for personnel, policy, procedures and follow-up. A report of the Heart Rhythm Society (HRS) Task Force on Catheter and Surgical Ablation of Atrial Fibrillation. Heart Rhythm. 2007;4(6):816–861.

11 Ponti RD, Marazzi R, Lumia D, et al. Role of three-dimensional imaging integration in atrial fibrillation ablation. World J Cardiol. 2010;2(8):215–222.

12 Govil A, Calkins H, Spragg DD. Fusion of imaging technologies: how, when, and for whom? J Interv Cardiac Electrophysiol. 2011;32(3):195–203.

13 Dong J, Dickfeld T, Dalal D, et al. Initial experience in the use of integrated electroanatomic mapping with three-dimensional MR/CT images to guide catheter ablation of atrial fibrillation. J Cardiovasc Electrophysiol. 2006;17(5):459–466.

14 Kistler PM, Rajappan K, Harris S, et al. The impact of image integration on catheter ablation of atrial fibrillation using electroanatomic mapping: a prospective randomized study. Eur Heart J. 2008;29(24):3029–3036.

15 Tang K, Ma J, Zhang S, et al. A randomized prospective comparison of CartoMerge and CartoXP to guide circumferential pulmonary vein isolation for the treatment of paroxysmal atrial fibrillation. Chin Med J. 2008;121 (6):508–512.

16 Della Bella P, Fassini G, Cireddu M, et al. Image integration-guided catheter ablation of atrial fibrillation: a prospective randomized study. J Cardiovasc Electrophysiol. 2009;20(3):258–265.

17 Caponi D, Corleto A, Scaglione M, et al. Ablation of atrial fibrillation: does the addition of three-dimensional magnetic resonance imaging of the left atrium to electroanatomic mapping improve the clinical outcome?: a randomized comparison of Carto-Merge vs. Carto-XP three-dimensional mapping ablation in patients with paroxysmal and persistent atrial fibrillation. Europace. 2010;12(8):1098–1104.

18 Ouyang F, Antz M, Ernst S, et al. Recovered pulmonary vein conduction as a dominant factor for recurrent atrial tachyarrhythmias after complete circular isolation of the pulmonary veins: lessons from double Lasso technique. Circulation 2005;111(2):127–135.

19 Verma A, Kilicaslan F, Pisano E, et al. Response of atrial fibrillation to pulmonary vein antrum isolation is directly related to resumption and delay of

pulmonary vein conduction. Circulation 2005;112(5): 627–635.

20 Weerasooriya R, Khairy P, Litalien J, et al. Catheter ablation for atrial fibrillation: are results maintained at 5 years of follow-up? J Am Coll Cardiol. 2011;57(2): 160–166.

21 Hussein AA, Saliba WI, Martin DO, et al. Natural history and long-term outcomes of ablated atrial fibrillation. Circ Arrhythmia Electrophysiol. 2011;4(3):271–278.

22 Ranjan R, Kato R, Zviman MM, et al. Gaps in the ablation line as a potential cause of recovery from electrical isolation and their visualization using MRI. Circ Arrhythmia Electrophysiol. 2011;4(3):279–286.

23 Wang XH, Liu X, Sun YM, et al. Early identification and treatment of PV re-connections: role of observation time and impact on clinical results of atrial fibrillation ablation. Europace. 2007;9(7):481–486.

24 Dickfeld T, Kato R, Zviman M, et al. Characterization of radiofrequency ablation lesions with gadolinium-enhanced cardiovascular magnetic resonance imaging. J Am Coll Cardiol. 2006;47(2):370–378.

25 Dickfeld T, Kato R, Zviman M, et al. Characterization of acute and subacute radiofrequency ablation lesions with nonenhanced magnetic resonance imaging. Heart Rhythm. 2007;4(2):208–214.

26 Kim RJ, Fieno DS, Parrish TB, et al. Relationship of MRI delayed contrast enhancement to irreversible injury, infarct age, and contractile function. Circulation. 1999;100(19):1992–2002.

27 Peters DC, Wylie JV, Hauser TH, et al. Detection of pulmonary vein and left atrial scar after catheter ablation with three-dimensional navigator-gated delayed enhancement MR imaging: initial experience. Radiology. 2007;243(3):690–695.

28 Taclas JE, Nezafat R, Wylie JV, et al. Relationship between intended sites of RF ablation and post-procedural scar in AF patients, using late gadolinium enhancement cardiovascular magnetic resonance. Heart Rhythm. 2010;7(4):489–496.

29 Badger TJ, Daccarett M, Akoum NW, et al. Evaluation of left atrial lesions after initial and repeat atrial fibrillation ablation: lessons learned from delayed-enhancement MRI in repeat ablation procedures. Circ Arrhythmia Electrophysiol. 2010;3(3):249–259.

30 Spragg DD, Khurram I, Zimmerman SL, et al. Initial experience with magnetic resonance imaging of atrial scar and co-registration with electroanatomic voltage mapping during atrial fibrillation: success and limitations. Heart Rhythm. 2012;9(12):2003–2009.

31 Bisbal F, Guiu E, Cabanas-Grandio P, et al. CMR-guided approach to localize and ablate gaps in repeat AF ablation procedure. JACC Cardiovasc Imaging. 2014;7 (7):653–663.

32 Nazarian S, Beinart R. CMR-Guided Targeting of Gaps After Initial Pulmonary Vein Isolation. JACC Cardiovasc Imaging. 2014;7(7):664–666.

33 Oakes RS, Badger TJ, Kholmovski EG, et al. Detection and quantification of left atrial structural remodeling with delayed-enhancement magnetic resonance imaging in patients with atrial fibrillation. Circulation. 2009;119 (13):1758–1767.

34 Marrouche NF, Wilber D, Hindricks G, et al. Association of atrial tissue fibrosis identified by delayed enhancement MRI and atrial fibrillation catheter ablation: the DECAAF study. JAMA. 2014;311(5):498–506.

35 Akoum N, Daccarett M, McGann C, et al. Atrial fibrosis helps select the appropriate patient and strategy in catheter ablation of atrial fibrillation: a DE-MRI guided approach. J Cardiovasc Electrophysiol. 2011;22(1):16–22.

36 McDowell KS, Vadakkumpadan F, Blake R, et al. Mechanistic inquiry into the role of tissue remodeling in fibrotic lesions in human atrial fibrillation. Biophysic J. 2013;104(12):2764–2773.

37 Jadidi AS, Cochet H, Shah AJ, et al. Inverse relationship between fractionated electrograms and atrial fibrosis in persistent atrial fibrillation: combined magnetic resonance imaging and high-density mapping. J Am Coll Cardiol. 2013;62(9):802–812.

38 Xerox. Merisight. 2014; merisight.com.

39 Higuchi K, Akkaya M, Koopmann M, et al. The effect of fat pad modification during ablation of atrial fibrillation: late gadolinium enhancement MRI analysis. Pacing Clin Electrophysiol. 2013;36(4):467–476.

40 Lardo AC, McVeigh ER, Jumrussirikul P, et al. Visualization and temporal/spatial characterization of cardiac radiofrequency ablation lesions using magnetic resonance imaging. Circulation. 2000;102(6):698–705.

41 Nazarian S, Kolandaivelu A, Zviman MM, et al. Feasibility of real-time magnetic resonance imaging for catheter guidance in electrophysiology studies. Circulation. 2008;118(3):223–229.

42 Hoffmann BA, Koops A, Rostock T, et al. Interactive real-time mapping and catheter ablation of the cavotricuspid isthmus guided by magnetic resonance imaging in a porcine model. Eur Heart J. 2010;31(4):450–456.

43 Ganesan AN, Selvanayagam JB, Mahajan R, et al. Mapping and ablation of the pulmonary veins and cavotricuspid isthmus with a magnetic resonance imaging-compatible externally irrigated ablation catheter and integrated electrophysiology system. Circ Arrhythmia Electrophysiol. 2012;5(6):1136–1142.

44 Ranjan R, Kholmovski EG, Blauer J, et al. Identification and acute targeting of gaps in atrial ablation lesion sets using a real-time magnetic resonance imaging system. Circ Arrhythmia Electrophysiol. 2012;5(6):1130–1135.

45 Eitel C, Piorkowski C, Hindricks G, Gutberlet M. Electrophysiology study guided by real-time magnetic resonance imaging. Eur Heart J. 2012;33(15):1975.

46 Sommer P, Grothoff M, Eitel C, et al. Feasibility of real-time magnetic resonance imaging-guided electrophysiology studies in humans. Europace 2013;15(1):101–108.

47 Grothoff M, Piorkowski C, Eitel C, et al. MR imaging-guided electrophysiological ablation studies in humans with passive catheter tracking: initial results. Radiology. 2014;271(3):695–702.

48 Dumoulin CL, Souza SP, Darrow RD. Real-time position monitoring of invasive devices using magnetic resonance. Magn Reson Med. 1993;29(3):411–415.

49 Dukkipati SR, Mallozzi R, Schmidt EJ, et al. Electro-anatomic mapping of the left ventricle in a porcine model of chronic myocardial infarction with magnetic resonance-based catheter tracking. Circulation. 2008; 118(8):853–862.

50 Schmidt EJ, Mallozzi RP, Thiagalingam A, et al. Electro-anatomic mapping and radiofrequency ablation of porcine left atria and atrioventricular nodes using magnetic resonance catheter tracking. Circ Arrhythmia Electrophysiol. 2009;2(6):695–704.

51 Oduneye SO, Biswas L, Ghate S, et al. The feasibility of endocardial propagation mapping using magnetic resonance guidance in a Swine model, and comparison with standard electroanatomic mapping. IEEE Trans Med Imaging. 2012;31(4):977–983.

52 Weiss S, Vernickel P, Schaeffter T, Schulz V, Gleich B. Transmission line for improved RF safety of interventional devices. Magn Reson Med. 2005;54(1): 182–189.

53 Weiss S, Wirtz D, David B, et al. *In vivo* evaluation and proof of radiofrequency safety of a novel diagnostic MR-electrophysiology catheter. Magn Reson Med. 2011;65 (3):770–777.

54 Rieke V, Butts Pauly K. MR thermometry. J Magn Reson Imaging. 2008;27(2):376–390.

55 Wansapura JP, Daniel BL, Vigen KK, Butts K. *In vivo* MR thermometry of frozen tissue using R2* and signal intensity. Academic Radiol. 2005;12(9):1080–1084.

56 Shmatukha A, Sethi B, Shurrab M, et al. Visualization of thermal ablation lesions using cumulative dynamic contrast enhancement MRI. Phys Med Biol. 2013;58 (10):3321–3337.

57 Shultz K, Pauly J, Scott G. Feasibility of full RF current-vector mapping for MR guided RF ablation. 15th Proceedings of the International Society for Magnetic Resonance In Medicine, Berlin, Germany, 2007.

58 Schmidt EJ, Fung MM, Ciris PA, et al. Navigated DENSE strain imaging for post-radiofrequency ablation lesion assessment in the swine left atria. Europace. 2014;16(1):133–141.

59 Badger TJ, Oakes RS, Daccarett M, et al. Temporal left atrial lesion formation after ablation of atrial fibrillation. Heart Rhythm. 2009;6(2):161–168.

60 McGann C, Kholmovski E, Blauer J, et al. Dark regions of no-reflow on late gadolinium enhancement magnetic resonance imaging result in scar formation after atrial fibrillation ablation. J Am Coll Cardiol. 2011;58 (2):177–185.

61 Celik H, Ramanan V, Barry J, et al. Intrinsic contrast for characterization of acute radiofrequency ablation lesions. Circ Arrhythmia Electrophysiol. 2014;7(4): 718–727.

62 Herzka D, Ding H, Pashakhanloo F, et al. Assessment of radiofrequency ablation lesions with 3D high-resolution free-breathing T2 mapping. Heart Rhythm 34th Annual Scientific Sessions, Denver, CO, 2013.

63 Vergara GR, Vijayakumar S, Kholmovski EG, et al. Real-time magnetic resonance imaging-guided radiofrequency atrial ablation and visualization of lesion formation at 3 Tesla. Heart Rhythm. 2011;8(2): 295–303.

64 Kolandaivelu A, Zviman MM, Castro V, Lardo AC, Berger RD, Halperin HR. Noninvasive assessment of tissue heating during cardiac radiofrequency ablation using MRI thermography. Circ Arrhythmia Electrophysiol. 2010;3(5):521–529.

65 Volland NA, Kholmovski EG, Parker DL, Hadley JR. Initial feasibility testing of limited field of view magnetic resonance thermometry using a local cardiac radiofrequency coil. Magn Reson Med. 2013;70(4): 994–1004.

66 Kocaturk O, Saikus CE, Guttman MA, et al. Whole shaft visibility and mechanical performance for active MR catheters using copper–nitinol braided polymer tubes. J Cardiovasc Magn Reson. 2009;11: 29.

67 Guttman MA, Ozturk C, Raval AN, et al. Interventional cardiovascular procedures guided by real-time MR imaging: an interactive interface using multiple slices, adaptive projection modes and live 3D renderings. J Magn Reson Imaging. 2007;26(6):1429–1435.

68 Elgort DR, Wong EY, Hillenbrand CM, Wacker FK, Lewin JS, Duerk JL. Real-time catheter tracking and adaptive imaging. J Magn Reson Imaging. 2003;18 (5):621–626.

69 Bock M, Muller S, Zuehlsdorff S, et al. Active catheter tracking using parallel MRI and real-time image reconstruction. Magn Reson Med. 2006;55(6):1454–1459.

70 Zhang Q, Wendt M, Aschoff AJ, Lewin JS, Duerk JL. A multielement RF coil for MRI guidance of interventional devices. J Magn Reson Imaging. 2001;14(1):56–62.

71 Zuehlsdorff S, Umathum R, Volz S, et al. MR coil design for simultaneous tip tracking and curvature delineation of a catheter. Magn Reson Med. 2004;52(1):214–218.

72 Nevo E, Inventor. Method and apparatus to estimate locatino and orientation of objects during magnetic resonance imaging. 2003.

73 Schmidt EJ, Tse ZT, Reichlin TR, et al. Voltage-based device tracking in a 1.5 Tesla MRI during imaging: initial validation in swine models. Magn Reson Med. 2014; 71(3):1197–1209.

74 Seiberlich N, Ehses P, Duerk J, Gilkeson R, Griswold M. Improved radial GRAPPA calibration for real-time free-breathing cardiac imaging. Magn Reson Med. 2011; 65(2):492–505.

75 Saybasili H, Herzka DA, Seiberlich N, Griswold MA. Real-time imaging with radial GRAPPA: implementation on a heterogeneous architecture for low-latency reconstructions. Magn Reson Imaging 2014;32(6):747–758.

76 Wech T, Gutberlet M, Greiser A, et al. High-resolution functional cardiac MR imaging using density-weighted real-time acquisition and a combination of compressed sensing and parallel imaging for image reconstruction. Fortschr Rontg Nuen. 2010;182(8):676–681.

77 Weiss S, Krueger S, Koken P, et al. Evaluation of an integrated MR-EP suite and catheter-navigated local MR lesion monitoring after RF ablation. 21st Proceedings of the International Society for Magnetic Resonance in Medicine, Salt Lake City, UT, 2013.

78 Sidebottom C, Rudolph H, Schmidt M, Eisner L. IEC 60601-1 - The Third Edition. J Med Dev Regul. 2006; May; 8–17.

79 Wu V, Barbash IM, Ratnayaka K, et al. Adaptive noise cancellation to suppress electrocardiography artifacts during real-time interventional MRI. J Magn Reson Imaging. 2011;33(5):1184–1193.

80 Tse ZT, Dumoulin CL, Clifford GD, et al. A 1.5T MRI-conditional 12-lead electrocardiogram for MRI and intra-MR intervention. Magn Reson Med. 2014;71(3): 1336–1347.

81 International Commission on Non-Ionizing Radiation Protection. Guidelines for limiting exposure to time-varying electric, magnetic, and electromagnetic fields (up to 300 GHz). International Commission on Non-Ionizing Radiation Protection. Health Phys. 1998;74 (4):494–522.

82 Shellock FG. Radiofrequency energy-induced heating during MR procedures: a review. J Magn Reson Imaging. 2000;12(1):30–36.

83 Knopp MV, Essig M, Debus J, Zabel HJ, van Kaick G. Unusual burns of the lower extremities caused by a closed conducting loop in a patient at MR imaging. Radiology 1996;200(2):572–575.

84 Nitz WR, Oppelt A, Renz W, Manke C, Lenhart M, Link J. On the heating of linear conductive structures as guide wires and catheters in interventional MRI. J Magn Reson Imaging. 2001;13(1):105–114.

85 Konings MK, Bartels LW, Smits HF, Bakker CJ. Heating around intravascular guidewires by resonating RF waves. J Magn Reson Imaging. 2000;12(1):79–85.

86 Atalar E. Radiofrequency safety for interventional MRI procedures. Academic Radiol. 2005;12(9):1149–1157.

87 White MJ, Thornton JS, Hawkes DJ, et al. Design, operation, and safety of single-room interventional MRI suites: practical experience from two centers. J Magn Reson Imaging. 2015;41(1):34–43.

88 Razavi R, Hill DL, Keevil SF, et al. Cardiac catheterisation guided by MRI in children and adults with congenital heart disease. Lancet. 2003;362(9399):1877–1882.

89 Tzifa A, Schaeffter T, Razavi R. MR imaging-guided cardiovascular interventions in young children. Magn Reson Imaging Clin North Am. 2012;20(1): 117–128.

90 Krueger S, Schmitz S, Weiss S, et al. An MR guidewire based on micropultruded fiber-reinforced material. Magn Reson Med. 2008;60(5):1190–1196.

91 Wolska-Krawczyk M, Rube MA, Immel E, Melzer A, Buecker A. Heating and safety of a new MR-compatible guidewire prototype versus a standard nitinol guidewire. Radiolog Phys Technol. 2014;7(1):95–101.

92 Bottomley PA, Kumar A, Edelstein WA, Allen JM, Karmarkar PV. Designing passive MRI-safe implantable conducting leads with electrodes. Med Phys. 2010;37 (7):3828–3843.

93 Ladd ME, Quick HH. Reduction of resonant RF heating in intravascular catheters using coaxial chokes. Magn Reson Med. 2000;43(4):615–619.

94 Susil RC, Yeung CJ, Halperin HR, Lardo AC, Atalar E. Multifunctional interventional devices for MRI: a combined electrophysiology/MRI catheter. Magn Reson Med. 2002;47(3):594–600.

95 Reiter T, Gensler D, Ritter O, et al. Direct cooling of the catheter tip increases safety for CMR-guided electrophysiological procedures. J Cardiovasc Magn Reson. 2012;14: 12.

96 Vernickel P, Schulz V, Weiss S, Gleich B. A safe transmission line for MRI. IEEE Trans Bio-Med Eng. 2005;52 (6):1094–1102.

97 Kreuger S, Lips O, Ruhl KM, et al. RF-safe intravascular imaging using self-visualizing transformer line. Paper presented at Joint Annual Meeting ISMRM-ESMRMB, Berlin. 2007.

98 Wong EY, Zhang Q, Duerk JL, Lewin JS, Wendt M. An optical system for wireless detuning of parallel resonant circuits. J Magn Reson Imaging. 2000;12(4): 632–638.

99 Yeung CJ, Susil RC, Atalar E. RF safety of wires in interventional MRI: using a safety index. Magn Reson Med. 2002;47(1):187–193.

100 Eryaman Y, Akin B, Atalar E. Reduction of implant RF heating through modification of transmit coil electric field. Magn Reson Med. 2011;65(5):1305–1313.

101 Celik H, Uluturk A, Tali T, Atalar E. A catheter tracking method using reverse polarization for MR-guided interventions. Magn Reson Med. 2007;58(6): 1224–1231.

102 Weiss S, David B, Luedkeke K-M, et al. Evaluation of a novel MR-RF Ablation Catheter with full clincal Functionality. 19th Proceedings of the International Society for Mangetic Resonance In Medicine, Montreal, Quebec, Canada, 2011.

103 Fandrey S, Weiss S, Muller J. A novel active MR probe using a miniaturized optical link for a 1.5-T MRI scanner. Magn Reson Med. 2012;67(1):148–155.

104 Arepally A, Karmarkar PV, Weiss C, Rodriguez ER, Lederman RJ, Atalar E. Magnetic resonance image-guided trans-septal puncture in a swine heart. J Magn Reson Imaging. 2005;21(4):463–467.

105 Raval AN, Karmarkar PV, Guttman MA, et al. Real-time MRI guided atrial septal puncture and balloon septostomy in swine. Catheter Cardiovasc Interv. 2006;67 (4):637–643.

106 Saikus CE, Ratnayaka K, Barbash IM, et al. MRI-guided vascular access with an active visualization needle. J Magn Reson Imaging. 2011;34(5):1159–1166.

107 Halabi M, Faranesh AZ, Schenke WH, et al. Real-time cardiovascular magnetic resonance subxiphoid pericardial access and pericardiocentesis using off-the-shelf devices in swine. J Cardiovasc Magn Reson. 2013; 15: 61.

108 Tzifa A, Krombach GA, Kramer N, et al. Magnetic resonance-guided cardiac interventions using magnetic resonance-compatible devices: a preclinical study and first-in-man congenital interventions. Circ Cardiovas Interv. 2010;3(6):585–592.

109 Sonmez M, Saikus CE, Bell JA, et al. MRI active guide-wire with an embedded temperature probe and providing a distinct tip signal to enhance clinical safety. J Cardiovasc Magn Reson. 2012;14: 38.

110 Etezadi-Amoli M, Stang P, Kerr A, Pauly J, Scott G. Interventional device visualization with toroidal transceiver and optically coupled current sensor for radiofrequency safety monitoring. Magn Reson Med. 2014.

111 Scott G, Stang P, Overall K, Kerr A, Pauly J. A Vector modulation transmit array system. 14th Proceedings of the International Society of Magnetic Resonance in medicine, Seattle, WA, 2006.

112 Etezadi-Amoli M, Stang P, Zanchi MG, Pauly J, Scott G, Kerr A. Controlling induced currents in guidewires using parallel transmitt. 18th Proceedings of the International Society of Magnetic Resonance in Medicine, Stockholm, Sweden, 2010.

CHAPTER 10

MRI definition of atrial substrate

Leenhapong Navaravong & Nassir F. Marrouche
Comprehensive Arrhythmia Research and Management Center (CARMA),
University of Utah School of Medicine, Salt Lake City, UT, USA

Introduction

Structural remodeling and fibrosis play significant role in cardiac arrhythmia including atrial fibrillation (AF). The deposition of fibrotic tissue inside LA wall correlates with structural changes and electrophysiological abnormalities of LA [1–3]. The novel development in delayed enhancement magnetic resonance imaging (DE-MRI) allows us to evaluate the structure change/fibrosis in LA wall and develops the personalized management of AF [4,5]. In this chapter, we will provide information about DE-MRI of LA in AF and its clinical implication.

Delayed enhancement MRI in atrial fibrillation

At the Comprehensive Arrhythmia Research and Management Center (CARMA), we developed DE-MRI sequence that can overcome the issue of spatial resolution of LA wall on conventional protocols. This allows better visualization of LA wall and abnormal enhancement within the wall. MRI scans are performed on a 1.5-Tesla (T) Avanto or a 3-T Trio scanner (Siemens Medical Solutions, Erlangen, Germany) with a total imaging matrix phased array receiver coil. Delayed enhancement MRI is obtained 15 min after a gadolinium bolus injection (0.1 mmol/kg Multihance; Bracco Diagnostic, Monroe Township, NJ) and a contrast-enhanced three-dimensional fast low-angle shot angiography sequence and a cine true fast imaging with steady-state precession sequence are used to define the anatomy of the left atrium and the pulmonary veins.

A three-dimensional inversion recovery gradient recalled, respiration triggered and navigated, electrocardiographically gated, gradient-echo and fat suppressed sequence is used for image acquisition. A transverse imaging volume with spatial resolution of $1.25 \times 1.25 \times 2.5$ mm results in images with two–four voxels across the LA wall in the imaging plane. The images are interpolated to $0.625 \times 0.625 \times 1.25$ mm voxel size using a zero-filled algorithm to reduce partial volume effects. For the 3-T and 1.5-T scanners, 13 and 20° flip angles are used, respectively. The inversion time ranges between 270 and 310 ms and 280–330 ms for a 1.5-T and 3-T scan, respectively. The echo time is optimized to ensure that fat and water are out of phase and to reduce the signal intensity of partial-volume fat-tissue voxels. Repetition time to echo time ratios are 5.24 : 2.3 (1.5-T scanner) and 3.3 : 1.4 (3-T scanner).

Preablation LA fibrosis quantification

DE-MRI images of LA will be processed by special software (Corview, Marrek Inc., Salt Lake City, UT). This includes delineation of endocardial and epicardial surface of LA to identify the LA wall, pixel intensity analysis with threshold selection, and fibrosis quantification. The percentage of LA fibrosis was calculated by using the area of LA wall with abnormal enhancement as numerator divided by total LA surface area. Additional information about the fibrosis quantification can be found on our previous publications [4–8]. This process is summarized in figure 1.

Relationship between LA fibrosis, LA enhancement, and AF

LA fibrosis is well described in AF patients [9–13]. Tissue biopsy of LA was obtained from 10 patients with abnormal enhancement of LA, who underwent

Practical Guide to Catheter Ablation of Atrial Fibrillation,
Second Edition. Edited by Jonathan S. Steinberg, Pierre Jaïs and Hugh Calkins.
© 2016 John Wiley & Sons, Ltd. Published 2016 by John Wiley & Sons, Ltd.

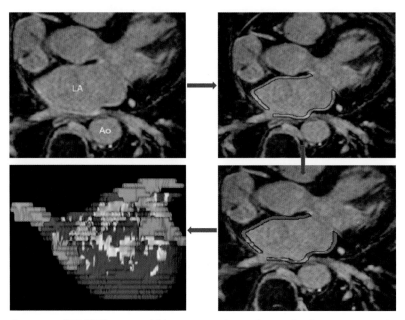

Figure 1 Stepwise process of DE-MRI image acquisition, segmentation, and processing for assessment and quantification of left atrial fibrosis. After DE-MRI images were acquired, epicardial and endocardial borders are contoured in each slice to define the left atrial wall. LA fibrosis is quantified for each segment based on relative intensity of abnormal delayed enhancement. Finally, three-dimensional model of LA was created and fibrosis was projected on the surface.

open heart surgery (9 with history of atrial fibrillation and 1 without history of atrial fibrillation) [7]. All tissue specimens from the area of abnormal enhancement demonstrated significant amount of interstitial fibrosis on Masson trichrome stain. Similarly, tissue specimen from nonenhanced area showed no or minimal fibrosis (Figure 2). This study confirms relationship between abnormal enhancement and histological proven fibrosis. Additionally, this study also compared atrial fibrosis using DE-MRI between AF and non-AF participants and showed that AF patients have a significantly higher percentage of abnormal enhancement compared to non-AF participants [7].

Left atrial fibrosis and clinical AF

AF is classified as paroxysmal (episodes of arrhythmia are self-terminating within 7 days), persistent (AF episode lasts longer than 7 days or that needs pharmacologic or electrical cardioversion to terminate), long-standing persistent (persistent AF with longer than 1 year duration), and permanent AF (no attempts are planned for restoration of sinus rhythm). Conventionally, we would predict positive correlation between higher degree of LA fibrosis and severity of AF phenotypes. However, there was significant overlap in the degree of fibrosis between patients with different AF phenotypes. The phenotype did not accurately predict

the degree of atrial fibrosis [6–8]. Moreover, the study done by our center demonstrated that lone AF patients have the same burden of atrial fibrosis as those with nonlone AF [8,14].

LA fibrosis and stroke

AF is associated with higher risk of stroke and thromboembolic events [15]. The stroke risk is commonly estimated by using CHADS2-VASC score and this was advocated in the recent national guideline [16]. Though this clinical scoring system is practical and easy to perform, it does not include significant information regarding LA structural remodeling/fibrosis. A cross-sectional study by our institution demonstrated that LA fibrosis by DE-MRI is an independent risk factor for stroke [17]. Patients with prior stroke had a significantly higher percentage of LA fibrosis than those without history of a previous stroke ($24.4 \pm 12.4\%$ versus $16.1 \pm 9.8\%$, $p < 0.001$). There was a significant difference in the rate of thromboembolism between patients in lowest quartile of LA fibrosis (<8.5%) and those in highest quartile (>21.1%) of LA. Patients with higher CHADS2 score had higher amounts of LA fibrosis. Akoum and colleagues also demonstrated that patients with LA fibrosis >20% were more likely to have a LAA thrombus (13.8% versus 3.3%, $p < 0.01$) and spontaneous echo contrast (17.2% versus 7.5%, $p = 0.04$) with

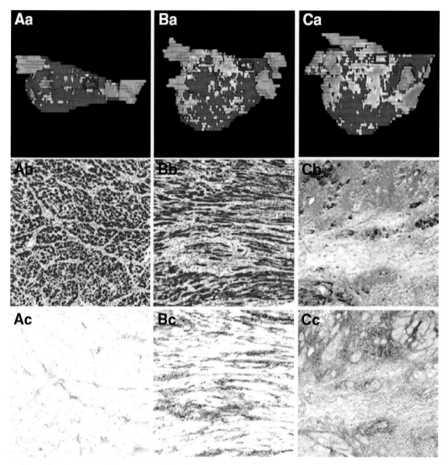

Figure 2 Left atrial wall structural remodeling (SRM) on delayed enhancement MRI correlates with surgical biopsy specimens. Examples from three surgical patients who underwent both three-dimensional (3D) DE-MRI scanning and biopsy of the LA wall. Control patient without atrial fibrillation shown in the left (Aa–Ac), AF patient with moderate amount of SRM in the middle (Ba–Bc), and AF patient with advanced SRM in the right (Ca–Cc) panels. Three-dimensional DE-MRI renderings show fibrosis/SRM in green with normal tissue in blue (top). Masson trichrome stains collagen blue and LA myocytes red (middle, standard staining; bottom, subtraction images). Red box shows biopsy location. *Source:* McGann et al., 2014 [7]. Reproduced with permission of Lippincott Williams & Wilkins.

odd ratio of 4.6 and 2.6, respectively [18]. Hence, data from DE-MRI helps clinicians in better risk stratification of AF patients.

LA fibrosis and AF management: Utah classification and management algorithm

Catheter ablation of AF is a standard of care for symptomatic patients, especially with those who failed antiarrhythmic drug therapy [16]. The success of ablation depends on patient characteristics and RFA strategies [19,20]. Prior to novel DE-MRI protocol, study demonstrated that the extent of low voltage on LA voltage mapping associated with a lower success

rate of AF ablation with pulmonary vein antrum isolation [21]. Prior work at our institution by Oakes et al. demonstrated a strong correlation between regions of enhancement on DE-MRI and low-voltage regions on electroanatomic maps and quantitative analysis of this relationship demonstrated a positive correlation of $R^2 = 0.61$ [4]. Later studies from our institution have shown that LA fibrosis from DE-MRI is a strong independent predictor of arrhythmia recurrence after RFA [6,7]. The Delayed-Enhancement MRI Determinant of Catheter Ablation of Atrial Fibrillation (DECAAF) study is a recently published, multicenter cohort study to evaluate the clinical utility of LA fibrosis from DE-MRI [8]. This DECAAF study demonstrated that for every 1% increases in atrial fibrosis, the hazard ratio of recurrence during one year was 1.06 (95% CI, 1.03–1.08; $P < 0.001$). When patients were divided into four groups based on the amount of LA fibrosis (group I, less than 10% of the atrial wall; group II, 10% or greater but less than20%; group III, 20% or greater but less than 30%; and group IV, 30% or greater), unadjusted cumulative incidence of arrhythmia recurrence for group I–IV were 15.3% (95% CI, 7.6%–29.6%), 35.8% (95% CI, 26.2%–47.6%), 45.9% (95% CI, 35.6%–57.5%), and 69.4% (95% CI, 48.6%–87.7%), respectively (Figure 3).

The ability to quantify the amount of LA fibrosis has allowed us to establish a direct correlation between the degree of LA fibrosis and the success of AF management. We have established a clinical staging system composed of four stages based on the amount of preablation delayed enhancement (fibrosis) as a percentage of the volume of the left atrial (LA) wall. This clinical staging system includes four stages that are Utah stage I (<10%), Utah stage II (10–20%), Utah stage III (20–30%), and Utah stage IV (>30%) (Figure 4).

Those patients with minimal preablation fibrosis (Utah stage I) did well with conventional pulmonary vein isolation [6]. In Utah stage 2, the number of pulmonary vein (PV) encircled by scar from ablation was found to be the most beneficial in reducing arrhythmia recurrent. These findings imply that pulmonary vein isolation is an appropriate ablation strategy for Utah stages I and II.

However, for Utah stages III and IV, pulmonary vein isolation alone is associated with a low success rate of ablation [6–8]. In the Utah stage III, the higher percentage of left atrial scar at 3 months postablation was associated with lower recurrence rate. In stage IV, which has highest recurrence rate after catheter ablation, neither LA scar after ablation nor PV encirclement reduced arrhythmia recurrent.

Our reports concur with other publications where PV isolation is not enough in advanced AF. Variable success rates have been reported with targeting areas of complex fractionated electrograms (CFAEs) and dominant frequency, adding linear lesions to PV circumferential isolation, as well as disrupting ganglionated plexi connections to the atrium [22–26].

LA posterior and septal walls play essential roles in harboring and maintaining atrial arrhythmias. Dominant frequency (DF) sites, complex fractionated electrograms (CFAE), ganglionic plexi, and fibrillatory activity tend to localize in posterior LA wall [22,23,26,27].

A study by Hunter et al. also demonstrated that PV ostium, appendage ridge, high posterior wall, and anterior and septal wall are regions inside LA that have high wall stress and the area with high wall stress correlates with low voltage on voltage maps [28]. Based on these findings, our group proposed additional substrate modification with posterior and septal wall debulking for patients and we found that progressive increases in postablation posterior and septal wall scarring did reduce recurrences rates [29].

On the basis of this staging system, we have developed a comprehensive MRI-based AF management algorithm (Figure 5). In Utah stages I and II, PV isolation is an appropriate strategy. Additional lesions in posterior and septal wall may be considered in Utah stage II. For Utah stage III, the most appropriate ablation strategy is PV isolation with posterior/septal

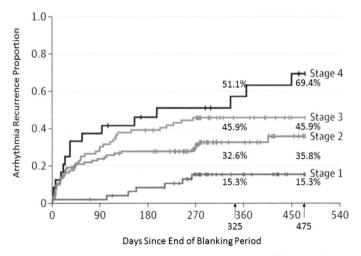

Figure 3 Cumulative incidence of arrhythmia recurrence according to baseline atrial fibrosis. Utah stage I, minimal (<10%); Utah stage II, mild (10%–20%); Utah stage III, moderate (20–30%); Utah stage IV (>30%). *Source:* Marrouche et al., 2014 [8]. Reproduced with permission from the American Medical Association.

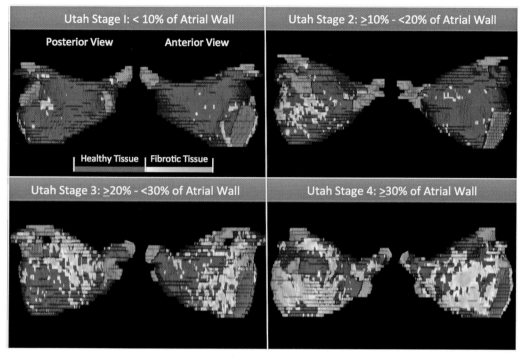

Figure 4 Four stages of left atrial tissue fibrosis based on DE-MRI.

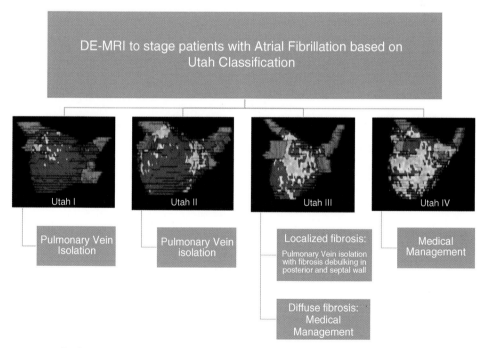

Figure 5 Personalized treatment of atrial fibrillation.

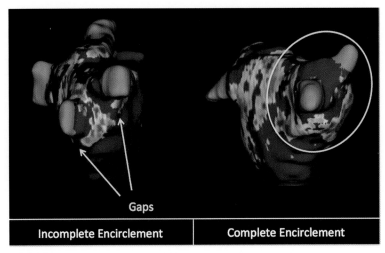

Figure 6 Post ablation DE-MRI evaluation of scarring in the pulmonary vein antral region demonstrating the presence (left panel) and the absence (right panel) of gaps around the right pulmonary veins.

wall and fibrosis debulking. Finally, we advise against catheter ablation in Utah stage IV patients due to high risk of recurrences.

Lesion assessment after ablation

DE-MRI can also be utilized in assessing atrial scarring resulting from radiofrequency ablation (Figure 6) [30,31]. As mentioned previously, patients with minimal fibrosis are likely to respond to PV isolation whereas patients with more advanced fibrosis require additional ablation to generate more atrial scar tissue for a lower recurrence [6]. Postablation DE-MRI is very useful in identifying gaps in the PV antral regions, which can facilitate redo ablation procedures.

Conclusions

Atrial substrates play a very crucial role in initiation and maintaining of AF. At our center, we have developed a novel DE-MRI sequence, which allows us to evaluate structural remodeling and fibrosis inside LA wall. DE-MRI is a very crucial tool not only in identifying atrial fibrosis but also in helping AF management. In addition to benefit regarding catheter ablation, DE-MRI can help us identify patients with higher risk of developing stroke and evaluate LA scar after ablation. Our understanding of atrial substrate and arrhythmia mechanism has been greatly enhanced with this technology. Further study in DE-MRI and its applications will advance the science and knowledge in cardiac electrophysiology and atrial fibrillation.

References

1 Anné W, Willems R, Roskams T, Sergeant P, Herijgers P, Holemans P, Ector H, Heidbüchel H. Matrix metalloproteinases and atrial remodeling in patients with mitral valve disease and atrial fibrillation. Cardiovasc Res. 2005;67(4):655–666.

2 Spach M, Miller WR, Dolber P, Kootsey J, Sommer J, Mosher CJ. The functional role of structural complexities in the propagation of depolarization in the atrium of the dog. Cardiac conduction disturbances due to discontinuities of effective axial resistivity. Circ Res. 1982;50 (2):175–191.

3 Tanaka K, Zlochiver S, Vikstrom KL, Yamazaki M, Moreno J, Klos M, Zaitsev AV, Vaidyanathan R, Auerbach DS, Landas S, Guiraudon G, Jalife J, Berenfeld O, Kalifa J. Spatial distribution of fibrosis governs fibrillation wave dynamics in the posterior left atrium during heart failure. Circ Res. 2007;101(8):839–847.

4 Oakes RS, Badger TJ, Kholmovski EG, Akoum N, Burgon NS, Fish EN, Blauer JJE, Rao SN, DiBella EVR, Segerson NM, Daccarett M, Windfelder J, McGann CJ, Parker D, MacLeod RS, Marrouche NF. Detection and quantification of left atrial structural remodeling with delayed-enhancement magnetic resonance imaging in patients with atrial fibrillation. Circulation 2009;119(13):1758–1767.

5 Vergara GR, Marrouche NF. Tailored Management of atrial fibrillation using a LGE-MRI based model: from the clinic to the electrophysiology laboratory. J Cardiovasc Electrophysiol. 2011;22(4):481–487.

6 Akoum N, Daccarett M, McGann C, Segerson N, Vergara G, Kuppahally S, Badger T, Burgon N, Haslam T, Kholmovski E, Macleod R, Marrouche N. Atrial fibrosis helps select the appropriate patient and strategy in catheter ablation of atrial fibrillation: a DEMRI guided approach. J Cardiovasc Electrophysiol. 2011;22(1):16–22.

7 McGann C, Akoum N, Patel A, Kholmovski E, Revelo P, Damal K, Wilson B, Cates J, Harrison A, Ranjan R, Burgon NS, Greene T, Kim D, Dibella EV, Parker D, Macleod RS, Marrouche NF. Atrial fibrillation ablation outcome is predicted by left atrial remodeling on MRI. Circ Arrhythm Electrophysiol. 2014;7(1):23–30.

8 Marrouche NF, Wilber D, Hindricks G, Jais P, Akoum N, Marchlinski F, Kholmovski E, Burgon N, Hu N, Mont L, Deneke T, Duytschaever M, Neumann T, Mansour M, Mahnkopf C, Herweg B, Daoud E, Wissner E, Bansmann P, Brachmann J. Association of atrial tissue fibrosis identified by delayed enhancement MRI and atrial fibrillation catheter ablation: the DECAAF study. JAMA 2014;311(5):498–506.

9 Spach MS, Boineau JP. Microfibrosis produces electrical load variations due to loss of side-to-side cell connections: a major mechanism of structural heart disease arrhythmias. Pacing Clin Electrophysiol. 1997;20:397–413.

10 Li D, Fareh S, Leung TK, Nattel S. Promotion of atrial fibrillation by heart failure in dogs: atrial remodeling of a different sort. Circulation 1999;100:87–95.

11 Chen MC, Chang JP, Liu WH, Yang CH, Chen YL, Tsai TH, Wang YH, Pan KL. Increased inflammatory cell infiltration in the atrial myocardium of patients with atrial fibrillation. Am J Cardiol. 2008;102:861–865.

12 Platonov PG, Mitrofanova LB, Orshanskaya V, Ho SY. Structural abnormalities in atrial walls are associated with presence and persistency of atrial fibrillation but not with age. J Am Coll Cardiol. 2011;58:2225–2232.

13 Kainuma S, Masai T, Yoshitatsu M, Miyagawa S, Yamauchi T, Takeda K, Morii E, Sawa Y. Advanced left-atrial fibrosis is associated with unsuccessful maze operation for valvular atrial fibrillation. Eur J Cardiothorac Surg. 2011;40:61–69.

14 Mahnkopf C, Badger TJ, Burgon NS, Daccarett M, Haslam TS, Badger CT, McGann CJ, Akoum N, Kholmovski E, Macleod RS, Marrouche NF. Evaluation of the left atrial substrate in patients with lone atrial fibrillation using delayed-enhanced MRI: implications for disease progression and response to catheter ablation. Heart Rhythm. 2010;7(10):1475–1481.

15 Dulli DA, Stanko H, Levine RL. Atrial fibrillation is associated with severe acute ischemic stroke. Neuroepidemiology. 2003;22(2):118–123.

16 January CT, Wann LS, Alpert JS, Calkins H, Cleveland JC Jr, Cigarroa JE, Conti JB, Ellinor PT, Ezekowitz MD, Field ME, Murray KT, Sacco RL, Stevenson WG, Tchou PJ, Tracy CM, Yancy CW. 2014 AHA/ACC/HRS Guideline for the Management of Patients With Atrial Fibrillation: a report of the American College of Cardiology/American Heart Association Task Force on Practice Guidelines and the Heart Rhythm Society. J Am Coll Cardiol. 2014; 64:2246–2280.

17 Daccarett M, Badger TJ, Akoum N, Burgon NS, Mahnkopf C, Vergara G, Kholmovski E, McGann CJ, Parker D, Brachmann J, Macleod RS, Marrouche NF. Association of left atrial fibrosis detected by delayed-enhancement magnetic resonance imaging and the risk of stroke in patients with atrial fibrillation. J Am Coll Cardiol. 2011;57: 831–838.

18 Akoum N, Fernandez G, Wilson B, McGann C, Kholmovski E, Marrouche N. Association of atrial fibrosis quantified using LGE-MRI with atrial appendage thrombus and spontaneous contrast on transesophageal echocardiography in patients with atrial fibrillation. J Cardiovasc Electrophysiol. 2013;24:1104–1109.

19 Wilber DJ, Pappone C, Neuzil P, De Paola A, Marchlinski F, Natale A, Macle L, Daoud EG, Calkins H, Hall B, Reddy V, Augello G, Reynolds MR, Vinekar C, Liu CY, Berry SM, Berry DA. ThermoCool AF Trial Investigators. Comparison of antiarrhythmic drug therapy and radiofrequency catheter ablation in patients with paroxysmal atrial fibrillation: a randomized controlled trial. JAMA. 2010;303(4):333–340.

20 Oral H, Scharf C, Chugh A, Hall B, Cheung P, Good E, Veerareddy S, Pelosi F Jr, Morady F. Catheter ablation for paroxysmal atrial fibrillation: segmental pulmonary vein ostial ablation versus left atrial ablation. Circulation 2003;108(19):2355–2360.

21 Verma A, Wazni OM, Marrouche NF, Martin DO, Kilicaslan F, Minor S, Schweikert RA, Saliba W, Cummings J, Burkhardt JD, Bhargava M, Belden WA, Abdul-Karim A, Natale A. Pre-existent left atrial scarring in patients undergoing pulmonary vein antrum isolation: an independent predictor of procedural failure. J Am Coll Cardiol. 2005;45(2):285–292.

22 Nademanee K, McKenzie J, Kosar E, Schwab M, Sunsaneewitayakul B, Vasavakul T, Khunnawat C, Ngarmukos T. A new approach for catheter ablation of atrial fibrillation: mapping of the electrophysiologic substrate. J Am Coll Cardiol. 2004;43:2044–2053.

23 Sanders P, Berenfeld O, Hocini M, Jäis P, Vaidyanathan R, Hsu L, Garrigue S, Takahashi Y, Rotter M, Sacher F, Scavee C, Ploutz-Snyder R, Jalife J, Haïssaguerre M. Spectral analysis identifies sites of high frequency activity maintaining atrial fibrillation in humans. Circulation 2005;112:789–797.

24 O'Neill M, Jäis P, Takahashi Y, Jonsson A, Sacher F, Hocini M, Sanders P, Rostock T, Rotter M, Pernat A, Clementy J, Haïssaguerre M. The stepwise ablation approach for chornic atrial fibrillation-evidence for accumulative effect. J Interv Card Electrophysiol. 2006;16:153–167.

25 Oral H, Scharf C, Chugh A, Hall B, Cheung P, Good E, Veerareddy S, Pelosi F Jr, Morady F. Catheter ablation for paroxysmal atrial fibrillation: segmental pulmonary vein ostial ablation versus left atrial ablation. Circulation. 2003;108:2355–2360.

26 Lu Z, Scherlag BJ, Lin J, Yu L, Guo J-H, Niu G, Jackman WM, Lazzara R, Jiang H, Po SS. Autonomic mechanism for initiation of rapid firing from atria and pulmonary veins: evidence by ablation of ganglionated plexi. Cardiovasc Res. 2009;84:245–252.

27 Morillo CA, Klein GJ, Jones DL, Guiraudon CM. Chronic rapid atrial pacing. Structural, functional, and electrophysiological characteristics of a new model of sustained atrial fibrillation. Circulation 1995;91:1588–1595.

28 Hunter RJ, Liu Y, Lu Y, Wang W, Schilling RJ. Left atrial wall stress distribution and its relationship to electrophysiologic remodeling in persistent atrial fibrillation. Circ Arrhythm Electrophysiol. 2012; 5(2):351–360.

29 Segerson NM, Daccarett M, Badger TJ, Shabaan A, Akoum N, Fish EN, Rao S, Burgon NS, Adjei-Poku Y, Kholmovski E, Vijayakumar S, DiBella EV, MacLeod RS, Marrouche NF. Magnetic resonance imaging-confirmed ablative debulking of the left atrial posterior wall and septum for treatment of persistent atrial fibrillation: rationale and initial experience. J Cardiovasc Electrophysiol. 2010;21(2):126–132.

30 Peters DC, Wylie JV, Hauser TH, Kissinger KV, Botnar RM, Essebag V, Josephson ME, Manning WJ. Detection of pulmonary vein and left atrial scar after catheter ablation with three-dimensional navigator-gated delayed enhancement MR imaging: initial experience. Radiology. 2007;243(3):690–695.

31 McGann CJ, Kholmovski EG, Oakes RS, Blauer JJ, Daccarett M, Segerson N, Airey KJ, Akoum N, Fish E, Badger TJ, DiBella EV, Parker D, MacLeod RS, Marrouche NF. New magnetic resonance imaging-based method for defining the extent of left atrial wall injury after the ablation of atrial fibrillation. J Am Coll Cardiol. 2008; 52(15):1263–1271.

CHAPTER 11

The utility of noninvasive mapping in persistent atrial fibrillation ablation

Han S. Lim,[1] Stephan Zellerhoff,[1] Nicolas Derval,[1,2] Seigo Yamashita,[1] Darren Hooks,[1] Benjamin Berte,[1] Saagar Mahida,[1] Arnaud Denis,[1,2] Ashok. J. Shah,[1] Frédéric Sacher,[1,2] Mélèze Hocini,[1,2] Pierre Jaïs,[1,2] & Michel Haïssaguerre[1,2]

[1]CHU de Bordeaux, Hopital Cardiologique Haut Leveque, Pessac, France
Université de Bordeaux, IHU LIRYC, Bordeaux, France
[2]INSERM U1045 - L'Institut de Rythmologie et Modeling Cardiaque, Bordeaux, France

Introduction

The elimination of pulmonary vein triggers remains the cornerstone of paroxysmal atrial fibrillation (AF) ablation [1,2]. In persistent AF, however, wider substrate involvement contributes to the sustenance of the arrhythmia. Multiple wavelets, re-entry, and focal sources have been proposed as mechanisms that sustain persistent AF [1,3–6]. Recent evidence suggest that persistent AF may be driven and maintained by localized reentrant and focal sources in the atria [7–11]. Moreover, initial studies targeting these localized sources have yielded promising results [9,10,12].

Atrial fibrillation is a dynamic rhythm. Although significant insights have been gleaned, previous attempts to map these AF-driving sources utilizing single-point catheters, regional invasive multielectrode catheters [11], and surgical plaques [8] have been limited by the inability to map the entire left and right atria simultaneously, contact issues, and

restricted surgical access [13]. Noninvasive mapping facilitates panoramic beat-to-beat mapping of this dynamic rhythm, providing simultaneous mapping of both atria during the arrhythmia to identify potential driving sources [10,12]. This article discusses the utility of noninvasive mapping in persistent AF ablation, including the methodology, the identification of localized AF reentrant and focal drivers, current experience and results, strengths and limitations, and future areas of study.

Methodology of noninvasive mapping

Body surface noninvasive mapping has been validated in numerous cardiac arrhythmias, including focal atrial tachycardias (ATs), macroreentrant ATs, Wolff–Parkinson–White syndrome, ventricular arrhythmias and AF [14–19]. It is based on the principle that the electric potential generated by the heart and its relation to the surrounding torso volume and the body surface follows Laplace's equation [15]. Body surface mapping applies an inverse solution to the forward problem of electrocardiography. Several computational algorithms are applied during this process to suppress potential errors [15].

Practical Guide to Catheter Ablation of Atrial Fibrillation, Second Edition. Edited by Jonathan S. Steinberg, Pierre Jaïs and Hugh Calkins.
© 2016 John Wiley & Sons, Ltd. Published 2016 by John Wiley & Sons, Ltd.

Two main sets of data are required during noninvasive mapping: (1) electrographic potentials recorded from the body surface and (2) geometries of the atria and torso. We use a commercially available noninvasive mapping system (ECVue™, Cardioinsight Technologies Inc., Cleveland, OH). A body vest consisting 252 electrodes is applied to the patient's torso to record surface potentials. The three-dimensional (3D) patient-specific atrial geometry is obtained from noncontrast thoracic computed tomography (CT) scan. The locations of the body surface electrodes on the patient's torso are also acquired during the CT scan. These two sets of data are then combined with the cardiac potentials derived from body surface potentials reconstructed during each beat and projected onto the epicardial shell of the individual patient [10]. Consecutive windows with R–R pauses ≥1000 ms during AF are recorded. The T-Q segments are selected for analysis to avoid QRST interference. In patients with rapid ventricular rates, atrioventricular (AV) conduction is slowed by the administration of diltiazem to create adequate recording windows. For patients presenting AF, mapping can be performed at the bedside before entering the electrophysiological laboratory, thus saving procedural time. For patients presenting sinus rhythm (SR), AF is induced in the electrophysiological laboratory by rapid atrial pacing, and AF drivers are analyzed after a predetermined waiting period (≈30 min in initial studies). During this time, other procedural steps may be undertaken, such as transseptal puncture and creation of the left atrial geometry using an electroanatomical mapping system.

Activation maps and phase maps can both be created for analysis [12,13]. Activation maps are computed by employing the traditional unipolar electrogram intrinsic deflection-based method ($-dV/dT$max). Specific filtering processes are applied to eliminate artifacts in signal morphology and to optimize phase transformation [10,13]. Phase mapping algorithms are utilized to create AF maps, whereby a representation of the depolarization and repolarization wave fronts are computed from the isophase values corresponding, respectively, to $\pi/2$ and $-\pi/2$ [12]. Color-coded movies of wave propagation patterns during AF are then displayed on the individualized 3D biatrial geometry of each patient.

A driver-density map is then created on each individual patient by summating all the drivers recorded in each window onto a cumulative map that is projected on the patient's biatrial geometry. Due to the meandering nature of the observed reentrant drivers, the CT-based biatrial geometry is divided into several anatomical driver domains, such as the (1) left pulmonary veins (PV)/left atrial appendage (LAA), (2) right PV/posterior septum, (3) posterior and inferior left atrium (LA) and the coronary sinus (CS), (4) superior right atrium (RA), (5) inferior RA, (6) anterior LA/roof, and (7) anteroseptal region.

Persistent AF ablation guided by noninvasive mapping

AF drivers revealed by noninvasive mapping

The use of noninvasive mapping and phase mapping techniques has provided new insight into the AF drivers in persistent AF. These drivers may be divided into two categories: (1) reentrant and (2) focal.

Localized AF drivers are classified as reentrant ("rotor") when a wave is observed to fully rotate around a functional core on phase progression. The reentrant drivers are verified by sequential activation of local unipolar electrograms covering the local cycle length around a pivot point. AF drivers are classified as focal when a wave front originates from a focal site with centrifugal activation. This is confirmed by a QS pattern on unipolar electrograms. In some studies, to avoid nonphysiological errors, drivers are classified only when ≥2 repeated events are recorded.

In a recent study by Haissaguerre et al. [12], 103 consecutive patients with persistent AF were mapped noninvasively during electrophysiological study and catheter ablation. A median of four driver regions was identified per patient. Of the observed AF drivers, 80.5% were reentrant and 19.5% were focal. Figure 1 demonstrates a reentrant driver identified by noninvasive mapping, meandering in the inferior LA. Figure 2 demonstrates a focal source arising from the PV, which in turn initiates several reentrant drivers. The median number of continuous rotations was 2.6 [2.3–3.3] for reentrant drivers. An average of six events was observed from a focal site. This short-lasting and periodic nature of reentrant driver activity matches rotor behavior described in optical mapping and animal studies [5,20].

The reentrant drivers were observed to meander in space and vary temporally. However, they would commonly recur at the same or adjacent site. In the entire cohort, reentrant drivers were commonly located in the right PV/septal region, left PV/LAA, left inferior wall/coronary sinus region and superior right atrium; however, this distribution varied amongst individuals. While enabling the operator to deliver a more individualized approach to the ablation of these AF drivers, noninvasive mapping has also revealed a higher proportion of drivers arising from less typical sites, such as the RA. Sixty-nine percent of reentrant driver activity and 71% focal activity were in

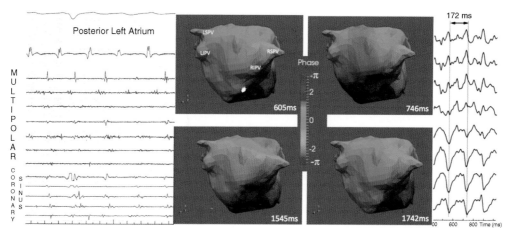

Figure 1 Intracardiac recordings (left) and noninvasive phase maps (middle), and reconstructed electrograms (right) of posterior left atrium during persistent AF. The four snapshots on the right show a rotor meandering in the inferior left atrium at different times. The blue wave indicating depolarizing front makes a full rotation in 170–180 ms. The core of the rotor (white star at the center of rainbow-colored phases of rotor) can be seen meandering in a small region. The phases of wave propagation are color-coded using rainbow scale. The blue color represents depolarizing wave and the green represents the end of repolarization. The wave front can be read by following the blue color. The time (milliseconds) at the bottom of each snapshot represents the moment in the time window when the snapshot was taken. Right: unipolar electrograms along the path of one rotor rotation, prior to any specific signal processing. Note the varying morphology of electrograms recorded within a small area surrounding the core and the presence of potentials covering the entire cycle length (172 ms). LIPV, left inferior PV; LSPV, left superior pulmonary vein; RIPV, right inferior PV; RSPV, right superior PV. *Source:* Haissaguerre et al., 2013 [10]. Reproduced with permission of Wiley.

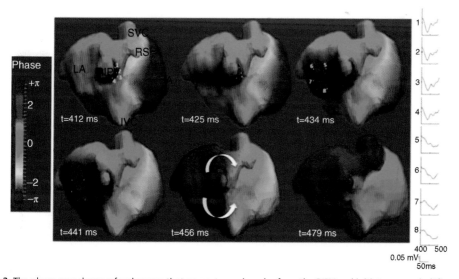

Figure 2 The phase map shows a focal source that emanates an impulse from the RIPV and initiates a couple ("figure of 8") of reentrant drivers. This phenomenon occurs consecutively for five beats (repetitive focal discharge and reentry events), the first of which is shown in the form of snapshots taken at successive time intervals. The blue color represents depolarization. The prephase electrograms taken at the site of focal source (1–4) and at a distance (5–8) show characteristic QS and rS patterns, respectively. The phases of wave propagation are color-coded using a rainbow scale. The deep blue color represents the depolarizing wave. The phase map can be appreciated by following the blue color. The time (ms) at the bottom of each snapshot represents the moment when the snapshot was taken. Abbreviations: SVC, superior vena cava; RA, right atrium; RIPV, right inferior pulmonary vein; RSPV, right superior pulmonary vein; LA, left atrium; IVC, inferior vena cava. *Source:* Haissaguerre et al., 2014 [12]. Reproduced with permission of Lippincott Williams & Wilkins.

the LA, and other driver activity was observed in the RA [12].

Electrogram characteristics of AF driver regions

Noninvasive mapping allows a panoramic overview of AF processes simultaneously in both atria. Due to the meandering and periodic nature of these detected AF drivers, identifying these drivers through conventional invasive catheter mapping methods yields inherent difficulties [13]. Although newer techniques are being developed, traditional point-to-point mapping and regional multielectrode mapping techniques are limited by the dynamicity of these drivers [21–24]. In the study by Haissaguerre et al., bipolar electrogram characteristics of driver versus nondriver regions detected by noninvasive mapping were compared in a smaller subset of patients [12]. Regions harboring reentrant AF drivers more frequently demonstrated prolonged fractionated electrograms, possibly indicative of local tissue heterogeneity anchoring reentry. Furthermore, electrograms recorded on a multispline catheter spanned across a large part of the AF cycle length, which is consistent with recordings of localized reentry. However, no significant differences in mean local cycle length and mean electrogram amplitude were found in the analysis of this initial subset of patients, perhaps due to the dynamic and periodic nature of these drivers. Furthermore, it is important to note that noninvasive and invasive maps were not acquired simultaneously and that synchronous recordings are currently being evaluated.

AF drivers, fractionation, and atrial fibrosis

Recent data indicate that reentrant drivers tend to harbor in the patchy zones and border zones of dense fibrosis detected by atrial magnetic resonance imaging (MRI) [25]. This is in light of the finding that most complex fractionated atrial electrograms (CFAE) sites were found in regions with patchy or no fibrosis, rather than in densely fibrotic regions [25]. However, although increased fractionation may signal proximity to a driver site, fractionation is not found to be a specific indicator [26,27]. Prolonged fractionated electrograms were found in 40% of regions not harboring an AF driver, compared to 62% in regions harboring an AF driver [12]. Furthermore, degree of fractionation may also be influenced by numerous other factors, such as anisotropic and slow conduction, the collision of multiple wave fronts, and contiguous anatomical structures [28].

Ablation strategy for AF drivers

The optimal ablation strategy for AF drivers is still under investigation. In our recent study, a cumulative driver density map was created for each patient following noninvasive mapping [12]. This cumulative summary map of all the drivers was projected onto the patient's CT-based biatrial geometry. This then served as a roadmap for ablation, starting with the region of highest density and progressing in a decreasing order. The median number of targeted driver regions was 4, which increased with longer AF duration. Radiofrequency point-by-point lesions were applied at the area covering the reentrant or focal drivers. Two end points were pursued during ablation: first, the regional end point of local cycle length slowing (see Figure 3); second, the overall procedural end point of AF termination. Importantly, complete elimination of regional electrograms was not desirable in order to avoid a potentially arrythmogenic scar. Pulmonary vein isolation was completed at the end of the procedure during sinus rhythm, if required. Patients were cardioverted into SR if they remained in AF at the end of the procedure. If AF terminated into AT, these ATs were subsequently mapped and ablated to achieve SR [12,29]. Figures 4 to 6 are various case examples of patients with persistent AF who underwent catheter ablation guided by noninvasive mapping.

Clinical outcomes

The above strategy yielded an acute AF termination rate of 80% [12]. Of these cases, about two-thirds (65.9%) terminated into an intermediate atrial tachycardia, while approximately one-third (34.1%) terminated directly into SR. Intermediate ATs were subsequently ablated into SR with this protocol. Twelve-month follow-up was completed in 90 patients, and 16 patients underwent redo procedures. During 12-month follow-up, 64% of patients were in stable SR, 22% in AT, and 20% in AF [12]. Patients who sustained AF termination during the procedure had a higher AF-free outcome during follow-up compared to those who did not [12].

Importantly, compared to the conventional stepwise ablation strategy for persistent AF ablation, the strategy of driver-based ablation guided by noninvasive mapping achieved similar 12-month clinical outcomes, but with half the amount of ablation (28 ± 17 min versus 65 ± 33 min for AF termination) [12]. This represents a significant improvement in our strategy toward persistent AF ablation, by minimizing ablation and therefore minimizing unnecessary damage to the atrial tissue and by avoiding linear ablation, which may be proarrhythmic in itself.

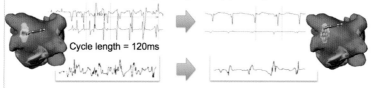

Ablation Method

Driver regions are ablated based on statistical prevalence

A) Increase in local cycle length beyond appendage CL

Cycle length = 120ms

B) Transformation of rapid complex signals into slower simple signals

C) Electrogram abolition is undue/excessive

TISSUE SCAR AFTER ABLATION

Figure 3 Strategy for driver ablation. Driver regions are ablated based on statistical prevalence. The local regional end points are increase in local regional cycle length and transformation of rapid complex signals to slower simple signals.

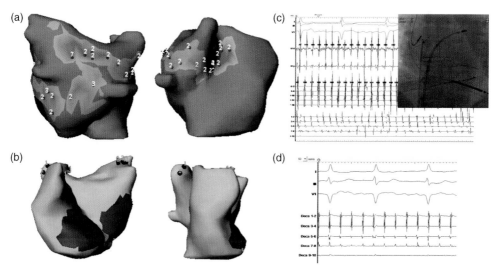

(a)

(b)

(c)

(d)

Figure 4 A 65 year-old gentleman with persistent AF of 7 months duration. (a) Cumulative driver-density maps demonstrating reentrant drivers concentrated around the right PV ostium/septum, posterior LA wall, left PV ostium, and inferior LA (left figure: posteroanterior view of the LA and RA; right figure, right lateral view). (b) Cumulative driver-density map of focal drivers originating from the left and right upper PVs (left figure, anteroposterior view of the LA and RA; right figure, right anterior oblique view). (c) Average baseline AF cycle length was 164 ms in the LA and 165 ms in the RA. Insert: the ablation catheter was positioned at the LA appendage and multispline catheter at the RA appendage. A decapolar catheter was positioned in the coronary sinus. (d) Following ablation of the first three driver regions: right PV/septum, left PV/LA appendage and inferoposterior LA, AF terminated into AT.

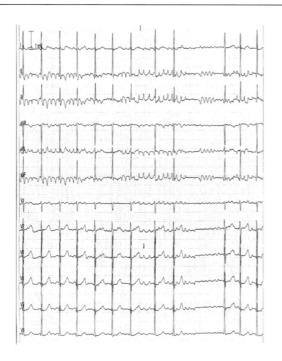

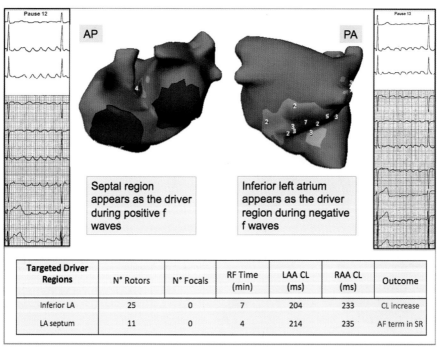

Targeted Driver Regions	N° Rotors	N° Focals	RF Time (min)	LAA CL (ms)	RAA CL (ms)	Outcome
Inferior LA	25	0	7	204	233	CL increase
LA septum	11	0	4	214	235	AF term in SR

Figure 5 (a) A 67 year-old patient with persistent AF of 5 months duration, LA size was 27 cm², baseline AF cycle length was 172 ms. Varying f-wave morphology was observed on the 12-lead surface electrocardiograph. (b) Noninvasive mapping revealed two separate driver regions: (i) reentrant activity was detected at the septal region during f waves of positive morphology (left panel) and (ii) reentrant activity was detected at the inferior LA during f waves of negative morphology (right panel). Ablation of the first driver region (inferior LA) resulted in AF cycle length prolongation. Ablation of the second driver region (septum) resulted in AF termination into sinus rhythm (total radiofrequency ablation time 11 min).

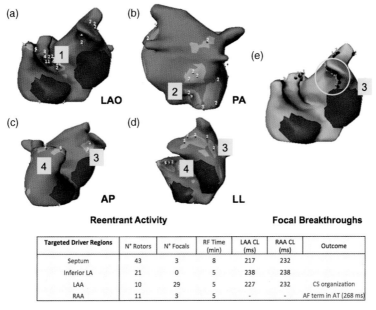

Targeted Driver Regions	N° Rotors	N° Focals	RF Time (min)	LAA CL (ms)	RAA CL (ms)	Outcome
Septum	43	3	8	217	232	
Inferior LA	21	0	5	238	238	
LAA	10	29	5	227	232	CS organization
RAA	11	3	5	-	-	AF term in AT (268 ms)

Figure 6 A 68 year-old patient with persistent AF of 7 months duration. Baseline AF cycle length was 215 ms (patient on amiodarone). Four driver regions were identified by noninvasive mapping. These driver regions were targeted sequentially, starting from the region of the highest density: (1) septum, (2) inferior LA, (3) LA appendage, and (4) RA appendage. (a–d) Demonstrate regions of reentrant activity. (e) Demonstrates sites of focal breakthrough. Ablation of these driver regions resulted in progressive AF cycle length prolongation, culminating in the organization of coronary sinus activity following the third driver region and AF termination into atrial tachycardia following ablation of the fourth driver region.

Noninvasive mapping of AT post-AF ablation

The utility of noninvasive mapping has also been validated in the scenario of post-AF ablation ATs. In a multicenter study of 52 patients with *de novo* and post-AF ablation ATs, noninvasive mapping correctly diagnosed the AT mechanism in 92% of the cases (85% of macroreentrant ATs and 100% of focal ATs) [14]. This technique is particularly useful when the AT is transient and only lasts for a few beats, and can also be applied at the bedside to capture ATs that only surface periodically.

Technical limitations of noninvasive mapping

By increasing the density of body surface electrodes and determining the exact locations of surface electrodes in relation to the individual patient's atrial geometry, spatial resolution is significantly improved from earlier versions. However, current approaches to noninvasive mapping remain bound by several limitations.

First, septal locations and areas with overlapping structures such as the PV/LAA ridge are difficult to image. A previous study estimated the localization

accuracy of noninvasive mapping in the atria at 6 mm [13]. Second, the current resolution of noninvasive mapping is unable to detect small signals less than 0.15 mV. Hence the deciphering of true potentials in scarred areas or areas previously targeted by ablation remains challenging (see Table 1). Third, a

Table 1 Strengths and limitations of noninvasive mapping in AF.

Strengths	Current limitations
Allows the following:	Adequate localization in the following:
1. Panoramic beat-to-beat mapping	
2. Simultaneous mapping of left and right atria	1. Septal locations
3. Mapping of a large atrial surface free from contact issues or surgical access issues	2. Areas with adjacent overlapping structures
4. Mapping close to normal physiological conditions, with minimal or no sedation (e.g., in-hospital or outpatient setting)	3. Scarred areas with diminished potentials

limited amount of radiation is required during the noncontrast CT scan to delineate atrial geometry (<2 mSv). Patients who undergo repeat noninvasive mapping do not require a repeat CT scan, as the previously acquired atrial geometry may be reused. While continuing technological advancement will further decrease the radiation dose, studies investigating the use of other imaging modalities such as MRI or rotational angiography to acquire atrial geometry are ongoing. Fourth, during data transformation to specific phase-based analyses, potential false positives may occur due to the interpolation of incomplete wave curvatures. This is addressed by validating the detected reentrant driver activity with the raw unipolar signals, ensuring a sequential pattern is observed that rotates around a pivot point and covers the local cycle length.

Future areas of investigation

Noninvasive mapping of AF drivers opens new avenues for advancing our understanding of AF pathophysiology and for catheter ablation. Remapping during the ablation procedure will identify dynamic changes occurring during ablation, such as the extinction or emergence of new drivers, allowing for adjustment of the ablation strategy to target new drivers or the use of linear lesions to improve results. The effect of chemical cardioversion in patients who remain in AF following the ablation of driver regions and the administration of antiarrhythmic agents and concurrent noninvasive mapping to identify dominant driver regions are areas worth investigating. Other questions include the role of preablation direct-current cardioversion to aid in reverse remodeling coupled with driver ablation. Noninvasive mapping also has the potential to serve as a risk-stratifying tool for AF, providing a noninvasive assessment of electrical remodeling and AF processes that complements MRI imaging of atrial fibrosis.

Conclusions

Noninvasive mapping allows unprecedented panoramic beat-to-beat mapping of AF and its underlying dynamic processes. This provides an individualized framework to guide catheter ablation of persistent AF. With the ablation of AF drivers guided by noninvasive mapping, the extent of ablation is approximately halved, while acute and long-term outcomes are maintained. Future studies using noninvasive mapping will shed light on the outcome of AF driver ablation with the concurrent use of antiarrhythmic agents and cardioversion.

Acknowledgments

This work was supported by the Agence Nationale de la Recherche (ANR) under grant ANR-10-IAHU-04, ANR Tempo, Leducq Foundation and European Frame Programme 7. Dr Lim is supported by the Neil Hamilton Fairley Early Career Fellowship from the National Health and Medical Research Council of Australia.

Relevant disclosures

Drs. Michel Haissaguerre, Meleze Hocini, and Pierre Jais are stock owners in and Drs. Ashok J. Shah and Remi Dubois are paid consultants to CardioInsight Inc., Cleveland, OH, USA.

References

1 Haissaguerre M, Jais P, Shah DC, Takahashi A, Hocini M, Quiniou G, Garrigue S, Le Mouroux A, Le Metayer P, Clementy J. Spontaneous initiation of atrial fibrillation by ectopic beats originating in the pulmonary veins. N Engl J Med. 1998;339:659–666.

2 Calkins H, Kuck KH, Cappato R, Brugada J, Camm AJ, Chen SA, Crijns HJ, Damiano RJ, Jr. Davies DW, DiMarco J, Edgerton J, Ellenbogen K, Ezekowitz MD, Haines DE, Haissaguerre M, Hindricks G, Iesaka Y, Jackman W, Jalife J, Jais P, Kalman J, Keane D, Kim YH, Kirchhof P, Klein G, Kottkamp H, Kumagai K, Lindsay BD, Mansour M, Marchlinski FE, McCarthy PM, Mont JL, Morady F, Nademanee K, Nakagawa H, Natale A, Nattel S, Packer DL, Pappone C, Prystowsky E, Raviele A, Reddy V, Ruskin JN, Shemin RJ, Tsao HM, Wilber D. Heart Rhythm Society Task Force on Catheter and Surgical Ablation of Atrial F. 2012 HRS/EHRA/ECAS Expert Consensus Statement on Catheter and Surgical Ablation of Atrial Fibrillation: recommendations for patient selection, procedural techniques, patient management and follow-up, definitions, end points, and research trial design: a report of the Heart Rhythm Society (HRS) Task Force on Catheter and Surgical Ablation of Atrial Fibrillation. Developed in partnership with the European Heart Rhythm Association (EHRA), a registered branch of the European Society of Cardiology (ESC) and the European Cardiac Arrhythmia Society (ECAS); and in collaboration with the American College of Cardiology (ACC), American Heart Association (AHA), the Asia Pacific Heart Rhythm Society (APHRS), and the Society of Thoracic Surgeons (STS). Endorsed by the governing bodies of the American College of Cardiology Foundation, the American Heart Association, the European Cardiac Arrhythmia Society, the European Heart Rhythm Association, the Society of Thoracic Surgeons, the Asia Pacific Heart Rhythm Society, and the Heart Rhythm Society. Heart Rhythm. 2012;9:632–696 e21.

3 Moe GK. On the multiple wavelet hypothesis of atrial fibrillation. Arch Int Pharmacodyn Ther. 1962;140: 183–188.

4 Allessie MA, Lammers WJEP, Bonke FIM, Hollen J. Experimental evaluation of Moe's multiple wavelet hypothesis of atrial fibrillation. In: Zipes DP, Jalife J. (eds), Cardiac Arrhtyhmias, New York, NY: Grune & Stratton, Inc, 1985, pp. 265–275.

5 Skanes AC, Mandapati R, Berenfeld O, Davidenko JM, Jalife J. Spatiotemporal periodicity during atrial fibrillation in the isolated sheep heart. Circulation. 1998;98:1236–1248.

6 Sanders P, Berenfeld O, Hocini M, Jais P, Vaidyanathan R, Hsu LF, Garrigue S, Takahashi Y, Rotter M, Sacher F, Scavee C, Ploutz-Snyder R, Jalife J, Haissaguerre M. Spectral analysis identifies sites of high-frequency activity maintaining atrial fibrillation in humans. Circulation. 2005;112:789–797.

7 Schuessler RB, Grayson TM, Bromberg BI, Cox JL, Boineau JP. Cholinergically mediated tachyarrhythmias induced by a single extrastimulus in the isolated canine right atrium. Circ Res. 1992;71:1254–1267.

8 Sahadevan J, Ryu K, Peltz L, Khrestian CM, Stewart RW, Markowitz AH, Waldo AL. Epicardial mapping of chronic atrial fibrillation in patients: preliminary observations. Circulation. 2004;110:3293–3299.

9 Narayan SM, Krummen DE, Shivkumar K, Clopton P, Rappel WJ, Miller JM. Treatment of atrial fibrillation by the ablation of localized sources: CONFIRM (Conventional Ablation for Atrial Fibrillation With or Without Focal Impulse and Rotor Modulation) trial. J Am Coll Cardiol. 2012;60:628–636.

10 Haissaguerre M, Hocini M, Shah AJ, Derval N, Sacher F, Jais P, Dubois R. Noninvasive panoramic mapping of human atrial fibrillation mechanisms: a feasibility report. J Cardiovasc Electrophysiol. 2013;24:711–717.

11 Haissaguerre M, Hocini M, Sanders P, Takahashi Y, Rotter M, Sacher F, Rostock T, Hsu LF, Jonsson A, O'Neill MD, Bordachar P, Reuter S, Roudaut R, Clementy J, Jais P. Localized sources maintaining atrial fibrillation organized by prior ablation. Circulation. 2006;113: 616–625.

12 Haissaguerre M, Hocini M, Denis A, Shah AJ, Komatsu Y, Yamashita S, Daly M, Amraoui S, Zellerhoff S, Picat M, Quotb A, Jesel L, Lim HS, Ploux S, Bordachar P, Attuel G, Meillet V, Ritter P, Derval N, Sacher F, Bernus O, Cochet H, Jais P, Dubois R. Driver domains in persistent atrial fibrillation. Circulation. 2014;130:530–538.

13 Cuculich PS, Wang Y, Lindsay BD, Faddis MN, Schuessler RB, Damiano RJ, Jr. Li L, Rudy Y. Noninvasive characterization of epicardial activation in humans with diverse atrial fibrillation patterns. Circulation. 2010;122: 1364–1372.

14 Shah AJ, Hocini M, Xhaet O, Pascale P, Roten L, Wilton SB, Linton N, Scherr D, Miyazaki S, Jadidi AS, Liu X, Forclaz A, Nault I, Rivard L, Pedersen ME, Derval N, Sacher F, Knecht S, Jais P, Dubois R, Eliautou S, Bokan R, Strom M, Ramanathan C, Cakulev I, Sahadevan J, Lindsay B, Waldo AL, Haissaguerre M. Validation of novel 3-dimensional electrocardiographic mapping of atrial tachycardias by invasive mapping and ablation: a multicenter study. J Am Coll Cardiol. 2013;62:889–897.

15 Rudy Y. Noninvasive electrocardiographic imaging of arrhythmogenic substrates in humans. Circ Res. 2013;112:863–874.

16 Wang Y, Cuculich PS, Woodard PK, Lindsay BD, Rudy Y. Focal atrial tachycardia after pulmonary vein isolation: noninvasive mapping with electrocardiographic imaging (ECGI). Heart Rhythm. 2007;4:1081–1084.

17 Wang Y, Schuessler RB, Damiano RJ, Woodard PK, Rudy Y. Noninvasive electrocardiographic imaging (ECGI) of scar-related atypical atrial flutter. Heart Rhythm. 2007;4:1565–1567.

18 Ghosh S, Rhee EK, Avari JN, Woodard PK, Rudy Y. Cardiac memory in patients with Wolff–Parkinson–White syndrome: noninvasive imaging of activation and repolarization before and after catheter ablation. Circulation. 2008;118:907–915.

19 Wang Y, Li L, Cuculich PS, Rudy Y. Electrocardiographic imaging of ventricular bigeminy in a human subject. Circ Arrhythm Electrophysiol. 2008;1:74–75.

20 Ryu K, Shroff SC, Sahadevan J, Martovitz NL, Khrestian CM, Stambler BS. Mapping of atrial activation during sustained atrial fibrillation in dogs with rapid ventricular pacing induced heart failure: evidence for a role of driver regions. J Cardiovasc Electrophysiol. 2005;16: 1348–1358.

21 Ganesan AN, Kuklik P, Lau DH, Brooks AG, Baumert M, Lim WW, Thanigaimani S, Nayyar S, Mahajan R, Kalman JM, Roberts-Thomson KC, Sanders P. Bipolar electrogram shannon entropy at sites of rotational activation: implications for ablation of atrial fibrillation. Circ Arrhythm Electrophysiol. 2013;6:48–57.

22 Ghoraani B, Dalvi R, Gizurarson S, Das M, Ha A, Suszko A, Krishnan S, Chauhan VS. Localized rotational activation in the left atrium during human atrial fibrillation: relationship to complex fractionated atrial electrograms and low-voltage zones. Heart Rhythm. 2013;10: 1830–1838.

23 Rostock T, Rotter M, Sanders P, Takahashi Y, Jais P, Hocini M, Hsu LF, Sacher F, Clementy J, Haissaguerre M. High-density activation mapping of fractionated electrograms in the atria of patients with paroxysmal atrial fibrillation. Heart Rhythm. 2006;3:27–34.

24 Lim HS, Yamashita S, Cochet H, Haissaguerre M. Delineating atrial scar by electroanatomic voltage mapping versus cardiac magnetic resonance imaging: where to draw the line? J Cardiovasc Electrophysiol. 2014;25: 1053–1056.

25 Jadidi AS, Cochet H, Shah AJ, Kim SJ, Duncan E, Miyazaki S, Sermesant M, Lehrmann H, Lederlin M, Linton N, Forclaz A, Nault I, Rivard L, Wright M, Liu X, Scherr D, Wilton SB, Roten L, Pascale P, Derval N, Sacher F, Knecht S, Keyl C, Hocini M, Montaudon M, Laurent F, Haissaguerre M, Jais P. Inverse relationship between fractionated electrograms and atrial fibrosis in persistent atrial fibrillation: combined magnetic resonance imaging and high-density mapping. J Am Coll Cardiol. 2013;62:802–812.

26 Konings KT, Smeets JL, Penn OC, Wellens HJ, Allessie MA. Configuration of unipolar atrial electrograms during

electrically induced atrial fibrillation in humans. Circulation. 1997;95:1231–1241.

27 Zlochiver S, Yamazaki M, Kalifa J, Berenfeld O. Rotor meandering contributes to irregularity in electrograms during atrial fibrillation. Heart Rhythm. 2008;5:846–854.

28 Lim HS, Haissaguerre M. Focused review: mapping human atrial fibrillation to guide catheter ablation.

Braunwald's heart disease: a textbook of cardiovascular medicine. 9th ed. (digital edition) 2013.

29 Ammar S, Hessling G, Reents T, Paulik M, Fichtner S, Schon P, Dillier R, Kathan S, Jilek C, Kolb C, Haller B, Deisenhofer I. Importance of sinus rhythm as endpoint of persistent atrial fibrillation ablation. J Cardiovasc Electrophysiol. 2013;24:388–395.

CHAPTER 12

Interpretation of circular mapping catheter recordings

Laurent Macle[1] & Jason G. Andrade[1,2]

[1]Electrophysiology Service, Montreal Heart Institute, Montreal, Canada and Department of Medicine, Université de Montréal, Montreal, Canada

[2]Department of Medicine, The University of British Columbia, Vancouver, Canada

Controversy: Differing energy sources – the use of radiofrequency energy
Suneet Mittal

Controversy: Differing energy sources/use of cryo-energy
Pipin Kojodjojo & D. Wyn Davies

Interpretation of circular mapping catheter recordings

The recognition that the majority of episodes of paroxysmal atrial fibrillation (AF) are triggered by ectopic beats arising in the vicinity of pulmonary veins (PVs) has led to the development of percutaneous procedures designed to electrically isolate the PV from the vulnerable substrate in the left atrium (LA) through the application of radiofrequency (RF) (or cryothermal) energy at the LA–PV junction or within the "antral" areas of the LA. Indeed, such is the central etiologic importance of the PVs in the invasive management of AF that the electrical isolation of the PVs is not only a key predictor of procedural success but also a cornerstone of all AF ablation procedures [1]. Unfortunately, distinguishing PV potentials (PVPs) from extrapulmonary vein electrograms (EGMs), or far-field signals, is not always straightforward. The purpose of this chapter is to discuss both the anatomic and electrophysiological bases for the interpretation of PV EGMs using a circular mapping catheter (CMC) and the pacing maneuvers relevant to PV isolation (PVI) procedures.

Role of the pulmonary veins

In the late 1990s, the pioneering work of Haissaguerre et al. demonstrated that AF (and in particular paroxysmal AF) was a triggered arrhythmia initiated by rapidly repetitive discharges originating predominantly in the pulmonary veins (PVs) [2]. Subsequent clinical and experimental research has demonstrated that the majority of human PVs (68–96%) contain sleeves of left atrial myocardium extending 13–25 mm beyond the LA–PV junction. These sleeves tend to be thickest in the PV carina and at the venoatrial junction (mean 1.1 mm) and longer in the superior PVs (with the left superior (11 ± 3 mm) being longer than the right (9 ± 3 mm)) [3,4]. While the PVs in patients with AF show only minor histopathological differences, it has

Practical Guide to Catheter Ablation of Atrial Fibrillation, Second Edition. Edited by Jonathan S. Steinberg, Pierre Jaïs and Hugh Calkins.

been demonstrated that the effective and functional refractory periods are much shorter in the PVs of those patients with AF (relative to the LA), whereas the opposite is true for non-AF controls [5]. Anatomically, these unique electrophysiological properties have been related to overlapping venoatrial tissue and complex myocardial fiber geometry. Specifically, the degree of conduction delay and heterogeneity has been related to sudden changes in fiber direction, with greater degrees of fiber rotation being correlated to longer degrees of the conduction delay. As a result, this nonuniform anisotropy and slowed conduction was proposed as the underlying mechanism for the initiation and maintenance of localized reentry. Enhanced automaticity and triggered activity has also been proposed as the etiologic cause of spontaneous PV ectopy.

Circular mapping catheters

The end point of electrical PV isolation is facilitated by the use of circular mapping catheters (CMC). CMCs can be divided into fixed and variable diameter catheters, and can contain 10 (decapolar) or 20 poles (icosapolar). Icosapolar catheters offer the advantage of improved differentiation between local PVPs and far-field atrial signals due to the use of 10 pairs of relatively closely coupled electrodes. Catheters with variable diameter offer the advantage of improved contact and stability at the ostium of the PV, as well as the ability to be used in variable PV sizes. However, when used in relatively smaller diameter PVs, there is a possibility of electrode overlap causing signal artifact. Irrespective of the catheter used, the standard nomenclature is to identify the distal electrode as 1, with increasing electrode numbers as the electrodes come more proximal (toward the CMC shaft). For fixed diameter decapolar circular catheters, mapping is usually performed with the shaft at the superior aspect of the vein. In this position, in the right-sided PVs, electrodes 1–5 are posterior and electrodes 6–10 are anterior. The opposite is true for the left-sided PVs. For variable-diameter CMCs, mapping is usually performed with the catheter shaft toward the posterior or superior aspect of the PV. The CMC should be positioned as proximal as possible within the venous ostia, without compromising catheter stability. Typically, the ostia and antra of the PVs are identified through a combination of pulmonary venography, 3D electroanatomic mapping, intracardiac echocardiography, as well as tactile catheter feedback, catheter impedance changes, and signal mapping.

PV electrogram interpretation

The interpretation of the complex signals recorded within the PV EGMs is not always straightforward

due to the anatomic proximity of the PVs to other electrically active structures. A typical electrogram sequence recorded with a CMC positioned in the venous ostia includes initial far-field EGM(s) followed by a sharp near-field deflection (PVP). In general, only the PVP itself will display near-field characteristics (sharp upstroke, narrow width, and a high dv/dt) with all other adjacent structures displaying far-field characteristics (lower amplitude, wider width, and lower dv/dt). In addition, PVPs tend to be more extensive or circumferential, whereas far-field signals tend to exist in a noncircumferential distribution. However, a reliance on morphologic criteria alone is insufficient in the differentiation of PVPs from far-field EGMs, which is critical in order to avoid excess unnecessary ablation.

For the right-sided PVs, the differential diagnosis of far-field potentials detected on the CMC include the right atrium (RA)/superior vena cava (SVC), the ipsilateral PV, and the posterior LA. For the left-sided PVs, the differential diagnosis includes the LA appendage (LAA), the LA myocardium, the ipsilateral PV, the vein of Marshall, and the left ventricle. With careful observation, anatomical understanding, and the performance of specific maneuvers, the PVPs can be differentiated from non-PV far-field signals (Figure 1).

The simplest maneuver to differentiate PV EGMs from far-field potentials is an interrogation of the PV activation sequence in sinus rhythm. As the PVs are an electrical dead-end, when traced from the venous ostium distally within the PV, the PVPs exhibit progressive temporal delay (proximal-to-distal activation) without losing their near-field characteristics. Comparatively, the non-PV potentials progressively reduce in amplitude (or disappear) without changing their timing as they are traced distally within the vein.

Pacing maneuvers

Pacing maneuvers are useful in the interpretation of PV EGMs when mapping is performed during sinus rhythm (Table 1). In general, they function by exploiting the unique anatomic and physiological characteristics of the LA–PV junction in order to separate the near-field PV EGMs from the far-field potentials (i.e. increase the conduction delay into the PV). In effect, these maneuvers take advantage of three complimentary observations: (1) the venous–atrial junction contains decremental conduction properties, (2) PV electrical activation can be altered based on wave front activation, and (3) pacing at a given site will result in the earlier occurrence of the EGM arising from that site.

Decremental pacing
Given the observation that decremental conduction properties frequently exist at the pulmonary venous–atrial

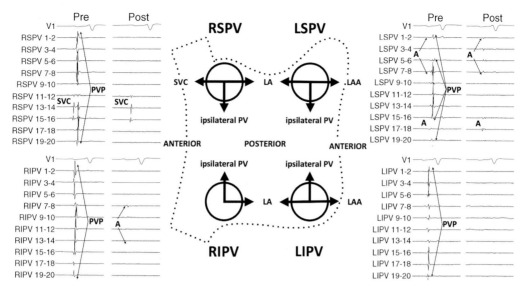

Figure 1 Shown are pulmonary vein recordings during sinus rhythm from the four standard PV ostia (pre- and post-PV isolation) along with a diagrammatic representation of potential far-field electrogram sources. A, atrial far-field signal; LA, left atrium; PVP, PV potential; LAA, left atrial appendage; LIPV, left inferior PV; LSPV, left superior PV; RSPV, right superior PV; RIPV, right inferior PV; SVC, superior vena cava.

junction, one simple maneuver to help elucidate true PVPs is to pace the atrium at an increasingly faster rate, or with a closely coupled extrastimulus. Specifically, if a potential is noted to occur progressively later than the far-field atrial EGM with increasing pacing rates or shorter coupling intervals, then it is likely a PV EGM (Figure 2). However, the usefulness of this pacing maneuver is limited by the observations that (1) not all PV ostia demonstrate decremental properties, (2) decremental conduction may be observed into the LAA with rapid pacing rates, and (3) AF may be induced by rapid pacing. Thus, further pacing maneuvers are almost always required.

Differential (CS) pacing

Differential pacing, with a goal of altering PV activation timing and sequence, has been shown to be extremely useful in the interpretation of PV EGMs. During sinus rhythm (or right atrial pacing), the activation of the left-sided PVs and LAA occurs almost simultaneously. This results in LAA and PV EGM signal overlap on the CMC positioned within the venous ostia. Atrial pacing from the distal coronary sinus (CS) will result in asynchronous LAA–PV activation, with the activation of the LAA occurring earlier. By moving the LAA activation forward, there

Table 1 Prevalence, morphology, distribution, and differentiating characteristics of extrapulmonary far-field electrogram sources.

	Prevalence of far-field EGMs	Far-field source	Distribution of far-field EGMs	Distinguishing pacing maneuver	Recognition in AF (compare PV with)
RSPV	~25%	SVC	Anterior–superior	Sinus rhythm or SVC pacing	Posterior SVC
		Adjacent LA	Posterior aspect	Perivenous pacing	Posterior LA
RIPV	rare	Adjacent LA	Posterior aspect	Perivenous pacing	Posterior LA/RA
LSPV	~100%	LAA	Anterior aspect	Distal CS or LAA pacing	LAA activation
		Adjacent LA	Posterior aspect	Perivenous pacing	Posterior LA
		Ipsilateral PV	Inferior aspect	Ipsilateral PV pacing	Superior LIPV
LIPV	~75%	LAA	Anterior aspect	Distal CS or LAA pacing	LAA activation
		Adjacent LA	Posterior aspect	Perivenous pacing	Posterior LA
		Ipsilateral PV	Superior aspect	Ipsilateral PV pacing	Interior LSPV

Abbreviations; A, atrial far-field; AF, atrial fibrillation; EGM. electrogram; LA, left atrium; LAA, left atrial appendage; PV, pulmonary vein; RSPV, right superior PV; LSPV, left superior PV; RIPV, right inferior PV; LIPV, left inferior PV; RA, right atrium; PVP, PV potential; SVC, superior vena cava.

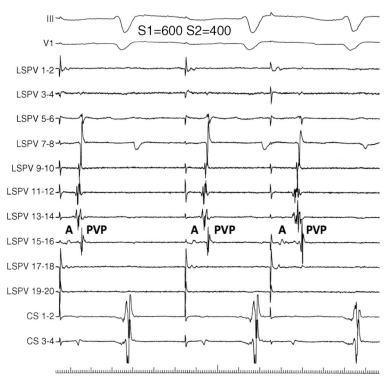

Figure 2 Decremental left atrial pacing. This tracing (100 mm/s) demonstrates the utility of decremental pacing to differentiate far-field left atrial appendage (LAA) electrograms (A) from pulmonary vein potential (PVP) when mapping the left superior PV. Programmed atrial stimulation is performed with a drive train of 600 ms. Following an atrial extrasystole ($S_2 = 400$ ms), the PVP is delayed and a wider separation between the far-field atrial potential and the PVP is observed on the circular mapping catheter positioned in the LSPV ostium (best seen on LSPV 13–14 and 15–16). CS, coronary sinus.

is an increase in the relative separation between the LAA and the local PV EGMs. While decremental conduction due to differential myocardial fiber orientation/activation has been proposed as an explanation for the observed PV conduction delay, it is most often simply due to an altered wave front activation of the PVs and a neighboring far-field source (Figure 3).

Site-specific pacing

Another pacing maneuver, which is complementary to those outlined above, is the use of site-specific pacing. This maneuver is usually performed with the ablation catheter, and unlike differential pacing cannot be performed during RF delivery. While conceptually similar to differential pacing, the idea behind site-specific pacing is that pacing directly at the proposed far-field source (i.e. LAA) will result in the local EGM being drawn in toward the pacing artifact (or even merge with the saturation artifact related to the pacing spike). In doing so the PV EGM is revealed, as the PVP timing will remain relatively unchanged on the CMC, or be further delayed as a result of the decremental conduction properties present at the LA–

PV junction (Figures 3c and 4). Common sites of pacing include (1) the LAA, (2) the ipsilateral PV, (3) the SVC, and (4) the atrial myocardium. Additionally, pacing can be performed from a bipole of the CMC positioned within the PV. In doing so the local PV EGM will be drawn into the pacing artifact and the far-field non-PV signal will be recorded later. However, when pacing from inside the PV, one should be careful to limit pacing outputs in order to avoid direct capture of the nearby non-PV far-field structure.

Simultaneous or combination pacing

An extension on the above maneuvers is to combine differential pacing with site-specific pacing in order to clearly differentiate the PV EGMs from the specific sources of the far-field signals. Most practically this would consist of combining differential pacing (to increase the separation of the PV EGM from the local far-field) with either perivenous pacing (for local atrial far-field EGM) or LAA pacing. The activation sequences would then be compared in order to identify the various components of the EGMs observed on the CMC placed within the PV (Figure 3).

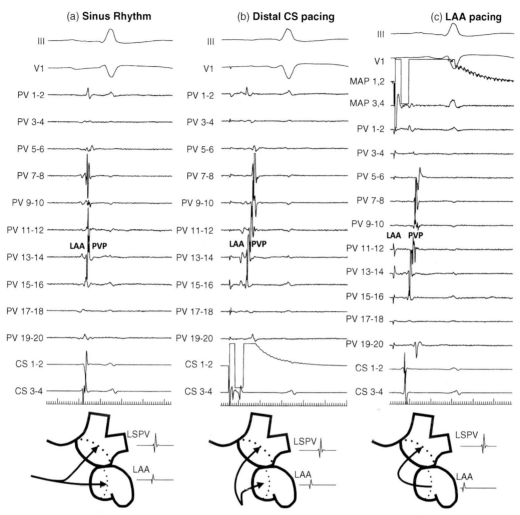

Figure 3 Differential pacing. This tracing (100 mm/s) illustrates the utility of differential pacing for the evaluation of PV electrograms (EGMs) recorded on a 20-pole circular mapping catheter positioned in the left superior PV. (a) In sinus rhythm, it is difficult to distinguish between pulmonary vein potentials and far-field LAA because they are activated synchronously. (b) During distal coronary sinus pacing, the activation of the LAA and LSPV becomes asynchronous resulting in the separation of the EGM recorded on the circular catheter. The first component (recorded on the anterior aspect of the circular catheter) represents a far-field deflection originating from the LAA. The second component represents the near-field PVP. (c) During direct LAA pacing using the ablation catheter (MAP 1,2) there is a wider separation between the two components, as the LAA electrogram is drawn into the stimulus artifact and the PVP is relatively delayed.

Pulmonary vein-specific electrogram interpretation

Left superior pulmonary vein

The left superior pulmonary vein (LSPV) is located posterior to the LAA and courses anterior to the plane of the coronary sinus. As such, the anterior aspect of the PV is opposed with the posterior wall of the proximal LAA. In sinus rhythm, a single PV EGM is usually observed at the ostium of the vein due to

simultaneous activation of the pulmonary vein and LAA. With differential pacing, double potentials are near universally observed, the first component of which is usually the posterior aspect of the LAA (which is observed on the anterior bipoles of the CMC) or posterior left atrial wall, followed by activation of the left superior PV (LSPV) myocardium [6]. It is important to note that the delay between the two components depends on the direction of the activating wave front. As the conduction delay is produced by

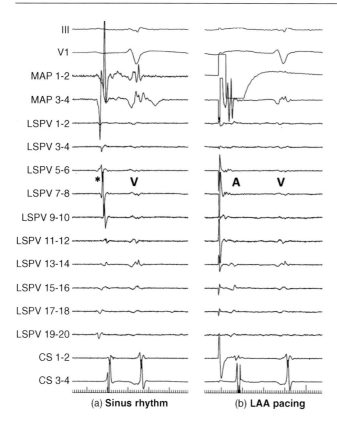

III

V1

MAP 1-2

MAP 3-4

LSPV 1-2

LSPV 3-4

LSPV 5-6

LSPV 7-8

LSPV 9-10

LSPV 11-12

LSPV 13-14

LSPV 15-16

LSPV 17-18

LSPV 19-20

CS 1-2

CS 3-4

(a) Sinus rhythm   (b) LAA pacing

Figure 4 These tracings (100 mm/s) show the utility of site-specific pacing to differentiate local atrial electrograms (EGMs) from pulmonary vein potentials. (a) During a repeat ablation procedure, there is a doubt about the origin of the EGMs recorded on the circular mapping catheter positioned at the ostium of the LSPV. In sinus rhythm, high-frequency EGMs are observed on LSPV 5–6, 7–8, 9–10 (asterisk). Activation timing is near simultaneous to the ablation catheter (MAP) positioned inside the LAA. (b) Demonstrates pacing is performed from the ablation catheter (MAP) in the LAA. The high-frequency EGMs are advanced by LAA pacing (A), immediately following the stimulus artifact and no PVPs are recorded on the circular mapping catheter indicating the vein remains isolated. A ventricular far-field signal (V) simultaneous to the QRS is also observed on the circular mapping catheter. CS: coronary sinus.

the change of activation at the anterior and inferior aspect of the LSPV, the delay between the potentials is maximized by pacing the LAA directly. When pacing the LAA directly, the activation of the LAA is anticipated, which then forces the wave front to change direction to activate the LSPV (Figure 3). When pacing progressively more proximal from within the CS (distal to proximal CS), the direction of LAA–LSPV activation is progressively more parallel, resulting in simultaneous LAA and LSPV activation and thus narrowing the interval between the two EGMs.

Left inferior pulmonary vein

The ostium of the left inferior pulmonary vein (LIPV) is located slightly anterior to that of the LSPV and lies posterior to the posteroinferior portion of the proximal LAA. In addition, the inferior wall of the LSPV and superior wall of the LIPV remain apposed for a short distance (3–5 mm) before the LIPV courses posterior and inferior. In sinus rhythm, a single PV EGM is usually observed due to simultaneous activation of the pulmonary vein and LAA (or low lateral LA). During distal CS, pacing double potentials are frequently observed (~75%), the first component of which is usually the posterior aspect of the LAA (which is observed on the anterior bipoles of the

CMC) or far-field posterior left atrial wall, followed by PVPs. Similar to the LSPV, the site of conduction delay is produced by the change of activation at the anterior and inferior aspect of the LIPV. In the case of the LIPV, the delay between the potentials is maximized by pacing from the low lateral left atrium inferior to the base of the LAA, with activation becoming progressively more simultaneous when pacing moves from the distal to proximal CS.

Right superior pulmonary vein

The right superior pulmonary vein (RSPV) courses posterior to the RA/SVC junction. In sinus rhythm, a single PV EGM is usually observed on the circular catheter within the vein, with double potentials spontaneously observed in up to 25% of cases. Most often, the first component is lower in amplitude and represents the SVC or posterior aspect of the right atrium. Thereafter, an intersignal interval of 20–50 ms is observed due to delayed conduction across the interatrial septum via Bachmann's bundle, followed by an abrupt change in activation wave front direction to reach the RSPV. In the case of SVC/RA origin, the first signal will occur within the initial 30 ms of P-wave onset given the proximity to the sinus node [7]. Given this anatomic proximity, pacing maneuvers are usually not helpful in the differentiation of the various components of the EGMs observed on the CMC as there is no pacing position that can further anticipate local activation in sinus rhythm. As such, the predominant method to identify the origin of the signals is to examine the location (far-field signals recorded on the anterior bipoles of the CMC) and the activation timing relative to the P wave during sinus rhythm.

Right inferior pulmonary vein

The right inferior pulmonary vein (RIPV) has the least electrically active neighbors as its more posterior course confers a greater anatomic separation from the adjacent atrial myocardium. As a result, when signals are observed on the CMC, they usually represent local PV EGMs. Rarely may a far-field posterior LA myocardial signal be observed. In these instances, pacing the LA myocardium close to the PV ostia is usually adequate to differentiate the etiology of the observed EGM.

Identifying arrhythmogenic veins

While the contemporary end point of AF ablation procedures is the electrical isolation of all PVs, it is important to identify the culprit arrhythmogenic vein when active during the PVI procedure. This allows the vein to be targeted first, thus facilitating the longest possible postisolation waiting period to observe for spontaneous acute reconnection. In addition, for patients with paroxysmal AF, it allows for AF termination to be achieved early in the case, and thus avoiding the need to pursue PV isolation during sustained AF, which may render the identification of PV EGMs more challenging. Arrhythmogenic veins may consist of isolated PV ectopy (which may be conducted (manifest) or nonconducted (concealed)), or PV "firing" leading to AF initiation (Figures 5 and 6).

PV recordings during ablation

Real-time PV EGM monitoring can help guide circumferential pulmonary vein isolation. For the left-sided PVs, we typically perform ablation during distal CS pacing in order to maximize the separation between the PV EGMs and the far-field potentials originating from the LAA. With progressive circumferential ablation (during sinus rhythm or CS pacing), an increasing conduction delay from the LA to the PV is observed, followed by eventual isolation (Figure 7). As sites of ablation-associated changes in PV activation or PV isolation are often the sites of PV reconnection, it is our practice to tag these locations on the electroanatomic 3D mapping system.

End points of ablation

The contemporary electrophysiological end point for AF ablation procedures is defined as the stable absence of any conduction into the pulmonary veins from the

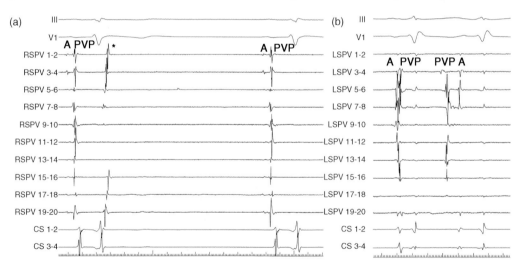

Figure 5 Arrhythmogenic veins. These tracings (100 mm/s) demonstrate examples of pulmonary vein arrhythmogenicity. (a) Demonstrates an example of concealed PV ectopy (first beat) recorded on a circular mapping catheter positioned at the ostium of the right superior PV (RSPV). During sinus rhythm, RA/SVC far-field signals synchronous with the onset of the P wave are observed (A) followed by PVPs. Following the first sinus beat, there is an ectopic beat originating from the PV (asterisk) that is not conducted to the left atrium. (b) Demonstrates an example of manifest PV ectopy. In contrast to the previous panel, the ectopic beat originating from the PV (in this case the LSPV is conducted into the left atrium after a slight delay. Note the reversal in activation sequence with PVP following the atrial signal (A) in sinus rhythm (passive activation of the vein), as during PV ectopy the PVP activity precedes the A. CS: coronary sinus.

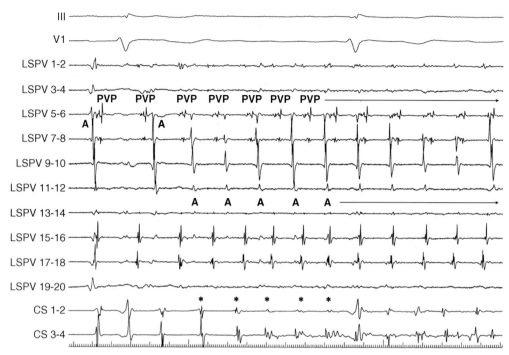

Figure 6 AF initiation. This tracing (100 mm/s) shows an initiation of AF. In sinus rhythm (first beat), an atrial far-field potential (A) is noted to precede local PV activation (PVP) on a circular mapping catheter positioned at the ostium of the LSPV. During the initiation of AF, a reversal of the activation sequence is observed with the PVP preceding the atrial electrogram. During AF, atrial far-field potentials can be distinguished from the PVP and are synchronous with the atrial activation recorded on the CS catheter (asterisks).

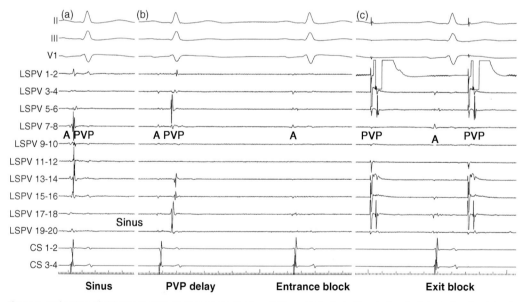

Figure 7 End points of ablation in sinus rhythm. These tracings (100 mm/s) illustrate the electrophysiological end points of pulmonary vein isolation. (a) Baseline recordings in sinus rhythm demonstrate synchronous activation of both the left atrial appendage far-field signals (A) and the PVP as recorded on a circular mapping catheter positioned at the ostium of the LSPV. (b) During radiofrequency delivery along the circumference of the PV, a change in PV activation sequence, with corresponding A-PV delay is observed (first beat). With ongoing ablation, the PVPs disappear indicating the presence of entrance block (PV disconnection). Post-PV isolation, only far-field atrial electrograms (A) are recorded on the circular catheter. (c) Demonstrates PV exit block. During PV pacing from LSPV 1–2, there is no evidence of conduction from the PV to the atrium despite persistent local PV capture (best seen on LSPV 3–4, 5–6, and 13–14 to 19–20). CS: coronary sinus.

left atrium (entrance block), as well as from the pulmonary vein into the left atrium (exit block) [1,8]. As this end point is a key predictor for a procedural success, it is important to clearly and rigorously document the achievement of pulmonary vein isolation.

Entrance block

With contemporary ablation tools, entrance conduction block, the cornerstone of contemporary PVI procedures, can be achieved in almost all cases. Unfortunately, the assessment entrance block is fraught with challenges. Under detection of PV EGMs (or pseudo-entrance block) may be observed with a relatively distal CMC position, poor CMC–PV tissue contact, and partial ablation. Conversely, over detection of neighboring electrically active structures (such as the LAA) may mimic, or mask, PV electrical activity leading to unnecessary ablation at or near the PV ostium. As such, optimal stable ostial CMC positioning and a careful verification of electrical PV isolation (often requiring the use of pacing maneuvers described above) is essential (Figure 7).

Exit block

While the demonstration of entrance conduction block is the standard end point of PV isolation procedures, it is PV exit conduction block (or the "stable absence of any conduction from the PV into the LA") that is the ultimate goal in the prevention of PV-induced atrial fibrillation. Exit block can be demonstrated either through the nonconduction of spontaneous PV discharges or by pacing the PV via the CMC (Figures 7c and 8). In the case of PV pacing, it is imperative to demonstrate local PV capture, otherwise it is impossible to determine whether exit block has been achieved (i.e., avoiding apparent exit block as a result of PV noncapture). In this case, the uneven distribution of PV myocardial sleeves necessitates pacing sequentially from multiple CMC bipoles around the circumference of the PV in order to ensure that all myocardial sleeves are adequately tested. Conversely, in some circumstances the documentation of local PV capture can be challenging due to the obscuring effect of the stimulus artifact on local PV EGMs. In this case, the use of programmed stimulation can take advantage of the decremental PV conduction properties to unmask local PV capture (Figure 9). Finally, it is important to use the minimum pacing output possible in order to avoid inadvertent capture of adjacent far-field structures, which results in misinterpretation of apparent exit conduction. Most often this takes the form of LAA capture during pacing from the anterior bipoles of a CMC positioned within the LSPV, LA capture during pacing from the

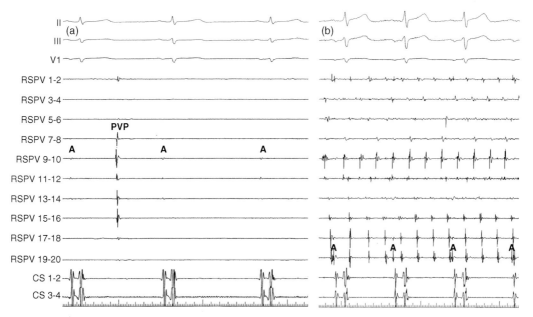

Figure 8 These tracings (100 mm/s) demonstrate examples of spontaneous exit block. (a) Demonstrates evidence of PVP dissociation after isolation of the RSPV by RF ablation. During sinus rhythm, there is a discharge from PV that has no relation to atrial (A) activation. PV dissociation is evidence of the attainment of PV exit block. (b) Demonstrates atrial fibrillation that is confined to the PV. During sinus rhythm (surface ECG), there is persistent focal AF noted in the PV that is dissociated from atrial activity recorded on the CS catheter. Small atrial far-field signals (A) are also noted on the circular mapping catheter.

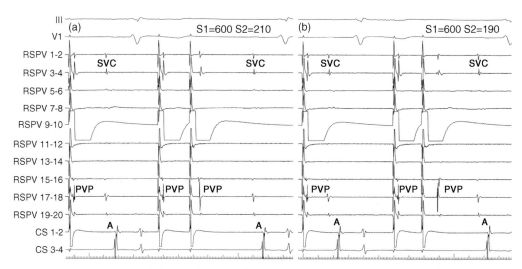

Figure 9 These tracings (100 mm/s) illustrate the utility of decremental pacing to unmask local PVPs and ensure PV capture during pacing maneuvers for the demonstration of exit block. In both tracings, an eight-beat drive train of 600 ms is delivered from the circular mapping catheter positioned within the ostium of the RSPV after isolation. During the drive train (PV pacing from RSPV 9–10), there is no evidence of conduction from the PV to the atrium (A) despite local PV capture. (a) An extrasystole is delivered at a coupling interval of 210 ms resulting in an increased separation between the pacing artifact and the subsequent PV activation. (b) The coupling interval is decreased to 190 ms resulting in an even greater separation between the pacing artifact and the local PV activation. Far-field signals from SVC are also observed on these tracings (synchronous with the p-wave onset on the surface ECG). CS: coronary sinus.

posterior bipoles of the LIPV CMC, and RA/SVC capture during pacing from the anterior bipoles of a CMC positioned within the RSPV.

PVI during sustained AF

The interpretation of circular mapping catheter recordings and the assessment of PVI is more challenging when ablation is performed during sustained AF. In contrast to sinus rhythm, the performance of pacing maneuvers to differentiate local PV EGMs from far-field signals is not possible during sustained AF. As such, the differentiation relieves on a combination of anatomic localization and activation timing. Similar to ablation during sinus rhythm, the timing of adjacent far-field structures should be compared with the EGMs recorded on the CMC positioned within the vein. For the LSPV, the LA far-field signals will be recorded anteriorly on the CMC and simultaneous with the atrial signals recorded on distal CS or on the ablation catheter placed in the LAA. For the LIPV, the EGMs recorded on the CMC should be compared with the atrial signals of the ablation catheter positioned in the low lateral LA. For the RSPV, the EGMs recorded anteriorly from the CMC should be compared with signals from the SVC or posterior LA wall.

The activation pattern of PVPs on the CMC during AF can be organized or disorganized. Once ablation is

commenced along the PV circumference, there will be a progressive organization of the local PV EGMs with eventual slowing (allowing for better differentiation between PV EGMs and far-field signals) and finally isolation (Figure 10) [9]. Once entrance block has occurred, it is possible that local PV ectopy will become manifest. In contrast to procedures performed in sinus rhythm, these dissociated potentials act as a confirmation of entrance block, as spontaneous PV firing can occur only once the PV is no longer inhibited (i.e. overdriven) by the conduction of electrical activity from the LA. Similarly, in the absence of spontaneous PV ectopy, the demonstration of local PV capture during ongoing AF may be used for the assessment of entrance block as the ability to capture the local PV myocardium during ongoing AF is possible only once the PV is no longer inhibited by the conduction of electrical activity from the LA (Figure 11). In all cases, electrical PV isolation must be confirmed after sinus rhythm has been restored.

Conclusions

Electrical isolation of the PVs is a key predictor for a procedural success and, therefore, the cornerstone of AF ablation procedures. The interpretation of PV EGMs is facilitated by the use of circular mapping catheters. It is important to distinguish PV EGMs

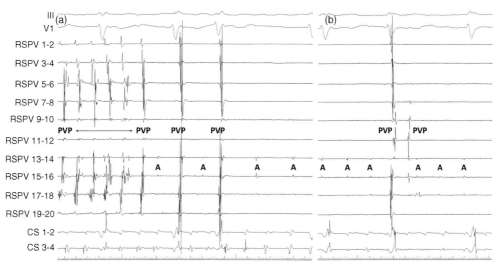

Figure 10 Ablation during AF. These tracings (100 mm/s) demonstrate the end points for pulmonary vein isolation when ablation is performed during AF. (a) Demonstrates PV disconnection during AF. In this tracing, the initial erratic PV activation organizes, is followed by high-degree LA–PV block, and finally PV disconnection. After isolation, only atrial far-field signals (A) are observed on the circular mapping catheter positioned in the RSPV. Of note, during organized PV activation the earliest activity indicates the remaining site of LA–PV connection (RSPV 1–2 and 19–20). (b) Demonstrates spontaneous PV ectopy in the same vein approximately 30 s after the attainment of PV isolation. In contrast to procedures performed in sinus rhythm, dissociated PVPs during AF are a manifestation of entrance (and not exit) block. In other words, they only become manifest once they are no longer inhibited by the ongoing conduction of LA electrical activity into the PV. In all cases, electrical PV isolation must be confirmed after sinus rhythm has been restored. CS: coronary sinus.

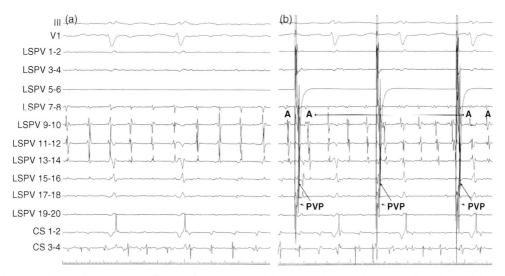

Figure 11 These tracings (100 mm/s) illustrate the assessment of signals recorded on a circular mapping catheter during ongoing AF. (a) After circumferential ablation was completed around the LSPV, there is a doubt about the origin of the remaining signals observed on LSPV 7–8 to 13–14. (b) In order to differentiate local PVP from far-field atrial activation (A), pacing was performed from the circular mapping catheter (LSPV 5–6) resulting in circumferential PV capture (PVP). Since the ability to capture the local PV myocardium during ongoing AF is possible only once entrance block is achieved, the signals observed on LSPV 7–8 to 13–14 represent atrial far-field signals (A). However, electrical PV isolation must be confirmed after sinus rhythm has been restored. CS: coronary sinus.

from extrapulmonary vein EGMs (or far-field signals) for safety and efficacy reasons. While not always straightforward, an understanding of anatomy and EGM timing and the use of pacing maneuvers enables one to solve most of the issues.

References

1 Calkins H, Kuck KH, Cappato R, et al. 2012 HRS/EHRA/ECAS Expert Consensus Statement on Catheter and Surgical Ablation of Atrial Fibrillation: recommendations for patient selection, procedural techniques, patient management and follow-up, definitions, endpoints, and research trial design: a report of the Heart Rhythm Society (HRS) Task Force on Catheter and Surgical Ablation of Atrial Fibrillation. Developed in partnership with the European Heart Rhythm Association (EHRA), a registered branch of the European Society of Cardiology (ESC) and the European Cardiac Arrhythmia Society (ECAS); and in collaboration with the American College of Cardiology (ACC), American Heart Association (AHA), the Asia Pacific Heart Rhythm Society (APHRS), and the Society of Thoracic Surgeons (STS). Endorsed by the governing bodies of the American College of Cardiology Foundation, the American Heart Association, the European Cardiac Arrhythmia Society, the European Heart Rhythm Association, the Society of Thoracic Surgeons, the Asia Pacific Heart Rhythm Society, and the Heart Rhythm Society. Heart Rhythm. 2012;9:632–696 e21.

2 Haissaguerre M, Jais P, Shah DC, et al. Spontaneous initiation of atrial fibrillation by ectopic beats originating in the pulmonary veins. N Engl J Med. 1998;339:659–666.

3 Ho SY, Cabrera JA, Tran VH, Farre J, Anderson RH, Sanchez-Quintana D. Architecture of the pulmonary veins: relevance to radiofrequency ablation. Heart 2001;86: 265–270.

4 Hassink RJ, Aretz HT, Ruskin J, Keane D. Morphology of atrial myocardium in human pulmonary veins: a postmortem analysis in patients with and without atrial fibrillation. J Am Coll Cardiol. 2003;42:1108–1114.

5 Jais P, Hocini M, Macle L, et al. Distinctive electrophysiological properties of pulmonary veins in patients with atrial fibrillation. Circulation 2002;106:2479–2485.

6 Shah D, Haissaguerre M, Jais P, et al. Left atrial appendage activity masquerading as pulmonary vein potentials. Circulation. 2002;105:2821–2825.

7 Shah D, Burri H, Sunthorn H, Gentil-Baron P. Identifying far-field superior vena cava potentials within the right superior pulmonary vein. Heart Rhythm. 2006;3:898–902.

8 Shah D. Electrophysiological evaluation of pulmonary vein isolation. Europace. 2009;11:1423–1433.

9 Macle L, Jais P, Scavee C, et al. Electrophysiologically guided pulmonary vein isolation during sustained atrial fibrillation. J Cardiovasc Electrophysiol. 2003;14:255–260.

Controversy: Differing energy sources – the use of radiofrequency energy

Suneet Mittal

Arrhythmia Institute of the Valley Hospital Health System, Ridgewood, NJ, USA

Case vignette: An overweight 43-year New York City police officer with history of hypertension and obstructive sleep apnea presented for evaluation of a complaint of palpitations and exertional dyspnea. Paroxysmal atrial fibrillation (AF) had been diagnosed 4 years ago; therapy with a β-blocker (Toprol XL 50 mg daily) and type IC antiarrhythmic drug (Rhythmol SR 325 mg twice daily) had been started and was initially successful in controlling symptoms. However, over the past year, AF had evolved into a persistent pattern. An exercise stress test with nuclear perfusion imaging showed compromised exercise tolerance, normal perfusion, and mild left ventricular dysfunction (calculated ejection fraction of 47%). He is referred for catheter ablation for more definitive management of symptomatic, drug refractory, persistent AF. What energy source is best for this patient?

Introduction

Current practice guidelines recommend catheter ablation to maintain sinus rhythm in patients with symptomatic, paroxysmal AF who failed treatment with an antiarrhythmic drug [1]. Based on the observation that triggers that initiate AF usually emanate from within the pulmonary veins (PVs), ablation strategies that target the PVs and/or PV antrum to an end point of PV isolation (PVI) are considered the cornerstone for most AF ablation procedures [2]. However, due to

the high recurrence rate observed in patients with persistent and long-standing persistent AF with PVI alone, additional ablation is typically performed. Common strategies include linear lesions across the left atrial roof and mitral isthmus, ablation of non-PV triggers (e.g., in superior vena cava, crista terminalis, and left atrial appendage), and ablation of complex fractionated atrial electrograms, targeting ganglionated plexi and/or targeting rotors [2]. The optimal techniques for achieving PVI, performing linear left atrial lesion, ablating ganglionated plexi, as well as mapping and ablating non-PV triggers and rotors are described in detail in other chapters in this book. In this chapter, I will attempt to identify the reasons why radiofrequency energy is the best single energy source to use in patients undergoing catheter ablation of AF (Box 1).

Mechanisms of action

During ablation with a standard 4-mm tip, nonirrigated radiofrequency energy catheter, the passage of current through tissue results in resistive heating. However, this type of heating decreases by the distance from the ablation electrode to the fourth power. As a result, the depth and geometry of the ablation lesion is more determined by conductive heating that occurs with continued energy delivery [3]. Currently, catheter ablation of AF is most commonly performed with an

---

Benefits of using a radiofrequency energy ablation catheter for catheter ablation of Atrial Fibrillation (AF)

1 Ability to target all putative mechanisms underlying the initiation and maintenance of AF
2 Proven efficacy
  a Long experience
  b Enormous numbers of patients treated and procedures performed using this technology
3 Ability to integrate with electroanatomic mapping, robotic navigation, and remote magnetic navigation systems

  a Increasing convenience
  b Reducing fluoroscopy
4 Impending ability to routinely assess for contact force
  a Eliminating delivery of lesions at sites with insufficient contact force
  b Minimizing complications

open irrigated ablation catheter. It has been demonstrated that irrigated applications of radiofrequency energy result in larger lesions than nonirrigated catheters. By delaying or eliminating an impedance rise despite boiling at the electrode–endocardial interface, it is possible to achieve higher tissue temperatures and thus deeper and more voluminous ablation lesions [4]. Importantly, irrigation consistently delays or eliminates coagulum on the ablation electrode, which reduces the risk of thromboembolism.

Efficacy

Pooled data from numerous single-center studies had shown that catheter ablation was associated with higher efficacy and a lower complication rate compared to antiarrhythmic drug therapy in patients with AF [5]. This was subsequently confirmed in the context of a randomized clinical trial [6]. In this study, 167 eligible patients with AF were randomized to undergo either catheter ablation ($n = 106$) or a trial of a new class I or III antiarrhythmic drug ($n = 61$). At the end of the 9-month effectiveness evaluation period, 66% of the catheter ablation group and 16% of the antiarrhythmic drug group remained free from protocol-defined treatment failure ($p < 0.001$; hazard ratio 0.30–95% CI: 0.19–0.47). In this study, all patients in the catheter ablation arm underwent PVI; however, an additional 36% underwent ablation of the cavo-tricuspid isthmus, 22% required at least one left atrial linear lesion, 17% had the superior vena cava targeted, and 17% had additional right or left atrial foci targeted. Importantly, no patients suffered a thromboembolic event. Radiofrequency energy is the only energy source suited to targeting all of these discrete arrhythmia mechanisms; the use of open irrigated catheters facilitates ablation while minimizing thromboembolism. The benefit of catheter ablation appears to persist over time. A recent review of outcomes ≥3 years postablation concluded that long-term success could be achieved in nearly 80% of patients, albeit with the need for a mean of 1.5 procedures per patient [7].

Integration with three-dimensional (3D) mapping

Although PVI and additional left atrial ablation can be accomplished using fluoroscopy alone, users of radiofrequency energy can also incorporate 3D mapping with or without integration of preacquired cardiac CT or MRI images of the left atrium. The benefits of this approach include a reduction in fluoroscopy and procedure time and an increase in long-term procedural efficacy [8]. There are two 3D systems available

– CARTO (Biosense Webster, Diamond Bar, CA) and NavX (St Jude Medical, St Pual, MN). Overall procedural times and clinical outcomes are similar with both systems [9].

Integration with remote navigation systems

Remote magnetic navigation (NIOBE^{TM}, Stereotaxis, St. Louis, MO) has been increasingly incorporated into clinical practice over the past decade. Putative benefits include the ability to manipulate the ablation catheter with increased precision, maintain constant contact against the tissue being targeted for ablation, a decreased risk of cardiac perforation, reduced fluoroscopy exposure for the patient and physician, and increased comfort for the operator who can be seated in a control room for the duration of a long procedure. The system consists of two neodymium–iron–boron magnets that generate a magnetic field, which can be manipulated to drive a specially designed ablation catheter (contains three small magnets in its distal tip). The acquired data are interfaced with a commercially available three-dimensional mapping system (CARTO). The ablation catheter is available in a nonirrigated and open irrigated design; however, both deliver only radiofrequency energy. Several studies have demonstrated the feasibility of using remote magnetic navigation to perform AF ablation [10].

An alternative approach for remote navigation is to use electromechanical guidance (Hansen Medical, Mountain View, CA). The Hansen system is a flexible, purely robotic platform, which combines 3D catheter control and anatomic visualization during catheter ablation of AF [11]. The hand motions at the workstation are transferred to the catheter inside the patient's heart. The visualization is achieved using an open irrigated radiofrequency ablation catheter coupled to either the CARTO or the NavX 3D mapping systems. Putative advantages of this system include catheter stability and an ability to monitor contract force using a proprietary IntelliSense Fine Force technology. A prospective, international, multicenter ("Man versus Machine") trial will enroll 258 patients with either paroxysmal or short-duration persistent AF; patients will be randomized to undergo PVI using either a manual or robotic ablation system [12]. An open irrigated ablation catheter and 3D mapping system will be used in all ablation procedures. The primary end point of the study is freedom from an atrial tachyarrhythmia without the use of an antiarrhythmic drug a year following ablation; secondary end points will include procedure time, fluoroscopy time, and the incidence of esophageal injury as assessed by endoscopy performed in all patients within 48 h of ablation. A more detailed description of electroanatomic, robotic, and magnetic navigation systems is available in other chapters in this book.

Future directions

A fundamental goal of left atrial catheter ablation for the management of AF is the ability to achieve durable PVI since failure of AF ablation is almost universally accompanied by recurrence of PV conduction and reisolation of PVs at the time of a repeat procedure results in an important increment in efficacy [13]. This observation suggests that there was insufficient lesion formation during the initial procedure. It is well recognized that tissue contact with the ablation catheter is the critical ingredient to lesion formation and thus conduction block. However, there is a fundamental trade-off that is faced by all operators. If insufficient contact is present, lesions will be smaller and more prone to reversibility; on the other hand, if excessive contact is present, there is greater risk for a steam pop, cardiac perforation, collateral damage, and thrombus formation (Figure 12).

Traditionally, catheter contact has been optimized by catheter manipulation, the use of steerable sheaths,

incorporating real-time imaging (e.g., intracardiac echocardiography), and monitored by a drop in impedance during ablation. More recently, it has been appreciated that the major determinant of lesion size is the electrode–tissue interface contact force (CF); improvements in catheter design have made it possible to measure the CF [14]. The TactiCath (St Jude Medical) is a 7 F, open irrigated, ablation catheter with a sensor integrated at the distal end, which is capable of measuring the CF (amplitude and orientation) between the tip electrode and the tissue (Figure 13). Preclinical studies confirmed that CF is a more important determinant of lesion size that power delivered; in addition, higher CF correlated with a greater likelihood of observing a steam pop or thrombus formation [14]. In clinical studies, a high variability in CF during mapping and ablation has been observed for individual investigators, among investigators, and for different ablation sites; this underscores the importance of routinely measuring CF [15] (Figure 14). This has recently been demonstrated in a small study of patients with paroxysmal AF undergoing PVI [16]. Low CF (< 10 g) was observed in 35% of all applications of radiofrequency energy delivered around the PVs. All patients treated

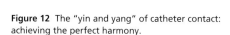

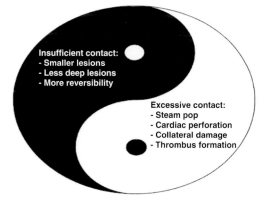

Figure 12 The "yin and yang" of catheter contact: achieving the perfect harmony.

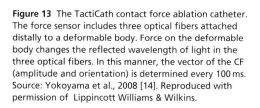

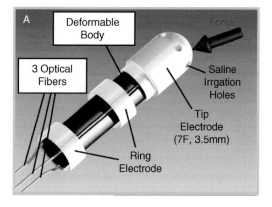

Figure 13 The TactiCath contact force ablation catheter. The force sensor includes three optical fibers attached distally to a deformable body. Force on the deformable body changes the reflected wavelength of light in the three optical fibers. In this manner, the vector of the CF (amplitude and orientation) is determined every 100 ms. Source: Yokoyama et al., 2008 [14]. Reproduced with permission of Lippincott Williams & Wilkins.

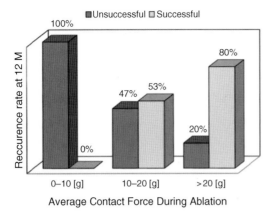

Average Contact Force During Ablation

Figure 14 The relationship between the average contact force during ablation and the 12-month recurrence rate of atrial fibrillation observed in the TOCCATA study. Patients with low CF (<10 g) universally experienced long-term failure from ablation, whereas patients with high CF (>20 g) had a very high likelihood of long-term freedom from AF. Source: Reddy et al., 2012 [16]. Reproduced with permission of Elsevier.

with a CF < 10 g experienced a recurrence of AF during follow-up; in contrast, 80% of patients treated with a CF > 20 g were free of AF.

Similar results have been observed with the ThermoCool® SmartTouch™ (Biosense Webster) CF catheter (Figures 15–17). Microdeformations of a precision spring connecting the tip and shaft of the ablation catheter are translated into a measure of CF; the CF and force orientation of the catheter are visualized directly on the CARTO system. The use of CF reduced ablation and procedure times compared to a standard open irrigated ablation catheter; in addition, total energy delivery was reduced substantially since lesions were not delivered at sites with insufficient surface contact [17]. These data highlight the future importance of routine assessment of CF prior to ablation to ensure the development of durable lesions.

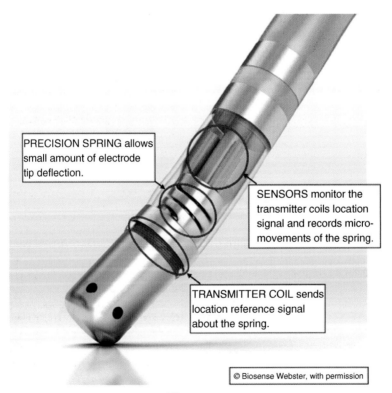

Figure 15 The design of the ThermoCool® SmartTouch™ force-sensing ablation catheter. Source: Martinek et al., 2012 [17]. Reproduced with permission of Wiley.

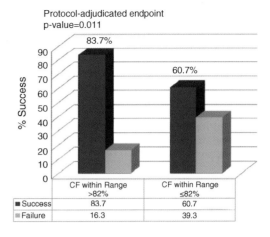

Figure 16 The relationship between contact force and clinical outcomes in the ThermoCool® SmartTouch™ trial. The study followed 172 patients for 1-year following catheter ablation. Patients in whom the CF was within an investigator's desired range >82% of the time had a significantly greater freedom from atrial fibrillation recurrence compared to patients in whom the CF was in range ≤82% of the time (83.7% versus 60.7%; $p = 0.011$). (Data presented as a Late Breaking Clinical Trial at the 2013 Annual Scientific Sessions of the Heart Rhythm Society.)

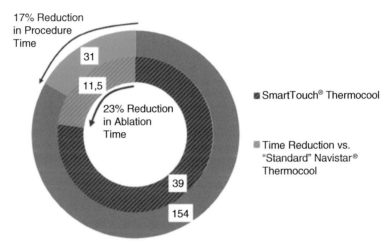

Figure 17 Absolute reduction in ablation (inner circle) and procedure duration (outer circle) in minutes and percentages using the ThermoCool® SmartTouch™ catheter (blue) as compared to a standard ThermoCool® catheter. Source: Martinek et al., 2012 [17]. Reproduced with permission of Wiley.

Case vignette: In our patient, Rhythmol SR was discontinued. The patient was then admitted for initiation of dofetilide; following the second dose he converted to sinus rhythm. The corrected QT interval remained stable during 72 h of in-patient hospitalization with continuous telemetry monitoring. At hospital discharge, the patient was fitted with an auto-triggered loop recorder, which showed continued paroxysms of AF. Three months later, allowing time for reverse atrial remodeling, PVI was also performed using a ThermoCool® open irrigated ablation catheter in conjunction with the CARTO 3 electroanatomic mapping system [18]. A year later, the patient has remained free of AF while off antiarrhythmic drugs.

References

1 Wann LS, Curtis AB, January CT, Ellenbogen KA, Lowe JE, Estes NAM 3rd, Page RL, Ezekowitz MD, Slotwiner DJ, Jackman WM, Stevenson WG, Tracy C.M. On behalf of the 2006 ACC/AHA/ESC Guidelines for the Management of Patients With Atrial Fibrillation Writing Committee. 2011 ACCF/AHA/HRS focused update on the management of patients with atrial fibrillation (updating the 2006 guideline): a report of the American College of Cardiology Foundation/American Heart Association Task Force on Practice Guidelines. J Am Coll Cardiol. 2011;57:223–242.

2 Calkins H, Kuck KH, Cappato R, Brugada J, Camm AJ, Chen SA, Crijns HJG, Damiano RJ, Jr. Davies DW, DiMarco J, Edgerton J, Ellenbogen K, Ezekowitz MD, Haines DE, Haissaguerre M, Hindricks G, Iesaka Y,

Jackman W, Jalife J, Jais P, Kalman J, Keane D, Kim YH, Kirchhof, Klein G, Kottkamp H, Kumagai K, Lindsay BD, Mansour M, Marchlinski FE, McCarthy PM, Mont JL, Morady F, Nademanee K, Nakagawa H, Natale A, Nattel S, Packer DL, Pappone C, Prystowsky E, Raviele A, Reddy V, Ruskin JN, Sheim RJ, Tsao HM, Wilber D. 2012 HRS/EHRA/ECAS Expert Consensus Statement on Catheter and Surgical Ablation of Atrial Fibrillation: Recommendations for Patient Selection, Procedural Techniques, Patient Management and Follow-up, Definitions, Endpoints, and Research Trial Design. Heart Rhythm. 2012;9:632–696.

3 Houmsse M, Daoud EG. Biophysics and clinical utility of irrigated-tip radiofrequency catheter ablation. Expert Rev Med Devices. 2012;9:59–70.

4 Demazumden D, Mirotznik MS, Schwartzmann D. Biophysics of radiofrequency ablation using an irrigated electrode. J Interv Card Electrophysiol. 2001;5:377–389.

5 Calkins H, Reynolds MR, Spector P, Sondhi M, Xu Y, Martin A, Williams CJ, Sledge I. Treatment of atrial fibrillation with antiarrhythmic drugs or radiofrequency ablation: two systematic literature reviews and meta analysis. Circ Arrhythm Electrophysiol. 2009;2:349–361.

6 Wilber DJ, Pappone C, Neuzil P, DePaola A, Marchlinski F, Natale A, Macle L, Daoud EG, Calkins H, Hall B, Reddy V, Augello G, Reynolds MR, Vinekar C, Liu CY, Berry SM, Berry DA, for the ThermoCool AF Trial Investigators. Comparison of antiarrhythmic drug therapy and radiofrequency catheter ablation in patients with paroxysmal atrial fibrillation. A randomized controlled trial. JAMA. 2010;303:333–340.

7 Ganesan AN, Shipp NJ, Brooks AG, Kuklik P, Lau DH, Lim HS, Sullivan T, Roberts-Thomson KC, Sanders P. Long-term outcomes of catheter ablation of atrial fibrillation: a systematic review and meta-analysis. J Am Heart Assoc. 2013; doi: 10.1161/JAHA.112.004549.

8 Della Bella P, Fassini G, Cireddu M, Riva S, Carbucicchio C, Giraldi F, Maccabelli G, Trevisi N, Moltrasio M, Pepi M, Galli CA, Andreini D, Ballerini G, Pontone G. Image integration-guided ablation of atrial fibrillation: a prospective randomized study. J Cardiovasc Electrophysiol. 2009;20:258–265.

9 Finlay MC, Hunter RJ, Baker V, Richmond L, Goromonzi F, Thomas G, Rajappan K, Duncan E, Tayebjee M, Dhinoja M, Sporton S, Earley MJ, Schilling RJ. A randomized comparison of Cartomerge vs. NaxV fusion in the catheter ablation of atrial fibrillation: The CAVERN Trial. J Interv Card Electrophysiol. 2012;33:161–169.

10 Bradfield J, Tung R, Mandapati R, Boyel NG, Shivkumar K. Catheter ablation utilizing remote magnetic navigation: a review of applications and outcomes. PACE. 2012;35:1021–1034.

11 Bai R, Di Biase L, Valderrabano M, Lorgat F, Mlcochova H, Tilz R, Meyerfeldt U, Hranitzky PM, Wazni O, Kanagaratnam P, Doshi RN, Gibson D, Pisapia A, Mohanty P, Saliba W, Ouyang F, Kautzner J, Gallinghouse GJ, Natale A. Worldwide experience with the robotic navigation system in catheter ablation of atrial fibrillation: methodology, efficacy, and safety. J Cardiovasc Electrophysiol. 2012;23:820–826.

12 Rillig A, Schmidt B, Steven D, Meyerfeldt U, Di Biase L, Wissner E, Becker R, Thomas D, Wohlmuth P, Gallinghouse GJ, Scholz E, Jung W, Willems S, Natale A, Ouyang F, Kuck KH, Tilz R. Design of the man and machine trial: a prospective trial international controlled noninferiority trial comparing manual with robotic catheter ablation for treatment of atrial fibrillation. J Cardiovasc Electrophysiol. 2013;24:40–46.

13 Shah AN, Mittal S, Sichrovsky TC, Cotiga D, Arshad A, Maleki K, Pierce WJ, Steinberg JS. Long-term outcome following successful pulmonary vein isolation: patterns and prediction of very late recurrence. J Cardiovasc Electrophysiol. 2008;19:661–667.

14 Yakoyama K, Nakagawa H, Shah DC, Lambert H, Leo G, Aeby N, Ikeda A, Pitha JV, Sharma T, Lazzara R, Jackman WM. Novel contact force sensor incorporated in irrigated radiofrequency ablation catheter predicts lesion size and incidence of steam pop and thrombus. Circ Arrrhythm Electrophysiol. 2008;1:354–362.

15 Kuck KH, Reddy VY, Schmidt B, Natale A, Neuzil P, Saoudi N, Kautzner J, Herrera C, Hindricks G, Jais P, Nakagawa H, Lambert H, Shah DC. A novel radiofrequency ablation catheter using contact force: TOCCATA study. Heart Rhythm. 2012;9:18–23.

16 Reddy VY, Shah D, Kautzner J, Schmidt B, Saoudi N, Herrera C, Jais P, Hindricks G, Peichl P, Yulzari A, Lambert H, Neuzil P, Natale A, Kuck KH. The relationship between contact force and clinical outcome during radiofrequency catheter ablation of atrial fibrillation in the TOCCATA study. Heart Rhythm. 2012;9:1789–1795.

17 Martinek M, Lemes C, Sigmund E, Derndorfer M, Aichinger J, Winter S, Nesser HJ, Purerfellner H. Clinical impact of an open-irrigated radiofrequency catheter with direct force measurement on atrial fibrillation ablation. PACE. 2012;35:1312–1318.

18 Khan A, Mittal S, Kamath GS, Garikipati NV, Marrero D, Steinberg JS. Pulmonary vein isolation alone in patients with persistent atrial fibrillation: an ablation strategy facilitated by antiarrhythmic drug induced reverse remodeling. J Cardiovasc Electrophysiol. 2011;22:142–148.

Controversy: Differing energy sources/use of cryo-energy

Pipin Kojodjojo & D. Wyn Davies
Department of General Medicine, St. Mary's Hospital, London, UK

Introduction

Electrical isolation of pulmonary veins is the cornerstone of atrial fibrillation (AF) ablation procedures. One such procedure is successful in preventing recurrence of paroxysmal AF (PAF) in 60–77% of patients [1,2]. In ablation of persistent AF, pulmonary venous isolation (PVI) is usually the first step in a stepwise approach to terminate AF [3]. In the search for the ideal source of energy for AF ablation, a variety of energy sources such as laser and focused ultrasound have been put into trial with radiofrequency energy being the most commonly used energy source [4]. This chapter details the evolution of cryo-energy as an alternative energy source for AF ablation.

Preclinical studies

Tissue injury to disrupt electrical conduction forms the basis for ablation therapy for arrhythmias. This can be achieved either by thermal heating by energy sources such as radiofrequency energy with conductive heating to deeper tissue layers resulting in denaturation of structural proteins and myocyte death or by freezing to achieve tissue destruction by the formation and dissolution of intracellular and extracellular ice.

Cryoablation and radiofrequency ablation (RFA) affect target tissues differentially. For instance, RFA disrupts tissue integrity and architecture. In an experiment using strips of porcine oesophageal tissue, Evonich, Nori, and Haines demonstrated that RFA delivered with a 8 mm tipped catheter at 20 W for 60 s resulted in a 24% reduction in tensile strength compared to controls, with widespread disruption of elastic tissue architecture microscopically [5]. On the other hand, cryoablation using a 6 mm tipped catheter for 300 s and a target temperature of −80 °C did not significantly affect tensile properties. This is, in part, due to relative resilience of the extracellular matrix to hypothermic injury. Thus, cryoablation could reduce inadvertent myocardial perforation, oesophageal injury, and the risk of atrio-esophageal fistulation. Similarly, cryothermal energy is less likely to cause coronary artery damage when ablating in the coronary sinus within 2 mm of the circumflex artery [6]. Maintenance of tissue integrity without the disruption and contraction of elastic lamina seen post-RFA could minimize the risk of pulmonary venous stenoses (PVS). Histologically, cryothermal lesions are typically well circumscribed, more homogeneous and associated with preservation of endothelial cell integrity [7] (Figure 18). The latter minimized activation of the coagulation cascade, resulting in cryoablation being 60% less thrombogenic than RFA in a canine preparation, with potential implications of lower embolic risk [7,8]. The precise, focused nature of cryoablation lesions may be less arrhythmogenic than the more ragged, patchy RFA lesions.

Importance of the energy delivery platform

Whilst preclinical findings would suggest safety and efficacy benefits of cryoablation over RFA, an important consideration when comparing these two energy sources in the clinical arena is the performance of the energy delivery platform.

The efficacy of cryo-lesions depends on various parameters such as surface area in contact with the myocardium, exposure time, rate of cooling, number of freeze/thaw cycles, and temperatures achieved by the ablation device [9]. In the early stages of development, cryo-energy was applied to the PV ostium initially using 8 mm tipped catheters (Freezor Max, Medtronic) and subsequently, self-expanding circular (Arctic Circler, Medtronic) cryoablation catheters. We also learnt from the early experience with cryo-energy of additional clinical benefits in the form of excellent catheter stability due to adhesiveness once ice had formed on the electrode–endocardial interface and comparative minimal discomfort to patients under conscious sedation. Unfortunately, PVI using these earlier platforms culminated in lengthy procedure times in excess of 6 h and was associated with unsatisfactory clinical outcomes [10–12]. This was largely due to the effects of competitive warming by PV, reducing cold transfer and limiting lesion sizes. This was substantially overcome

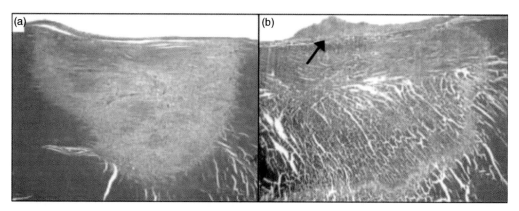

Figure 18 Histology of cryo-energy (a) and radiofrequency lesions (b) stained with Masson's trichome. The cryo-lesion is more homogeneous and well demarcated. In contrast, the radiofrequency lesion is well circumscribed with serrated edges and overlying endocardial thrombus. Source: Khairy et al., 2003 [8]. Reproduced with permission of Lippencott, Williams & Wilkins.

with the development of the cryoballoon to obstruct blood flow from the treated vein, forming a more efficient delivery platform to deliver contiguous lesions around the PV antra.

The cryoballoon (Arctic Front or Arctic Front Advance, Medtronic) is a deflectable 10.5 Fr "balloon within a balloon" catheter utilizing nitrous oxide as the refridgerant in the inner balloon [13]. A central lumen allows for the catheter to be introduced over a standard 0.035″ guidewire into the PV ostia via a 15 Fr deflectable sheath (Flexcath, Medtronic) (Figure 19). This assembly is introduced under fluoroscopy sequentially into each targeted PV. The cryoballoon is inflated in the body of the left atrium before it is advanced over-the-wire into the PV antrum. Fifty percent contrast is injected distally via the central

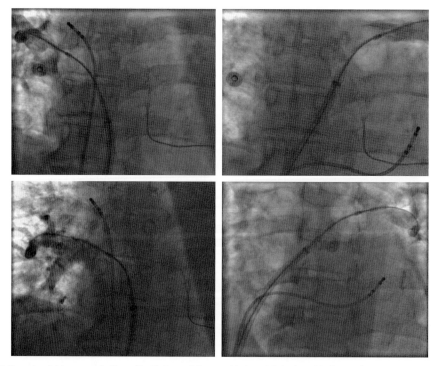

Figure 19 Twenty-eight mm cryoballoon (Arctic Front Advance, Medtronic) deployed in four pulmonary veins in a patient with paroxysmal AF.

lumen of the catheter to confirm a good seal between the balloon and PV antra. Ideally, contrast is completely trapped within the PV indicating perfect balloon to antral contact around the entire circumference of the PV antrum. Once a good seal is achieved, at least two separate 5-min cryoballoon applications are applied to each PV, aiming for a trough temperature of less than −40 °C during each application. A lower trough temperature during cryoballoon application as well as a tighter PV occlusion by the balloon increases the likelihood of achieving PVI. Once cryoablation is commenced, any point of contact between the endocardium and the balloon will be treated, although an optimal zone of cooling exists around the equator of the balloon. The cryoballoon is the only device approved by the European Union and Food and Drug Administration (FDA) for percutaneous cryotherapy for AF. Therefore, the remainder of this chapter will focus on the clinical outcomes and complications of the cryoballoon for AF therapy.

Acute procedural outcomes

The electrophysiological end point during PVI is the presence of entrance block into each PV. In our institution, after each PV antrum has been treated with two 5-min cryoballoon applications, entrance block is confirmed by a separate curvilinear mapping catheter. The cryoballoon is available in two sizes, 23 mm and 28 mm, but the latter is used in virtually all our cases as the larger balloon allows for electrical isolation at a more antral level and is less likely to injure the right phrenic nerve during applications to the right pulmonary veins and traumatize early branching PV [14–16]. Other operators prefer a more tailored approach using a combination of both balloons with sizing based on preprocedural CT and MRI scans. Retrospective analysis suggest routine "oversizing" of the cryoballoon may result in higher AF recurrence rates due to PV–balloon mismatch and more heterogeneous cooling over the larger surface area of the 28 mm cryoballoon [13,17]. Routinely using a 28 mm first-generation cryoballoon and only two 5-min cryo-applications per vein, 83% of targeted PVs can be isolated [16]. Residual gaps can be treated with further balloon applications with cryoballoon of a different size or focal cryoablation using 8 mm tipped cryoablation catheters. Design modifications incorporated into the second-generation cryoballoon (Arctic Front Advance) to distribute refrigerant more homogeneously, allowing for a larger zone of optimal cooling that extends over the entire frontal hemisphere of the balloon, should enhance single-shot PV isolation using the cryoballoon alone,

with fewer applications and shorter cryotherapy times [18]. Procedural times typically average less than 2 h with a mean fluoroscopic time of less than 25 min [16,18]. According to a systematic review of cryoballoon ablation (CBA) for AF, 98.5% of targeted PVs were isolated [19]. In case series of more than 100 patients, acute procedural success rates defined by isolation of all targeted PVs range from 97.06 to 100% [15–17,20–22].

Long-term clinical outcomes

Based on pooled data from 5 studies comprising 519 paroxysmal AF patients, 72.8% were free from recurrent AF at 1 year, largely after a single procedure [19]. In a much smaller data set of 62 persistent AF subjects, a substantially lower 1-year success rate of 45.2% was seen.

Robust direct comparisons between cryoballoon therapy and conventional radiofrequency ablation is limited. In single-center case series using either matched controls or consecutive patients undergoing PVI, freedom from AF recurrence up to 1 year was statistically similar between nonrandomized groups receiving CBA or RFA [16,23,24]. Analysis of data from the German Ablation Registry identified 2256 consecutive PAF patients who have completed 1-year follow-up after their first index ablation [25]. Of these, 604 (26.8%) patients underwent CBA, whereas the remaining 1652 (73.2%) received RFA. AF recurrence rates at 1 year were similar between the groups (45.8% after CBA and 45.4% after RFA). To prospectively examine this issue, the ongoing Fire and Ice Study will randomize 572 patients undergoing paroxysmal AF ablation using either the cryoballoon or conventional irrigated tipped RFA.

The Sustained Treatment for Paroxysmal AF (STOP AF) trial is the only randomized study that compared treatment efficacy of CBA versus antiarrhythmic agents for PAF (20). For this, 245 symptomatic PAF patients refractory to one or more membrane-active antiarrhythmic agents were randomized across 26 American centers in a 2: 1 ratio to receive either CBA or drug therapy. Exclusion criteria included left atrial dimensions exceeding 50 mm, left ventricular ejection fraction of less than 40%, and congestive heart failure with New York Heart Association functional class III or IV. The desired electrophysiological end point was entrance block with additional focal cryoablation delivered at the physician's discretion with a 8 mm tipped catheter if conduction gaps persisted after repeated cryoballoon applications. One repeat cryoablation procedure was permissible during the 3-month blanking period. Isolation of all four PVs was achieved in 97.6% of subjects undergoing ablation. PVI was achieved with

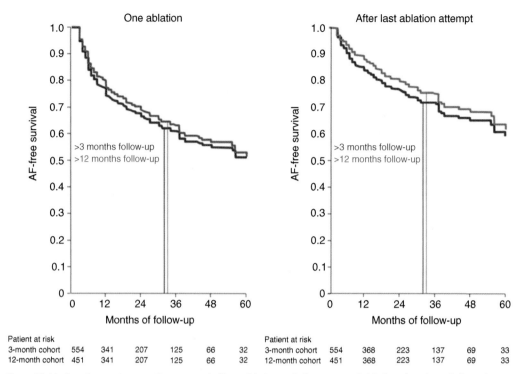

Figure 20 Medium-term outcomes after one cryoballoon ablation and after repeated ablations, in cohorts followed up for >3 months (solid gray lines) and >12 months (gray lines). Source: Vogt et al., 2013 [17]. Reproduced with permission of Elsevier.

the balloon alone in 83%. After 12 months of follow-up, 114 out of 163 (69.9%) of patients treated with the cryoballoon remained free from AF (this includes 8 patients on previously ineffective antiarrhythmic agents and 31 patients who underwent repeated cryoablation during the blanking period) compared to only 6 out of 82 (7.3%) randomized to drug therapy. Arrhythmic symptoms and SF-36 quality of life scores were significantly improved by CBA. Over the course of the study, 79% of drug-treated patients crossed over to receive CBA due to drug treatment failure, subsequently attaining similar clinical outcomes to intent-to-treat ablation patients. This data led to FDA approval for the cryoballoon to be used in the treatment of drug-refractory PAF.

The cryoballoon had received regulatory approval in the European Union in 2005 and hence several large German registries have recently published clinical outcomes of CBA after extended follow-up of up to 5 years. Out of 163 patients who underwent their first PAF ablation using the cryoballoon between 2005 and 2007, 86 (53%) remained free from atrial arrhythmias after 5 years with a single CBA procedure [26] (only 6 required antiarrhythmic therapy). Left atrial dilatation in this cohort, largely free from structural heart disease, was the sole predictor of PAF recurrence. A

separate, larger cohort of 451 patients (95.7% PAF) treated with CBA between 2005 and 2011were prospectively followed up over a median 30 months [17]. Of these, 61.6% patients remained free of AF without the need for repeat procedures after a 3-month blanking period. Allowing for repeated ablations, 74.9% of patients were free from AF. In both series, whilst most AF recurrences occurred within the first 12 months, freedom from AF did not plateau but instead continued with a gradual decline after the first year (Figure 20). Overall, these results are probably better, or at least noninferior, to clinical results of postradiofrequency ablation (Table 2).

Safety of cryoballoon ablation

Preclinical studies implied that cryoablation may be the safer energy source compared to RFA. Does this translate into lesser procedural complications? As mentioned above, there are no direct comparisons between CBA and RFA. By aggregating more than 1300 patients from 22 studies, the incidence of vascular access complications, pericardial effusion, and tamponade were 1.79%, 1.46%, and 0.57%, comparable to post-RFA results [19]. In this systematic review, no cases of atrio-oesophageal fistulation were found

Table 2 Comparison between efficacy and safety end points for cryoballoon ablation and radiofrequency ablation

	Cryoballoon ablation		Radiofrequency ablation		
	Systematic review [19]	High-volume single center [17]	Worldwide survey [4]	Systematic review [32]	High-volume single center [33,34]
Number of subjects	1221	605	6580	2800	1000[b]
Efficacy end points					
Freedom from recurrent AF at 12 months off antiarrhythmics	72.83%	77.6%	74.9%	57%	75.7%
Mean procedural times (min)	206.3	156	NA	NA	156
Mean fluoroscopy times (min)	46.0	25.2	NA	NA	23.7
Safety end points					
Vascular access complications	1.79%	NA	1.47%	1.0%	1.3%
Pericardial effusion	1.46%	0.2%	NA	1.4%	NA
Tamponade	0.57%	0.2%	1.31%	0.8%	1.3%
Symptomatic PV stenosis	0.17%	0%	0.29%	1.6%[a]	0.1%
TIA/stroke	0.32%	0.3%	0.94%	0.5%	0.4%
Phrenic nerve palsy	6.38%	2%	NA	0%	0%
Atrio-esophageal fistulation	0%	0%	0.04%	0%	0.2%

[a] Uncertain what proportion is symptomatic.
[b] Out of 674 patients for efficacy end points.

but there has been at least one such case reported in the literature [27].

Some centers routinely performed noninvasive imaging within the first year after cryoablation to screen for PVS. From such data, the incidence of radiographic PVS after CBA was 0% (none out of 545 patients), but this figure rises to 0.9% (7 out of 773 patients) if results of the STOP AF trial were included. In the latter study, magnetic resonance imaging was performed post-CBA and PVS was uniquely defined by a greater than 75% reduction in cross-sectional area from baseline. Thus, out of 228 patients (including drug therapy patients who crossed over), 10 stenotic PVs were observed in 7 patients, of which only 2 patients were symptomatic. Only one required PV stenting whilst respiratory symptoms resolved spontaneously within 12 months in the other. Overall, the risk of sympomatic PV stenosis is 0.17% (2 out of 1163).

The most common complication of cryoballoon ablation is the development of right phrenic nerve palsy (PNP). From pooled data, the incidence of PNP is 6.38% (86 out of 1349 procedures) [19]. Only 4.73% persisted after the ablation procedure, but only 0.37% (5 out of 1349 procedures) persisted beyond 1 year. Right phrenic nerve is most frequently injured during right upper PV cryoablation and during the use of the smaller 23 mm balloon [15]. Hence, it is essential to pace the phrenic nerve via a deflectable catheter in the superior vena cava when treating the right PV, with immediate cessation of cryoablation with any reduction in the intensity of right hemi-diaphragmatic contractions. In our institution, the incidence of phrenic nerve palsy is reduced to less than 1.6% by routinely only using the 28 mm balloon, limiting cryoballoon applications to two per vein, pacing the right phrenic nerve at a higher frequency of 40 contractions per minute during cryoablation of the right PV and by palpating for a reduction in the strength of diaphragmatic contractions in the right hypochondria, which in our experience heralds the onset of complete right PNP [16]. In the STOP AF trial, 11.2% of procedures were complicated by right PNP, although the higher detection rate is, in part, due to routine inspiration/expiration chest radiographs taken after each ablation. Another factor that may account for the higher PNP and PVS rates in the STOP AF study, apart from the more stringent screening investigations and definitions of complications, could be that many subjects were treated during the initial learning experience with the cryoballoon, with even the most experienced operators in this trial having only performed between 12 and 23 cryoballoon ablations.

Periprocedural stroke occurred in 0.32 % of cryoballoon cases, rates comparable to the radiofrequency ablation experience. Considerable attention has also focused on the appearance of subclinical cerebral microemboli following AF ablation, detected by diffusion-weighted magnetic resonance imaging [28]. Based on results of two prospective observational studies, the choice of technology used for AF ablation strongly

influences the appearance of cerebral microemboli [29,30]. A stepwise increase in proportion of
patients with new cerebral lesions is described, with
cryoballoon carrying the lowest risk (4.3–5.6%), irrigated RFA with intermediate risk (7.4–8.3%), and
finally with more than one-third of patients
(37.5–38.9%) developing new lesions after multielectrode phased RFA with the PV ablation catheter
(PVAC, Medtronic). Whilst 94% of these new lesions
are no longer detectable during follow-up scans and
resolve without scarring, the long-term sequelae of
these asymptomatic cerebral lesions are unknown [31].

Conclusions

To date, more than 35,000 cryoballoon ablation procedures have been performed worldwide. Whilst the
ongoing Fire and Ice Study will provide direct, comparative data for radiofrequency ablation and cryoablation, the growing body of evidence presented
demonstrates that cryo-energy delivered by an efficient platform in the form of a veno-occlusive balloon
is a valid and at least comparative alternative to point-
by-point radiofrequency ablation for therapy of paroxysmal AF. Furthermore, PVI using the cryoballoon
is technically easier and can be accomplished in less
than 2 h. Technical modifications made to the second-
generation cryoballoon will further enhance capability
to isolate all targeted veins using the cryoballoon
alone. Close monitoring of right phrenic nerve function during right-sided cryoablation is essential,
although recovery from right phrenic nerve palsy is
nearly complete in most cases within 12 months.

References

1 Bhargava M, Di Biase L, Mohanty P, Prasad S, Martin
  DO, Williams-Andrews M, et al. Impact of type of atrial
  fibrillation and repeat catheter ablation on long-term
  freedom from atrial fibrillation: results from a multicenter
  study. Heart Rhythm. 2009;6(10):1403–12.
2 Jais P, Hocini M, Sanders P, Hsu LF, Takahashi Y, Rotter
  M, et al. Long-term evaluation of atrial fibrillation ablation guided by noninducibility. Heart Rhythm. 2006;3
  (2):140–5.
3 O'Neill MD, Wright M, Knecht S, Jais P, Hocini M,
  Takahashi Y, et al. Long-term follow-up of persistent
  atrial fibrillation ablation using termination as a procedural endpoint. Eur Heart J. 2009;30(9):1105–1112.
4 Cappato R, Calkins H, Chen SA, Davies W, Iesaka Y,
  Kalman J, et al. Updated worldwide survey on the methods, efficacy, and safety of catheter ablation for human
  atrial fibrillation. Circ Arrhythm Electrophysiol. 2010;3
  (1):32–38.
5 Evonich RF, III Nori DM, Haines DE. A randomized trial
  comparing effects of radiofrequency and cryoablation on

the structural integrity of esophageal tissue. J Interv Card
  Electrophysiol. 2007;19(2):77–83.
6 Aoyama H, Nakagawa H, Pitha JV, Khammar GS,
  Chandrasekaran K, Matsudaira K, et al. Comparison of
  cryothermia and radiofrequency current in safety and
  efficacy of catheter ablation within the canine coronary
  sinus close to the left circumflex coronary artery.
  J Cardiovasc Electrophysiol. 2005;16(11):1218–1226.
7 Sarabanda AV, Bunch TJ, Johnson SB, Mahapatra S,
  Milton MA, Leite LR, et al. Efficacy and safety of circumferential pulmonary vein isolation using a novel cryothermal balloon ablation system. J Am Coll Cardiol.
  2005;46(10):1902–1912.
8 Khairy P, Chauvet P, Lehmann J, Lambert J, Macle L,
  Tanguay JF, et al. Lower incidence of thrombus formation
  with cryoenergy versus radiofrequency catheter ablation.
  Circulation. 2003;107(15):2045–2050.
9 Andrade JG, Khairy P, Dubuc M. Catheter cryoablation:
  biology and clinical uses. Circ Arrhythm Electrophysiol.
  2013;6(1):218–227.
10 Wong T, Markides V, Peters NS, Wright AR, Davies DW.
  Percutaneous isolation of multiple pulmonary veins using
  an expandable circular cryoablation catheter. Pacing Clin
  Electrophysiol. 2004;27(4):551–554.
11 Wong T, Markides V, Peters NS, Davies DW. Percutaneous pulmonary vein cryoablation to treat atrial
  fibrillation. J Interv Card Electrophysiol. 2004;11
  (2):117–126.
12 Tse HF, Reek S, Timmermans C, Lee KL, Geller JC,
  Rodriguez LM, et al. Pulmonary vein isolation using
  transvenous catheter cryoablation for treatment of atrial
  fibrillation without risk of pulmonary vein stenosis. J Am
  Coll Cardiol. 2003;42(4):752–758.
13 Andrade JG, Dubuc M, Guerra PG, Macle L, Mondesert
  B, Rivard L, et al. The biophysics and biomechanics of
  cryoballoon ablation. Pacing Clin Electrophysiol. 2012;35
  (9):1162–1168.
14 Reddy VY, Neuzil P, d'Avila A, Laragy M, Malchano ZJ,
  Kralovec S, et al. Balloon catheter ablation to treat
  paroxysmal atrial fibrillation: what is the level of pulmonary venous isolation? Heart Rhythm. 2008;5(3):353–360.
15 Neumann T, Vogt J, Schumacher B, Dorszewski A,
  Kuniss M, Neuser H, et al. Circumferential pulmonary
  vein isolation with the cryoballoon technique results from
  a prospective 3-center study. J Am Coll Cardiol. 2008;52
  (4):273–278.
16 Kojodjojo P, O'Neill MD, Lim PB, Malcolm-Lawes L,
  Whinnett ZI, Salukhe TV, et al. Pulmonary venous
  isolation by antral ablation with a large cryoballoon for
  treatment of paroxysmal and persistent atrial fibrillation:
  medium-term outcomes and non-randomised comparison with pulmonary venous isolation by radiofrequency
  ablation. Heart. 2010;96(17):1379–1384.
17 Vogt J, Heintze J, Gutleben KJ, Muntean B, Horstkotte D,
  Nolker G. Long-term outcomes after cryoballoon pulmonary vein isolation: results from a prospective study in
  605 patients. J Am Coll Cardiol. 2013;61(16):1707–1712.
18 Furnkranz A, Bordignon S, Schmidt B, Gunawardene M,
  Schulte-Hahn B, Urban V, et al. Improved procedural

efficacy of pulmonary vein isolation using the novel second-generation cryoballoon. J Cardiovasc Electrophysiol. 2013;24(5):492–497.

19 Andrade JG, Khairy P, Guerra PG, Deyell MW, Rivard L, Macle L, et al. Efficacy and safety of cryoballoon ablation for atrial fibrillation: a systematic review of published studies. Heart Rhythm. 2011;8(9):1444–1451.

20 Packer DL, Kowal RC, Wheelan KR, Irwin JM, Champagne J, Guerra PG, et al. Cryoballoon ablation of pulmonary veins for paroxysmal atrial fibrillation: first results of the North American Arctic Front (STOP AF) pivotal trial. J Am Coll Cardiol. 2013;61(16): 1713–1723.

21 Van Belle Y, Janse P, Theuns D, Szili-Torok T, Jordaens L. One year follow-up after cryoballoon isolation of the pulmonary veins in patients with paroxysmal atrial fibrillation. Europace. 2008;10(11):1271–1276.

22 Kuck KH, Furnkranz A. Cryoballoon ablation of atrial fibrillation. J Cardiovasc Electrophysiol. 2010;21 (12):1427–1431.

23 Linhart M, Bellmann B, Mittmann-Braun E, Schrickel JW, Bitzen A, Andrie R, et al. Comparison of cryoballoon and radiofrequency ablation of pulmonary veins in 40 patients with paroxysmal atrial fibrillation: a case–control study. J Cardiovasc Electrophysiol. 2009;20 (12):1343–1348.

24 Tayebjee MH, Hunter RJ, Baker V, Creta A, Duncan E, Sporton S, et al. Pulmonary vein isolation with radiofrequency ablation followed by cryotherapy: a novel strategy to improve clinical outcomes following catheter ablation of paroxysmal atrial fibrillation. Europace. 2011;13(9):1250–1255.

25 Schmidt M, Dorwarth U, Andresen D, Brachmann J, Kuck K, Kuniss M, et al. German Ablation Registry I: one-year outcome in RF versus cryoballoon atrial fibrillation ablation. Heart Rhythm. 2013;10(S5):POO1–115.

26 Neumann T, Wojcik M, Berkowitsch A, Erkapic D, Zaltsberg S, Greiss H, et al. Cryoballoon ablation of paroxysmal atrial fibrillation: 5-year outcome after single procedure and predictors of success. Europace. 2013.

27 Stockigt F, Schrickel JW, Andrie R, Lickfett L.

Atrioesophageal fistula after cryoballoon pulmonary vein isolation. J Cardiovasc Electrophysiol. 2012;23 (11):1254–1257.

28 Gaita F, Caponi D, Pianelli M, Scaglione M, Toso E, Cesarani F, et al. Radiofrequency catheter ablation of atrial fibrillation: a cause of silent thromboembolism? Magnetic resonance imaging assessment of cerebral thromboembolism in patients undergoing ablation of atrial fibrillation. Circulation. 2010;122(17):1667–1673.

29 Herrera SC, Deneke T, Hocini M, Lehrmann H, Shin DI, Miyazaki S, et al. Incidence of asymptomatic intracranial embolic events after pulmonary vein isolation: comparison of different atrial fibrillation ablation technologies in a multicenter study. J Am Coll Cardiol. 2011;58(7):681–688.

30 Gaita F, Leclercq JF, Schumacher B, Scaglione M, Toso E, Halimi F, et al. Incidence of silent cerebral thromboembolic lesions after atrial fibrillation ablation may change according to technology used: comparison of irrigated radiofrequency, multipolar nonirrigated catheter and cryoballoon. J Cardiovasc Electrophysiol. 2011;22(9):961–968.

31 Deneke T, Shin DI, Balta O, Bunz K, Fassbender F, Mugge A, et al. Postablation asymptomatic cerebral lesions: long-term follow-up using magnetic resonance imaging. Heart Rhythm. 2011;8(11):1705–1711.

32 Calkins H, Reynolds MR, Spector P, Sondhi M, Xu Y, Martin A, et al. Treatment of atrial fibrillation with antiarrhythmic drugs or radiofrequency ablation: two systematic literature reviews and meta-analyses. Circ Arrhythm Electrophysiol. 2009;2(4):349–361.

33 Arya A, Hindricks G, Sommer P, Huo Y, Bollmann A, Gaspar T, et al. Long-term results and the predictors of outcome of catheter ablation of atrial fibrillation using steerable sheath catheter navigation after single procedure in 674 patients. Europace. 2010;12(2):173–180.

34 Dagres N, Hindricks G, Kottkamp H, Sommer P, Gaspar T, Bode K, et al. Complications of atrial fibrillation ablation in a high-volume center in 1000 procedures: still cause for concern? J Cardiovasc Electrophysiol. 2009;20(9):1014–1019.

CHAPTER 13

Circumferential ablation with pulmonary vein isolation guided by lasso catheter

Andreas Metzner, Kazuhiro Satomi, Karl-Heinz Kuck, &
Feifan Ouyang
Department of Cardiology, Asklepios Klinik St. Georg, Hamburg, Germany

Controversy: Circumferential versus segmental pulmonary vein isolation/circumferential PVI
Riccardo Proietti, Luigi Di Biase, Pasquale Santangeli, Prasant Mohanty, Conor Barrett, Stephan Danik, Sanghamitra Mohanty, Rong Bai, Chintan Trivedi, John David Burkhardt, & Andrea Natale

Controversy: Circumferential versus segmental pulmonary vein isolation/segmental PVI
Gregory K. Feld

Introduction

Recent studies have demonstrated that myocardium around the pulmonary vein (PV) ostia plays an important role in the initiation and perpetuation of atrial fibrillation (AF) [1]. This important finding has led to the development of segmental PV ostial isolation [2,3], circumferential ablation [4], or isolation around the PVs guided by 3D electroanatomic mapping [5]. Also, substrate modification with the deployment of limited linear ablation (such as roof line, anterior line, and left isthmus line) [6,7] or ablations of areas characterized by complex fractionated electrograms [8,9] have been demonstrated to improve the clinical outcome after PV isolation in patients with persistent or long-standing persistent AF. However, these lesions after circumferential PV isolation are limited with regard to clinical outcome in patients with paroxysmal atrial fibrillation [10,11].

Practical Guide to Catheter Ablation of Atrial Fibrillation,
Second Edition. Edited by Jonathan S. Steinberg, Pierre Jaïs and Hugh Calkins.
© 2016 John Wiley & Sons, Ltd. Published 2016 by John Wiley & Sons, Ltd.

The most established method in the majority of ablation centers is PV isolation aiming for segmental ablation of the ipsilateral PV or wide area circumferential ablation (WACA) around the ipsilateral PVs guided by 3D mapping. In these procedures, the recordings of one or two Lasso catheters positioned within the PV has an important role in identifying electrical connections between the PV and the left atrium (LA). Also, electroanatomical mapping provides more precise information both on the anatomy of the atrial chambers and on the electrical characteristics of the atrial tissue and contributes to shorter fluoroscopic time.

In this chapter, we will describe circumferential ablation technique for PV isolation guided by the Lasso catheter and electroanatomical mapping in patients with paroxysmal or persistent AF.

Complete PV isolation using 3D mapping and Lasso technique

The ablation procedure is routinely performed under deep sedation with boluses of midazolam and fentanyl and a continuous infusion of propofol in our center.

Transesophageal echocardiography is routinely performed prior to the procedure to rule out LA thrombi in all patients. Anticoagulation treatment with warfarin is continued targeting an INR of 2.0–3.0. In case of an INR <2.0 at admission, low molecular weight heparin (LMWH) adapted to individual body weight is applied. Novel oral anticoagulants (NOACs) are stopped the day before ablation and continued the day after ablation. In between, LWMH is given as described. The anticoagulation therapy after ablation is continued for 3 months and eventually continued based on the individual CHA_2DS_2-VASc score.

All procedures consist of the steps described in the next section [5].

Transseptal puncture

Two 8.5 F SL1 sheaths (St Jude Medical, Inc., Minnetonka, MN, USA) are advanced to the LA by a modified Brockenbrough technique using fluoroscopy and pressure monitoring in all patients. One transseptal puncture targets an infero-posterior site of the foramen ovale allowing easy access to the right inferior PV and the antral myocardium near the right inferior PV (Figure 1). After transseptal catheterization, intravenous unfractionated heparin is administered to maintain an activated clotting time ≥300 s. Additionally, continuous infusions of heparinized saline are connected to the transseptal sheaths (flow rate of 10 ml/h) to avoid thrombus formation or air embolism.

LA reconstruction

Electroanatomical mapping and ablation is performed using an irrigated 3.5-mm-tip catheter (ThermoCool Navi-Star or ThermoCool, Biosense-Webster,

Diamond Bar, CA, USA) in sinus rhythm (SR) or AF by using the CARTO™ system (Biosense-Webster, Diamond Bar, CA, USA) or the NavX™ system (St Jude Medical, Inc., Minneapolis, USA). Only the mapping points of the LA surface are collected, all mapping points within the PVs or the left ventricle are deleted to ensure an adequate LA anatomy characterized by a posterior wall that is flat in the right lateral and left lateral views (Figures 2–4).

Selective PV angiography and identification of PV ostium

After LA reconstruction, each PV ostium is individually identified by selective venography using a 7-F multipurpose catheter and carefully tagged on the electroanatomical map. (Figures 5 and 6) We arbitrarily defined any point with clear PV–LA inflection and marked the opposite points with perpendicularity to the PV on the RAO 30° or LAO 40° (Figures 2 and 3). This step is essential for successful PV isolation. In our experience, the misunderstanding of the PV ostium may sometimes make the ablation and thus the isolation of the PVs more difficult or bears a potential risk for PV stenosis. For example, the isolation of the left-sided PVs in the setting of a narrow ridge between the left atrial appendage and the left PVs can be very difficult if the anterior edge of the left PV ostia is inappropriately marked in the left atrial appendage. On the other hand, severe PV stenosis can be produced if the PV ostium is tagged and consequently ablated inside the PVs [12].

Single and double Lasso technique

Before 2005, one 15 mm or 20 mm decapolar Lasso catheter (Biosense-Webster, Inc.) was commonly

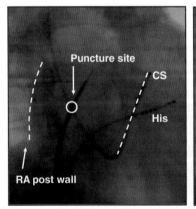
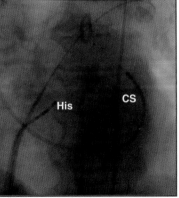

Figure 1 The right and left images show, respectively, fluoroscopic right and left anterior oblique views (LAO and RAO) during transseptal puncture. One puncture is always performed at the inferoposterior site of the foramen ovale for easy access to the right inferior vein and the atrial myocardium. CS, coronary sinus; His, His bundle; RAO, right oblique view; LAO, left oblique view.

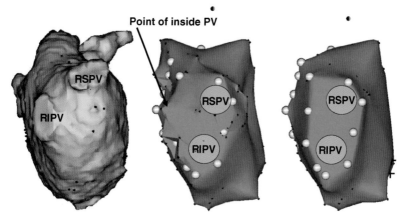

Figure 2 The left image shows a right lateral MR view of the left atrium (LA). The middle and right images show, respectively, electroanatomical maps of the LA in the right lateral view before and after correction of the map in the same patient. The pulmonary vein (PV) ostia (identified by angiography) were tagged by white dots. Note that (1) in the MR imaging view the ostium of right superior pulmonary vein (RSPV) is more anterior than the ostium of the right inferior pulmonary vein (RIPV); (2) in the original map (middle image) the LA posterior wall is not flat due to many mapped points within the right- and left-sided PVs, whereas in the corrected map in the right image, the LA posterior wall is very flat after the deletion of the points within the PVs on both sides; and (3) the anterior wall is prominent due to points obtained with excessive pressure on the LA anterior wall in the original map in the middle image, whereas the anterior wall is smooth after the deletion of these points in the corrected map in the right image. RSPV, right superior pulmonary vein; RIPV, right inferior pulmonary vein.

placed within the ipsilateral superior PV or within the common trunk or a branch of a common PV before radiofrequency (RF) delivery (Figures 7 and 8). The Lasso catheter should be placed in a stable ostial position to obtain a good signal during the procedure. If the Lasso catheter is placed too distally, the PV potential might be too small or even unrecordable especially in patients with a damaged atrium. If the Lasso catheter is located in the LA outside of the PV, it could result in misunderstanding of the LA and PV signal. In addition to the exact identification and tagging of the respective PV ostium on the CARTO map, keeping in mind the Lasso catheter position and the location of its electrodes enables one to perform

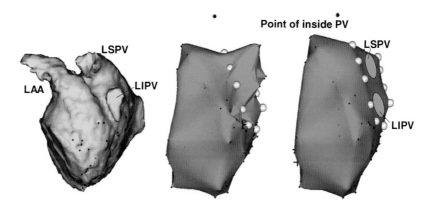

Figure 3 The left image shows a left lateral MR view of the left atrium (LA). The middle and right images show electroanatomical maps by CARTO of the LA in the left lateral view in same patient. The pulmonary vein (PV) ostia (identified by angiography) were tagged by white dots. Note that in the original map (middle image), the LA posterior wall is not flat due to many mapped points within the right- and left-sided PVs; in the corrected map in the upper middle image, the LA posterior wall is very flat after the deletion of the points within the PVs on both sides, whereas the anterior wall is smooth after the deletion of these points in the corrected map in the right image. RSPV, right superior pulmonary vein; RIPV, right inferior pulmonary vein; LSPV, left superior pulmonary vein; LIPV, left inferior pulmonary vein.

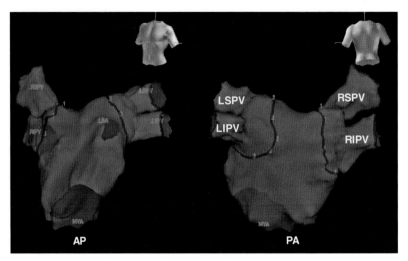

Figure 4 The left and right images show electroanatomical maps by NavX of the left atrium in the anteroposterior and posteroanterior view. The pulmonary vein ostia (identified by angiography) were marked by black lines. RSPV, right superior pulmonary vein; RIPV, right inferior pulmonary vein; LSPV, left superior and inferior pulmonary vein; LIPV, left inferior pulmonary vein; LAA, left atrial appendage.

mapping and ablation by using only the electroanatomical map without frequent use of fluoroscopy during the procedure, which contributes to further reduction of fluoroscopic and procedure times.

CCLs surrounding the ipsilateral PVs

Irrigated RF energy is delivered with a target temperature of 43 °C, a maximal power limit of 25–40 W, and an infusion rate of 17 or 25 mL/min. In all patients,

maximal power of 30 W is delivered along the posterior wall to avoid the potential risk of esophageal thermal injury or LA–esophageal fistula. RF ablation sites are tagged simultaneously on the reconstructed 3D LA. RF energy is applied for 20–30 s until the maximal local electrogram amplitude decreases to <70% or double potentials appear, and/or the sequence of PV activation recorded from the Lasso catheter changes. RF ablation is performed along the

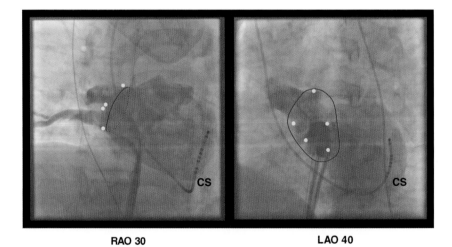

Figure 5 The right and left images show, respectively, fluoroscopic right and left anterior oblique views (LAO and RAO) of the left atrium. The right superior and inferior PV ostia are marked by yellow points. The red lines indicate the ablation line around the right PVs. RAO, right oblique view; LAO, left oblique view; CS, coronary sinus.

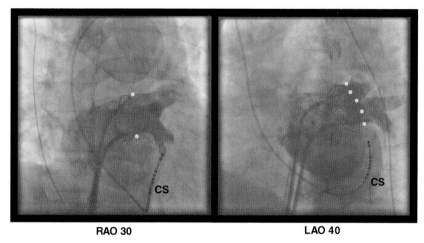

RAO 30　　　　　　　　　**LAO 40**

Figure 6 The right and left images show, respectively, fluoroscopic right and left anterior oblique views (LAO and RAO) of the left atrium. The left superior and inferior PV ostia are marked by yellow points. The red lines indicate the ablation line around the right PVs. RAO, right oblique view; LAO, left oblique view; CS, coronary sinus.

posterior wall for more than 10 mm and along the anterior wall for ≈5 mm from the previously angiographically defined PV ostia (Figures 9 and 10).

Procedural end point

In our experience, more than 90% of the septal PVs are isolated by completing anatomical CCLs alone, whereas about 50% of lateral PVs are still not isolated with one or multiple conduction gaps due to inappropriate lesion formation after completion of CCLs even when performed by experienced physicians (Figure 11). However, the remaining conduction gaps can easily be detected with 3D mapping in conjunction with the respective activation sequence provided by the Lasso catheter.

In patients with paroxysmal or short persistent AF, the ablation end point of CCLs is defined as the absence of all PV spikes during SR as assessed by the Lasso catheter sequentially placed in the ipsilateral superior and inferior PVs at least 30 min after PV isolation. Termination of AF is not included in the end point in our procedure. Electrical cardioversion is performed after complete electrical isolation of the

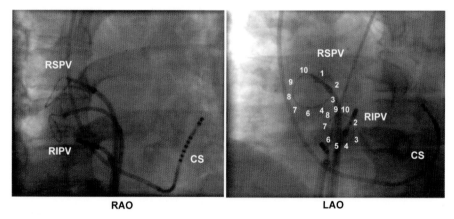

RAO　　　　　　　　　**LAO**

Figure 7 Fluoroscopic right and left anterior oblique views show two Lasso catheters within right superior pulmonary vein (RSPV) and right inferior pulmonary vein (RIPV), mapping catheter (Map) in left atrium, catheter inside coronary sinus (CS), and catheter at His bundle region (His) in left panel. RAO, right oblique view; LAO, left oblique view; Map, mapping catheter; CS, coronary sinus; His, His bundle region; RSPV, right superior pulmonary vein; RIPV, right inferior pulmonary vein.

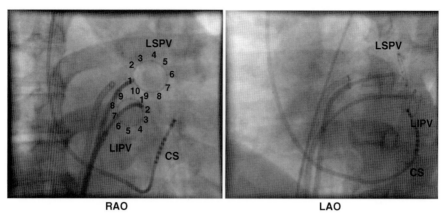

Figure 8 Fluoroscopic right and left anterior oblique views show two Lasso catheters within the left superior pulmonary vein (LSPV) and the left inferior pulmonary vein (LIPV), a mapping catheter (Map) in the LA, a catheter inside the coronary sinus (CS), and a catheter at the His bundle region (His) in the left panel. Numbers indicate the location of the electrodes of the Lasso catheter. RAO, right oblique view; LAO, left oblique view; Map, mapping catheter; CS, coronary sinus; His, His bundle region; LSPV, left superior pulmonary vein; LIPV, left inferior pulmonary vein.

bilateral PVs in case of AF persistence. However, AF was terminated before or immediately after circumferential PV isolation in the majority of patients with paroxysmal AF and normal LA diameter [13]. Even in patients with persistent AF and an AF duration of <6 months and normal atria, in about 50–60% of patients AF is converted to stable sinus rhythm or macroreentrant atrial tachycardia, which is predominantly a common-type atrial flutter or perimitral flutter [14].

(a)

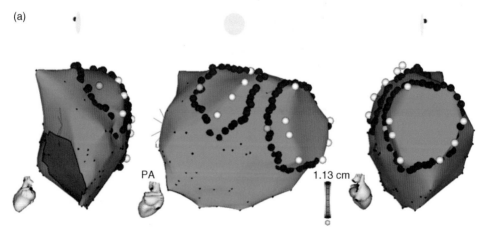

Figure 9 (a) 3D anatomical maps of the left atrium (LA) in a posteroanterior and right lateral view are shown. Note that (1) the angiographic ostia of all PVs are tagged with white points, (2) the right and left continuous circular lesions are marked by multiple red dots around the PVs, (3) the two sites with brown dots located in the right posterosuperior continuous circular lines (CCLs) and in the left antero-inferior CCLs, indicate simultaneous isolation of the ipsilateral PV when both CCLs are complete. RSPV, right superior pulmonary vein; RIPV, right inferior pulmonary vein; LSPV, left superior pulmonary vein; LIPV, left inferior pulmonary vein. (b) Right lateral, posteroanterior, and left lateral views of CARTO merge combined with CARTO maps and MR imaging of the left atrium are shown. Note that the right and left continuous circular lesions are marked by red points around PV ostia. (c) An MRI-derived, virtual endoscopic view of the junction of the right- and left-sided pulmonary veins and LA on CARTO merge imaging is shown. The ostia of the RSPV and RIPV are shown in the left panel and LSPV, LIPV, and left atrial appendage (LAA) in the right panel. Note that (1) the right and left CCLs are marked by multiple red dots around the PVs in left and right panel and (2) CCLs are located on the ridge between left PV and LAA in right panel.

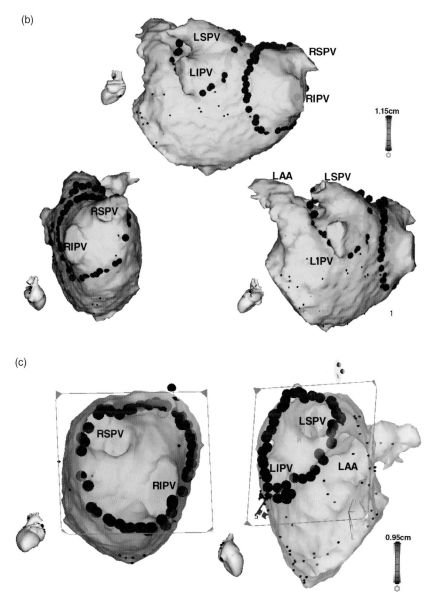

Figure 9 (*Continued*)

Lasso catheter findings during CCLs

In our initial studies, the use of the double Lasso technique provided important information concerning LA–PV conduction and interesting electrophysiological findings about the PV activation. This technique was also helpful for complete PV isolation by CCLs. Comprehension of the electrophysiological information provided by the Lasso catheter recordings is essential for electrical PV isolation. Careful analysis of the signals at the LA–PV junction is required to avoid misleading interpretation.

Complete PV isolation by CCLs

Our studies have demonstrated that CCLs can be performed both during SR or CS pacing and during AF [5,15]. During SR or CS pacing, CCLs resulted in progressive delay of the PV activation and in sequence change of PV activation recorded from the Lasso catheter within the respective ipsilateral PV. Finally,

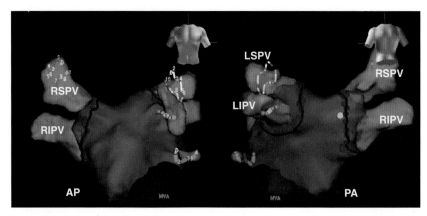

Figure 10 3D anatomical maps of the left atrium by NavX in posteroanterior and anterior–posterior views are shown. The angiographic ostia of all pulmonary veins are tagged with black lines. The right and left continuous circular lesions are marked by multiple red dots around the PVs. Two Lasso catheters are located in left and right PV to confirm isolation of both PVs. RSPV, right superior pulmonary vein; RIPV, right inferior pulmonary vein; LSPV, left superior and inferior pulmonary vein; LIPV, left inferior pulmonary vein; LAA, left atrial appendage.

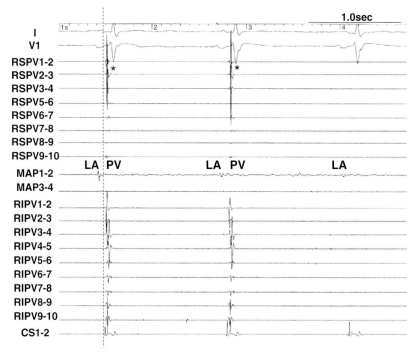

Figure 11 Tracings during sinus rhythm are ECG leads I, V1, and intracardiac electrograms recorded from two Lasso catheters within the left superior and inferior pulmonary veins (LSPV and LIPV), a mapping catheter (Map), a catheter inside the coronary sinus (CS) during RF application in a patient with paroxysmal AF. Note a simultaneous isolation of both LSPV and LIPV when the right continuous circular lesions are complete.

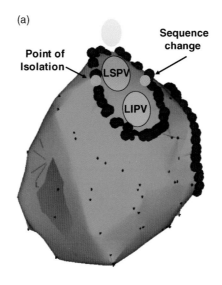

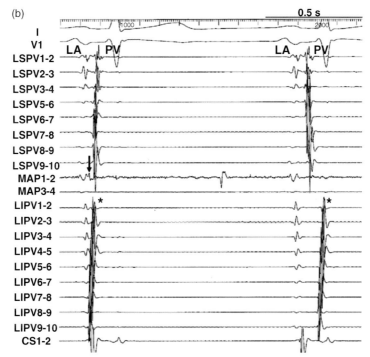

Figure 12 (a) 3D anatomical maps of the left atrium in a left lateral view are shown. Note that (1) the left continuous circular lesions are marked by multiple red dots around the pulmonary veins (PVs), (2) the two sites with a brown dot located in the left posterosuperior continuous circular lesions (CCLs) indicate the change of PV sequence and another brown dot in the left anterior CCLs indicates simultaneous isolation of the ipsilateral PVs. (b) Tracings during sinus rhythm are ECG leads I, V1, and intracardiac electrograms recorded from two Lasso catheters within the left superior and inferior pulmonary veins (LSPV and LIPV), a mapping catheter (Map), a catheter inside the coronary sinus during RF application in a patient with paroxysmal atrial fibrillation. Note (1) the earliest activation of pulmonary vein recorded by Map (marked by yellow), (2) a sequence change of both LSPV and LIPV and all LIPV signals significantly delayed in the second beat compared to the first beat during the RF application at left anterior continuous circular lesion. (c) Note (1) a simultaneous isolation of both LSPV and LIPV when the left CCLs are complete at the left posterior region, (2) the earliest activation of pulmonary vein recorded by Map (marked by yellow). LSPV, left superior pulmonary vein; LIPV, left inferior pulmonary vein; LA, left atrium; PV, pulmonary vein.

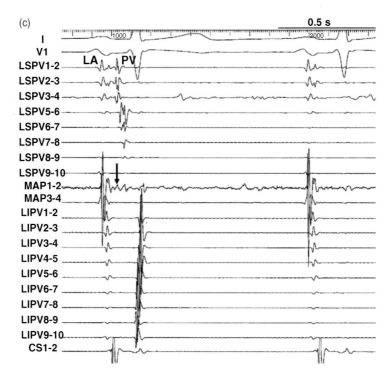

Figure 12 *(Continued)*

the isolation of the ipsilateral PVs is achieved without amplitude reduction of the PV spike (Figure 12). RF application should be immediately stopped in case of ablation catheter dislodgement into the PV to avoid the potential risk of PV stenosis. In our previous experiences without using the lasso technique, RF application inside the PV may cause attenuation of the PV signals or isolation of only the distal part of the PV and subsequently makes identification of the ostial PV activation sequence more difficult (Figure 13).

During AF, the disorganized activation within PVs becomes progressively organized keeping the same or similar PV activation sequence and prolonged CL until final isolation of the PVs. The fibrillatory CL recorded from the CS was also progressively longer after ablation than before ablation in patients without termination of AF during CCLs (Figure 14). Using the double Lasso technique, the ipsilateral PV spikes disappeared simultaneously in more than 95% of patients at completion of the respective CCL during SR or AF. This important finding provides the scientific evidence that complete electrical PV isolation by CCL can be achieved and confirmed in clinical practice by using a single Lasso catheter in one of the ipsilateral PVs.

Automatic activity and tachycardia in PVs

After complete electrical isolation of the ipsilateral PVs, regular or irregular automatic activity dissociated from the atrial activity was observed in ≈95% patients (Figure 15). Also, induced or spontaneous sustained fast PV tachyarrhythmias were observed within the isolated PVs after complete electrical isolation in ≈45% patients (Figure 16). In our methodology, both findings of automaticity and PV tachycardia within the isolated area were much higher compared to the incidence of automacitiy and PV tachycardia after segmental PV isolation [16]. The high incidence of automatic activity and fast PV tachyarrhthmias within the isolated PVs may be due to the increased mass of myocardium within the isolated area compared to previous studies using a segmental PV isolation approach.

AF termination during CCLs

In one of our initial studies, 51 patients with paroxysmal AF underwent complete PV isolation during AF as previously described. After complete PV isolation, external cardioversion (CV) was required to terminate AF in only 5 patients (9.8%); in the remaining 46 patients (90.2%), AF termination occurred before or

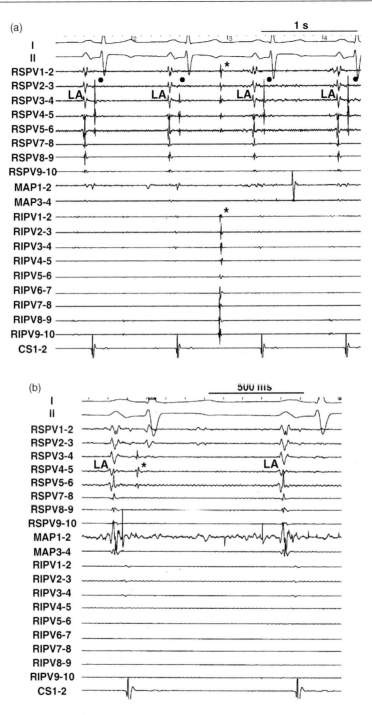

Figure 13 Tracings are ECG leads I and II and intracardiac electrograms recorded from two Lasso catheters within the right superior pulmonary vein (RSPV) and right inferior pulmonary vein (RIPV), a mapping catheter (Map), and a catheter inside the coronary sinus (CS) in a patient with paroxysmal AF. (a) Note that (1) significantly delayed second potential (PV) following the left atrial (LA) potential only recorded by Lasso catheter in RSPV and (2) automatic activity dissociated from the atrial and PV activity (marked by asterisk) in both RSPV and RIPV, suggesting that a distal part of CCLs of the right PVs is isolated. (b) Note the elimination of the second potential by a single application at the posterior region of RSPV. This phenomenon suggests that a junctional region between LA and RSPV was separately isolated.

(a)

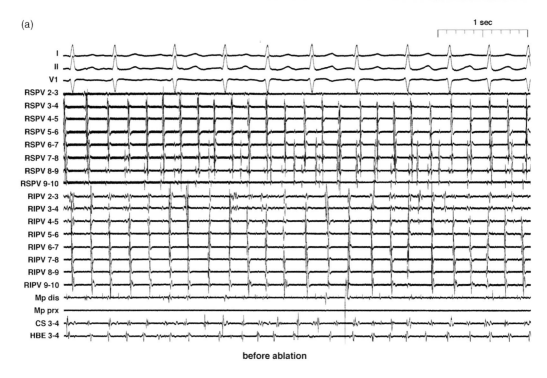

before ablation

(b)

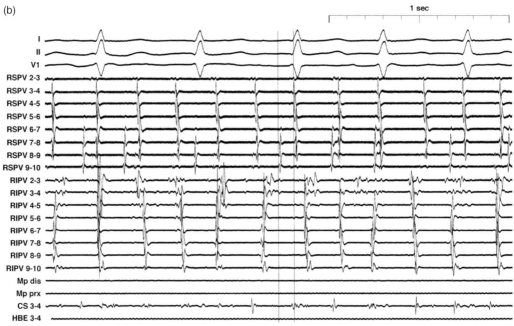

Figure 14 Tracings are ECG leads I, II, and V1 and intracardiac electrograms recorded from two Lasso catheters within the RSPV and RIPV, a mapping catheter (Mp), a catheter inside the CS, and a catheter at the His bundle region (HBE) in a patient with persistent AF. In (a), note that the PV spikes recorded within the RSPV and RIPV are disorganized, with beat-to-beat variation of PV activation sequences and cycle length (CL) before the right-sided continuous circular lesions (CCLs). In (b), note that the PV spikes within the RSPV and RIPV become organized with a similar beat-to-beat PV activation and a variation of CL during RF application on the CCLs. In (c), note that the slow PV spikes with identical activation sequence (marked by asterisk) suddenly disappear when CCLs are completed during RF application.

(c)

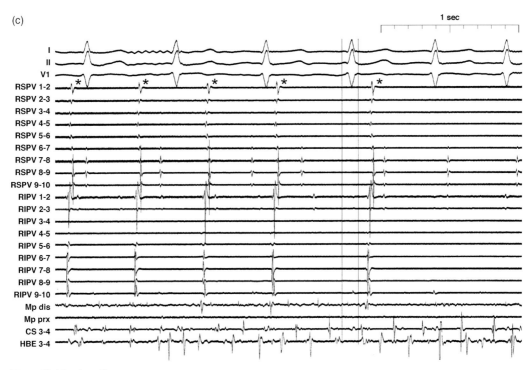

Figure 14 (*Continued*)

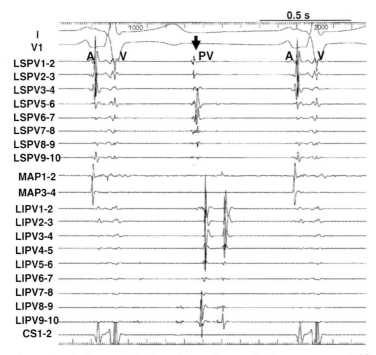

Figure 15 Tracings during sinus rhythm are ECG leads I and V1 and intracardiac electrograms recorded from two Lasso catheters within the left superior and inferior pulmonary veins (LSPV and LIPV), a catheter inside the coronary sinus (CS) and mapping catheter (MAP) after PV isolation. Note automatic activity dissociated from the atrial activity (PV) in both LSPV and LIPV. A, atrial signal; V, ventricular signal; PV, dissociated pulmonary vein signal.

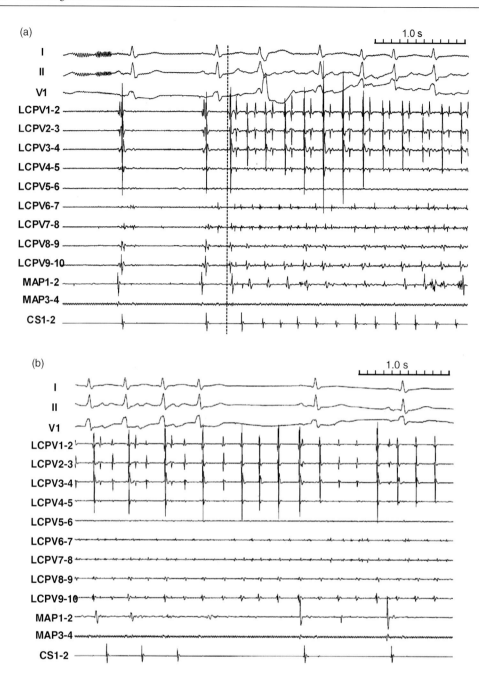

Figure 16 Tracings during sinus rhythm are ECG leads I, II, and V1 and intracardiac electrograms recorded from a Lasso catheter within the left common pulmonary vein (LCPV), a catheter inside the coronary sinus (CS), and a mapping catheter (MAP) in a patient with paroxysmal AF. In (a), note that the initiation of AF by pulmonary vein tachycardia (marked by "PV") originating from the LCPV before pulmonary vein isolation. In (b), note that (1) AF termination by complete CCLs around LCPV and (2) continuous pulmonary vein tachycardia within the LCPV and sinus rhythm (SR) in the atrium. A, LA activation; PV, pulmonary vein activation.

immediately after complete PV isolation [17]. Importantly, a single PV as trigger for AF was demonstrated in five patients (9.8%) in whom sustained PV fibrillation or tachycardia was always observed within the PV before isolation during AF and after isolation during SR. However, in patients with persistent AF lasting more than 7 days and less than 1 year, AF termination occurred only in 30% of the cases [15]. AF termination in patients with paroxysmal or persistent AF may be explained by the fact that CCLs eliminate a number of random reentries and consequently result in inability of AF perpetuation. Based on our data, AF termination should not be the end point for catheter ablation since AF terminated in a reasonable number of patients before complete isolation of the PVs.

Electrical cardioversion is performed after the complete isolation of the bilateral PVs in case of AF persistence. Interestingly, in some patients the PV is still conducted with marked conduction delay immediately after cardioversion during SR. The conduction through CCLs between LA and PV may depend on the cycle length (Figure 17). Therefore the complete PV isolation should be confirmed during SR according to our experience.

Separating PV potentials from far-field atrial potentials

Correct identification of the PV signals and far-field atrial potentials on the Lasso recording is essential for successful and safe PV isolation. As an anatomical fact, the superior vena cava (SVC) is located anterior and in close proximity to the right superior PV. Also, a myocardial sleeve from the RA can extend deeply into the SVC and thus produce a discrete spike potential within the SVC [18]. Therefore, the far-field potentials originating from the SVC can be recorded within the RSPV in patients undergoing PV ablation [19]. Generally, these far-field potentials are small and sharp and recorded on the Lasso catheter only along the anterior portion of the RSPV (Figures 18 and 19).

On the other hand, PV signals from both left PVs are generally fused with the activation from the left atrial appendage (LAA) during SR [20]. However, the fused components can be separated by pacing from a catheter within the CS or the LAA [21]. The PV potential follows the far field LAA potential during pacing in the LAA or from the CS. The amplitude of each potential depends on the location of the Lasso catheter. An ostial Lasso catheter position will demonstrate a high voltage far field potential (Figure 20).

For the ablation of the left-sided PVs we usually start RF applications at the roof and the anterior superior part of the ridge between the left superior

PV and the LAA during SR. In case of continuous and transmural lesions the PV signals will separate from the LAA potential and become visible in almost all patients (Figure 22). This can easily facilitate correct identification of the ridge and RF ablation along the ridge between the LPVs and the LAA. After RF lesions along the ridge, triple potentials consisting of double LAA potentials and the PV potential were occasionally observed from the Lasso catheter due to the conduction delay in some patients (Figure 21). However, it is more difficult to distinguish the PV and far-field LAA potentials during AF. Careful judgment of activation sequence during ablation (such as organized PV activation or prolonged CL of PV activation) may help to identify both components. Furthermore, it might be difficult to assess the reduction of local signals caused by RF applications during AF. This may result in inadequate application numbers in some areas. In our experience, stable SR can be maintained after isolation of the right-sided PVs in most patients with failed cardioversion before ablation. Consequently, ablation of the lateral PVs can be performed in SR in a high percentage of patients with diagnosis of persistent AF.

Recovered PV conduction after the initial ablation procedure

The recurrence rate after the initial PV isolation seems to be different depending on the ablation technique and the follow-up. In our experience, the recurrence rate of atrial tachyarrhythmias was 25% in patients with ablation during stable sinus rhythm and 37.5% in patients with ablation during AF during more than 6 months follow-up without a blanking period. Interestingly, recovered PV conduction has been demonstrated in 80-90% of patients with recurrent tachyarrhythmia after previous successful CCLs. The recovered PV conduction was mostly characterized by a significant delay during SR as compared to the conduction before ablation (Figure 23). During the 2nd procedure, the conduction gaps were randomly distributed in all regions of the previous CCLs. However, the majority of recovered gaps within CCLs around the left-sided PVs is located along the ridge between the LAA and the left-sided PVs due to low contact force between the ablation catheter and myocardium. All conduction gaps were easily identified in the previous CCLs by using initially two Lasso catheters within the ipsilateral PVs and later using only a single Lasso catheter sequentially placed in the superior and inferior ipsilateral PVs, and could be successfully closed with few RF applications.

Interestingly, the surface ECG showed a constant P-wave morphology and an identical atrial activation

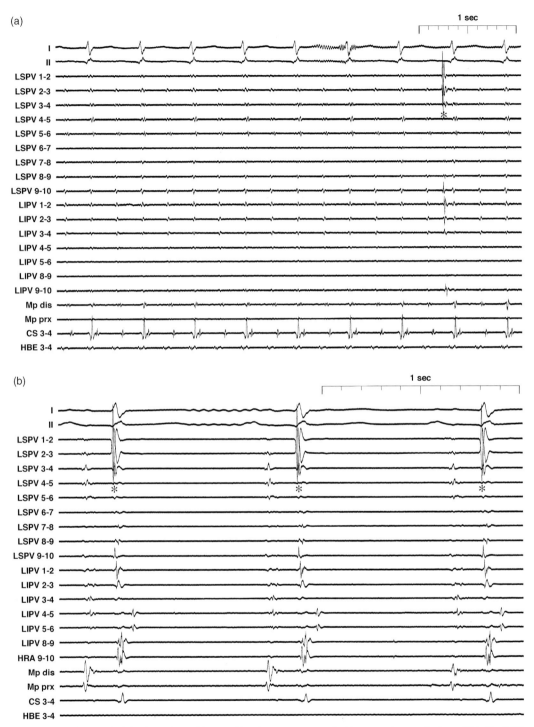

Figure 17 Tracings are ECG leads I and II and intracardiac electrograms recorded from two Lasso catheters within the LSPV and LIPV, a mapping catheter (Mp), a catheter inside the CS, and a catheter at the His bundle region (HBE) in a patient with persistent AF. (a) Note that (1) persistent tachycardia demonstrated by surface ECG and CS catheter, (2) automatic activity dissociated from the atrial activity (marked by asterisk) in both LSPV and LIPV, resulting from complete left PV isolation. (b) Note that (1) sinus rhythm is recovered after external cardioversion and (2) marked delayed PV signals (asterisk) in LSPV and LIPV, showing that PVs still have conduction during sinus rhythm. (c) Note a simultaneous isolation of both LSPV and LIPV by a single application.

(c)

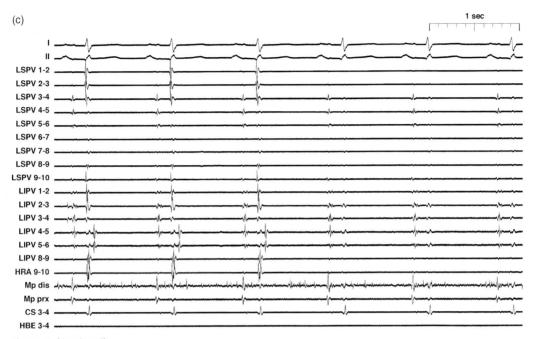

Figure 17 (*Continued*)

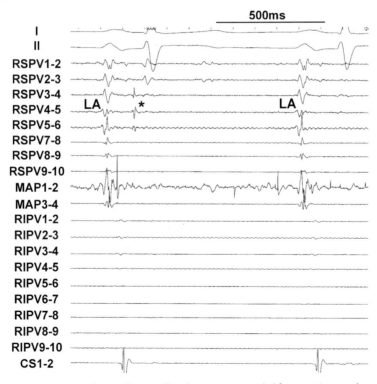

Figure 18 Tracings are ECG leads I and V1 and intracardiac electrograms recorded from two Lasso catheters within the RSPV and RIPV, mapping catheter (MAP), and a catheter inside the CS in a patient with paroxysmal AF. Note that the local potential recorded by the mapping catheter placed at the anterior region of the RIPV shows three components of signals before isolation, indicating the right atrium far-field potential (RA), the left atrial potential (LA) and the pulmonary vein potential (PV).

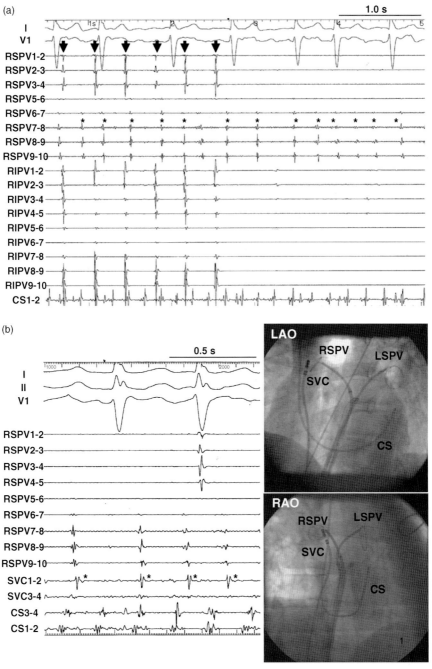

Figure 19 (a) Tracings are ECG leads I and V1 and intracardiac electrograms recorded from two Lasso catheters within the right superior pulmonary vein (RSPV) and right inferior pulmonary vein (RIPV) and a catheter inside the coronary sinus (CS) in a patient with persistent AF. Ipsilateral right pulmonary vein tracings are shown during AF. Note that the slow PV spikes with identical activation sequence (marked by asterisk) suddenly disappear when CCLs are completed during RF application. Sharp potentials still persist in RSPV 6–7 to 9–10 (marked by "*"). (b) In the left panel, tracings are ECG leads I, II, and V1 and intracardiac electrograms recorded from a Lasso catheter within the RSPV, a mapping catheter in the superior vena cava (SVC), and a catheter inside the CS in the left panel. Fluoroscopic right and left anterior oblique views are shown in the right panel. Note (1) the dissociated PV activation recorded by Lasso catheter within the RSPV (marked by asterisk) and (2) the ablation catheter placed in the SVC opposite to RSPV 7–8 to 9–10 (catheter positions shown on the right panel) records sharp potentials (marked by "*") with a timing identical to the residual potentials in the RSPV (despite AF). CS, coronary sinus, RSPV, right superior pulmonary vein; SVC, superior vena cava; LAO, left anterior oblique view, RAO, right anterior oblique view.

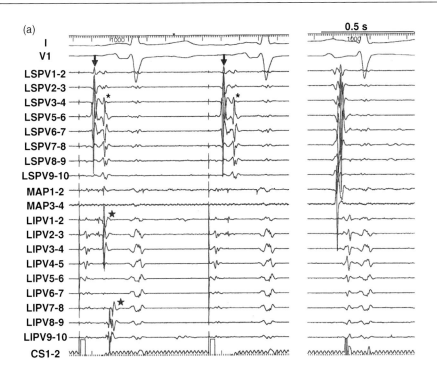

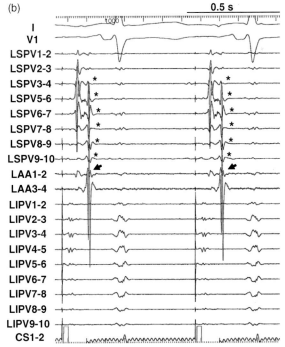

Figure 20 (a–b) Tracings are ECG leads I and V1 and intracardiac electrograms recorded from two Lasso catheters within the left superior pulmonary vein (LSPV) and left inferior pulmonary vein (LIPV), a mapping catheter (Map), and a catheter inside the coronary sinus (CS) during RF application for the left pulmonary veins. (a) In the left panel note that during CS pacing RF application eliminates spiky potentials recorded by Lasso catheters in the LIPV (marked by "*") and two separate components of signals are still recorded in the LSPV (marked by asterisk). In the right panel, during sinus rhythm the two components of the signal in LSPV are fused. (b) A mapping catheter placed in the left atrial appendage records sharp potentials (marked by arrow) with timing identical to the residual potentials in the LSPV (marked by asterisk). This phenomenon shows that CS pacing could lead to misunderstanding of a delayed LAA potential as PV potential.

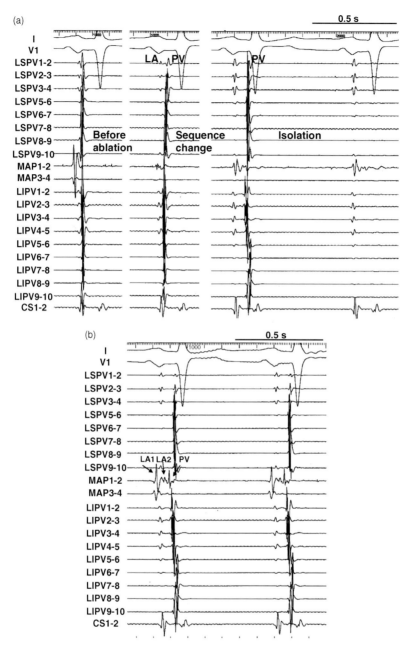

Figure 21 (a–b) Tracings are ECG leads I and V1 and intracardiac electrograms recorded from two Lasso catheters within the left superior pulmonary vein (LSPV) and left inferior pulmonary vein (LIPV), a mapping catheter (Map), and a catheter inside the coronary sinus (CS) during RF application for the left pulmonary vein (PV). (a) Note that the signals on the Lasso catheters in LSPV and LIPV are isolated simultaneously after a sequence change of Lasso recordings without any applications at the anterior part of LSPV. (b) Note that the local potential of recorded by a mapping catheter placed on the anterior region of the LSPV shows three components of signals before isolation, indicating double potentials of left atrium (LA) and PV potential (LA1, LA2, and PV). This phenomenon may suggest a spontaneous block at the anterior region of left PV (between left PV and left atrial appendage). (c) 3D anatomical maps of the left atrium in a posteroanterior view are shown. Note that (1) the left PV ostium was marked by white dots, (2) the left continuous circular lesions are marked by multiple red dots around the PVs, (3) the region showing triple potential by a mapping catheter was marked by a green dot, and (4) the two sites with a brown dot located in the left posterior continuous circular lesions (CCLs) indicate the change of PV activation sequence and another brown dot in the left anterior inferior CCLs indicates simultaneous isolation of the ipsilateral PV without any applications at the anterior region of left PV.

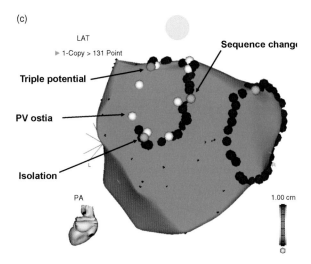

(c)

LAT

▶ 1-Copy > 131 Point

Sequence change

Triple potential

PV ostia

Isolation

PA

1.00 cm

Figure 21 (*Continued*)

sequence before complete PV isolation in some patients with recurrence of PV tachycardia. The AT with irregular or regular CL resulted from PV tachycardias, sometimes from PV fibrillation, conducting through gaps between PV and LA, which was demonstrated by Lasso catheters within the respective ipsilateral PVs. After complete PV isolation, SR occurred in the setting of continuous PV tachyarrhythmias within ipsilateral PVs (Figure 24). The PV tachyarrhythmias required external cardioversion for termination during SR, strongly suggesting that the PV tachyarrhythmia is due to reentry [17]. This interesting finding suggests that a single PV can act as AF substrate.

Our data were consistent with previous studies showing that recovered PV conduction is a dominant finding in patients with recurrent atrial tachyarrhythmias after previous PV isolation [22,23]. Importantly, the majority of patients was free from recurrence after the second procedure. The clinical success was ≈95% after permanent complete PV isolation including the 2nd ablation procedure in patients with paroxysmal and persistent AF. These data strongly support the concept that permanent PV isolation should be the defined end point of CCLs.

In patients without recovered PV conduction, we attempt to uncover non PV foci triggering AF by stimulation and provoked maneuvers and to abolish all non PV foci by irrigated RF ablation. In patients with recovered conduction frequently non PV extrasystoles activated the PV and induced fast PV tachycardia, which then activated the atria

via the conduction gaps and resulted in atrial tachycardia and AF. The atrial extra beats persisted but could not induce AF after the recovered PV conduction was abolished (Figure 25). Consequently, in our ablation strategy extra beats were not targeted in the majority of patients. Based on our data, the incidence of 10–20% triggers being non-PV foci from previous reports could be an overestimation.

Inducibility of AF after CCL-based PV Isolation

It has been reported that sustained AF could be induced by burst stimulation after segmental PV isolation or circumferential ablation around the PVs in 46% to 60% of patients with paroxysmal AF [6,25]. Also, it has been demonstrated that additional linear lesions in the LA can improve clinical outcome and reduce inducibility [7]. However, in one of our initial studies with 60 patients after complete isolation of the ipsilateral PVs due to paroxysmal AF, sustained AF lasting more than 10 min was induced in only 13% of patients by burst pacing with 2 : 1 capture with maximum output (2.9 ms pulse duration and 20 mV output). Interestingly, there was no statistically significant difference in the recurrence rate of tachyarrhythmias between patients with paroxysmal AF with inducible and noninducible AF during 5.7 ± 2.0 months follow-up after complete CCLs [26]. These data may support the hypothesis that the circumferentially isolated areas using our technique are much larger than in previous studies based on a much higher

(a)   Visible PV spike by application at superior LPV

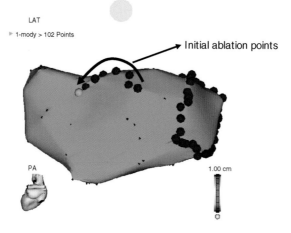

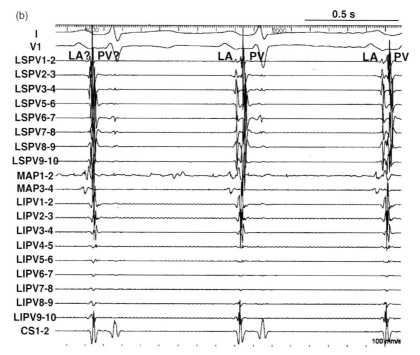

Figure 22 (a) 3D anatomical maps of the left atrium in a posteroanterior view are shown. Note that (1) the left PV ostium was marked by white dots, (2) the left continuous circular lesions are marked by multiple red dots around the PVs, (3) the one site with a brown dot located in the left anterior–superior CCLs indicates the change of PV activation sequence. (b) Tracings are ECG leads I and V1 and intracardiac electrograms recorded from two Lasso catheters within the left superior pulmonary vein (LSPV and left inferior pulmonary vein (LIPV), a mapping catheter (Map), and a catheter inside the coronary sinus (CS) during RF application for the left pulmonary veins. The change of activation sequence of both the LSPV and the LIPV and the marked delay of all LSPV signals in the second beat compared with the first beat during RF application at the left antero-superior continuous circular lesion indicates that conduction block created by the ablation has made the PV spike visible.

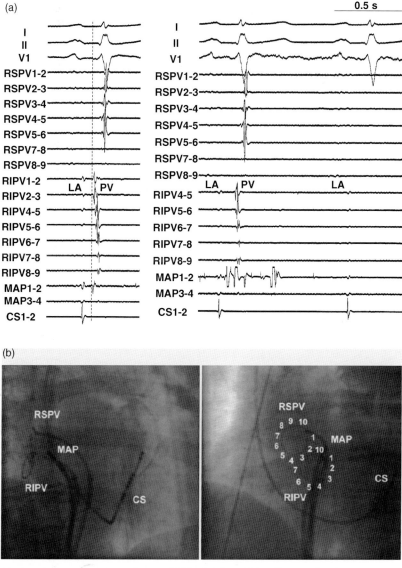

Figure 23 (a) Tracings during a repeat procedure are ECG leads I, II, and V1 and intracardiac electrograms recorded from one Lasso catheter within the right superior and inferior pulmonary vein (RSPV and RIPV), a mapping catheter (MAP dis and MAP prx) in the left atrium, and a catheter within the CS. Note that (1) there is a recovered PV conduction with a significant conduction delay during sinus rhythm in left panel and (2) a simultaneous isolation of both RSPV and RIPV by a single application at the conduction in right posterior region in the right panel. (b) Fluoroscopic right and left anterior oblique views are shown. Note that the catheters position at the posterior region of right the PV.

(a)

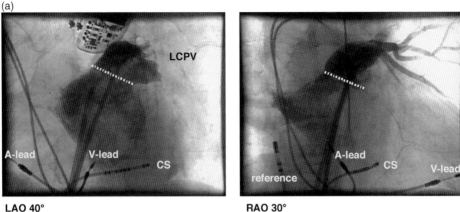

LAO 40°   RAO 30°

(b)

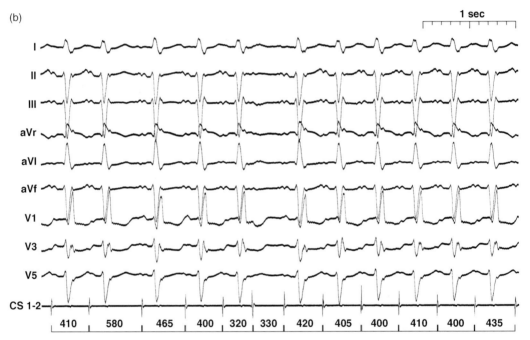

Figure 24 (a) Fluoroscopic right and left anterior oblique views in a patient with recurrent tachycardia are shown. Note a dual chamber pacemaker with an atrial and a ventricular lead, a Lasso catheter within the left common pulmonary vein (LCPV), a catheter inside the coronary sinus (CS), and contrast in the left veins showing a common ostium. RAO, right anterior oblique view; LAO, left anterior oblique view; Map, mapping catheter; CS, coronary sinus; His, His bundle region; LCPV, left common pulmonary vein. (b) Tracings are 12 surface ECG leads and intracardiac electrograms recorded from a catheter within the coronary sinus (CS). Note that tachycardia presents with the same P wave morphology on the surface ECG and irregular cycle length recorded from the CS catheter. (c) Tracings are ECG leads I, II, and V1 and intracardiac electrograms recorded from one Lasso catheter within the left common pulmonary vein (LCPV), a mapping catheter (Mp dis and Mp prx) at the inferior gap of the previous continuous circular lesions (CCLs) around the left-sided PVs in the patient during clinical tachycardia. Note that (1) LCPV fibrillation with continuous change in cycle length (CL) and activation sequence activating the left atrium via an inferior conduction gap and resulting in irregular CL of the tachycardia; (2) the local left atrial potential following fractionated electrogram recorded by mapping catheter. (d) Fluoroscopic right and left anterior oblique views are shown. Note that a mapping catheter was located at the inferior conduction gap of the previous CCLs. In (e), note (1) atrial tachycardia termination by closing the inferior gap of the previous left-sided CCLs; (2) continuous PV fibrillation within the LCPV and paced rhythm in the atrium. In (f), note that the PV fibrillation persists within the LCPV more that 30 min after the complete isolation, and is terminated by external cardioversion with 200 J.

(c)

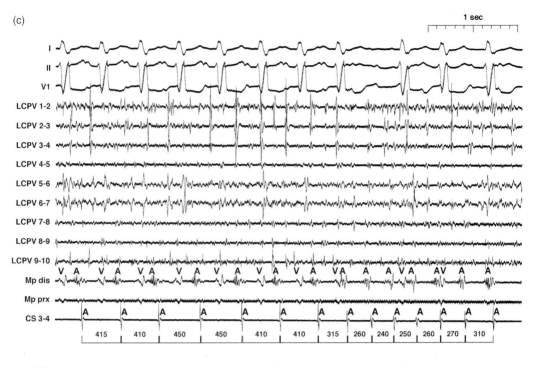

(d)

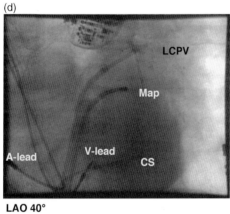

LAO 40°

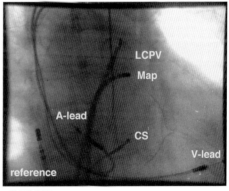

RAO 30°

Figure 24 (*Continued*)

(e)

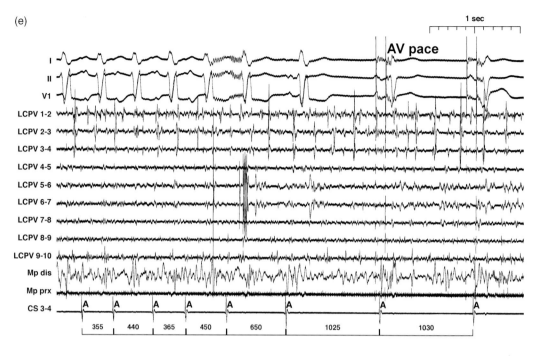

(f)

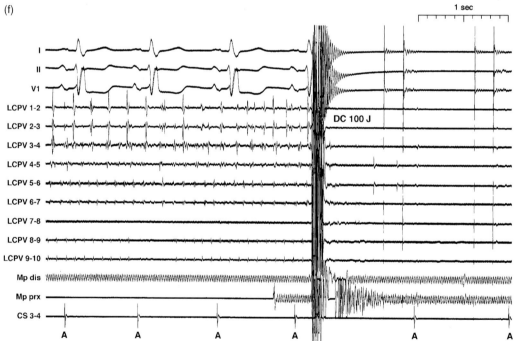

Figure 24 (*Continued*)

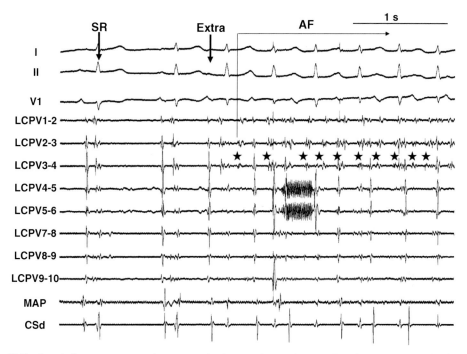

Figure 25 Tracings during a repeat procedure are ECG leads I, II, and V1 and intracardiac electrograms recorded from one Lasso catheter within the left common PV (LCPV), a mapping catheter (MAP) in the left atrium, and a catheter within the coronary sinus (CS), in a patient with recurrent atrial tachycardia after the initial ablation. Note that (1) there is a recovered PV conduction with a significant delay during sinus rhythm, (2) the initial atrial extrasystole (marked by an arrow) has similar P-wave morphology and atrial activation to the sinus rhythm, which indicates non-PV origin most likely from the right atrium after exclusion of recovered PV conduction to the right-sided PVs, (3) the non-PV atrial extrasystole activates the LCPV and initiates a fast PV tachycardia with a cycle length of 144–238 ms within the LCPV; and (4) the fast PV tachycardia activates the atria via a conduction gap with two-to-one conduction.

incidence of AF termination during ablation in patients with paroxysmal and persistent AF, a higher incidence of spontaneous automatic activity and induced PV tachyarrhythmias within isolated areas, and a lower incidence of induced AF after complete PV isolation. This might be explained by the elimination of triggered activity and/or mother waves outside the PV ostia that may initiate and/or perpetuate AF. More importantly, based on our experience of more than 1300 AF ablation procedures guided by double lasso and 3-D mapping, only permanent PV isolation can achieve long-term success in patients with normal LA regardless of whether the AF is paroxysmal or persistent.

Circumferential PV isolation with single Lasso

In our initial experience, simultaneous isolation of the ipsilateral right-sided or left-sided PVs was achieved in >95% of patients by experienced

physicians using the double-lasso technique. This important finding of simultaneous isolation recorded in the majority of ipsilateral PVs by the double-lasso approach provided scientifically important information and led to the use of only a single lasso (Figure 26a–c). In addition, the double-lasso technique demands three transseptal sheaths, which may cause difficulties in manipulation of the ablation catheter within the left atrium and potentially increases the procedure costs.

Complications

In an initial series with >1300 AF ablations using irrigated ablation in conjunction with a 3-D mapping system, cardiac tamponade occurred only in 5 patients (0.4%), and minor embolism occurred in one patient, with complete recovery 3 days after ablation. Most frequent complications were local hematomas in ≈2% patients.

(a)

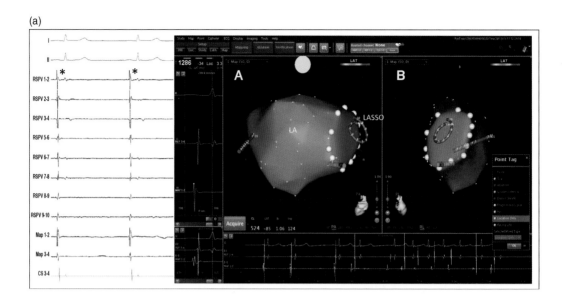

(b)

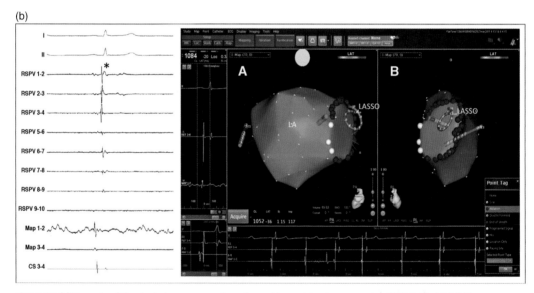

Figure 26 (a) Example of the single-Lasso approach performed in septal pulmonary veins (PVs). Left atrial (LA) reconstruction in a posterior (a) and a right lateral (b) view (left panel). Surface (I, II) and intracardiac leads (RSPV 1–10; Map 1–2 and Map 3–4) during ablation of septal PVs. After LA reconstruction and tagging of the ipsilateral PVs (white dots) based on selective PV angiographies a single 20 mm Lasso catheter (Lasso) is positioned in a stable position inside the septal superior PV. Before ablation the far-field atrial potential and the PV potential are fused (*). (b) Ablation of the septal PVs is started inferior followed by a counterclockwise direction along the previously tagged ostium of the ipsilateral PVs (red dots). After completion of the roof ablation, the PV potentials recorded from the superior PV delay and separate from the far-field atrial potential (*). (c) After completion of the circumferential ablation line (yellow dot) along the posterior–inferior segment near the septal inferior PV, the PV potential recorded from the superior PV suddenly disappears (*), indicating simultaneous isolation of the ipsilateral superior and inferior PVs.

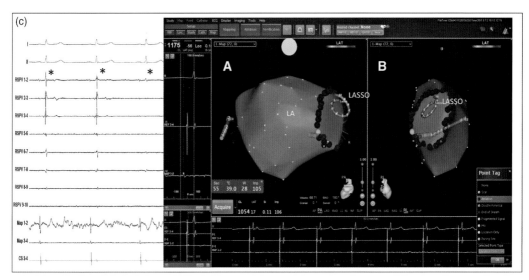

Figure 26 (Continued)

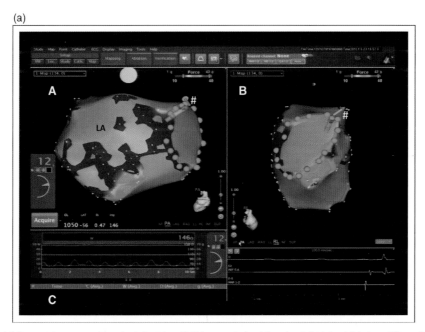

Figure 27 (a) Contact force mapping of a left atrium (LA) in a posterior (a) and a right lateral (b) view. After selective pulmonary vein (PV) angiographies, the septal PVs are tagged (green dots). The contact force (CF) at each individual mapping point is color-coded: red = low CF (<10 g); purple = high CF (>40 g); other colors code for CF >10 g and <40 g. The force–time interval (FTI) is displayed on a graph (c). The CF vector is shown as an arrow. (b) The septal pulmonary veins (RPVs) and the lateral PVs (LPVs) are divided into six segments (roof, anterior superior, anterior inferior, inferior, posterior inferior, and posterior superior). The different colors show the different characteristic contact force (CF) levels at each individual segment (red: average CF >30 g; yellow: average CF >20 g and <30 g; green: average CF >10 g and <20 g; blue: average CF <10 g). Note that lowest CF is achieved along the anterior segment of the lateral PVs and along the inferior segment of the lateral and the septal PVs.

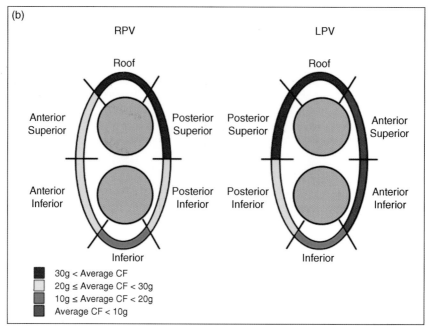

Figure 27 (*Continued*)

Long-term clinical outcome after CCLs in patients with paroxysmal AF

In a series of 161 patients with paroxysmal AF ablated in 2003 and 2004 long-term follow-up was recently assessed and published [24]. After a median follow-up of 4.8 years (0.33–5.5 years), sinus rhythm was present in 75 patients (46.6%) after the initial procedure. During reablation performed in 66 patients, electrical reconduction of initially isolated PVs was detected in 62 patients (94%) and the gaps were closed. A third procedure was performed in 12 patients and PV reconduction was present in 8 patients (66.7%). After a median of 1 (1–3) procedure, stable sinus rhythm was finally achieved in 128 of 161 patients (79.5%). In another 21/161 patients (13.0%) clinical improvement occurred during a median follow-up of 4.6 years (0.33–5.5 years) (Figure 27).

Conclusions

Based on our experience with high clinical success and low procedural complication rates, the recommended ablation strategy in patients with paroxysmal or persistent AF is PV isolation by CCLs. The complete circumferential PV isolation is the preferable end point for catheter ablation of paroxysmal and persistent atrial fibrillation

Acknowledgments

We thank Detlef Hennig for his assistance.

References

1 Haissaguerre M, Jais P, Shah DC, et al. Spontaneous initiation of atrial fibrillation by ectopic beats originating in the pulmonary veins. N Engl J Med. 1998;339: 659–666.

2 Haissaguerre M, Shah DC, Jais P, et al. Electrophysiological breakthroughs from the left atrium to the pulmonary veins. Circulation. 2000;102:2463–2465.

3 Oral H, Knight BP, Tada H, et al. Pulmonary vein isolation for paroxysmal and persistent atrial fibrillation. Circulation. 2002;105:1077–1081.

4 Pappone C, Rosanio S, Oreto G, et al. Circumferential radiofrequency ablation of pulmonary vein ostia: a new anatomic approach for curing atrial fibrillation. Circulation. 2000;102:2619–2628.

5 Ouyang F, Bänsch D, Ernst S, et al. Complete isolation of left atrium surrounding the pulmonary veins: new insights from the double-Lasso technique in paroxysmal atrial fibrillation. Circulation. 2004;110:2090–2096.

6 Haissaguerre M, Sanders P, Hocini M, et al. Changes in atrial fibrillation cycle length and inducibility during catheter ablation and their relation to outcome. Circulation. 2004;109:3007–3013.

7 Jais P, Hocini M, Sanders P, et al. Long-term evaluation of atrial fibrillation ablation guided by noninducibility. Heart Rhythm. 2006;3:140–145.

8 Nademanee K, McKenzie J, Kosar E, et al. A new approach for catheter ablation of atrial fibrillation: mapping of the electrophysiologic substrate. J Am Coll Cardiol. 2004;43:2044–2053.

9 Oral H, Chugh A, Good E, et al. A tailored approach to catheter ablation of paroxysmal atrial fibrillation. Circulation. 2006;113:1824–1831.

10 Chen M, Yang B, Chen H, Ju W, Zhang F, Tse HF, Cao K. Randomized comparison between pulmonary vein antral isolation versus complex fractionated electrogram ablation for paroxysmal atrial fibrillation. J Cardiovasc Electrophysiol. 2011;22(9):973–981.

11 Mun HS, Joung B, Shim J, Hwang HJ, Kim JY, Lee MH, Pak HN. Does additional linear ablation after circumferential pulmonary vein isolation improve clinical outcome in patients with paroxysmal atrial fibrillation? Prospective randomized study. Heart. 2012;98(6):480–484.

12 Schmidt B, Ernst S, Ouyang F, et al. External and endoluminal analysis of left atrial anatomy and the pulmonary veins in three-dimensional reconstructions of magnetic resonance angiography: the full insight from inside. J Cardiovasc Electrophysiol. 2006;17:957–964.

13 Huang H, Wang X, Chun J, Ernst S, Satomi K, Ujeyl A, Chu H, Shi H, Bänsch D, Antz M, Kuck KH, Ouyang F. A single pulmonary vein as electrophysiological substrate of paroxysmal atrial fibrillation. J Cardiovasc Electrophysiol. 2006;17(11):1193–1201.

14 Ouyang F, Ernst S, Chun J, Bänsch D, Li Y, Schaumann A, Mavrakis H, Liu X, Deger FT, Schmidt B, Xue Y, Cao J, Hennig D, Huang H, Kuck KH, Antz M. Electrophysiological findings during ablation of persistent atrial fibrillation with electroanatomic mapping and double Lasso catheter technique. Circulation. 2005;112(20): 3038–3048.

15 Ouyang F, Ernst S, Chun J, et al. Electrophysiological findings during ablation of persistent atrial fibrillation with electroanatomic mapping and double Lasso catheter technique. Circulation. 2005;112:3038–3048.

16 Takahashi Y, O'Neill MD, Sanders P, Rotter M, Rostock T, Jonsson A, Sacher F, Clementy J, Jais P, Haissaguerre M. Sites of focal atrial activity characterized by endocardial mapping during atrial fibrillation. J Am Coll Cardiol. 2006;47(10):2005–2012.

17 Huang H, Wang X, Chun J, et al. A single pulmonary vein as electrophysiological substrate of paroxysmal atrial fibrillation. J Cardiovasc Electrophysiol. 2006;17: 1193–1201.

18 Marrouche NF, Natale A, Wazni OM, et al. Left septal atrial flutter: electrophysiology, anatomy, and results of ablation. Circulation. 2004;109:2440–2447.

19 Shah D, Burri H, Sunthorn H, et al. Identifying far-field superior vena cava potentials within the right superior pulmonary vein. Heart Rhythm. 2006;3:898–902.

20 Ho SY, Sanchez-Quintana D, Cabrera JA, et al. Anatomy of the left atrium: implications for radiofrequency ablation of atrial fibrillation. J Cardiovasc Electrophysiol. 1999;10:1525–1533.

21 Shah D, Haissaguerre M, Jais P, et al. Left atrial appendage activity masquerading as pulmonary vein potentials. Circulation. 2002;105:2821–2825.

22 Cappato R, Negroni S, Pecora D, et al. Prospective assessment of late conduction recurrence across radiofrequency lesions producing electrical disconnection at the pulmonary vein ostium in patients with atrial fibrillation. Circulation. 2003;108:1599–1604.

23 Ouyang F, Antz M, Ernst S, et al. Recovered pulmonary vein conduction as a dominant factor for recurrent atrial tachyarrhythmias after complete circular isolation of the pulmonary veins: lessons from double Lasso technique. Circulation. 2005;111:127–135.

24 Ouyang F, Tilz R, Chun J, Schmidt B, Wissner E, Zerm T, Neven K, Köktürk B, Konstantinidou M, Metzner A, Fuernkranz A, Kuck KH. Long-term results of catheter ablation in paroxysmal atrial fibrillation: lessons from a 5-year follow-up. Circulation. 2010;122(23):2368–2377.

25 Oral H, Chugh A, Lemola K, et al. Noninducibility of atrial fibrillation as an end point of left atrial circumferential ablation for paroxysmal atrial fibrillation: a randomized study. Circulation. 2004;110:2797–2801.

26 Satomi K, Tilz R, Takatsuki S, Chun J, Schmidt B, Bänsch D, Antz M, Zerm T, Metzner A, Köktürk B, Ernst S, Greten H, Kuck KH, Ouyang F. Inducibility of atrial tachyarrhythmias after circumferential pulmonary vein isolation in patients with paroxysmal atrial fibrillation: clinical predictor and outcome during follow-up. Europace. 2008;10(8):949–954.

Controversy: Circumferential versus segmental pulmonary vein isolation/circumferential PVI

Riccardo Proietti,[1,2] Luigi Di Biase,[3,4,5,6] Pasquale Santangeli,[6,7] Prasant Mohanty,[3] Conor Barrett,[8] Stephan Danik,[8] Sanghamitra Mohanty,[3] Rong Bai,[3,9] Chintan Trivedi,[3] John David Burkhardt,[3] & Andrea Natale[3,5,10,11,12,13]

[1]University of Milan, Ospedale Sacco, Milan, Italy
[2]McGill University Health Centre, Montreal, Canada
[3]Texas Cardiac Arrhythmia Institute at St. David's Medical Center, Austin, Texas, USA
[4]Albert Einstein College of Medicine, at Montefiore Hospital, New York, USA
[5]Department of Biomedical Engineering, University of Texas, Austin, Texas, USA
[6]Department of Cardiology, University of Foggia, Foggia, Italy
[7]University of Pennsylvania, Philadelphia, Pennsylvania, USA
[8]Al-Sabah Arrhythmia Institute (AI), St. Luke's Hospital, New York, NY, USA
[9]Department of Cardiology, Beijing Anzhen Hospital, Capital Medical University, Beijing, China
[10]Division of Cardiology, Stanford University, Palo Alto, California
[11]Case Western Reserve University, Cleveland, Ohio
[12]Scripps Clinic, San Diego, California, USA
[13]Dell Medical School, Austin, Texas, USA

The practice of catheter ablation for atrial fibrillation (AF) has been extensively evolved in recent years, following the seminal concept of pulmonary vein isolation (PVI). The cornerstone approach of AF ablation is the disconnection of rapidly firing myocardial sleeves located inside or close to the pulmonary vein from the left atrial myocardium. These are responsible for initiating and maintaining AF. Alongside PVI, new targets of ablation inside the left atrium (LA) are widely contested and difficult to be validate. Significant technological advances in AF ablation have improved the feasibility and safety of the intervention. However, the desired success rate remains elusive; despite technological improvements, a high recurrence rate of atrial tachyarrhythmias following AF ablation is still occurring. Therefore, it is of utmost importance to incorporate a well-developed ablative strategy for PVI in order to obtain effective clinical results.

At present, two main approaches are utilized for PVI: ostial isolation, which is a selective ablation of PV potentials at the ostium of pulmonary veins, and wide antral isolation, which involves the isolation of a wider area encompassing part of the left atrial posterior wall.

Pulmonary vein isolation as initially described by Haissaguerre et al. [1] targets myocardial cells inside pulmonary veins and is referred to as focal ablation. Over the last decade, PVI rapidly advanced to deliver radiofrequency energy around the individual ostium of the four pulmonary veins to achieve electrical disconnection of pulmonary activity from the atrial myocardial fibers.

While the ostium can be easily detected with atrial radiography, and electrically mapped with the use of a mapping catheter, ostial PVI presents the added difficulty of not violating the inside of the pulmonary veins with radiofrequency lesions capable of causing potentially serious complications such as pulmonary vein stenosis. An early study [2] of patients in whom ablation was performed relatively deeply within the PV states that 42.4% of ablated PV veins had stenosis.

Early on, the target of radiofrequency ablation shifted from the ostium to the antrum of pulmonary veins, including a larger part of the atrial myocardium. Natale et al. [3] initially described a protocol for pulmonary antral isolation. Afterward, antral ablation was defined as a lesion performed at least 1.5 cm away from the pulmonary vein ostium as identified by angiography or 3D electroanatomical reconstruction (Figure 28). The antrum resulted in an easily achievable location for the ablation catheter, even though it became harder to identify using only the radiographic images. The end point of the procedure is the isolation of PV antra, defined as entrance and exit blocks into and from the PV antra. Exit block is demonstrated by the presence of dissociated PV potentials that do not conduct into the LA. Entrance block is demonstrated by lack of potential inside the PV antrum and not by voltage amplitude reduction. If PV isolation is not achieved, breakthrough conduction gaps are checked along the PV antrum–LA

(a)

(b)

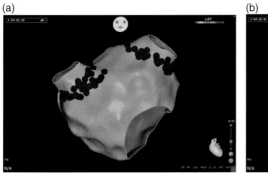
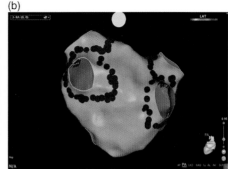

Figure 28 Carto 3D mapping map of PVI using an antral isolation. Red dots indicate RF lesions at the antrum of the PVs. (A = AP, antero-posterior view), B = PA, postero-anterior view.

junction as sites of earliest local activity or sites of reversal of local electrocardiogram.

The antral approach recalls the principles of Cox maze surgical ablation that aimed to compartmentalize the atrium into small regions by the creation of wide encirclement lines. The rationale of this approach lies in reducing total excitable atrial mass, impacting either on mechanisms of arrhythmias maintenance such as" rotor" generations or on tachycardia recurrence postatrial fibrillation ablation.

The main advantages attributed to PV antrum isolation over other ablative strategies include a higher clinical success rate and a lower incidence of postprocedural atrial arrhythmias and PV stenosis.

Increasingly, a different approach consisting of the encirclement of both ispilaterals veins with a continuous radiofrequency lesion has been proposed. Ouyang [4] first described the achievement of PVI through the single encirclement of both ispilateral pulmonary veins guided by a 3D mapping system and double-Lasso technique. Arentz et al. [5] described a simplified approach in which only one Lasso catheter was used requiring only two transseptal punctures instead of three. Notably, the authors demonstrated that verification of electrical isolation was crucial for the outcomes of the procedure. In 36% of the cases, the completion of PV anatomical encirclement did not correspond to electrical isolation of the lesion performed.

With this approach, lesions were easily performed even in the presence of anatomical variations such as the presence of middle pulmonary veins. This procedure does not include the involvement of the carina region in the ablation, which has been shown in previous studies to be an important trigger source for AF induction [6]. However, the completion of electrical isolation removes the necessity for radiofrequency erogation in this area. As stated before, an anatomical approach aiming to perform a large lesion

between the veins without checking electrical conduction could present major limitations.

The catheter ablation of AF moving from the PVI ostial isolation toward antral ablation – either single or multiple encirclement – covers a progressively extensive part of the left atrium myocardium. A more extensive debulking of the left atrium implies important pathophysiological mechanisms. PV antra are funnel-like structures. As the atrial walls expand during the early embryologic stages, the smooth tissue of the PVs becomes incorporated into the walls of the left atrium, which later becomes the posterior wall and some of the roof of the LA. This incorporated portion of the LA along with the PVs defines the PV antra.

The anterior border of the left PV antrum coincides with the anterior aspect of the PV ostia. However, the antrum diverges posteriorly to encompass a significant, if not all, portion of the LA posterior wall.

On the other hand, the right PV antrum encompasses the right PVs, with further extensions anteriorly and superiorly into the anterior interatrial septum. Posteriorly, the right and left PV antra form most, if not all, of the LA posterior wall.

Studies carried out in animal hearts have shown that microreentry localized at the PV–LA junction plays a critical role in maintaining AF [7–10]. The changing orientation of myocardial fiber and ionic differences in the channel distribution around pulmonary veins are responsible, respectively, for nonuniform anisotropy and shorter action potential duration. These anatomical and molecular characteristics favor reentry and may help to explain the preferential anchoring of venous waves at the PV–LA junction, which are capable of maintaining atrial fibrillation. Previously, Jaïs et al. [11] demonstrated the decremental conduction properties of pulmonary veins in humans. More recently, Kumagai et al. [12], using a 64-pole basket catheter, showed exit and entry of the activation front at the PV–LA junction, thus providing further evidence for a reentrant mechanism of atrial fibrillation. Atienza et al. [13] showed an acceleration of activation frequency at the PV–LA junction after adenosine infusion, suggesting that reentry is the mechanism for AF maintenance.

Wide antral PV isolation, through the inclusion of a larger area of the PV–LA junction, has the potential to remove the heterogeneous electrophysiological milieu capable of sustaining reentry in humans.

Conflicting evidence exists about the automaticity of animal isolated PV myocytes, and most studies on PV preparations indicate that the PVs are not spontaneously active under normal conditions, but spontaneous and triggered activity can be induced by sympathomimetic activity [14]. Thus, the critical role of PV in AF seems to be more attributive to the heterogeneous electrical properties of the PV–LA junction than to the trigger activity of cells within the PVs [15]. Moreover, antrum ablation may include structures such as the posterior wall of left atrium, which seems to play a critical role in AF maintenance.

Several findings support this hypothesis: (i) the same embryologic origin of PVs and posterior wall, previously discussed, (ii) AF termination during ablation prior to complete electrical isolation of the vein, and (iii) the interruption of AF after ablation of short cycle length activity in the posterior left atrium.

In addition, pilot studies have documented the successful ablation of ganglionic plexi by PV antrum isolation, which are located at the border of the PVs [16]. These plexi usually are located at the border of the PV antra at the following locations: anterior to the right PVs, inferior to the right inferior PV, superior and medial to the left superior PV, and inferior to the left inferior PV.

Therefore, several factors may explain the potential advantage of wide antral PVI: (i) the elimination of reentry wavelets localized around the PV antrum, (ii) autonomic denervation, (iii) pulmonary vein isolation, (iv) extensive debulking of the left atrium, and (v) ablation of non-PV foci localized in the posterior left atrium wall.

Triggering activity of posterior LA wall and roof has been recently demonstrated by a study that mapped ectopic activity initiating atrial fibrillation with EnSite array system. In a cohort of 65 patients, 11% presented non-PV triggered atrial fibrillation. In half the patients studied, the ectopic activity was localized in the LA roof and posterior wall [17].

Several studies pointed out the role played by the LA posterior wall in triggering and driving atrial fibrillation. Voeller et al. [18] tested in a large cohort of patients a variant of Cox maze procedure that aimed to completely electrically isolate the posterior left atrium, by adding a second ablation line between the superior right and the left pulmonary veins. The group treated with complete box isolation showed a higher freedom from atrial fibrillation recurrence and lower use of antiarrhythmic drugs at 6 months follow-up.

During the human heart development, the primordial embryonic PV grows to progressively incorporate the entire LAPW. The embryological homogeneity of the PVs and the LAPW gives the anatomical basis that suggests these two structures may equally contribute to the development of AF. As compared to the other parts of the LA, the LAPW myocytes present with larger intracellular Ca^{2+} transient and sarcoplasmic reticulum Ca^{2+} contents but a smaller protein expression of Na–Ca exchanger, leading to a high arrhythmogenic potential and distinctive electrophysiological characteristics that may contribute to the pathophysiology of AF.

Tamborero et al. [19] assessed the benefit of a box lesion in the LA posterior wall in patients undergoing transcatheter radiofrequency ablation. In this study, the isolation of the LA posterior wall did not increase the success rate of wide antral circumferential encirclement of ispilateral veins. The authors of this study reported the results suggesting that antral ablation already target the critical points of LA posterior wall capable of triggering and sustaining arrhythmias and no further lesion lines were required.

We disagree with the authors' opinion because the verification of posterior wall isolation was not confirmed with the circular mapping catheter and at follow-up many of the redo posterior did not show isolation.

The theoretical advantage of antral ablation has been criticized by the possibilities of recurrence of adverse left atrial tachycardia following an extensive ablation.

Several studies tried to compare ostial versus antral PVI. Of the more than 80 papers published concerning this topic, only 12 studies [5,20–30] (Table 1) compared in cohort studies these two ablation strategies, with no conclusive evidence.

In a subanalysis of different approaches to catheter ablation, a better outcome with wide antral versus ostial PVI was detected, but the AF recurrence was the only end point [31].

Recently, a meta-analysis was performed by our group on the available literature data. The cumulative recurrence rate of atrial tachyarrhytmias among the two different ablation strategies at long-term follow-up was considered a primary outcome. One year recurrence, left atrial tachyarrhythmia recurrence, and procedural safety, including postopertive mortality, PV stenosis, and embolic events were assessed as secondary outcomes [32].

Table 1 Cohort studies comparing segmental and ostial PVI.

Study	Year	Country	Number of participants	Mean age (years)	Male	Paroxysmal AF %	Additional line	Follow-up length (month)
Arentz et al. [5]	2007	Germany	110	55 ± 10	83	60	None	15
Fiala et al. [26]	2008	Czech Republic	110	52 ± 10	86	100%	None	48
Hwang et al. [25]	2008	South Korea	81	51 ± 11	70	83%	TI	9
Lo et al. [24]	2007	Taiwan	73	53 ± 11	59	79%	Roof, TI, MI	15
Liu et a. [23]	2006	China	110	58 ± 9	72	100%	Roof, TI, MI	9
Mansour, Ruskin, and Keane [22]	2004	US	80	54 ± 10	68	85%	MI	21
Nilsson et al. [21]	2006	Denmark	100	56 ± 10	71	51%	None	12
Oral et al. [20]	2003	US	80	53 ± 10	62	100%	Roof, MI	6
Sawhney et al. [27]	2010	US	66	57 ± 10	48	100%	Roof, MI, TI	24
Tan, Yang, and Wen [29]	2009	China	85	60 ± 10	54	71%	None	9
Yamada et al. [28]	2009	Japan	101	59 ± 10	78	100%	None	12
Yamane et al. [30]	2007	Japan	187	53 ± 10	144	65%	None	12

The primary finding was that PVI performed with a wide antral approach is more effective than ostial PVI in achieving freedom from total atrial tachyarrhythmia recurrence at the long-term follow-up (Figure 29), which is driven by a striking reduction of AF recurrences (Figure 30). The efficacy of a more extensive ablation approach is also evident when the outcome is assessed after the first procedure (Figure 31). A subanalysis including only studies with patients affected by paroxysmal AF confirmed a better outcome with antral versus ostial PVI. The same analysis could not be repeated for patients with persistent AF due to the lack of data. Since PVI is essential for the treatment of all types of AF (paroxysmal, persistent, and chronic),

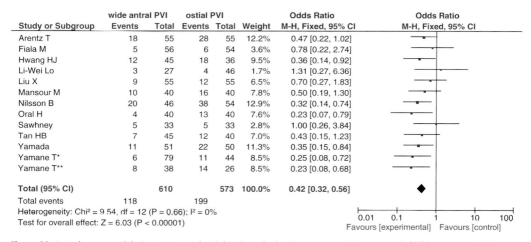

Figure 29 Antral versus ostial. Outcome: total atrial tachyarrhythmia recurrence. Yamane et al. [30] have reported these data separately for paroxysmal atrial fibrillation* and persistent atrial fibrillation**. *Source:* Proietti et al., 2014 [32]. Reproduced with permission of Lippincott Williams & Wilkins.

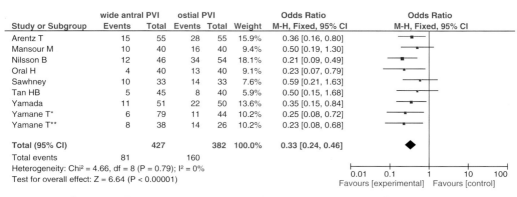

Figure 30 Antral versus Ostial. Outcome: recurrence AF only. (Reproduced with permission from [32]). Yamane et al. [30] have reported these data separately for paroxysmal atrial fibrillation* and persistent atrial fibrillation**.)

the antral approach is largely adopted in the treatment of long-lasting AF because it guarantees a greater impact on substrate modification

Few studies have assessed the occurrence of left atrial tachycardia as a separate outcome, not revealing any significant difference in patients undergoing wide antral ablation versus segmental PVI (Figure 32). However, these results are based on the analysis of few events reported in only a subgroup of the included studies and thus cannot be viewed as definite. With regard to the incidence of major complications, no difference was detected among the two ablation strategies (Figure 33).

In conclusion, when dealing with AF catheter ablation, selecting the appropriate approach to PVI isolation is critical for the clinical success

rate. PVI began as a selective ablation at the ostium of the pulmonary veins, but has evolved into a more extensive ablation debulking of the PV antrum. The aim of the latter strategy is to eliminate the arrhythmogenic substrate of the PV–LA junction maintaining AF. The antrum encirclement is best executed with a single encirclement of both pulmonary ipsilateral veins guided by 3D mapping. Electrical assessment of PVI should remain of paramount importance, regardless of the chosen technique (ostial or antral). Recent scientific evidence outlines that a more extensive ablation of the LA performed with the antral approach is associated with better clinical results. Finally, the incidence of left atrial tachycardia is not significantly greater when a wide antral ablation strategy is used.

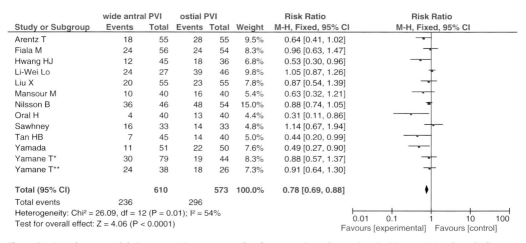

Figure 31 Antral versus ostial. Outcome: AF recurrence after first procedure. (Reproduced with permission from [32]). Yamane et al. [30] have reported these data separately for paroxysmal atrial fibrillation* and persistent atrial fibrillation**.)

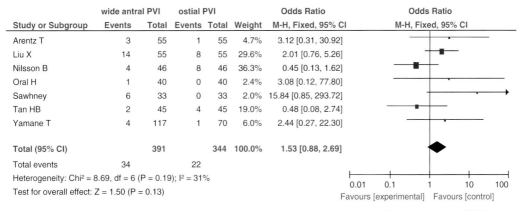

Figure 32 Antral versus Ostial. Outcome: left atrial tachycardia recurrence. (Reproduced with permission from [32].)

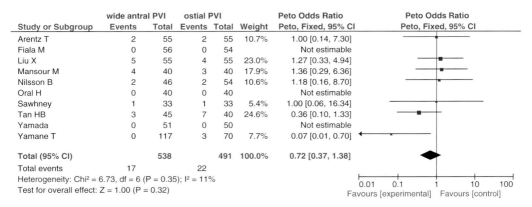

Figure 33 Antral versus Ostial. Outcome: complications.

References

1 Haissaguerre, M, Jaïs P, Shah DC, Takahashi A, Hocini M, Quiniou G, Garrigue S, Le Mouroux A, Le Métayer P, Clémenty J. Spontaneous initiation of atrial fibrillation by ectopic beats originating in the pulmonary veins. N Engl J Med, 1998. 339(10):659–666.

2 Chen SA, Hsieh MH, Tai CT. Initiation of atrial fibrillation by ectopic beats originating from the pulmonary veins: electrophysiologic characteristics, pharmacological response and effects of radiofrequency ablation. Circulation. 1999;100:1879–1886.

3 Kanj M, Wazni O, Natale A. Pulmonary vein antrum isolation. 2007;4:S73–S79.

4 Ouyang F, Ernst S, Chun J, Bänsch D, Li Y, Schaumann A, Mavrakis H, Liu X, Deger FT, Schmidt B, Xue Y, Cao J, Hennig D, Huang H, Kuck KH, Antz M, Ouyang F, Ernest S, Julian C. et al. Electrophysiological findings during ablation of persistent atrial fibrillation with electroanatomic mapping and double Lasso catheter technique. Circulation. 2005, 112:3038–3048.

5 Arentz T, Weber R, Bürkle G, Herrera C, Blum T, Stockinger J, Minners J, Neumann FJ, Kalusche D. Small or large isolation areas around the pulmonary veins for the treatment of atrial fibrillation? Results from a prospctive randomized study. Circulation. 2007;115: 3057–3063.

6 Valles E, Fan R, Roux JF, Liu CF, Harding JD, Dhruvakumar S, Hutchinson MD, Riley M, Bala R, Garcia FC, Lin D, Dixit S, Callans DJ, Gerstenfeld EP, Marchlinski FE. Localization of atrial fibrillation triggers in patients undergoing pulmonary vein isolation: importance of the carina region. J Am Coll Cardiol. 2008;52 (17):1413–1420.

7 Skanes AC, Mandapati R, Berenfeld O, Davidenko JM, Jalife J. Spatiotemporal periodicity during atrial fibrillation in the isolated sheep heart. Circulation. 1998;98: 1816–1821.

8 Arora R, Verheule S, Scott L, Navarrete A, Katari V, Wilson E, Vaz D, Olgin JE. Arrhythmogenic substrate of the pulmonary veins assessed by high resolution optical mapping. Circulation. 2003;107:1816–1821.

9 Hocini M, Ho SY, Kawara T, Linnenbank AC, Potse M, Shah D, Jaïs P, Janse MJ, Haïssaguerre M, De Bakker JM. Electrical conduction in canine pulmonary veins: electrophysiological and anatomic correlation. Circulation. 2002;105:2442–2448.

10 Hamabe A, Okuyama Y, Miyauchi Y, Zhou S, Pak HN, Karagueuzian HS, Fishbein MC, Chen PS. Correlation between anatomy and electrical activation in canine pulmonary veins. Circulation. 2003;107:1550–1555.

11 Jaïs P, Hocini M, Macle L, Choi KJ, Deisenhofer I, Weerasooriya R, Shah DC, Garrigue S, Raybaud F, Scavee C, Le Metayer P, Clémenty J, Haïssaguerre M. Distinctive electrophysiological properties of pulmonary veins in patients with atrial fibrillation. Circulation. 2002;106:2479–2485.

12 Kumagai K, Ogama N, Noguchi H, Yasuda T, Nakashima H, Saku K. Electrophysiologic properties of pulmonary veins assessed using a multielectrode basket catheter. JACC 2004;43:2281–2289.

13 Atienza F, Almendral J, Moreno J, Vaidyanathan R, Talkachou A, Kalifa J, Arenal A, Villacastín JP, Torrecilla EG, Sánchez A, Ploutz-Snyder R, Jalife J, Berenfeld O. Activation of inward rectifier potassium channels accelerates atrial fibrillation in humans: evidence for a reentrant mechanism. Circulation. 2006;114:2434–2442.

14 Schotten U, Verheule S, kirchhof P and Goette A. Pathophysiological mechanisms of atrial fibrillation: a translational appraisal. Physiol Rev. 2011, 91:265–235.

15 Atienza F and Jalife J. Reentry and atrial fibrillation. Heart Rhythm. 2007;4:S13–S16.

16 Verma A, Saliba W, Lakkireddy D, Burkhadrt JD, Cummings JE, Wazni OM, Belden WA, Thal S, Schweikert RA, Martin DO, Tchou PJ, Natale A. Vagal responses induced by endocardial left atrial autonomic ganglia stimulation before and after pulmonary vein antrum isolation for atrial fibrillation. Heart Rhythm. 2007;4:1177–1182.

17 Yamaguchi T, Tsuchiya T, Miyamoto K, Nagamoto Y, Takahashi N. Characterization of non-pulmonary vein foci with an EnSite array in patients with paroxysmal atrial fibrillation. Europace. 2010;12:1698–1706.

18 Voeller RK, Bailey MS, Zierer A, Lall SC, Sakamoto S, Aubuchon K, Lawton JS, Moazami N, Huddleston CB, Munfakh NA, Moon MR, Schuessler RB, Damiano RJ. Isolating the entire posterior left atrium improves surgical outcomes after the Cox maze procedure. J Thorac Cardiovasc Surg. 2008;135:870–877.

19 Tamborero D, Mont L, Berruezo A, Matiello, Benito B, Sitges M, Vidal B, de Caralt TM, Perea RJ, Vatasescu R, Brugada J. Left atrial posterior wall isolation does not improve the outcome of circumferential pulmonary vein ablation for atrial fibrillation: a prospective randomized study. Circ arrhythm Electrophysiol. 2009;2:35–40.

20 Oral H, Scharf C, Chugh A, Hall B, Cheung P, Good E, Veerareddy S, Pelosi F Jr, Morady F. Catheter ablation for paroxysmal atrial fibrillation: segmental pulmonary vein ostial ablation versus left atrial ablation. Circulation. 2003;108:2355–2360.

21 Nilsson B, Chen X, Pehrson S, Køber L, Hilden J, Svendsen JH. Recurrence of pulmonary vein conduction and atrial fibrillation after pulmonary vein isolation for atrial fibrillation: a randomized trial of the ostial versus the extraostial ablation strategy. Am Heart J. 2006;152:537 e1–e8.

22 Mansour M, Ruskin J, Keane D. Efficacy and safety of the segmental ostial versus circumferential extra-ostial pulmonary vein isolation for atrial fibrillation. J Cardiovasc Electrophysiolog. 2004;15:532–537.

23 Liu X, Long D, Dong J, Hu F, Yu R, Tang R, Fang D, Hao P, Lu C, Liu X, He X, Liu X, Ma C. Is circumferential pulmonary vein isolation preferable to stepwise segmental pulmonary vein iolation for patients with paroxysmal atrial fibrillation? A randomized study. Circulation J. 2006;70:1392–1397.

24 Lo LW, Tai CT, Lin YJ, Chang SL, Wongcharoen W, Hsieh MH, Tuan TC, Udyavar AR, Hu YF, Chen YJ, Tsao HM, Chen SA. Mechanism of recurrent atrial fibrillation: comparison between segmental ostial versus circumferential pulmonary vein isolation. J Cardiovasc Electrophysiol. 2007;18:803–807.

25 Hwang H, Myung Lee J, Joung B, Lee BH, Kim JB, Lee MH, Jang Y, Kim SS. Atrial electroanatomical remodelling as a determinant of different outcomes between two current ablation strategies: circumferential pulmonary vein isolation vs pulmonary vein isolation. Clin Cardiol. 2010;33:E69–E74.

26 Fiala M, Chovancík J, Nevralová R, Neuwirth R, Jiravský O, Nykl I, Sknouril L, Dorda M, Januska J, Branny M. Pulmonary vein isolation using segmental versus electroanatomical circumferential ablation for paroxysmal atrial fibrillation. Over 3-year results of a prospective randomized sutdy. J Interv Card Electrophysiol. 2008, 22:13–21.

27 Sawhney N, Anousheh R, Chen W, Feld GK. Circumferential pulmonary vein ablation with additional linear ablation results in an increased incidence of left atrial flutter compared with segmental pulmonary vein isolation as an initial approach to ablation of paroxysmal atrial fibrillation. Circ Arrhythm Electrophysiol. 2010;3:243–248.

28 Yamada T, Yoshida N, Murakami Y, Okada T, Yoshida Y, Muto M, Inden Y, Murohara T. The difference in autonomic denervetion and its effect on atrial fibrillation recurrence between the standard segmental and circumferential pulmonary vein isolation techniques. Europace. 2009;11:1612–1619.

29 Tan HB, Yang XL, Wen XT. Efficacy and safety of segmental pulmonary isolation and circumferential pulmonary vein isolation in patients with atrial fibrillation: a comparative study. Nan Fang Yi Ke Da Xue Xue Bao. 2009;29:128–132.

30 Yamane T, Date T, Kanzaki Y, Inada K, Matsuo S, Shibayama K, Miyanaga S, Miyazaki H, Sugimoto K, Mochizuki S. Segmental pulmonary vein antrum isolation using the "large-size" Lasso catheter in patients with atrial fibrillation. Circ J. 2007;71:753–760.

31 Parkash R, Tang A, Sapp JL and Wells G. Approach to the catheter ablation technique of paroxysmal and persistent atrial fibrillation: a meta-analysis of the rnadomized controlled trials. J Cardiovasc Electrophysiol. 2011.

32 Proietti R, Santangeli P, Di Biase L, Joza J, Bernier ML, Wang Y, Sagone A, Viecca M, Essebag V, Natale A. Comparative effectiveness of wide antral versus ostial pulmonary vein isolation: a systematic review and meta-analysis. Circ Arrhythm Electrophysiol. 2014;7(1):39–45.

Controversy: Circumferential versus segmental pulmonary vein isolation/segmental PVI

Gregory K. Feld

Department of Medicine, Division of Cardiology, Electrophysiology Program at the University of California and the Sulpizio Family Cardiovascular Center, La Jolla, CA, USA

Introduction

With the recognition that pulmonary vein ectopic triggers atrial fibrillation (AF), pulmonary vein isolation (PVI) with radiofrequency catheter ablation has become the predominating approach for the treatment of symptomatic, drug refractory AF, over the past decade [1–7]. During this period though [1–7], the methodology used to achieve PVI has evolved from an electrophysiologically guided segmental ostial catheter ablation (SOCA) approach (Figures 34 and 35) to a combined anatomically and electrophysiologically guided circumferential pulmonary vein ablation approach (CPVA) using electroanatomical mapping (Figures 36 and 37a and b). One possible factor leading to the wider use of CPVA has been the suggestion that SOCA may be associated with a greater risk of PV stenosis [8]. In addition, at least one earlier study suggested CVPA may provide better durability of PVI and long-term success in the prevention of AF recurrence [9]. The CPVA approach to PVI has also been combined in many electrophysiology laboratories with additional left atrial linear ablation (LALA) to improve success rates in persistent AF [7,10,11]. However, there has been growing concern that CPVA and LALA are associated with greater risk of iatrogenic atrial tachyarrhythmias compared to SOCA. This concern has been borne out in several recent studies, demonstrating that atypical left atrial flutter (AFL) occurs more commonly after CPVA plus LALA than after more limited SOCA for the treatment of paroxysmal AF [12–15]. There are also disparate results with respect to the prevention of AF recurrence between these two approaches [16–19]. This chapter will review the literature that addresses the efficacy and safety of these two approaches for the ablation of AF.

AF suppression after SOCA versus CPVA for PVI

Several studies have been published comparing SOCA with CPVA for PVI for treatment of AF. In one such study by Karch et al. [16], 100 patients with symptomatic AF were randomized to either CPVA ($n = 50$) or SOCA ($n = 50$), and freedom from atrial tachyarrhythmias was assessed using a 7-day Holter monitor at 6 months follow-up. Twenty-one patients (42%) were free from any atrial tachyarrhythmias after CPVA and thirty-three patients (66%) after SOCA ($p = 0.02$), and twenty-seven patients (54%) remained free from symptomatic arrhythmias after CPVA and forty-one patients (82%) after SOCA ($p < 0.01$). In contrast, Oral et al. [17] studied 80 consecutive patients with symptomatic paroxysmal AF, of whom 40 underwent PVI by SOCA and 40 underwent CPVA. Addition of LALA was performed at the mitral isthmus connecting the mitral valve annulus to the left circumferential lesion and at the posterior left atrium connecting the left and right circumferential ablation lesions. Conduction block across the posterior and mitral isthmus lines was not routinely evaluated. At 6 months, 67% of patients who underwent SOCA and 88% of patients who underwent CPVA plus LALA were free of symptomatic PAF when not taking antiarrhythmic drug therapy ($p = 0.02$). Multivariate analysis revealed only an increased left atrial size and the SOCA technique was independent predictors of recurrent PAF.

Mansour et al. [18] performed a similar study in 80 consecutive patients with symptomatic paroxysmal AF, of whom 40 patients underwent PVI by SOCA and 40 patients underwent CPVA. Additional LALA was performed at the mitral isthmus in patients presenting in AF. At 11 ± 2.5 months, 24 (60%) patients who underwent SOCA and 30 (75%) patients who underwent CPVA plus LALA were free of symptomatic PAF off antiarrhythmic drug therapy ($p = $ NS). There was no statistically significant difference between the two approaches for PVI, but there was a trend favoring CPVA.

Fiala et al. [19] tested the hypothesis that CPVA would improve the outcome of PVI for treatment of symptomatic paroxysmal AF compared to SOCA. Fifty-four patients underwent SOCA (group 1) and

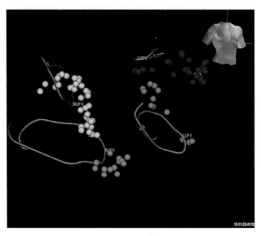

Figure 34 St Jude NavX map showing method for SOCA with Lasso™ catheter shadowed at the ostium of all four pulmonary veins and ablation lesions (colored dots) at pulmonary vein ostia resulting in isolation. (From Sawhney N, Anousheh R, Chen W, Feld GK.) Circumferential pulmonary vein ablation with additional linear ablation results in an increased incidence of left atrial flutter compared to segmental pulmonary vein isolation as an initial approach to ablation of paroxysmal atrial fibrillation. *Source:* Sawhney et al., 2010 [25]. Reproduced with permission of Lippincott Williams & Wilkins.

fifty-six patients underwent CPVA (group 2), in a randomized study. Following a single ablation procedure, at 48 ± 8 months follow-up, 30 (56%) patients in group 1 and 32 (57%) patients in group 2 remained free of arrhythmia ($p = 0.41$). After repeat ablation, 43 (80%) in group 1 and 45 (80%) group 2 were free of arrhythmia off antiarrhythmic drugs, and 48 (89%) in group 1 and 51 (91%) in group 2 did not have arrhythmia recurrence without or with antiarrhythmic drugs. The authors concluded from this study that there was no advantage in long-term arrhythmia-free clinical outcome after CPVA versus SOCA for PV isolation in patients with paroxysmal AF.

There may also be a difference in the outcome of these two approaches to PVI, depending on the duration of AF prior to ablation. For example, Nilsson et al. [20] showed that in a total of 100 consecutive

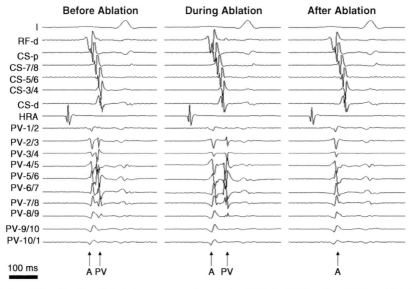

Figure 35 Surface ECG and endocardial electrogram recordings during SOCA for PVI. I, surface ECG lead I; RF-d, distal radiofrequency catheter electrode; CSp-CSd, coronary sinus catheter electrodes from proximal to distal; HRS, high right atrium electrode; PV 1/2–PV 10/1, distal to proximal electrodes on the circular pulmonary vein mapping catheter (Lasso™). Reproduced with permission of Wiley.

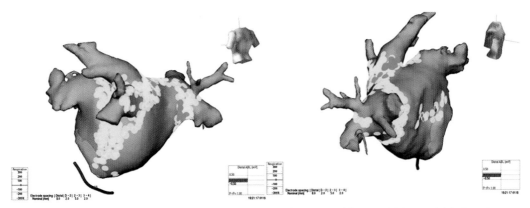

Figure 36 St Jude ESI 3D electroanatomical map view (left panel left posterior oblique and right panel right lateral projections) demonstrating CPVA plus LALA at the LA roof and mitral isthmus.

patients with symptomatic AF (51 paroxysmal and 49 persistent), randomized to SOCA ($n = 54$) or CPVA ($n = 46$), 84% of the patients had recurrent arrhythmias after initial PVI, including 72% with AF and 12% with organized left atrial tachycardia. In patients undergoing repeat ablation for recurrent AF, all but two patients had recurrence of PV conduction (>95%). During a mean follow-up of 12 months without antiarrhythmic drugs, 57% of patients who underwent CPVA were free of arrhythmia symptoms compared to 31% of patients who underwent SOCA ($p < .05$). This difference in success rate between the two ablation strategies was mainly seen, however, in patients with known persistent AF (52% versus 15%; $p = .02$), as opposed to patients with paroxysmal AF (65% versus 46%; $p = 0.26$).

Analysis of the data on cryoballoon ablation for PVI [21–23], which is essentially a hybrid between SOCA and CPVA, in other words ostial circumferential PVI, reveals similar results in long-term suppression of AF to radiofrequency ablation, with better results in patients with paroxysmal AF (approximately 70% suppression of AF at 12 months) compared to persistent AF (approximately 40% suppression of AF at 12 months). However, cryoballoon ablation for PVI has its own inherent problems, including increased cost and increased risk of phrenic nerve injury compared to the standard radiofrequency ablation [21–23].

Thus, to date there has been no clear evidence that either SOCA or CVPA with or without LALA is more effective in preventing recurrent paroxysmal AF during follow-up, although there is a trend for better outcome in patients with persistent AF. A randomized trial of these two approaches needs to be done in an adequate population size of both paroxysmal and persistent AF patients, over a long enough period of follow-up (i.e., preferably 24 months), and with

adequate monitoring (e.g., mobile cardiac outpatient telemetry or MCOT) to determine if there is a statistically significant difference in the recurrence rates of AF, requirement for antiarrhythmic drugs, and complications including pulmonary vein stenosis, mortality or repeat hospitalization, and stroke rate.

Atrial tachyarrhythmias after SOCA versus CPVA for treatment of AF

For many of the reasons noted above, most electrophysiology laboratories currently perform CPVA for treatment of AF, and in some cases LALA is added to reduce AF recurrence, especially in patients with persistent AF. However, CPVA with or without LALA has been associated with development of left atrial tachyarrythmias [12–14], which is rarely seen after SOCA alone [15].

For example, Knecht et al. [24] performed ablation in 180 consecutive patients with persistent AF, in whom termination was achieved in 154 cases. Patients were divided into two groups: (group A) those who did not require LALA to terminate AF (85 patients) and (group B) those who did (69 patients). There was no difference in clinical and echocardiographic characteristics. After 28 months follow-up, the incidence of left atrial tachyarrhythmias necessitating repeat or additional linear ablation was higher in group A (76%) compared to group B (33%) ($p = 0.002$). When complete conduction block across lines could not be achieved during the index procedure, the incidence of subsequent roof ($p = 0.008$) or mitral isthmus-dependent ($p = 0.010$) macro reentrant atrial tachycardia was higher.

In a randomized, prospective study by Sawhney et al. [25], 66 consecutive patients with paroxysmal AF were prospectively randomized to undergo SOCA versus CPVA + LALA (i.e., a roof line and a mitral

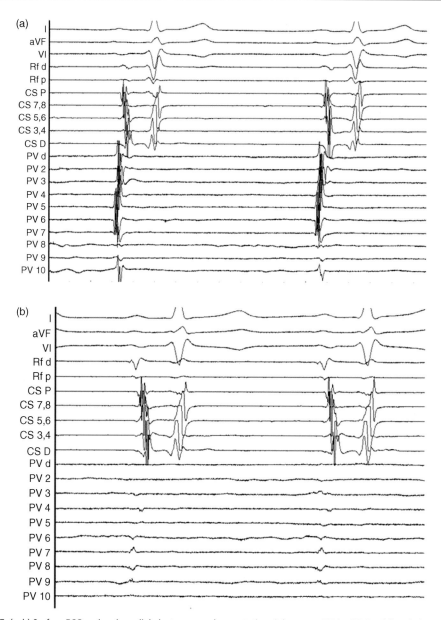

Figure 37 (a–b) Surface ECG and endocardial electrograms demonstating right upper PVI by CPVA. Abbreviations the same as in Figure 2, plus additional surface ECG leads aVF and V1 and RFp, radiofrequency proximal electrode.

isthmus line with documentation of bidirectional mitral isthmus block). All patients were seen at 1, 3, 6, and every 12 months after ablation, with 14-day continuous ECG monitoring every 6 months. At 16.4 ± 6.3 months after 1 ablation procedure (Figure 38), 19 patients (58%) remained free of atrial arrhythmias after PVI versus 17 patients (51%) after CPVA + LALA ($p = 0.62$). After SOCA, 14 patients had recurrent paroxysmal AF, whereas after CPVA +

LALA, 8 patients had recurrent AF, 6 had atypical left atrial flutter, and 2 had both AF and atypical left atrial flutter (Figure 39, $p = 0.002$ between SOCA versus CPVA + LALA for atypical left atrial flutter). Twenty-eight patients (85%) remained arrhythmia-free after 1.3 ± 0.5 SOCA procedures versus 28 patients (85%) after 1.4 ± 0.6 CPVA + LALA procedures ($p = \text{NS}$). Fluoroscopy time was longer after CPVA + LALA versus SOCA (91 versus 73 min, $p = 0.04$). It was

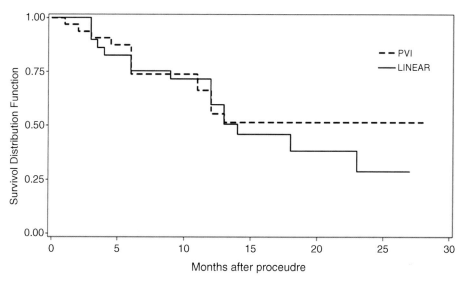

Figure 38 Kaplan–Meier curve showing the probability of developing any atrial arrhythmias over time (in months) in the SOCA (broken line) versus CPVA plus LALA (solid line) groups ($p = 0.62$). (From Sawhney N, Anousheh R, Chen W, Feld GK.) Circumferential pulmonary vein ablation with additional linear ablation results in an increased incidence of left atrial flutter compared to segmental pulmonary vein isolation as an initial approach to ablation of paroxysmal atrial fibrillation. *Source:* Sawhney et al., 2010 [25]. Reproduced with permission of Lippincott Williams & Wilkins.

concluded that as an initial ablation approach in patients with paroxysmal AF, more atypical left atrial flutter occurred after CPVA + LALA and fluoroscopy times were longer, compared to SOCA.

In a study by Anousheh et al. [26], 60 consecutive patients with persistent ($n = 25$) or paroxysmal ($n = 35$) AF, undergoing CPVA plus LALA at the MI and LA roof, were evaluated in a prospective, nonrandomized study. PVI was achieved in all patients, but bidirectional MI block was achieved in only 50 of 60 patients (83%). During 18 ± 5 months follow-up, 12 patients (20%) developed recurrent AF

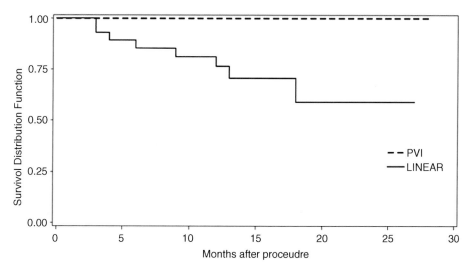

Figure 39 Kaplan–Meier curve showing the probability of developing atypical left AFL over time (in months) in the SOCA (broken line) versus CPVA plus LALA (solid line) groups ($p = 0.002$). (From Sawhney N, Anousheh R, Chen W, Feld GK.) Circumferential pulmonary vein ablation with additional linear ablation results in an increased incidence of left atrial flutter compared to segmental pulmonary vein isolation as an initial approach to ablation of paroxysmal atrial fibrillation. *Source:* Sawhney et al., 2010 [25]. Reproduced with permission of Lippincott Williams & Wilkins.

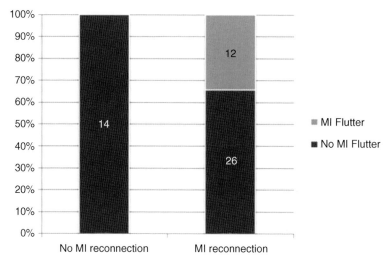

Figure 40 Bar plot demonstrating the incidence of mitral isthmus-dependent left atrial tachycardia in patients by mitral isthmus reconnection status. Recovery of mitral isthmus conduction is associated with the development of mitral isthmus-dependent left atrial tachycardia. *Source:* Sawhney et al., 2011 [27]. Reproduced with permission of Lippincott Williams & Wilkins.

and 15 (25%) developed atrial tachyarrhythmias. Patients in whom mitral isthmus block was not achieved at initial ablation had a four times higher risk of developing atrial tachyarrhythmias ($p = 0.008$, 95% CI 1.43–11.48) versus patients with mitral isthmus block. In 12 patients with atrial tachyarrhythmias undergoing repeat ablation, 22 atrial tachyarrhythmias were identified, with reentry involving the mitral isthmus in 9 patients, the LA roof in 6 and the ridge between the LA appendage and left PVs in 7. In patients with mitral isthmus block at initial ablation, the recovery of mitral isthmus conduction was seen in 8 of 13 patients undergoing repeat ablation.

In another study by Sawhney et al. [27], of 163 patients with AF who underwent CPVA plus LALA, in whom mitral isthmus and cavo-tricuspid isthmus (CTI) ablation produced bidirectional conduction block, 52 underwent repeat ablation for recurrent atrial tachyarrhythmias (AF or atypical left atrial flutter). Of these 52 patients, coronary sinus ablation was required in 48 to achieve bidirectional mitral isthmus block at the index ablation. During repeat ablation, mitral isthmus and CTI conduction was assessed in sinus rhythm. At repeat ablation, mitral isthmus conduction had recovered in 38 of 52 patients, compared to CTI conduction that recovered in only 12 of 52 patients ($p = 0.001$). At repeat ablation (Figure 40), the recurrent clinical arrhythmia in 12 patients was mitral isthmus-dependent left atrial tachycardia. The recovery of mitral isthmus conduction was associated with development of mitral isthmus-dependent left atrial tachycardia ($p = 0.01$). The authors concluded that despite using bidirectional

conduction block as a procedural end point, recovery of mitral isthmus conduction is common and may lead to atypical left atrial flutter after linear ablation for AF. The reason for greater recovery of mitral isthmus versus CTI conduction is unknown but could be due to differences in isthmus anatomy [28,29] or the lower power used for ablation in the left versus right atrium.

Summary

The role of premature atrial contractions originating in the pulmonary veins and triggering AF has been well established, as has the importance of PVI as a treatment of AF over the past 15 years. Other sources of premature beats triggering AF have certainly been described (i.e., superior vena cava, nonpulmonary vein foci in the LA, etc.), but are far less common. The methods to achieve PVI have also evolved during this time period from a SOCA approach initially to a CPVA approach with or without additional LALA. However, there is controversy in the literature regarding the most effective approach (i.e., SOCA versus CPVA) to achieve durable PVI and ensure long-term success in preventing recurrence of AF. In fact, there is no definitive, prospective, randomized study published to date, with a large enough population of patients, over an acceptable duration of follow-up, and with adequate monitoring to ensure identification of AF recurrence, which convincingly proves one method (i.e., SOCA versus CPVA) as being superior to achieve durable PVI and long-term suppression of AF. Therefore, at present it would seem prudent to perform the minimal amount of ablation necessary in patients with paroxysmal AF, in order to achieve durable PVI, minimize the risk of iatrogenic atrial tachyarrhythmias, and reduce procedure and fluoroscopy exposure time. In patients with long-standing persistent AF, performing more extensive ablation including CPVA, plus additional linear ablation, CFAE, or other driver ablation may be necessary to terminate AF and improve long-term outcome in preventing AF recurrence. However, the most appropriate approach to ablation should also be studied in this patient population, in order to prove that more extensive ablation is really necessary to achieve adequate long-term outcomes, similar to those seen in patients with paroxysmal AF.

References

1 Haïssaguerre M, Jaïs P, Shah DC, et al. Spontaneous initiation of atrial fibrillation by ectopic beats originating in the pulmonary veins. N Engl J Med. 1998;339: 659–666.

2 Haïssaguerre M, Jaïs P, Shah DC, et al. Catheter ablation of chronic atrial fibrillation targeting the reinitiating triggers. J Cardiovasc Electrophysiol. 2000;11:2–10.

3 Haïssaguerre M, Shah DC, Jaïs P, et al. Electrophysiological breakthroughs from the left atrium to the pulmonary veins. Circulation. 2000;102:2463–2465.

4 Ouyang F, Bänsch D, Ernst S, et al. Complete isolation of left atrium surrounding the pulmonary veins. Circulation. 2004;110:2090–2096.

5 Pappone C, Rosanio S, Oreto G, et al. Circumferential radiofrequency ablation of pulmonary vein ostia: a new anatomic approach for curing atrial fibrillation. Circulation. 2000;102:2619–2628.

6 Oral H, Pappone C, Chugh A, et al. Circumferential pulmonary-vein ablation for chronic atrial fibrillation. N Engl J Med. 2006;354:934–941.

7 Calkins H, Kuck KH, Cappato R, et al. Heart Rhythm Society Task Force on Catheter and Surgical Ablation of Atrial Fibrillation. 2012 HRS/EHRA/ECAS Expert Consensus Statement on Catheter and Surgical Ablation of Atrial Fibrillation: recommendations for patient selection, procedural techniques, patient management and follow-up, definitions, endpoints, and research trial design: a report of the Heart Rhythm Society (HRS) Task Force on Catheter and Surgical Ablation of Atrial Fibrillation. Developed in partnership with the European Heart Rhythm Association (EHRA), a registered branch of the European Society of Cardiology (ESC) and the European Cardiac Arrhythmia Society (ECAS); and in collaboration with the American College of Cardiology (ACC), American Heart Association (AHA), the Asia Pacific Heart Rhythm Society (APHRS), and the Society of Thoracic Surgeons (STS). Endorsed by the governing bodies of the American College of Cardiology Foundation, the American Heart Association, the European Cardiac Arrhythmia Society, the European Heart Rhythm

Association, the Society of Thoracic Surgeons, the Asia Pacific Heart Rhythm Society, and the Heart Rhythm Society. Heart Rhythm. 2012;9:632–696.

8 Tamborero D, Mont L, Nava S, et al. Incidence of pulmonary vein stenosis in patients submitted to atrial fibrillation ablation: a comparison of the selective segmental ostial ablation vs the circumferential pulmonary veins ablation. J Interv Card Electrophysiol. 2005;14: 21–25.

9 Arentz T, Weber R, Bürkle Jochem Stockinger B, et al. Small or large isolation areas around the pulmonary veins for the treatment of atrial fibrillation? Results from a prospective randomized study. Circulation. 2007;115: 3057–3063.

10 Jais P, Hocini M, Hsu LF, et al. Technique and results of linear ablation at the mitral isthmus. Circulation. 2004;110:2996–3002.

11 Hocini M, Jais P, Sanders P, et al. Techniques, evaluation, and consequences of linear block at the left atrial roof in paroxysmal atrial fibrillation: a prospective randomized study. Circulation. 2005;112:3688–3696.

12 Chugh A, Oral H, Lemola K, et al. Prevalence, mechanisms, and clinical significance of macroreentrant atrial tachycardia during and following left atrial ablation for atrial fibrillation. Heart Rhythm 2005;2:464–471.

13 Chae S, Oral H, Good E, Dey S, et al. Atrial tachycardia after circumferential pulmonary vein ablation of atrial fibrillation: mechanistic insights, results of catheter ablation, and risk factors for recurrence. J Am Coll Cardiol. 2007;50:1781–1787.

14 Matsuo S, Wright M, Knecht S, et al. Peri-mitral atrial flutter in patients with atrial fibrillation ablation. Heart Rhythm. 2010;7:2–8.

15 Oral H, Knight BP, Morady F. Left atrial flutter after segmental ostial radiofrequency catheter ablation for pulmonary vein isolation. Pacing Clin Electrophysiol. 2003;26:1417–1419.

16 Karch MR, Zrenner B, Deisenhofer I, et al. Freedom from atrial tachyarrhythmias after catheter ablation of atrial fibrillation: a randomized comparison between 2 current ablation strategies. Circulation. 2005;111:2875–2880.

17 Oral H, Scharf C, Chugh A, Hall B, et al. Catheter ablation for paroxysmal atrial fibrillation: segmental pulmonary vein ostial ablation versus left atrial ablation. Circulation. 2003;108:2355–2360.

18 Mansour M, Ruskin J, Keane D. Efficacy and safety of segmental ostial versus circumferential extra-ostial pulmonary vein isolation for atrial fibrillation. J Cardiovasc Electrophysiol. 2004;15:532–537.

19 Fiala M, Chovancík J, Nevralová R, et al. Pulmonary vein isolation using segmental versus electroanatomical circumferential ablation for paroxysmal atrial fibrillation: over 3-year results of a prospective randomized study. J Interv Card Electrophysiol. 2008;22:13–21.

20 Nilsson B, Chen X, Pehrson S, et al. Recurrence of pulmonary vein conduction and atrial fibrillation after pulmonary vein isolation for atrial fibrillation: a randomized trial of the ostial versus the extrastial ablation strategy. Am Heart J. 2006;152:537. e1–e8.

21 Kojodjojo P, O'Neill MD, Lim PB, et al. Pulmonary venous isolation by antral ablation with a large cryoballoon for treatment of paroxysmal and persistent atrial fibrillation: medium-term outcomes and non-randomised comparison with pulmonary venous isolation by radiofrequency ablation. Heart. 2010;96:1379–1384.

22 Packer DL, Kowal RC, Wheelan KR, et al. for the STOP AF Cryoablation Investigators. Cryoballoon ablation of pulmonary veins for paroxysmal atrial fibrillation: first results of the North American Arctic Front (STOP AF) pivotal trial. J Am Coll Cardiol. 2013;61:1713–1723.

23 Neumann T, Vogt J, Schumacher B, et al. Circumferential pulmonary vein isolation with the cryoballoon technique results from a prospective 3-center study. J Am Coll Cardiol. 2008;52:273–278.

24 Knecht S, Hocini M, Wright M, et al. Left atrial linear lesions are required for successful treatment of persistent atrial fibrillation. Eur Heart J. 2008;29:2359–2366.

25 Sawhney N, Anousheh R, Chen W, et al. Circumferential pulmonary vein ablation with additional linear ablation results in an increased incidence of left atrial flutter compared with segmental pulmonary vein isolation as an initial approach to ablation of paroxysmal atrial fibrillation. Circ Arrhythm Electrophysiol. 2010;3: 243–248.

26 Anousheh R, Sawhney NS, Panutich M, et al. Effect of mitral isthmus block on development of atrial tachycardia following ablation for atrial fibrillation. PACE (Pacing and Clinical Electrophysiology) 33:460–468;2010.

27 Sawhney N, Anand K, Robertson CE, et al. Recovery of mitral isthmus conduction leads to the development of macro-reentrant tachycardia after left atrial linear ablation for atrial fibrillation. Circ Arrhythm Electrophysiol. 2011;4:832–837.

28 Cabrera JA, Ho SY, Climent V, et al. The architecture of the left lateral atrial wall: a particular anatomic region with implications for ablation of atrial fibrillation. Eur Heart J. 2008;29:356–362.

29 Wongcharoen W, Tsao HM, Wu MH, et al. Morphologic characteristics of the left atrial appendage, roof, and septum: implications for the ablation of atrial fibrillation. J Cardiovasc Electrophysiol. 2006;17:951–956.

CHAPTER 14

How to select target sites in electrogram-guided ablation: options, techniques, and results

Anand N. Ganesan, Dennis H. Lau, &
Prashanthan Sanders

Centre for Heart Rhythm Disorders (CHRD), South Australian Health and Medical Research Institute (SAHMRI), University of Adelaide and Royal Adelaide Hospital, Adelaide, SA, Australia

Controversy: Electrogram-guided ablation: valuable technique
Naoya Oketani & Koonlawee Nademanee

Controversy: Electrogram-guided ablation: limited contribution to successful outcome
Hatice Duygu Bas, Kazim Baser & Hakan Oral

Introduction

Catheter ablation has become established as a potential curative therapy for the treatment of atrial fibrillation (AF) [1] with pulmonary vein isolation (PVI) emerging as the most consistent and important ablative strategy [1]. PVI targets the dominant source of triggers that in some cases also represents the substrate maintaining AF. The most commonly used approaches rely on the circumferential application of radiofrequency lesions around the pulmonary vein ostia [2–5]. With a defined electrophysiological approach, this has been a successful approach in most patients with paroxysmal AF [6].

Electrogram (EGM)-guided approaches to AF ablation have emerged as a significant alternative conceptual paradigm over the past decade [7,8]. In contrast to

Practical Guide to Catheter Ablation of Atrial Fibrillation, Second Edition. Edited by Jonathan S. Steinberg, Pierre Jaïs and Hugh Calkins.
© 2016 John Wiley & Sons, Ltd. Published 2016 by John Wiley & Sons, Ltd.

targeting a fixed anatomical structure – the pulmonary veins – the aim of these EGM-guided ablation is to modify the fibrillatory substrate of the atrium to prevent the maintenance of fibrillation, eluding to the potential for an individualized approach [7]. EGM-guided ablation techniques may be broadly classified into strategies aimed to target signals with specific characteristics in the time domain (complex fractionated atrial electrograms (CFAE)) [7] or in the frequency domain (dominant frequency (DF)) [8]. In this chapter, we discuss the genesis, technique, and clinical results of EGM-guided ablation approaches and their influence on contemporary clinical practice.

Mechanisms of atrial fibrillation

The ongoing debate regarding the AF mechanism is relevant insofar as it provides the theoretical framework to the clinical practice of EGM-guided ablation. AF has been considered to be the consequence of a complex interplay of triggers and substrate [9]. Clinical and experimental evidence has suggested that the predominant triggers for AF episodes arise via ectopic impulses from the pulmonary veins [2,4,10,11], with a subsidiary role for AF triggering from other structures including the superior vena cava [12,13], and coronary sinus [14]. It is also clear that AF arises in the context of electrophysiological and structural remodelling arising from clinical risk factors including aging [15], heart failure [16], valvular heart disease [17,18], sinus node disease [19,20], coronary artery disease [21], hypertension [22,23], atrial septal defects, obesity [24], and obstructive sleep apnoea [25,26].

A number of theoretical mechanisms have been proposed to explain cardiac electrical wave propagation in AF [27]. The multiple wavelet theory postulates that AF is maintained by the precession of a discrete number of electrical waves, which arise as a consequence of inhomogeneities in electrical refractoriness [28–30]. The principal alternative hypothesis has been that AF is maintained by predominantly focal drivers, whereby arrhythmia maintenance occurs by a single or small number of sources that drive ongoing AF [31]. A series of studies by Jalifé and coworkers have demonstrated that these focal drivers are rapidly spinning local reentrant circuits called *rotors* that emit curved *spiral waves* [32,33]. In this theory, the disorganization and irregularity that are the hallmarks of AF arise as a consequence of the interaction of these waves with functional or anatomical boundaries [34,35].

A paradox of the clinical practice of EGM guided ablation is that ablation techniques have largely evolved in the clinical electrophysiology laboratory ahead of mechanistic understanding, because the complexity of AF has until recently prevented direct understanding of the arrhythmia mechanism in individual patients. Contemporary EGM-guided ablation has thus developed as a collection of substrate-based approaches implemented empirically around the common end point of achieving AF termination [36].

The clinical importance of AF termination

The goal of EGM-guided strategies in AF ablation is to achieve intraprocedural AF termination [37,38]. AF termination has been regarded as a critical end point of EGM-guided approaches because (i) AF termination has been interpreted to be occurring as a consequence of the destruction of regions important to the maintenance of arrhythmia [39,40] and (ii) AF termination during ablation has been associated with improved clinical outcomes [41], although this finding is not uniform in the literature [42]. O'Neill et al. in a prospective study utilizing a stepwise approach with the aim of achieving AF termination in 153 persistent AF patients found a dramatically lower incidence of recurrent AF at long-term follow-up in patients achieving intraprocedural AF termination (5% recurrence in AF termination patients versus 39% recurrence in those without AF termination, $P < 0.001$) [41].

AF termination has been interpreted to imply that either critical driving sources [40] or regions of critical substrate [7] have been targeted. Analysis of electrograms at sites of AF termination has influenced EGM-guided ablation strategies. Takahashi et al. systematically analyzed EGMs at sites of AF termination in 40 ablation patients [43]. A number of variables were assessed including (1) the percentage of continuous electrical activity, (2) the bipolar voltage, (3) the dominant frequency, (4) the fractionation index, (5) the mean absolute value of derivatives of electrograms, (6) the local cycle length, and (7) the presence of a temporal gradient of activation [43]. Of these, only the percentage and the presence of a continuous electrical activity and the presence of a temporal gradient of activation were independent predictors of AF slowing and/or termination ($P = 0.016$ and $P = 0.038$, respectively).

Complex fractionated atrial electrogram ablation

Definitions and Development of the CFAE technique

The definition of CFAE as originally developed as ablation technique included "atrial electrograms that are: (1) fractionated and composed of two deflections or more and/or have a perturbation of the baseline with continuous deflections from a prolonged activation complex as shown in the atrial septum in Figure 1A; or (2) atrial electrograms with a very short cycle length ($\leq$120 ms) Figure 1B [7]." An additional criterion considered important by Nademanee was that CFAEs were typically low-voltage signals with an amplitude range between 0.06 and 0.250 mV [7].

CFAE mapping was originally implemented as the biatrial nonfluoroscopic mapping in spontaneous or induced AF using the electroanatomic mapping system CARTO (CARTO, Biosense Webster Inc, CA, USA) [7]. This series included $n = 121$ patients, with $n = 64$ chronic AF patients [7]. Selected CFAE sites meeting the empirically defined selection criteria were tagged and targeted for ablation, although the order of ablation was not prespecified Figure 2 [7]. Ablation confined solely to the area of CFAE resulted in termination of AF in 95% (115/121) of patients (although 32% received concomitant intraprocedural ibutilide). In follow-up, 91% of patients were reported as free of atrial arrhythmia and symptoms 1 year after the index ablation procedure [7].

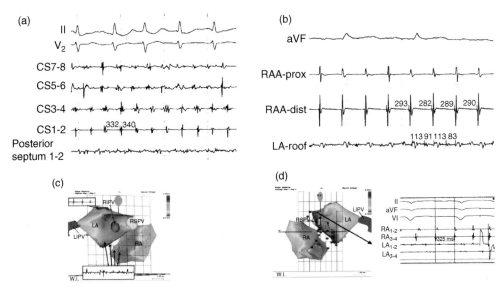

Figure 1 Definition and example of complex fractionated atrial electrogram (CFAE) ablation. (a) Example of CFAE EGM from over the posterior septum meeting CFAE criteria due to continuous fractionation. (b) Example CFAEEGM from LA roof with EGMs with short cycle length compared to rest of atrium. (c) Example EGMs and CARTO electroanatomic maps from a permanent AF patient. CFAE electrograms are seen at RA septum electrodes 1–2 and 3–4. The pink dots on the CARTO map correspond to tagged areas of CFAE, which in this case are along the septum. LAO view electroanatomic map showing ablation points in the region corresponding to high CFAE. LA 3–4 represents CFAE along the left side of the septum. *Source:* Nademanee et al., 2004 [7]. Reproduced with permission of Elsevier.

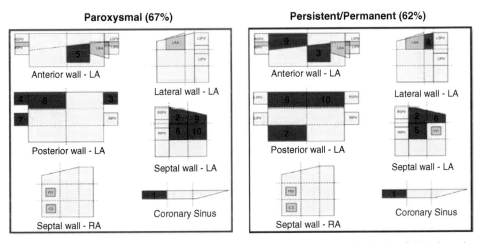

Figure 2 Locations of CFAE. Nademanee and coworkers have suggested a nonrandom distribution of CFAE throughout the atria, with specifically a preponderance of CFAE not being noted at the following sites: proximal coronary sinus, SVC–RA junction, septal wall anterior to right superior pulmonary vein and right inferior pulmonary vein, anterior wall medial to left atrial appendage, and posterosuperior wall medial to left superior pulmonary vein [62,99].

Mechanisms of CFAE

The remarkable clinical results achieved with empirical CFAE ablation spurred significant basic science interest in potential mechanisms for CFAE, to explain the high rates of termination observed by the Nademanee group. The original postulated rationale for CFAE was that these signals were the analogs of fractionated EGMs identified during intraoperative mapping studies [7], where CFAEs were found to occur in areas of slow conduction and/or pivot points where wavelets turn around at the end of arcs of a functional block [30]. To this original explanation for CFAE, additional putative mechanisms have been postulated, including (i) CFAE occurring as a consequence of action potential shortening as a consequence of activation of cholinergic local ganglionated plexi of the autonomic nervous system [44,45] and (ii) CFAE forming at the boundary zones of regions activated by high-frequency rotors [34,35,46] or in relation to the area of meander of a locally stable rotor [47,48].

Implementation of the CFAE in the electrophysiology laboratory

Technical considerations

An issue that needs to be considered in the analysis of studies utilizing CFAE mapping in AF is that of CFAE definition and recording conditions [49]. The original CFAE description utilized a definition with hybrid of subjectively defined qualitative and quantitative elements. The original implementation of CFAE involved sequential mapping of patients in AF [7]. For patients arriving in sinus rhythm to the electrophysiology laboratory, AF was induced with rapid pacing, if necessary, supplemented by isoproterenol infusion. Electrophysiology was in the bipolar mode with bandpass filtered from 30–500 Hz [7]. Mapping was performed in the CARTO navigation system, with sites visually assessed by the operator as conforming to CFAE definition tagged, which the operator then utilized for the purposes of ablation [7].

Techniques for automated identification of CFAE

A number of alternative algorithms have been implemented to automate the process of CFAE site selection during AF ablation, with the objective of improving the consistency and reproducibility. To achieve this goal, automated algorithms to assist identification and targeting of CFAE sites have been integrated into the two electroanatomic mapping systems in widespread clinical use (CARTO or EnSite Navx, St Jude Medical, MN, USA). Each of these algorithms has been systematically validated by expert observers and evaluated in clinical studies of AF ablation [50–53].

The CFAE identification algorithm implemented in the CARTO system measures a number of parameters. The interval confidence level (ICL) measures the number intervals between tagged local intrinsic deflections within a defined recording period, in a 2.5 s recording period [54]. The algorithm operates by initially identifying all peaks falling within a prespecified voltage range (typically 0.05–2 mV), followed by taking an average of time intervals in the range of 50 m–120 ms [54]. The assumption of the algorithm is that the greater number of tagged deflections, the more reliable its categorization as CFAE [54]. As an alternative algorithm, the average interpotential interval refers to the average of intervals between successive tagged deflections exceeding 50 ms. CFAE is typically defined by $ICL \geq 5$ and $AIPI < 100$ ms [54]. Another alternative is the shortest coupling length (SCI), which measures the shortest interval in milliseconds of all intervals between consecutive CFAE complexes [54].

CFE mean measures fractionation as the average time duration between consecutive deflections and is implemented in the NavX system (St Jude Medical). For detection, the deflection must (1) exceed an adaptive "peak-to-peak sensitivity" noise threshold (typically 0.03–0.05 mV) [52,55], (2) possess a "downstroke" morphology in which the leading local maximum and the trailing local minimum amplitude occurs within a time "duration" set to avoid far-field event detection [52,55], and (3) exceed a "refractory" period from the previous detection (typically 30 ms) [52,55]. When all criteria are met, a yellow "tick-mark" is placed at the instant of maximum negative slope. The mean local cycle length is calculated and plotted onto an atrial anatomical map as a color-coded shell [52].

CFAE ablation as primary strategy or adjunctive to PVI

CFAE ablation was originally implemented as a standalone alternative strategy to PVI for AF ablation [7]. In general, however, CFAE ablation has often been implemented as an adjunctive strategy to PVI, either performed before or after PVI in patients with nonparoxysmal AF [56]. In terms of patient selection, Nademanee has advocated CFAE as the primary ablation technique for both paroxysmal and persistent AF [54]. For paroxysmal AF, ablation elimination of CFAE with the end point of noninducibility has been the nominated end point [54]. For nonparoxysmal AF, the end point of ablation has been considered as AF termination [54].

Spatiotemporal stability of CFAE locations

A number of studies have examined the issue of spatial and temporal stability of mapped CFAE location [49]. These studies have used a number of different approaches to examine the evolution of CFAE sites over time, with a variety of results and interpretations. Temporal stability is critical from a practical point of view because it enables sequential mapping of CFAE sites prior to ablation. Approaches to examine temporal stability have predominantly utilized sequentially acquired maps during AF. Some studies have concluded that temporal stability is present during sequentially acquired CFAE maps [57–59]. On the other hand, others have concluded that significant variability exists in CFAE sites over time [49,60].

In terms of spatial stability, Nademanee and cow-orkers have specified several key regions as having increased preponderance of CFAE. These include proximal coronary sinus, SVC–RA junction, septal wall anterior to the right superior pulmonary vein and the right inferior pulmonary vein, anterior wall medial to the left atrial appendage, and posterosuperior wall medial to the left superior pulmonary vein [29].

An additional consideration is of differences in CFAE between paroxysmal and nonparoxysmal AF. CFAE in persistent AF tends to be morphologically more fractionated and complex compared to persist-ent AF. Stiles et al. identified a significantly lower CFE mean in persistent AF patients compared to paroxys-mal AF [55]. Ciaccio et al. similarly identified shorter interdeflection intervals in persistent AF CFAEs, although there was greater intrinsic morphologic EGM variation during paroxysmal than persistent AF [61].

Refining relevant CFAE subsets

A number of studies have utilized different approaches to differentiate subsets of CFAE poten-tially responsible for greater clinical effect, in an attempt to distinguish the so-called "passive" CFAE from "active" CFAE involved in the AF driving mech-anism. Drug therapy including intraprocedural ibuti-lide, flecainide, or nifekalant has been described as an empirical approach by Nademanee [62] and system-atically studied by others as an approach to distinguish potential "nondriver" passive CFAE regions [63,64]. Antiarrhythmic drugs have been shown to decrease maximum and mean cycle lengths and proportion of left atrial CFAE [64]. This has been postulated to enable more targeted CFAE ablation in persistent AF, potentially leading to rapid termination, and the use of intravenous ibutilide to facilitate persistent AF termi-nation by CFAE ablation is the subject of randomized investigation [65].

Hunter et al. used a qualitative scale to subcatego-rize CFAE over a five-level scale, where grade 1 represented the most fractionated and grade 5 the least fractionated CFAE [66,67]. In a small trial with $n = 20$ patients randomized to the order of CFAE ablation, AF cycle length increased significantly more for grade 1 CFAE compared to lower grades of CFAE, suggesting an intrinsic hierarchy of CFAE in terms of clinical effect [66].

Nonetheless, residual challenges remain with respect to identification of the optimal CFAE subsets. It seems likely that a multitude of factors and

mechanisms may contribute to CFAE that can be identified in practice. Narayan et al. using monophasic action potential recordings coregistered with CFAE suggested a variety of aetiologies for CFAE including localized drivers, short-term heart rate accelerations, and far-field signals [68]. It is also clear that in many instances, although CFAE is regarded as a form of "substrate" ablation, myocardium associated with CFAE may have relatively normal or preserved elec-trophysiological properties in sinus rhythm [69,70], suggesting that these signals may in many cases have a functional origin.

Clinical results of CFAE ablation

Wide variation in the clinical results of CFAE ablation has been noted in clinical studies. After the initial positive results of Nademanee, Oral et al. reported the results of adjunctive CFAE ablation in 100 patients with chronic AF [71]. The study protocol involves sequential CFAE ablation in the pulmonary veins and their antra, followed by CFAE elimination in the left atrial septum, roof, anterior and posterior left atrial walls, and posterior mitral annulus [71]. Acute AF termination was achieved in 16/100 patients, with only 33/100 patients in sinus rhythm at a mean of 14 ± 7 months of follow-up [71]. In patients with recurrent arrhythmia, the lack of isolation of the pulmonary veins was considered to be an important mechanism by the authors [71].

Following on from this study, today CFAE ablation is predominantly implemented as an adjunctive strat-egy to PVI, with or without linear left atrial abla-tion [72]. STAR-AF, the single randomized study examining the role of adjunctive CFAE ablation plus PVI, PVI alone, or CFAE alone suggested improved outcomes with PVI plus CFAE ablation together [56].

A number of clinical studies have investigated the clinical impact of adjunctive CFAE ablation on PVI. Two systematic reviews collating results of random-ized controlled trials utilizing adjunctive CFAE have had positive results in nonparoxysmal AF [73,74]. Li et al. performed a meta-analysis including 7 trials with 622 patients comparing PVI plus CFAE to PVI alone [73]. The overall results of the study showed that adjunctive CFAE ablation yielded a small but statistically significant increase in the relative risk (RR) of sinus rhythm maintenance (RR 1.17, $P = 0.03$) [73]. In the three trials including paroxysmal AF patients, no benefit was seen in terms of increasing sinus rhythm maintenance (RR 1.04 95%CI 0.92–1.18) [73]. In the five trials reporting nonpar-oxysmal AF outcome, there was significant benefit with adjunctive CFAE ablation (RR 1.35 95%CI: 1.04–1.75) [73]. However, this finding of net benefit was not uniform, with at least two trials showing no benefit of adjunctive CFAE ablation in NPAF [75,76]. The results of a meta-analysis by Hayward et al. yielded very similar results to that of Li et al. [74]. This study also identified that adjunctive CFAE ablation with PVI came at the cost of increased fluoroscopy time (14 ± 8 min, $P < 0.001$) and procedure time (43 ± 19 min, $P = 0.001$) [74].

CFAE ablation: conclusions

The role of CFAE ablation as an EGM-guided ablation strategy is an area of ongoing scientific and clinical debate. In the recently published Consensus Statement on the Catheter and Surgical Ablation of AF, CFAE ablation was routinely employed by 50% of Task Force writing committee members [1]. Significant questions remain as to the utility and reproducibility and specificity of this form of EGM-guided ablation, and ongoing investigation will be necessary to determine the optimal role of this technique in AF ablation patients.

Dominant frequency ablation

Spectral analysis and dominant frequency (DF) mapping has been the major alternative EGM-guided approach that has significantly influenced AF ablation. Dominant frequency analysis utilizing the Fast Fourier transform (FFT) has been applied to AF to understand the pathophysiology of the arrhythmia and as a potential mapping tool to assist localization of the drivers of AF. In contrast to CFAE, which is considered as a form of time domain analysis, DF mapping is a frequency domain analysis.

The fundamental concept of DF mapping as applied to AF is that the bipolar EGM signals recorded can be considered as the sum of sinusoids with different frequencies, amplitude, and phase [77]. The dominant frequency is the frequency of the most prominent sinusoidal waveform, and can be considered as the surrogate for the fastest local activation rate [77].

Dominant frequency analysis was first applied to AF in the seminal studies of Jalifé and coworkers. FFT applied to optical action potential and bipolar voltage recordings demonstrated a left atrium-to-right atrium frequency gradient in the cholinergic sheep AF model [78], a finding replicated in humans [79]. In the same model, DF analysis was able to localize a single driving source in the posterior left atrium [33]. In optical mapping studies, there was a strong correlation between the angular frequency of driving rotors and the DF on the pseudo-ECG of corresponding AF episodes [33]. This critical finding laid the foundation for clinical studies using DF mapping to localize drivers in human AF.

Sanders et al. applied the technique of DF mapping in $n = 32$ AF ablation patients [8]. Fast Fourier transform was retrospectively applied to bipolar EGMs acquired in AF patients prior to ablation. DF was defined as the frequency with the maximum amplitude in the EGM's power spectrum Figure 3 [8]. The study identified clear differences in the spatial distribution of DF between paroxysmal and persistent AF patients Figure 4. In PAF, DF sites were predominantly localized to the pulmonary veins [8]. In nonparoxysmal AF, DF sites were more widely distributed throughout the body of the atrium. In PAF patients, in this retrospective analysis, ablation localized at sites of high DF was associated with AF slowing and termination [8]. The association between high DF sites and AF slowing or termination was not clearly observed in nonparoxysmal AF patients [8].

Techniques for dominant frequency analysis in the electrophysiology laboratory

Fourier analysis has been highly influential in the study of clinical AF recordings in the electrophysiology laboratory. The most common application has been for the determination of DF as an estimate of the local activation rate in AF. The mathematical background to the utilization of Fourier analysis in AF recordings has previously been reviewed [77]. The Fast Fourier transform is most commonly utilized to bipolar EGM recordings acquired prior to ablation. In DF studies, bipolar EGMs are commonly acquired at a high sampling frequency (≥ 1 kHz), bandpass filtered (typically 30–500 Hz).

The first preprocessing step that is usually applied is rectification that converts the multiphasic bipolar EGMs to monophasic signals [77]. Signals are then typically edge tapered by multiplication with a Hanning window to minimize the effects of edge segments on the Fourier power spectrum [77]. The next step is the application of the Fast Fourier transform. The Sanders et al. study used a 4096 point transform, yielding a frequency resolution of 0.24 Hz, a standard that has been widely used in DF mapping in AF [8].

The Fourier transform yields a power spectrum, in which the frequency is plotted on the x-axis against signal amplitude on the y-axis [77]. The Sanders et al. study used a second bandpass step to limit frequencies of interest to 3–15 Hz, as these were considered the frequencies corresponding to physiological activation rates [8]. The last step used to select the dominant frequency is to limit DF sites to those where the ratio

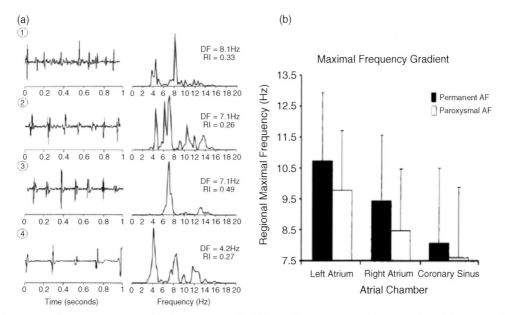

Figure 3 Dominant frequency analysis. (a) Spectral analysis of bipolar electrogram signals from a patient with paroxysmal AF. The left panels show example bipolar electrograms. The right panels show corresponding power spectra. Each site has a distinct dominant frequency (DF) and regularity index (RI). The highest dominant frequency occurs in the top panel, which was from an electrode in the right inferior pulmonary vein. Panels 2 and 3 are from the DF sites in the right superior pulmonary vein and left superior pulmonary vein. Panel 4 is from the posterior right atrium. (b) Frequency gradient. A left-to-right frequency gradient is present across atrial chambers in paroxysmal and persistent AF. Source: Sanders et al., 2005 [8]. Reproduced with permission of Lippincott Williams & Wilkins.

of the spectral power at the DF and its adjacent frequencies to overall spectral power in the 3–15 Hz band (the regularity index) exceeds 0.2 [8].

Dominant frequency analysis in AF
Dominant frequency analysis has a tremendous influence on the analysis of AF. DF analysis was utilized to demonstrate a left-to-right gradient suggestive of a predominance of drivers in the left atrium, particularly in paroxysmal AF [79]. Circumferential pulmonary vein and CFAE ablation have both been associated with a decrease in DF, with decreased DF associated with reduced AF recurrence after ablation [36,80]. DF has been correlated with LA pressure [81], epicardial fat [82], and the locations of cardiac ganglionated plexi [83].

Relationship of DF sites to CFAE
The relationship between sites of CFAE and DF sites in AF is at present incompletely understood. Basic experiments have suggested that electrogram fractionation may occur at the edge of regions of high dominant frequency [35] or adjacent to the central region of meandering in the vicinity of locally stable rotors [47,48]. Clinical studies have suggested a

modest correlation within individual patients between CFAE and DF [55,84], but not when analyzed on a point-by-point basis [55,65,85].

Spatiotemporal stability of DF locations
In terms of applicability to mapping during ablation, a significant issue for consideration is that of spatiotemporal stability of mapped DF locations, and the presence of a surrounding centrifugal gradient around putative AF drivers. Sanders et al. showed that DF was stable for short periods during comparisons of the first and second segments of short (10 s) recordings. Krummen et al. were able to demonstrate centrifugal gradients surrounding the sites of high DF [86]. Others, however, have identified significant instability of DF during prolonged basket catheter recordings [60,87], as well as the absence of a centrifugal gradient around DF sites [87].

Limitations of dominant frequency analysis
Dominant frequency analysis is vulnerable to changes in EGM properties other than activation rate. Dominant frequencies analysis may be significantly

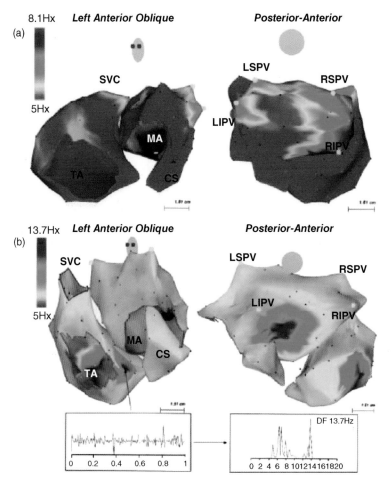

Figure 4 Example dominant frequency maps in paroxysmal and permanent AF. (a) Dominant frequency map of a patient in paroxysmal AF. The maximal DF in blue is in the right inferior pulmonary vein, which was the site of eventual termination of AF during ablation. (b) DF of a patient in permanent AF. The dominant frequencies are higher than in paroxysmal AF patient, with many sites of high DF located in the body of the atrium. Example high DF electrogram and power spectrum are shown in the lower panels. *Source:* Sander et al., 2005 [8]. Reproduced with permission of Lippincott Williams & Wilkins.

impacted by frequency variation, combined amplitude and frequency variation, and changes in phase [88]. Other factors, such as split potentials and far-field ventricular potentials, may interfere with results. Some studies have suggested that dominant frequency analysis may not accurately correlate with AF cycle length in time domain analysis [89]. The Jalifé group has, however, suggested that the failure to find an accurate correlation between AF cycle length and dominant frequency analysis may be related to methodological considerations [90].

Impact of ablation at high DF sites

Although DF mapping has been tremendously influential in terms of informing the mechanistic understanding of AF, in fact, only two studies have prospectively evaluated the impact of DF-targeted ablation. These have had widely discrepant results. Atienza et al. utilized real-time DF mapping to target sites during ablation of persistent AF patients, followed by circumferential pulmonary vein isolation. Ablation of high DF regions was associated with a reduction in the left-to-right DF gradient, and reduction in DF following ablation was associated with a reduced risk of AF recurrence [91]. AF termination was achieved in 72% of paroxysmal AF patients, but only 11% of persistent AF patients [91]. In contrast, Verma and coworkers prospectively applied DF mapping in 30 persistent AF patients. AF termination occurred in only 2/30 patients [65].

Table 1 Studies applying different approaches for electrogram-guided ablation.

Study	Patient population/study design	Approach	Results
Nademanee et al. 2004 [7]	Paroxysmal ($n = 57$) and chronic ($n = 64$) AF, case series	Intervention/comparator: Ablation of CFAE according to operator-defined criteria. No PVI performed End point: Freedom from atrial arrhythmia Follow-up: 1 year Monitoring for recurrence: 3 monthly clinic follow-up	91% 1-year freedom from atrial arrhythmia including patients with multiple procedures
Verma et al. [75]	Paroxysmal ($n = 120$) and nonparoxysmal AF ($n = 80$), case: control	Intervention/comparator: with or without adjuvant ablation of anterior LA CFAEs. End point: Freedom from AF or atypical flutter Follow-up: 12 months Monitoring for recurrence: Rhythm transmitters for 3 months, then clinic visit and Holter monitoring every 3 months	Adjunctive CFAE offered no benefit in paroxysmal AF (87% success with CFAE, 85% without CFAE, $p =$ NS). Adjunctive CFAE offered benefit in NPAF, (82% success with CFAE versus 72% without CFAE, $P = 0.047$)
Nademanee and coworker [99]	AF patients with high-risk substrate ($n = 674$), Paroxysmal AF ($n = 254$), NPAF ($n = 420$)	Intervention/comparator: Ablation of operator defined CFAE sites on nonfluoroscopically acquired CARTO maps, with end point of conversion to sinus rhythm or elimination of CFAE End point: Freedom from atrial tachyarrhythmia Follow-up: Mean follow-up 836 days Monitoring for recurrence: 3 monthly clinic follow-up with annual Holter monitoring	517/654 patients were in sinus rhythm (81.4%) with 310 patients undergoing more than 1 procedure
Verma et al. [52]	Paroxysmal ($n = 42$ and persistent ($n = 28$) AF, case: control	Intervention/comparator: PVAI with or without CFAE ablation End point: Freedom from atrial arrhythmia Follow-up: 13 months	Adjunctive CFAE led to single-procedure 83% success versus 71% in matched controls who had PVAI alone ($P = 0.045$)
Elayi et al. [96]	Permanent AF ($n = 144$), randomized controlled trial	Intervention/comparator: CPVA or PVAI with or without CFAE ablation End point: Freedom from AF/AT Follow-up: Mean 16 months Monitoring for Recurrence:	Ablation strategy combining PVAI with CFAE maintained highest success (61% in sinus rhythm versus 40% with PVAI versus 11% with CPVA, $P < 0.001$
Oral et al. 2009 [76]	Persistent AF not terminated by PVAI ($n = 119$), randomized controlled trial	Intervention/Comparator: PVAI with or without CFAE ablation End point: Freedom from atrial arrhythmia Follow-up: Mean 10 months. Monitoring for Recurrence:	No benefit of adjunctive CFAE versus PVAI alone ($P = 0.84$)

(continued)

Table 1   (*Continued*)

Study	Patient population/study design	Approach	Results
Lin et al. [72]	Nonparoxysmal AF, consecutive trial (*n* = 60)	Clinic visits with event monitor at 6 months Intervention/comparator: PVI plus linear ablation with or without CFAE End point: Freedom from atrial arrhythmia Monitoring for recurrence: Clinic visits with an event monitor at 6 months	Adjunctive CFAE ablation did offer clinical benefit over PVI plus linear ablation (*P* = 0.035)
Deisenhofer et al. [97]	Paroxysmal AF (*n* = 98)	Intervention/comparator: PVI with or without CFAE End point: Freedom from atrial tachyarrhythmia Follow-up: Mean 19 months Monitoring for recurrence: 7 day Holter at 3 months	Adjunctive CFAE did not reach statistical significance in this population (*P* = 0.08)
Di Biase et al. [98]	Paroxysmal AF	Intervention comparator: PVAI with or without CFAE End point: Freedom from atrial arrhythmia Follow-up: 12 months Monitoring for recurrence: Event recorder for 5 months, 48 h Holter every 3 months	No difference observed between PVAI and PVAI plus CFAE (*P* = NS) in terms of freedom from atrial arrhythmia
Verma et al. [56]	Paroxysmal AF (high burden, *n* = 43) and persistent AF (*n* = 23)	Intervention/comparator: PVI with or without CFAE End point: Freedom from AF > 30 s, freedom from atrial arrhythmia Follow-up: 12 months Monitoring for recurrence: ECG and 48 h Holter at 3,6,12 months, with additional monitoring if symptomatic	PVI plus CFAE had a higher freedom from AF (74%) compared to PVI alone (48%) and CFE alone (29%) (*P* = 0.004)

Source: Adapted with permission from Ref. [74].

DF ablation: conclusions

Dominant frequency ablation has emerged as a potential ablation strategy from basic studies demonstrating the utility of this technique in identification of AF sources in experimental models. The technique has been widely used as an analytical tool to understand clinical AF, but to date limited investigation has been prospectively performed to determine the utility of this form of EGM-guided ablation in the clinical electrophysiology laboratory. At present, DF ablation remains an investigational tool in AF ablation (see Tables 1 and 2).

Emerging techniques in EGM-guided ablation

Shannon entropy mapping

Shannon entropy (ShEn) mapping is a new technique utilizing the bipolar EGM to enable localization of AF rotors [92]. ShEn mapping utilizes a fundamental property of the bipolar EGM, namely, its direction dependence. The basic hypothesis of ShEn mapping is that the spatial uncertainty of wave front direction in the pivot zone could lead to information uncertainty in bipolar EGMs from this region [92]. To quantify information certainty, Shannon entropy is utilized.

Table 2 Results of selected studies utilizing DF ablation.

Study	Patient population/ study design	Approach	Results
Atienza et al. 2004	Paroxysmal ($n = 32$), persistent ($n = 18$)	Intervention/comparator: Ablation of dominant frequency sites ablated real-time in CARTO-XP, with sequential PVI performed. End point: Freedom from atrial arrhythmia Follow-up: 1 year Monitoring for recurrence: 3 monthly clinic follow-up	1-year freedom from atrial arrhythmia 75% for paroxysmal AF and 50% for persistent AF
Verma et al. 2011	Persistent AF ($n = 50$)	Intervention/comparator: DF ablation plus PVAI compared to PVAI ablation End point: Freedom from atrial arrhythmia Follow-up: 12 months Monitoring for recurrence: Clinic visit and Holter monitor every 3 months	Adjunctive DF ablation (57% success) offered no benefit to PVAI alone (60% success). 2/30 patients in DF ablation group had acute AF termination

ShEn quantifies the distribution of information within a bipolar EGM's amplitude histogram [93]. The paradigm involved is that high ShEn is associated with the pivot of the rotor and low ShEn with regions away from the pivot [92]. To date, ShEn has been shown to localize rotors in simulated model rotors and experimental systems, but is awaiting clinical evaluation [92].

Waveform similarity indices

Waveform coherence techniques have developed by Ravelli et al. [94]. These methods calculate the morphological similarity between all bipolar atrial activation deflections in a bipolar EGM recording. Using this method, Ravelli et al. identified repetitive sources of activation in the pulmonary veins, SVC, and anterior right atrium in persistent AF patients [94]. Lin et al. utilized a modified similarity index-based approach for selective CFAE targeting in $n = 119$ persistent AF patients, with an association between high CFAE EGM similarity and AF termination [95].

Conclusions

EGM-guided ablation has had a tremendous influence on contemporary clinical ablation practice in AF ablation, although it has not been universally adopted by all centers. A number of techniques have been utilized for EGM-guided ablation, with significant

divergence in clinical results. The mechanistic underpinnings for CFAE are similarly unclear, with a variety of explanations postulated to explain CFAE. The optimal technique and strategy for EGM-guided ablation in AF ablation procedures will require further investigations.

References

1 Calkins H, Kuck KH, Cappato R, Brugada J, Camm AJ, Chen SA, et al. HRS/EHRA/ECAS expert consensus statement on catheter and surgical ablation of atrial fibrillation: recommendations for patient selection, procedural techniques, patient management and follow-up, definitions, end points, and research trial design: a report of the Heart Rhythm Society (HRS) Task Force on Catheter and Surgical Ablation of Atrial Fibrillation. Heart Rhythm. 2012;9(4):632–696 e21.

2 Haissaguerre M, Jais P, Shah DC, Arentz T, Kalusche D, Takahashi A, et al. Catheter ablation of chronic atrial fibrillation targeting the reinitiating triggers. J Cardiovasc Electrophysiol. 2000;11(1):2–10.

3 Haissaguerre M, Jais P, Shah DC, Garrigue S, Takahashi A, Lavergne T, et al. Electrophysiological end point for catheter ablation of atrial fibrillation initiated from multiple pulmonary venous foci. Circulation. 2000; 101(12):1409–1417.

4 Haissaguerre M, Jais P, Shah DC, Takahashi A, Hocini M, Quiniou G, et al. Spontaneous initiation of atrial

fibrillation by ectopic beats originating in the pulmonary veins. N Engl J Med. 1998;339(10):659–666.

5 Kanj MH, Wazni O, Fahmy T, Thal S, Patel D, Elay C, et al. Pulmonary vein antral isolation using an open irrigation ablation catheter for the treatment of atrial fibrillation: a randomized pilot study. J Am Coll Cardiol. 2007;49(15):1634–1641.

6 Ganesan AN, Shipp NJ, Brooks AG, Kuklik P, Lau DH, Lim HS, et al. Long-term outcomes of catheter ablation of atrial fibrillation: a systematic review and meta-analysis. J Am Heart Assoc. 2013;2(2):e004549.

7 Nademanee K, McKenzie J, Kosar E, Schwab M, Sunsaneewitayakul B, Vasavakul T, et al. A new approach for catheter ablation of atrial fibrillation: mapping of the electrophysiologic substrate. J Am Coll Cardiol. 2004; 43(11):2044–2053.

8 Sanders P, Berenfeld O, Hocini M, Jais P, Vaidyanathan R, Hsu LF, et al. Spectral analysis identifies sites of high-frequency activity maintaining atrial fibrillation in humans. Circulation. 2005;112(6):789–797.

9 Nattel S, Burstein B, Dobrev D. Atrial remodeling and atrial fibrillation: mechanisms and implications. Circ Arrhythm Electrophysiol. 2008;1(1):62–73.

10 Haissaguerre M, Shah DC, Jais P, Hocini M, Yamane T, Deisenhofer I, et al. Electrophysiological breakthroughs from the left atrium to the pulmonary veins. Circulation. 2000;102(20):2463–2465.

11 Haissaguerre M, Shah DC, Jais P, Hocini M, Yamane T, Deisenhofer I, et al. Mapping-guided ablation of pulmonary veins to cure atrial fibrillation. Am J Cardiol. 2000;86(9A):9K–19K.

12 Arruda M, Mlcochova H, Prasad SK, Kilicaslan F, Saliba W, Patel D, et al. Electrical isolation of the superior vena cava: an adjunctive strategy to pulmonary vein antrum isolation improving the outcome of AF ablation. J Cardiovasc Electrophysiol. 2007;18(12): 1261–1266.

13 Huang BH, Wu MH, Tsao HM, Tai CT, Lee KT, Lin YJ, et al. Morphology of the thoracic veins and left atrium in paroxysmal atrial fibrillation initiated by superior caval vein ectopy. J Cardiovasc Electrophysiol. 2005;16(4): 411–417.

14 Haissaguerre M, Hocini M, Takahashi Y, O'Neill MD, Pernat A, Sanders P, et al. Impact of catheter ablation of the coronary sinus on paroxysmal or persistent atrial fibrillation. J Cardiovasc Electrophysiol. 2007;18(4): 378–386.

15 Kistler PM, Sanders P, Fynn SP, Stevenson IH, Spence SJ, Vohra JK, et al. Electrophysiologic and electroanatomic changes in the human atrium associated with age. J Am Coll Cardiol. 2004;44(1):109–116.

16 Sanders P, Morton JB, Davidson NC, Spence SJ, Vohra JK, Sparks PB, et al. Electrical remodeling of the atria in congestive heart failure: electrophysiological and electroanatomic mapping in humans. Circulation. 2003;108 (12):1461–1468.

17 John B, Stiles MK, Kuklik P, Brooks AG, Chandy ST, Kalman JM, et al. Reverse remodeling of the atria after treatment of chronic stretch in humans: implications for

the atrial fibrillation substrate. J Am Coll Cardiol. 2010;55(12):1217–1226.

18 John B, Stiles MK, Kuklik P, Chandy ST, Young GD, Mackenzie L, et al. Electrical remodelling of the left and right atria due to rheumatic mitral stenosis. Eur Heart J. 2008;29(18):2234–2243.

19 Sanders P, Morton JB, Kistler PM, Spence SJ, Davidson NC, Hussin A, et al. Electrophysiological and electroanatomic characterization of the atria in sinus node disease: evidence of diffuse atrial remodeling. Circulation. 2004;109(12):1514–1522.

20 Roberts-Thomson KC, John B, Worthley SG, Brooks AG, Stiles MK, Lau DH, et al. Left atrial remodeling in patients with atrial septal defects. Heart Rhythm. 2009;6 (7):1000–1006.

21 Alasady M, Abhayaratna WP, Leong DP, Lim HS, Abed HS, Brooks AG, et al. Coronary artery disease affecting the atrial branches is an independent determinant of atrial fibrillation after myocardial infarction. Heart Rhythm. 2011;8(7):955–960.

22 Medi C, Kalman JM, Spence SJ, Teh AW, Lee G, Bader I, et al. Atrial electrical and structural changes associated with longstanding hypertension in humans: implications for the substrate for atrial fibrillation. J Cardiovasc Electrophysiol. 2011;22(12):1317–1324.

23 Lau DH, Mackenzie L, Kelly DJ, Psaltis PJ, Brooks AG, Worthington M, et al. Hypertension and atrial fibrillation: evidence of progressive atrial remodeling with electrostructural correlate in a conscious chronically instrumented ovine model. Heart Rhythm. 2010;7 (9):1282–1290.

24 Munger TM, Dong YX, Masaki M, Oh JK, Mankad SV, Borlaug BA, et al. Electrophysiological and hemodynamic characteristics associated with obesity in patients with atrial fibrillation. J Am Coll Cardiol. 2012;60(9):851–860.

25 Gami AS, Hodge DO, Herges RM, Olson EJ, Nykodym J, Kara T, et al. Obstructive sleep apnea, obesity, and the risk of incident atrial fibrillation. J Am Coll Cardiol. 2007;49(5):565–571.

26 Dimitri H, Ng M, Brooks AG, Kuklik P, Stiles MK, Lau DH, et al. Atrial remodeling in obstructive sleep apnea: implications for atrial fibrillation. Heart Rhythm. 2012;9 (3):321–327.

27 Schotten U, Verheule S, Kirchhof P, Goette A. Pathophysiological mechanisms of atrial fibrillation: a translational appraisal. Physiol Rev. 2011;91(1):265–325.

28 Moe GK, Rheinboldt WC, Abildskov JA. A computer model of atrial fibrillation. Am Heart J. 1964;67:200–220.

29 Ravelli F, Mase M, Cristoforetti A, Del Greco M, Centonze M, Marini M, et al. Anatomic localization of rapid repetitive sources in persistent atrial fibrillation: fusion of biatrial CT images with wave similarity/cycle length maps. JACC Cardiovasc Imaging. 2012;5(12):1211–1220.

30 Konings KT, Kirchhof CJ, Smeets JR, Wellens HJ, Penn OC, Allessie MA. High-density mapping of electrically induced atrial fibrillation in humans. Circulation. 1994;89(4):1665–1680.

31 Jalife J. Deja vu in the theories of atrial fibrillation dynamics. Cardiovasc Res. 2011;89(4):766–775.

32 Skanes AC, Mandapati R, Berenfeld O, Davidenko JM, Jalife J. Spatiotemporal periodicity during atrial fibrillation in the isolated sheep heart. Circulation. 1998;98 (12):1236–1248.

33 Mandapati R, Skanes A, Chen J, Berenfeld O, Jalife J. Stable microreentrant sources as a mechanism of atrial fibrillation in the isolated sheep heart. Circulation. 2000;101(2):194–199.

34 Berenfeld O, Zaitsev AV, Mironov SF, Pertsov AM, Jalife J. Frequency-dependent breakdown of wave propagation into fibrillatory conduction across the pectinate muscle network in the isolated sheep right atrium. Circ Res. 2002;90(11):1173–1180.

35 Kalifa J, Tanaka K, Zaitsev AV, Warren M, Vaidyanathan R, Auerbach D, et al. Mechanisms of wave fractionation at boundaries of high-frequency excitation in the posterior left atrium of the isolated sheep heart during atrial fibrillation. Circulation. 2006;113 (5):626–633.

36 Lemola K, Ting M, Gupta P, Anker JN, Chugh A, Good E, et al. Effects of two different catheter ablation techniques on spectral characteristics of atrial fibrillation. J Am Coll Cardiol. 2006;48(2):340–348.

37 Haissaguerre M, Hocini M, Sanders P, Sacher F, Rotter M, Takahashi Y, et al. Catheter ablation of long-lasting persistent atrial fibrillation: clinical outcome and mechanisms of subsequent arrhythmias. J Cardiovasc Electrophysiol. 2005;16(11):1138–1147.

38 Haissaguerre M, Sanders P, Hocini M, Takahashi Y, Rotter M, Sacher F, et al. Catheter ablation of long-lasting persistent atrial fibrillation: critical structures for termination. J Cardiovasc Electrophysiol. 2005;16 (11):1125–1137.

39 Haissaguerre M. In search of the sources of cardiac fibrillation. EMBO Mol Med. 2010;2(4):117–119.

40 Haissaguerre M, Hocini M, Sanders P, Takahashi Y, Rotter M, Sacher F, et al. Localized sources maintaining atrial fibrillation organized by prior ablation. Circulation. 2006;113(5):616–625.

41 O'Neill MD, Wright M, Knecht S, Jais P, Hocini M, Takahashi Y, et al. Long-term follow-up of persistent atrial fibrillation ablation using termination as a procedural endpoint. Eur Heart J. 2009;30(9):1105–1112.

42 Elayi CS, Di Biase L, Barrett C, Ching CK, al Aly M, Lucciola M, et al. Atrial fibrillation termination as a procedural endpoint during ablation in long-standing persistent atrial fibrillation. Heart Rhythm. 2010;7(9): 1216–1223.

43 Takahashi Y, O'Neill MD, Hocini M, Dubois R, Matsuo S, Knecht S, et al. Characterization of electrograms associated with termination of chronic atrial fibrillation by catheter ablation. J Am Coll Cardiol. 2008;51(10): 1003–1010.

44 Scherlag BJ, Hou YL, Lin J, Lu Z, Zacharias S, Dasari T, et al. An acute model for atrial fibrillation arising from a peripheral atrial site: evidence for primary and secondary triggers. J Cardiovasc Electrophysiol. 2008;19(5): 519–527.

45 Chaldoupi SM, Linnenbank AC, Wittkampf FH, Boldt LH, VAN Wessel H, VAN Driel VJ, et al. Complex fractionated electrograms in the right atrial free wall and the superior/posterior wall of the left atrium are affected by activity of the autonomic nervous system. J Cardiovasc Electrophysiol. 2012;23(1):26–33.

46 Atienza F, Calvo D, Almendral J, Zlochiver S, Grzeda KR, Martinez-Alzamora N, et al. Mechanisms of fractionated electrograms formation in the posterior left atrium during paroxysmal atrial fibrillation in humans. J Am Coll Cardiol. 2011;57(9):1081–1092.

47 Zlochiver S, Yamazaki M, Kalifa J, Berenfeld O. Rotor meandering contributes to irregularity in electrograms during atrial fibrillation. Heart Rhythm. 2008;5(6): 846–854.

48 Umapathy K, Masse S, Kolodziejska K, Veenhuyzen GD, Chauhan VS, Husain M, et al. Electrogram fractionation in murine HL-1 atrial monolayer model. Heart Rhythm. 2008;5(7):1029–1035.

49 Lau DH, Maesen B, Zeemering S, Verheule S, Crijns HJ, Schotten U. Stability of complex fractionated atrial electrograms: a systematic review. J Cardiovasc Electrophysiol. 2012 May 3;23:980–987.

50 Scherr D, Dalal D, Cheema A, Cheng A, Henrikson CA, Spragg D, et al. Automated detection and characterization of complex fractionated atrial electrograms in human left atrium during atrial fibrillation. Heart Rhythm. 2007;4(8):1013–1020.

51 Calo L, De Ruvo E, Sciarra L, Gricia R, Navone G, De Luca L, et al. Diagnostic accuracy of a new software for complex fractionated electrograms identification in patients with persistent and permanent atrial fibrillation. J Cardiovasc Electrophysiol. 2008;19(10): 1024–1030.

52 Verma A, Novak P, Macle L, Whaley B, Beardsall M, Wulffhart Z, et al. A prospective, multicenter evaluation of ablating complex fractionated electrograms (CFEs) during atrial fibrillation (AF) identified by an automated mapping algorithm: acute effects on AF and efficacy as an adjuvant strategy. Heart Rhythm. 2008;5(2):198–205.

53 Wu J, Estner H, Luik A, Ucer E, Reents T, Pflaumer A, et al. Automatic 3D mapping of complex fractionated atrial electrograms (CFAE) in patients with paroxysmal and persistent atrial fibrillation. J Cardiovasc Electrophysiol. 2008;19(9):897–903.

54 Nademanee K, Schwab M, Porath J, Abbo A. How to perform electrogram-guided atrial fibrillation ablation. Heart Rhythm. 2006;3(8):981–984.

55 Stiles MK, Brooks AG, Kuklik P, John B, Dimitri H, Lau DH, et al. High-density mapping of atrial fibrillation in humans: relationship between high-frequency activation and electrogram fractionation. J Cardiovasc Electrophysiol. 2008;19(12):1245–1253.

56 Verma A, Mantovan R, Macle L, De Martino G, Chen J, Morillo CA, et al. Substrate and Trigger Ablation for Reduction of Atrial Fibrillation (STAR AF): a randomized, multicentre, international trial. Eur Heart J. 2010;31(11):1344–56.

57 Roux JF, Gojraty S, Bala R, Liu CF, Hutchinson MD, Dixit S, et al. Complex fractionated electrogram distribution and temporal stability in patients undergoing atrial fibrillation ablation. J Cardiovasc Electrophysiol. 2008;19(8):815–820.

58 Scherr D, Dalal D, Cheema A, Nazarian S, Almasry I, Bilchick K, et al. Long- and short-term temporal stability of complex fractionated atrial electrograms in human left atrium during atrial fibrillation. J Cardiovasc Electrophysiol. 2009;20(1):13–21.

59 Lin YJ, Tai CT, Kao T, Chang SL, Wongcharoen W, Lo LW, et al. Consistency of complex fractionated atrial electrograms during atrial fibrillation. Heart Rhythm. 2008;5(3):406–412.

60 Habel N, Znojkiewicz P, Thompson N, Muller JG, Mason B, Calame J, et al. The temporal variability of dominant frequency and complex fractionated atrial electrograms constrains the validity of sequential mapping in human atrial fibrillation. Heart Rhythm. 2010;7 (5):586–593.

61 Ciaccio EJ, Biviano AB, Whang W, Gambhir A, Garan H. Different characteristics of complex fractionated atrial electrograms in acute paroxysmal versus long-standing persistent atrial fibrillation. Heart Rhythm. 2010;7(9):1207–1215.

62 Nademanee K, Lockwood E, Oketani N, Gidney B. Catheter ablation of atrial fibrillation guided by complex fractionated atrial electrogram mapping of atrial fibrillation substrate. J Cardiol. 2010;55(1):1–12.

63 Singh SM, D'Avila A, Kim SJ, Houghtaling C, Dukkipati SR, Reddy VY. Intraprocedural use of ibutilide to organize and guide ablation of complex fractionated atrial electrograms: preliminary assessment of a modified step-wise approach to ablation of persistent atrial fibrillation. J Cardiovasc Electrophysiol. 2010;21(6):608–616.

64 Kumagai K, Toyama H. Usefulness of ablation of complex fractionated atrial electrograms using nifekalant in persistent atrial fibrillation. J Cardiol. 2013;61(1):44–48.

65 Verma F, Likkireddy D, Wulffhart Z, et al. Relationship Between Complex Fractionated Electrograms (CFE) and Dominant Frequency (DF) Sites and Prospective Assessment of Adding DF-Guided Ablation to Pulmonary Vein Isolation in Persistent Atrial Fibrillation (AF). J Cardiovasc Electrophysiol 2011;22:1309–1316.

66 Singh SM, D'Avila A, Kim YH, Aryana A, Mangrum JM, Michaud GF, et al. The Modified Ablation Guided by Ibutilide Use in Chronic Atrial Fibrillation (MAGIC-AF) Study: clinical background and study design. J Cardiovasc Electrophysiol. 2012;23(4):352–358.

67 Hunter RJ, Diab I, Tayebjee M, Richmond L, Sporton S, Earley MJ, et al. Characterization of fractionated atrial electrograms critical for maintenance of atrial fibrillation: a randomized, controlled trial of ablation strategies (the CFAE AF trial). Circ Arrhythm Electrophysiol. 2011;4(5):622–629.

68 Hunter RJ, Diab I, Thomas G, Duncan E, Abrams D, Dhinoja M, et al. Validation of a classification system to grade fractionation in atrial fibrillation and correlation

with automated detection systems. Europace. 2009;11 (12):1587–1596.

69 Narayan SM, Wright M, Derval N, Jadidi A, Forclaz A, Nault I, et al. Classifying fractionated electrograms in human atrial fibrillation using monophasic action potentials and activation mapping: evidence for localized drivers, rate acceleration, and nonlocal signal etiologies. Heart Rhythm. 2011;8(2):244–253.

70 Teh AW, Kistler PM, Lee G, Medi C, Heck PM, Spence SJ, et al. The relationship between complex fractionated electrograms and atrial low-voltage zones during atrial fibrillation and paced rhythm. Europace. 2011;13 (12):1709–1716.

71 Jadidi AS, Duncan E, Miyazaki S, Lellouche N, Shah AJ, Forclaz A, et al. Functional nature of electrogram fractionation demonstrated by left atrial high-density mapping. Circ Arrhythm Electrophysiol. 2012;5(1):32–42.

72 Oral H, Chugh A, Good E, Wimmer A, Dey S, Gadeela N, et al. Radiofrequency catheter ablation of chronic atrial fibrillation guided by complex electrograms. Circulation. 2007;115(20):2606–2612.

73 Lin YJ, Tai CT, Chang SL, Lo LW, Tuan TC, Wongcharoen W, et al. Efficacy of additional ablation of complex fractionated atrial electrograms for catheter ablation of nonparoxysmal atrial fibrillation. J Cardiovasc Electrophysiol. 2009;20(6):607–615.

74 Li WJ, Bai YY, Zhang HY, Tang RB, Miao CL, Sang CH, et al. Additional ablation of complex fractionated atrial electrograms after pulmonary vein isolation in patients with atrial fibrillation: a meta-analysis. Circ Arrhythm Electrophysiol. 2011;4(2):143–148.

75 Hayward RM, Upadhyay GA, Mela T, Ellinor PT, Barrett CD, Heist EK, et al. Pulmonary vein isolation with complex fractionated atrial electrogram ablation for paroxysmal and nonparoxysmal atrial fibrillation: a meta-analysis. Heart Rhythm. 2011;8(7):994–1000.

76 Verma A, Patel D, Famy T, Martin DO, Burkhardt JD, Elayi SC, et al. Efficacy of adjuvant anterior left atrial ablation during intracardiac echocardiography-guided pulmonary vein antrum isolation for atrial fibrillation. J Cardiovasc Electrophysiol. 2007;18(2):151–156.

77 Oral H, Chugh A, Yoshida K, Sarrazin JF, Kuhne M, Crawford T, et al. A randomized assessment of the incremental role of ablation of complex fractionated atrial electrograms after antral pulmonary vein isolation for long-lasting persistent atrial fibrillation. J Am Coll Cardiol. 2009;53(9):782–789.

78 Ng J, Goldberger JJ. Understanding and interpreting dominant frequency analysis of AF electrograms. J Cardiovasc Electrophysiol. 2007;18(6):680–685.

79 Mansour M, Mandapati R, Berenfeld O, Chen J, Samie FH, Jalife J. Left-to-right gradient of atrial frequencies during acute atrial fibrillation in the isolated sheep heart. Circulation. 2001;103(21):2631–2636.

80 Lazar S, Dixit S, Marchlinski FE, Callans DJ, Gerstenfeld EP. Presence of left-to-right atrial frequency gradient in paroxysmal but not persistent atrial fibrillation in humans. Circulation. 2004;110(20):3181–3186.

81 Yoshida K, Chugh A, Good E, Crawford T, Myles J, Veerareddy S, et al. A critical decrease in dominant frequency and clinical outcome after catheter ablation of persistent atrial fibrillation. Heart Rhythm. 2010; 7(3):295–302.

82 Yoshida K, Ulfarsson M, Oral H, Crawford T, Good E, Jongnarangsin K, et al. Left atrial pressure and dominant frequency of atrial fibrillation in humans. Heart Rhythm. 2011;8(2):181–187.

83 Nagashima K, Okumura Y, Watanabe I, Nakai T, Ohkubo K, Kofune M, et al. Does location of epicardial adipose tissue correspond to endocardial high dominant frequency or complex fractionated atrial electrogram sites during atrial fibrillation? Circ Arrhythm Electrophysiol. 2012;5(4):676–683.

84 Lu Z, Scherlag BJ, Lin J, Niu G, Ghias M, Jackman WM, et al. Autonomic mechanism for complex fractionated atrial electrograms: evidence by fast fourier transform analysis. J Cardiovasc Electrophysiol. 2008;19 (8):835–842.

85 Chang SH, Ulfarsson M, Chugh A, Yoshida K, Jongnarangsin K, Crawford T, et al. Time- and frequency-domain characteristics of atrial electrograms during sinus rhythm and atrial fibrillation. J Cardiovasc Electrophysiol.   2011; 22(8):851–857.

86 Lee G, Roberts-Thomson K, Madry A, Spence S, Teh A, Heck PM, et al. Relationship among complex signals, short cycle length activity, and dominant frequency in patients with long-lasting persistent AF: a high-density epicardial mapping study in humans. Heart Rhythm. 2011;8(11):1714–1719.

87 Krummen DE, Anawati M, Ahn D, Peng KA, Briggs C, Rappel WJ, et al. Correlation of electrical rotors and focal sources with sites of centrifugal stepdown in dominant frequency in human atrial fibrillation. Heart Rhythm. 2011;8(5):S176.

88 Jarman JW, Wong T, Kojodjojo P, Spohr H, Davies JE, Roughton M, et al. Spatiotemporal behavior of high dominant frequency during paroxysmal and persistent atrial fibrillation in the human left atrium. Circ Arrhythm Electrophysiol. 2012;5(4):650–658.

89 Ng J, Kadish AH, Goldberger JJ. Effect of electrogram characteristics on the relationship of dominant frequency to atrial activation rate in atrial fibrillation. Heart Rhythm. 2006;3(11):1295–1305.

90 Elvan A, Linnenbank AC, van Bemmel MW, Misier AR, Delnoy PP, Beukema WP, et al. Dominant frequency of atrial fibrillation correlates poorly with atrial fibrillation cycle length. Circ Arrhythm Electrophysiol. 2009;2(6): 634–644.

91 Berenfeld O, Jalife J. Letter by Berenfeld and Jalife regarding article "Dominant frequency of atrial fibrillation correlates poorly with atrial fibrillation cycle length." Circ Arrhythm. 2010;3(1):e1; author reply e2–e3.

92 Atienza F, Almendral J, Jalife J, Zlochiver S, Ploutz-Snyder R, Torrecilla EG, et al. Real-time dominant frequency mapping and ablation of dominant frequency sites in atrial fibrillation with left-to-right frequency gradients predicts long-term maintenance of sinus rhythm. Heart Rhythm. 2009;6(1):33–40.

93 Ganesan AN, Kuklik P, Lau DH, Brooks AG, Baumert M, Lim WW, et al. Bipolar electrogram shannon entropy at sites of rotational activation: implications for ablation of atrial fibrillation. Circ Arrhythm Electrophysiol. 2013;6(1):48–57.

94 Shannon C. A mathematical theory of communication. Bell Syst Tech J. 1948;27:379–423, 623–656.

95 Ravelli F, Faes L, Sandrini L, Gaita F, Antolini R, Scaglione M, et al. Wave similarity mapping shows the spatiotemporal distribution of fibrillatory wave complexity in the human right atrium during paroxysmal and chronic atrial fibrillation. J Cardiovasc Electrophysiol. 2005;16(10):1071–1076.

96 Lin YJ, Lo MT, Lin C, Chang SL, Lo LW, Hu YF, et al. Nonlinear analysis of fibrillatory electrogram similarity to optimize the detection of complex fractionated electrograms during persistent atrial fibrillation. J Cardiovasc Electrophysiol. 2013;24(3): 280–289.

97 Elayi CS, Verma A, Di Biase L, Ching CK, Patel D, Barrett C, et al. Ablation for longstanding permanent atrial fibrillation: results from a randomized study comparing three different strategies. Heart Rhythm. 2008;5 (12): 1658–1664.

98 Deisenhofer I, Estner H, Reents T, Fichtner S, Bauer A, Wu J, et al. Does electrogram guided substrate ablation add to the success of pulmonary vein isolation in patients with paroxysmal atrial fibrillation? A prospective, randomized study. J Cardiovasc Electrophysiol. 2009;20(5):514–521.

99 Di Biase L, Elayi CS, Fahmy TS, Martin DO, Ching CK, Barrett C, et al. Atrial fibrillation ablation strategies for paroxysmal patients: randomized comparison between different techniques. Circ Arrhythm Electrophysiol. 2009;2(2):113–119.

100 Lockwood E, Nademanee, K. Electrogram-guided ablation. In: Calkins H, Steinberg JS, (eds), A Practical Approach to Catheter Ablation of Atrial Fibrillation. Philadelphia, PA: Lipincott & Williams, 2008.

Controversy: Electrogram-guided ablation: valuable technique

Naoya Oketani[1] & Koonlawee Nademanee[2]

[1]Department of Cardiovascular Medicine and Hypertension, Graduate School of Medical and Dental Sciences, Kagoshima University, Kagoshima, Japan
[2]Pacific Rim Electrophysiology Research Institute, Los Angeles, CA, USA

Introduction

In 2004, we introduced electrogram-guided ablation for treatment of atrial fibrillation (AF) without pulmonary vein isolation (PVI) [1]. We described electroanatomical mapping of both atria including coronary sinus with a 3D reconstruction of atrial chambers integrated with electrical information obtained from an atrial electrogram recording of voltage and complex fractionated atrial electrograms. We demonstrated that substrates serving as "AF perpetuators" can be identified by searching for areas that have CFAEs [1]. During sustained AF, CFAEs are often recorded in specific areas of the atria and exhibit temporal and spatial stability [1,2]. By ablating areas that harbor persistent stable CFAE recording, AF was terminated in over 85% of patients and associated with an excellent long-term outcome in both paroxysmal and persistent AF [1–5].

Our observation that CFAEs might represent AF substrate has sparked the interest of clinical electrophysiologists, basic scientists, and computational biologists, and continues to do so even after a decade has passed. Controversy is still rife, however, when it comes to CFAE-guided ablations, because several elite investigators from world-class laboratories have not been able to replicate our results. These investigators have cast doubts to many in the scientific community as to whether CFAE areas truly represent AF substrates and could serve as good targets for AF ablation [6–10].

Given the complexity and heterogeneity of AF, confounding variables associated with ablation tools and techniques, as well as operator-related factors, make the underpinning causes of these different outcomes among different operators of CFAE ablation unclear [11]. However, we have performed AF ablations for over a decade with this technique and continue to observe excellent long-term clinical outcomes that are comparable, if not better than, the anatomical approach based on PVI as a cornerstone of the procedure [4,5,12].

Of particular significance, high-risk patients and the elderly who maintain normal sinus rhythm (NSR) after CFAE ablations have lower mortality and stroke risk, allowing for possible discontinuation of anticoagulation in the majority of these patients [4,5]. In this chapter, we explain important nuances of CFAE ablation based on our experience and discuss some areas of controversy.

Electrophysiologic mechanisms underlying CFAEs

It has been long established that CFAEs are likely to represent an area of focal reentry using pathological or functional anisotropic propagation; this phenomenon is commonly observed in ischemic myocardium or around the border zone of the scarred myocardium [13]. Konings et al. were the first to acknowledge the significance of CFAEs during intraoperative observation of patients in AF. They found CFAEs mostly in the areas of slow conduction and/or pivot points where the wavelets turn around the end of the arch of the functional block [14].

On the other hand, Kalifa et al. identified a key relationship between areas of dominant frequency and areas of fractionation. Mapping of sustained AF in sheep models has demonstrated that CFAEs are found in the boundaries of high-frequency excitation (mother rotors), suggesting that CFAE areas may not be the main driving source that perpetuates AF but are in a location that abuts the driver [15]. In another study, Zlochiver et al., by using singular value decomposition, were able to show that the recorded complex electrograms could be divided into strictly periodic and residual components. The periodic components probably occurred due to underlying rotor wave activity, whereas residual components were probably related to the meandering of the spiral wave source [16].

The most prominent theory underlying the occurrence of CFAE involves the complex interplay of the intrinsic cardiac nervous system on atrial tissues. In animal models, the stimulation of parasympathetic fibers within the ganglionic plexi (GP) has been shown to decrease atrial effective refractory periods and allow AF to perpetuate. Simultaneously, stimulation of sympathetic fibers may occur in similar areas, which can initiate PV ectopy [17–20]. Ongoing research has identified a close relationship between the location of CFAEs and the GP in animal models. CFAE-targeted ablation may provide a surrogate for modification of the GP if this relationship can be confirmed in humans. Indeed, ablation in areas that have resulted in a vagal response has shown excellent results in the treatment of AF.

Electrogram-guided ablation: which CFAE to be ablated?

We define CFAE based on voltage and cycle length: the typical CFAEs that are a good target for ablations are those that have low-voltage (ranging from 0.04–0.25 mV) and are often composed of two or more deflections and/or have a perturbation of the baseline with continuous deflection of a prolonged activation complex. The cycle length should be short, between 50–120 ms (Figure 5a).

In our original publication [1], we also define atrial electrograms that have a very short cycle length (≤100 ms) with or without multiple potential as CFAEs (Figure 5b). These types of short cycle length atrial electrograms are usually located around the antrum of the PV, superior vena cava (SVC) or coronary sinus ostium and their cycle lengths, when compared to the rest of the atria, are often the shortest – the so-called "AF drivers." The other key component of the primary CFAE target site is that CFAEs recorded at that site should have temporal and spatial

stability and do not meander. We do not recommend ablating CFAE sites that are fleeting, with an exception that the appearance of the electrograms could change when AF is organized or changed to atrial tachycardia (AT) or flutter (AFL).

The criticism of the above definition of CFAE is that it involves inherent subjectivity and has several weaknesses [21–27]. First, the definition of CFAE using cycle length and morphology is too broad and will result in imprecise quantification of CFAE, resulting in unnecessarily ablating wide areas of the atrium. This can lead to incorrect detection of target sites for ablation, mistaking electrograms that are fractionated and functional in nature [22]. Second, it fails to describe the wide range of electrogram fractionation that occurs in specific cases. In addition, inconsistent results have been found using the above CFAE definition. Third, CFAE is a nonlinear phenomenon, which is not accounted for using the above criteria [23].

For this reason, several investigators have proposed that CFAE is best analyzed by nonlinear dynamics such as Shannon entropy [22], recurrence quantification analysis (RQA) [25], and entropy index, rather than using the time domain and cycle length definition. Some investigators also use the organization index (OI) and regularity index (RI), and/or amplitude analysis and wavelet transform (WT) [25,27–29]. All these computational/mathematical transformations of atrial electrograms are created with the goal of being more precise and avoiding subjectivity of the analysis to precisely define the properties of CFAE in atrial tissue in order to reduce the size of ablated areas.

However, it is important to recognize that the above proposed nonlinear analysis of CFAE has not been tested in humans, with respect to the method of

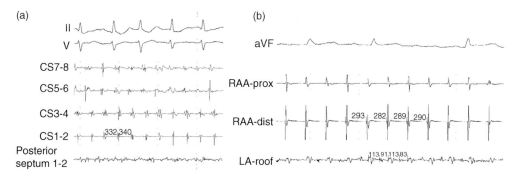

Figure 5 Example of CFAE electrograms. (a) Shows CFAE recorded from the posterior septum (posterior septum 1–2). Note that the electrograms from this site are composed of two or more deflections and/or have a perturbation of the baseline with continuous deflections from a prolonged activation complex with a very short cycle length. (b) Shows CFAE electrogram from the left atrial roof, an example of CFAE that has very short cycle length, which is much shorter than those recorded from the rest of atria, despite having no multiple prolonged potential.

guidance to the correct target that will consistently result into AF termination. In contrast, our visualization and time domain approach, albeit with some degree of subjectivity and interoperator variability, has served us well as far as selecting primary CFAE target sites leading to AF termination (see discussion below). In any event, we agree that further improvement in software algorithm, including integrated nonlinear dynamic analysis along with repetitive electrogram pattern recognition, is needed in order to better classify CFAE sites that are AF perpetuators.

Ablation end points and AF termination by CFAE ablation

Unlike the anatomical approach with PVI, one of the key end points for CFAE ablation is AF termination; the others are elimination of all primary CFAE sites and noninducible AF in paroxysmal AF patients. The typical response of AF ablations by targeting CFAE is that tachycardia cycle length will progressively increase and tachycardia becomes more and more organized and often changes to AT or AFL, which will be mapped and ablated until the rhythm is converted to NSR.

Typical continuous CFAEs are easy to recognize, but when AF is organized or changed to AT/AFL, the electrograms at that site also change. And low-voltage electrograms around the areas previously ablated are also important. CFAEs exist not as sparse points, but in some dense areas. After ablating the areas of CFAEs, the electrograms would be changed: voltage lowered, less fractionated, and/or more organized. There may be concern about how we find the residual CFAE sites. Since CFAEs have temporal and spatial stability, we tried to find the residual CFAE sites around the tagged and/or previously ablated areas, occasionally with ibutilide in the United States and nifekalant in Japan to highlight the residual CFAEs while increasing the AF cycle length.

The typical example of how CFAE ablation terminates AF is shown in Figure 6. The patient in this Figure 6 is a 66-year-old man who has persistent AF. After ablations over the roof of the left atrium and antra of the left and right superior pulmonary vein, AF became organized with an increase in the tachycardia cycle length from 170–190 ms to 210–230 ms (Figure 6a). Cavotricuspid isthmus ablation was performed further increasing the cycle length from 210 to 270 ms but did not terminate the tachycardia (Figure 6b). Additional ablations along the roof and anterior aspect of the left atrium further increased the tachycardia cycle length and eventually terminated the tachycardia (Figure 6c, a, d; figure legends).

We analyzed our data from 616 patients (206 paroxysmal AF and 410 persistent AF) who had undergone CFAE-guided AF ablation from January 2006 to December 2007 at Pacific Rim EP Research Institute Center in Los Angeles, all by the same operator [30]. In this group, we were able to terminate AF to NSR during ablation of CFAE target sites in 203/206 (99%) of paroxysmal AF and 328/410 (80%) of persistent AF patients, occasionally with ibutilide. The remaining patients required external cardioversion to restore and maintain sinus rhythm. The common areas of CFAE were at the anterior aspect of the right PV antra, the posterior aspect of the left PV antra, the ridge of the left atrial appendage, the proximal coronary sinus, and the posterior septum of the right atrium.

We then prospectively evaluated the reproducibility of the above findings in Kagoshima, Japan, by studying 670 patients (356 paroxysmal AF, 314 persistent AF including 69 long-standing AF) who had undergone CFAE-guided AF ablation from September 2008 to September 2014 in our institution in Kagoshima by 5 operators [31]. In this group, we were able to terminate AF to NSR during ablation of CFAE target sites with or without PVI in 96% of paroxysmal and 81% of persistent AF patients, occasionally with nifekalant (a class III drug similar to ibutilide).

Seitz et al. from Marseille, France, studied 121 patients with paroxysmal ($n = 19$; 15.7%), persistent ($n = 77$; 63.6%), or long-standing persistent ($n = 25$; 20.7%) AF, who underwent electrogram-based substrate ablation by targeting CFAE with an AF termination end point [31]. They were able to terminate AF to NSR in 80.2% without concomitant use of any antiarrhythmic drugs.

Our findings, along with those of Seitz et al., confirmed our original observation that CFAE ablation is effective in terminating AF to sinus rhythm. This is in sharp contrast to several studies in recent years showing that, in their experience, CFAE ablation yielded a very low AF termination rate (<20%). The possible explanation for the differences between the studies has been discussed in detail elsewhere. Importantly, both our patients and those in Seitz's study did well during long-term follow-up. Thus, to perform electrogram-guided ablations for a better long-term result, the total outcome of AF termination should be around ≥80%.

Relationship between CFAE and rotor

Narayan et al. have recently published studies using impulse and rotor modulation to guide ablation with

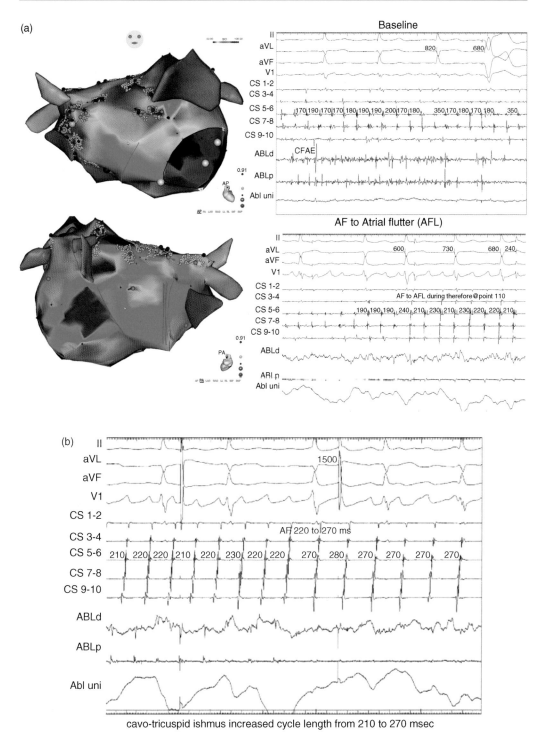

Figure 6 (a) Shows effects of ablations at CFAE sites along the left atrial roof, antra of the left and right superior pulmonary veins, around the mouth of left atrial appendage resulting in changing AF to atrial flutter (AFL) with a significant increase in cycle length from the range of 170–190 ms to 210–230 ms. (b) Cycle length further increased from 220 to 270 ms after ablations were performed at the cavotricuspid isthmus of the right atrium. (c) More ablations were performed over the roof of the left atrium and anterior aspect of the left atrium from the roof to mitral annulus and resulted in further increase in the cycle length from 280 to 300 ms after RF application was applied at the blue dot. (d) Termination of the tachycardia after RF application was applied to the second blue dot slightly above the first one from (c). After the last ablations, no inducible tachycardia could be provoked.

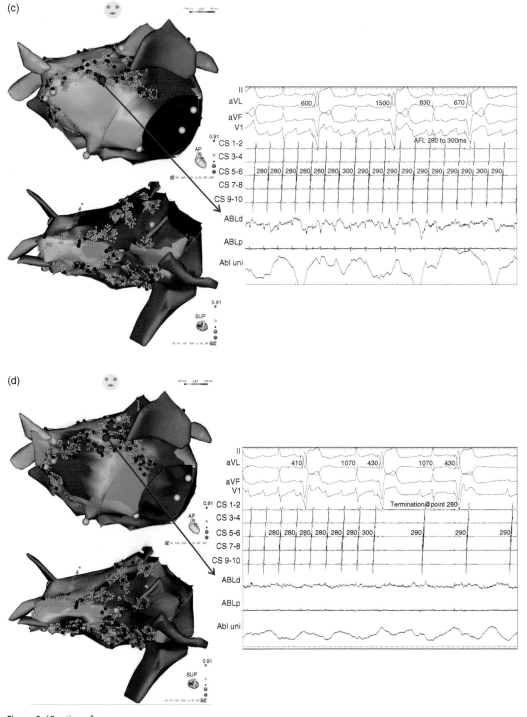

Figure 6 (*Continued*)

better results than when using ablation without this approach, generating excitement and interest in using rotor mapping to guide AF ablation [32]. The rotor hypothesis proposes that in a significant number of patients, a rotor or a small number of rotors are drivers that maintain AF. A rotor is a vortex of a spiral wave rotating around an unexcitable core. Narayan et al. have shown that human AF can be sustained by localized rotors [32,33]. They found that rotors that serve as the stable source of AF correlated poorly with CFAE.

On the other hand, several other studies have shown some relationship between rotors and fractionation. As mentioned earlier, Zlochiver et al. found that the periodic component of recorded complex electrograms is caused by underlying rotor wave activity, but the residual components are related to the meandering of the spiral wave source [16]. These findings suggest that sustained AF depends on uninterrupted periodic activity of the discrete reentrant site and on the evidence that a high degree of irregularity is present in electrogram signals at the rotor tip.

Haissaguerre et al. recently reported their observation of the relationship between reentrant drivers and focal drivers with CFAE [34]. They compared bipolar electrogram characteristics at 21 driver regions harboring reentrant activities with 85 without any driver activity. Prolonged fractionated electrograms were more frequently recorded at the reentrant driver (repetitive rotor) regions (62% versus 40%; odds ratio, 3.41; 95% confidence interval (CI), 1.07–10.95; $p = 0.04$). The difference between the Narayan and Haissaguerre study results remains unclear. We speculate, however, that the difference in methodology of identifying rotors and the difference in the definition of CFAE may be the reason for their differences.

It should be noted that most of the studies evaluating the relationship between CFAE and rotors utilize an automatic software algorithm (with the exception of Haissaguerre's study mentioned above), either from Biosense Webster or from St Jude Medical, which is imperfect and too sensitive in sourcing out CFAE areas without specificity in identifying primary CFAE sites for an AF ablation. This software tends to call too many areas as CFAE sites, which would not be considered as good target sites for AF ablations in our laboratory. Thus, it remains unclear if there is any relationship between primary CFAE sites and the rotor source of AF. It is clear, however, that more work is needed to better understand the relationship between rotors that serve as drivers of AF maintenance and CFAE.

Relationship between clinical outcomes and unintentional pulmonary vein isolation during substrate ablation of AF guided solely by CFAE mapping

We reported a study to evaluate the effectiveness of AF ablation guided solely by targeting CFAE areas, and to determine whether its clinical efficacy has any relationship with unintentionally isolating the PV [35]. We studied 100 consecutive patients (ages 59 ± 11 years; 54 with paroxysmal, 35 persistent, and 11 longstanding persistent AF), who underwent CFAE ablation. PV potential (PVP) was recorded before and after ablation. After excluding 39 patients in whom sinus rhythm could not be maintained before ablation by an internal cardioversion and/or who had a history of PVI(s), PVPs were analyzed. AF was terminated during ablation in 98% of paroxysmal, 80% of persistent, and 55% of long-standing persistent AF patients. Nifekalant (0.3–0.6 mg/kg) was administered in 30, 57, and 83%, respectively. The common areas of CFAE around the PVs were anterior to the right PVs, posterior to the left PVs, and at the ridge of the left atrial appendage. Among 215 PVs in 61 patients (42 paroxysmal, 19 persistent), only 17 PVs (8%) were unintentionally isolated. The atrial potential to PVP was prolonged (>30 ms) in 13% of PVs. After at least 12 months of follow-up (23 ± 5 months), 65% of paroxysmal (11% with drug), 54% of persistent (37% with drug), and 45% of long-standing (60% with drug) AF patients were free from atrial arrhythmia after one session. In 26 of 61 (43%) patients, the interval from the local atrial potential to the PVP was prolonged or at least 1 of the 4 PVs was isolated. There was no difference in the outcome whether PVP was affected by CFAE ablation or not in this study. Thus, we concluded that CFAE ablation terminated AF without isolating PVs in a high percentage of patients, and yielded good clinical outcomes.

Clinical outcomes of electrogram-guided ablation

Since we have employed our ablation approach for more than a decade, we have had an opportunity to have long follow-up of our clinical outcomes in our study patients. One has to evaluate important clinical outcomes beyond maintenance of NSR: mortality and stroke risk reduction are two such important clinical end points. And this reduction is a major reason that our technique of electrogram-guided CFAE ablation is appealing and valuable; we have demonstrated excellent clinical outcomes of catheter substrate ablation for patients with high risk for stroke with AF [4,5].

We performed AF substrate ablation guided by CFAE mapping in 674 high-risk AF patients. Our study cohort consisted of patients who were at least 65 years old or had at least 1 or more risk factors for stroke including hypertension, diabetes, structural heart disease, a prior history of stroke, transient ischemic attack, congestive heart failure, or ejection fraction of $\leq$40% from March 2000 to May 2007. The clinical end points were NSR, death, stroke, or bleeding. Of these 674 patients, 635 were available for follow-up and made up the study cohort. The patients were relatively old (mean age 67 ± 12 years, $\geq$75 years 169, 26.6%), and 129 (22.8%) had an ejection fraction $\leq$40%.

After a mean follow-up period of 836 ± 605 days, 517 were in NSR (81.4%). There were 15 deaths among the patients who stayed in NSR compared with 14 deaths among those who remained in AF (5-year survival rate, 92% versus 64%, respectively; $p < 0.0001$). SR was the most important independent favorable parameter for survival (hazard ratio (HR), 0.14; 95% CI, 0.06–0.36; $p < 0.0001$), whereas old age was unfavorable. Warfarin therapy was discontinued in 434 of the 517 patients in NSR post-ablation (84%) whose annual stroke rate was only 0.4% compared to 2% in those with continuing warfarin treatment ($p = 0.004$).

We concluded that CFAE-targeted ablation of AF is effective in maintaining SR in selected high-risk AF patients and might allow patients to stop warfarin therapy. NSR after AF ablation is a marker of relatively low mortality and stroke risk. Our findings support conducting further randomized studies to determine whether AF ablation is associated with mortality and/or stroke reduction.

The above findings were confirmed by our recent study showing the benefits of catheter ablation for elderly patients with AF with respect to mortality and stroke reductions [5]. Specifically, we evaluated the safety and efficacy including long-term outcomes of catheter ablation for maintaining NSR in elderly with AF. We evaluated 587 elderly patients with AF ($\geq$75 years old). Of the 324 who were eligible for ablation, 261 (group 1) underwent ablation guided by CFAE. The remaining 63 patients (group 2) either declined or were not suitable for ablation. The end points were NSR, stroke, death, and major bleeding. In the results, 216 patients (83%) remained in NSR compared to only 14 group 2 patients (22%) (mean follow-up, 3 ± 2.5 years; $p < 0.001$). The 1- and 5-year survival rates for group 1 with NSR, group 1 with AF, and group 2 patients were 98% and 87%, 86% and 52%, and 97% and 42%, respectively ($p < 0.0001$; Figure 7). NSR was an independent favorable parameter for

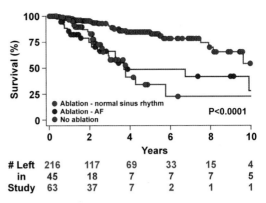

# Left	216	117	69	33	15	4
in	45	18	7	7	7	5
Study	63	37	7	2	1	1

Figure 7 Kaplan–Meier curve demonstrating improved survival in patients who remained in sinus rhythm after atrial fibrillation ablation from all-cause mortality compared to patients who remained in atrial fibrillation after ablation and patients who did not undergo catheter ablation.

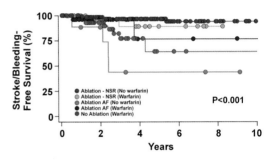

Figure 8 Multiple overlay Kaplan–Meier stroke-/bleeding-free survival curves among five groups of patients: (1) successful ablation, normal sinus rhythm (NSR) on no warfarin; (2) successful ablation, NSR on warfarin; (3) unsuccessful ablation, atrial fibrillation (AF) on no warfarin; (4) unsuccessful ablation, AF on warfarin; and (5) no ablation, NSR on warfarin (group 2).

survival (HR, 0.36; 95% CI, 0.02–0.63; $p = 0.0005$), whereas older age (HR, 1.09; 95% CI, 1.01–1.16; $p = 0.02$) and depressed ejection fraction <40% (HR, 2.38; 95% CI, 1.28–4.4; $p = 0.006$) were unfavorable. Warfarin therapy was discontinued in 169 of the 216 group 1 patients (78%) who maintained NSR and had only 3% 5-year stroke/bleeding rates compared to 16% in group 2 ($p < 0.001$; Figure 8). We concluded that elderly patients with AF benefit from AF ablation, which is safe and effective in maintaining SR and is associated with lower mortality and stroke risk.

Conclusions

Electrogram-guided CFAE ablation for treatment of AF is quite effective not only for long-term maintenance of NSR but also for excellent clinical outcomes with respect to stroke and mortality reduction. The shortcoming of this approach is that many centers worldwide have not been able to fully replicate our results, perhaps due to subjectivity involved in how one selects primary CFAE targets for ablation and the confounding factors of the ablation technique. The technique needs a better way to define, classify, and identify primary CFAE targets.

Future development of nonlinear dynamic analysis of fractionation, in conjunction with conventional visualization and pattern recognition, may help to uniformly establish criteria for primary CFAE target sites for AF ablation so that investigators and electrophysiologists can relate their results from one to the other and have a clear picture as to the role of electrogram-guided ablation in AF treatment. More studies of the relationship between reentrant rotors and CFAE are needed. However, we believe, based on over a decade of experience with CFAE ablation, that the technique is useful and should be incorporated in AF ablation strategy.

Disclosures

Dr. Nademanee has consulting agreements with Biosense Webster Inc. and receives research grants and royalties from Biosense Webster Inc. Dr. Oketani reports no conflicts.

References

1 Nademanee K, McKenzie J, Kosar E, et al. A new approach for catheter ablation of atrial fibrillation: mapping of the electrophysiologic substrate. J Am Coll Cardiol. 2004;43:2044–2053.

2 Nademanee K, Lockwood E, Oketani N, Gidney B. Catheter ablation of atrial fibrillation guided by complex fractionated atrial electrogram mapping of atrial fibrillation substrate. J Cardiol. 2010;55:1–12.

3 Oketani N, Ichiki H, Iriki Y, et al. Catheter ablation of atrial fibrillation guided by complex fractionated atrial electrogram mapping with or without pulmonary vein isolation. J Arrhythm. 2012;28:311–323.

4 Nademanee K, Schwab MC, Kosar EM, et al. Clinical outcomes of catheter substrate ablation for high-risk patients with atrial fibrillation. J Am Coll Cardiol. 2008;51:843–849.

5 Nademanee K, Amnueypol M, Lee F, et al. Benefits and risks of catheter ablation in elderly patients with atrial fibrillation. Heart Rhythm. 2014; in press.

6 Oral H, Chugh A, Good E, et al. Radiofrequency catheter ablation of chronic atrial fibrillation guided by complex electrograms. Circulation. 2007;22;115:2606–2612.

7 Dixit S, Marchlinski FE, Lin D, et al. Randomized ablation strategies for the treatment of persistent atrial fibrillation:

RASTA study. Circ Arrhythm Electrophysiol. 2012; 5:287–294.

8 Oral H, Chugh A, Yoshida K, et al. A randomized assessment of the incremental role of ablation of complex fractionated atrial electrograms after pulmonary vein isolation for long-lasting persistent atrial fibrillation. J Am Coll Cardiol. 2009;53:782–789.

9 Di Biase L, Elayi CS, Fahmy TS, et al. Atrial fibrillation ablation strategies for paroxysmal patients: randomized comparison between different techniques. Circ Arrhythm Electrophysiol. 2009;2:113–119.

10 Deisenhofer I, Estner H, Reents T, et al. Does electrogram guided substrate ablation add to the success of pulmonary vein isolation in patients with paroxysmal atrial fibrillation? A prospective, randomized study. J Cardiovasc Electrophysiol. 2009;20:514–521.

11 Nademanee K. Trials and travails of electrogram-guided ablation of chronic atrial fibrillation. Circulation. 2007; 115:2592–2594.

12 Nademanee, K, Oketani N. The role of complex fractionated atrial electrograms in atrial fibrillation: moving to the beat of a different drum. J Am Coll Cardiol. 2009; 53:790–791.

13 De Bakker J, Wittkampf F. The pathophysiologic basis of fractionated and complex electrograms and the impact of recording techniques on their detection and interpretation. Circ Arrhythm Electrophysiol. 2010;3:204–213.

14 Konings KT, Smeets JL, Penn OC, Wellens HJ, Allessie MA. Configuration of unipolar atrial electrograms during electrically induced atrial fibrillation in humans. Circulation. 1997;95:1231–1241.

15 Kalifa J, Tanaka K, Zaitsev AV, et al. Mechanisms of wave fractionation at boundaries of high-frequency excitation in the posterior left atrium of the isolated sheep heart during atrial fibrillation. Circulation. 2006;113:626–633.

16 Zlochiver S, Yamazaki M, Kalifa J, Berenfeld O. Rotor meandering contributes to irregularity in electrograms during atrial fibrillation. Heart Rhythm. 2008;5: 846–854.

17 Armour JA, Murphy DA, Yuan BX, Macdonald S, Hopkins DA. Gross and microscopic anatomy of the human intrinsic cardiac nervous system. Anat Rec. 1997;247: 289–298.

18 Pauza DH, Skripka V, Pauziene N, Stropus R. Morphology, distribution, and variability of the epicardiac neural ganglionated subplexuses in the human heart. Anat Rec. 2000;259:353–382.

19 Lockwood E, Nademanee K. Electrogram-guided ablation. In: Calkins H, Jais P, Steinberg JS, (eds), A Practical Approach to Catheter Ablation of Atrial Fibrillation, Philadelphia: Lippincott Williams & Wilkins, 2008.

20 Scherlag BJ, Yamanashi W, Patel U, Lazzara R, Jackman WM. Autonomically induced conversion of pulmonary vein focal firing into atrial fibrillation. J Am Coll Cardiol. 2005;45:1878–1886.

21 Reddy V. Atrial fibrillation: unanswered questions and future directions. Cardiol Clin. 2009;27:201–216.

22 Jadidi AS, Duncan E, Miyazaki S, et al. Functional nature of electrogram fractionation demonstrated by left atrial

high-density mapping. Circ Arrhythm Electrophysiol. 2012;5:32–42.

23 Ciaccio E, Biviano A, Whang W, Garan H. Identification of recurring patterns in fractionated atrial electrograms using new transform coefficients. BioMed Eng OnLine 2012;11:4.

24 Ganesan A, Kuklik P, Lau D, Brooks A, Baumert M, et al. Bipolar electrogram Shannon entropy at sites of rotational activation: implications for ablation of atrial fibrillation. Circ Arrhythm Electrophysiol. 2013;6:48–57.

25 Navoret N, Jacquir S, Laurent G, Binczak S. Detection of complex fractionated atrial electrograms using recurrence quantification analysis. IEEE Trans Bio-Med Eng. 2013; 60:1975–1982.

26 Skanes A, Mandapati R, Berenfeld O, Davidenko J, Jalife J. Spatiotemporal periodicity during atrial fibrillation in the isolated sheep heart. Circulation. 1998;98:1236–1248.

27 Navoret N, Jacquir S, Laurent G, Binczak S. Relationship between complex fractionated atrial electrogram patterns and different heart substrate configurations. Comput Cardiol. 2012;39:893–896.

28 Umapathy K, Masse S, Kolodziejska K, Veenhuyzen G, Chauhan V, Husain M, et al. Electrogram fractionation in murine HL-1 atrial monolayer model. Heart Rhythm. 2008;5:1029–1035.

29 Grzeda KR, Noujaim SF, Berenfeld O, Jalife J. Complex fractionated atrial electrograms: properties of time-domain versus frequency-domain methods. Heart Rhythm. 2009;6:1475–1482.

30 Okitani N, Nademanee K. Incidence and mode of AF termination during substrate ablation of AF guided solely by complex fractionated atrial electrogram mapping. Circulation. 2008;118(Suppl):S925. [Abstract].

31 Seitz J, Horvilleur J, Curel L, Lacotte J, Maluski A, Ferracci A, et al. Active or passive pulmonary vein in atrial fibrillation: is pulmonary vein isolation always essential? Heart Rhythm. 2014;11:579–586.

32 Narayan SM, Krummen DE, Shivkumar K, et al. Treatment of atrial fibrillation by the ablation of localized sources: CONFIRM (Conventional Ablation for Atrial Fibrillation With or Without Focal Impulse and Rotor Modulation) Trial. J Am Coll Cardiol. 2012;60:628–636.

33 Narayan SM, Shivkumar K, Krummen DE, Miller JM, Rappel WJ. Panoramic electrophysiological mapping but not electrogram morphology identifies stable sources for human atrial fibrillation. Stable atrial fibrillation rotors and focal sources relate poorly to fractionated electrograms. Circ Arrhythm Electrophysiol. 2013; 6:58–67.

34 Haissaguerre M, Hocini M, Denis A, et al. Driver domains in persistent atrial fibrillation. Circulation. 2014;130: 530–538.

35 Iriki Y, Ishida S, Oketani N, et al. Relationship between clinical outcomes and unintentional pulmonary vein isolation during substrate ablation of atrial fibrillation guided solely by complex fractionated atrial electrogram mapping. J Cardiol. 2011;58:278–286.

Controversy: Electrogram-guided ablation: limited contribution to successful outcome

Hatice Duygu Bas, Kazim Baser, & Hakan Oral
Division of Cardiovascular Medicine, University of Michigan, Ann Arbor, MI, USA

Following the seminal observation that arrhythmogenic foci within the pulmonary veins (PV) and their antrum trigger atrial fibrillation (AF) [1], antral PV isolation (PVI) has become an essential step during catheter ablation of AF. However, despite a high efficacy in patients with paroxysmal AF, antral PVI had a rather modest efficacy in patients with persistent AF in whom atrial electroanatomical remodeling promotes additional drivers of AF beyond PV arrhythmogenicity. Therefore, other ablation strategies including linear ablation, targeting complex fractionated atrial electrograms (CFAEs) alone or in combination as a stepwise approach often in conjunction with PVI have been pursued to improve clinical outcomes in patients with persistent AF [2].

Ablation of CFAEs was proposed by Nademanee et al. [3], who targeted CFAEs as a stand-alone ablation strategy and reported sinus rhythm in 70% of patients at 1 year after a single ablation procedure [3]. However, in a subsequent study, sinus rhythm was maintained in only 33% of the patients with persistent and long-standing persistent AF after a single ablation procedure. The efficacy improved to ~60% after repeat ablation procedures in 40% of the patients to eliminate recurrent AF and *de novo* atypical atrial flutter [4]. Similar findings were also observed in other studies [5,6], suggesting that CFAEs ablation alone can be insufficient in patients with nonparoxysmal AF.

As recurrent AF originating from residual PV foci was often observed after targeting CFAEs as the sole ablation strategy, CFAE ablation was considered as an adjuvant to PVI in patients with paroxysmal AF and particularly in patients with persistent AF whose AF persisted after PVI. The incremental role of CFAE ablation after PVI has been investigated in several controlled studies. In patients with paroxysmal AF, CFAE ablation has not been demonstrated to be incremental to PVI [6–9], suggesting that PV arrhythmogenicity is the primary mechanism of AF and in the absence of extensive atrial electroanatomical remodeling PVI is often sufficient to achieve good clinical outcomes. However, in patients with persistent and long-standing persistent AF, the results of several

studies on the incremental role of CFAEs ablation have not been consistent [10–13]. The variability in outcomes can be explained by the heterogeneity of study populations, the definitions of CFAE, the extent of mapping and ablation and procedural end points such as termination of AF and the number of repeat ablation procedures performed.

A recent meta-analysis of seven controlled studies suggested that additional CFAEs ablation after PVI increases the likelihood of maintaining sinus rhythm at 1 year without antiarrhythmic drugs in patients with nonparoxysmal AF (relative risk: 1.35; $P = 0.02$), but not in patients with paroxysmal AF (relative risk: 1.04; $P = 0.5$, Figure 9) [14]. Similar findings were reported in another meta-analysis that reported added benefit of CFAE ablation at the expense of longer procedure and fluoroscopy times [15]. However, these meta-analyses should be evaluated with caution because of the small sample size and variable follow-up period of individual studies. Furthermore, definition and mapping technique of CFAEs (visual or with automated systems), acute procedural end points, and additional right atrial ablation were often not uniform among these studies.

To be able to accurately interpret the role of CFAE ablation in AF, several points warrant further consideration. First, CFAEs have often been identified visually using subjective criteria, and can be highly operator-dependent. CFAEs have been defined as fractionated electrograms with two or more deflections or with continuous activity over a 10-s period or as electrograms with a very short cycle length (mean cycle length of <120 ms over a 10 s, Figure 10) [4]. However, each of these definitions may reflect a different mechanism since fractionated electrograms can be observed at sites of wavebreak [16], summation of electrograms from underlying overlapping layers of myocardium or due to anisotropy, and can indicate sites of passive activation. On the other hand, electrograms with a rapid activation rate may point to a potential driver of AF; however, the rate can be quite variable among different drivers. A poor anatomic overlap between definitions of CFAE was shown in a

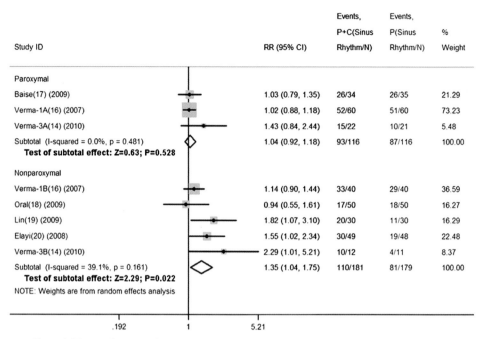

Figure 9 Effects of ablation of CFAEs on long-term maintenance of sinus rhythm in patients with paroxysmal and nonparoxysmal atrial fibrillation. P indicates pulmonary vein antrum isolation; C, complex fractionated atrial electrogram. (Reproduced with permission from Ref. [14].)

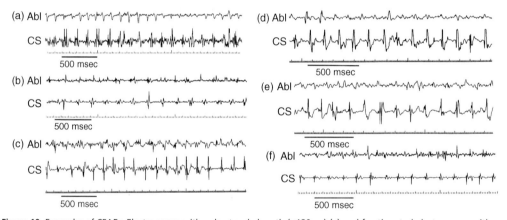

Figure 10 Examples of CFAEs. Electrograms with a short cycle length (≤120 ms) (a) and fractionated electrograms with continuous electrical activity (b–f) are shown. Abl indicates distal bipole of the ablation catheter; CS, distal bipole of coronary sinus catheter. (Reproduced with permission from Ref. [4].)

recent study that utilized epicardial mapping of the posterior left atrium [17].

Another limitation is the subjective identification of CFAE based on visual analysis. Automated algorithms (with different recording systems) have been developed in an attempt to provide more objective and standard identification of CFAEs [18,19]. Catheter electrode size, length of recording, unipolar versus bipolar recording, and sampling frequency may also influence CFAE identification [20]. Automated detection of CFAEs has not been unequivocally demonstrated to improve clinical outcomes [18,19].

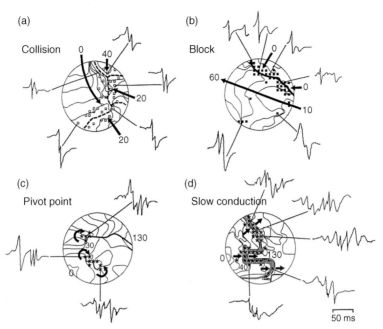

Figure 11 Comparison of the electrogram morphology and the underlying pattern of activation as recorded during AF. (a) Four wave fronts (arrows) invade the mapping area from different directions and collide along the dashed line. Along either side of this line of collision, short double potentials were recorded (□). (b) Long double electrograms (■) are shown to be recorded at a line of functional conduction block (thick line). Fragmented electrograms (★) were recorded both at pivot points (c) and from areas with slow conduction (d; crowding of isochrones). Isochrones were drawn at 10-ms interval. Arrows indicate the direction of activation. Numbers indicate activation times in milliseconds. (Reproduced with permission from Ref. [21].)

In addition to a lack of consensus upon the definition and identification of CFAEs, sensitivity and specificity of CFAE in identifying critical sites to perpetuation of AF is also questionable. Prior studies suggested that CFAEs might represent anchor points for reentrant circuits, areas of slow conduction, collision, or indicate sites of rotor meandering and autonomic innervation (Figure 11) [21–23]. CFAEs were also observed at sites of wavebreak and fibrillatory conduction at the periphery of a rotor [16]. Therefore, CFAEs may be nonspecific markers of critical target sites as they can be identified at the vicinity of a driver rotor. A recent study investigated whether CFAEs represented true drivers of AF or far-field signals by examining the monophasic action potentials and activation sequences [24]. The majority of CFAE sites were due to far-field activity [24]. Ubiquitous distribution of CFAEs in the atria and coronary sinus [25] and their relative nonspecificity may lead to extensive ablation of noncritical areas and thereby an increase in the risk of proarrhythmia, atrial contractile dysfunction as well as the procedure and fluoroscopy duration. In a prior study, ablation of CFAE sites with continuous activity or a temporal activation gradient

was associated with slowing or termination of AF [26,27]. In another study, PVI was found to reduce the prevalence of CFAEs, and had eliminated the need for a more extensive left atrial ablation [28].

CFAEs have been frequently observed in the right atrium as well. The role of right atrial ablation of CFAEs after left atrial ablation has been investigated in few studies. In a prior randomized study, AF terminated in only 3% of the patients during right atrial ablation, suggesting a limited contribution of the right atrial CFAEs as the critical drivers of AF [29]. However, in other studies, right atrial ablation was required in up to 20–30% of the patients to terminate AF after left atrial ablation [30].

Current definition of CFAEs include a variety of electrogram characteristics that may indicate both active, such as focal sources, rotors, or immediate vicinity of rotors with high activation rates, and passive sites such as sites with anisotropic conduction, wave front collision, fibrillatory conduction of areas of overlapping myocardial layers. Therefore, there is a need to better define CFAEs and improve both the sensitivity and the specificity. Mapping using monophasic action potentials has been suggested to more

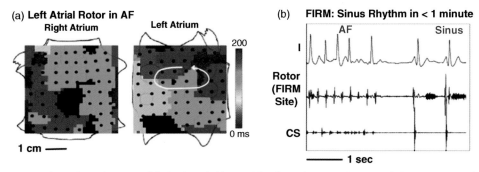

Figure 12 Focal impulse and rotor modulation (FIRM) ablation. (a) Left atrial rotor with counterclockwise activation (red to blue) and disorganized right atrium during atrial fibrillation (AF) in a 60-year-old man. (b) FIRM ablation at left atrial rotor terminated AF to sinus rhythm in <1 min, with ablation artifact recorded at rotor center. (Reproduced with permission from Ref. [32].) (Please see the color version of this figure in the color plate section.)

accurately identify the drivers of AF [24,31]. Pharmacologic intervention using ibutilide was also utilized to discern sites of passive activation and fibrillatory conduction from active drivers of AF in a small early study [31]. Whether these approaches will improve the utility of CFAE mapping remains to be confirmed in larger controlled studies.

More recently, using specific algorithms primarily based on extensive signal processing and phase mapping techniques with Hilbert transformation, drivers of AF both in the form of focal drivers and in rotors have been successfully mapped in human subjects with AF. Ablation of these sites was associated with a remarkable improvement in the likelihood of maintaining sinus rhythm (Figure 12) [32,33]. As signal processing techniques and real-time mapping of drivers of AF continue to evolve, and are used to guide ablation, it remains unclear whether CFAEs will still be considered as targets during catheter ablation due to their limited sensitivity and specificity.

References

1 Haissaguerre M, Jais P, Shah DC, et al. Spontaneous initiation of atrial fibrillation by ectopic beats originating in the pulmonary veins. N Engl J Med. 1998;339: 659–666.

2 Calkins H, Kuck KH, Cappato R, et al. HRS/EHRA/ECAS Expert Consensus Statement on Catheter and Surgical Ablation of Atrial Fibrillation: recommendations for patient selection, procedural techniques, patient management and follow-up, definitions, endpoints, and research trial design: a report of the Heart Rhythm Society (HRS) Task Force on Catheter and Surgical Ablation of Atrial Fibrillation. Developed in partnership with the European Heart Rhythm Association (EHRA), a registered branch of the European Society of Cardiology (ESC) and the European Cardiac Arrhythmia Society (ECAS); and in collaboration with the American College of Cardiology (ACC), American Heart Association (AHA), the Asia Pacific Heart Rhythm Society (APHRS), and the Society of Thoracic Surgeons (STS). Endorsed by the governing bodies of the American College of Cardiology Foundation, the American Heart Association, the European Cardiac Arrhythmia Society, the European Heart Rhythm Association, the Society of Thoracic Surgeons, the Asia Pacific Heart Rhythm Society, and the Heart Rhythm Society. Heart Rhythm. 2012;9:632–696 e621.

3 Nademanee K, McKenzie J, Kosar E, et al. A new approach for catheter ablation of atrial fibrillation: mapping of the electrophysiologic substrate. J Am Coll Cardiol. 2004;43:2044–2053.

4 Oral H, Chugh A, Good E, et al. Radiofrequency catheter ablation of chronic atrial fibrillation guided by complex electrograms. Circulation. 2007;115:2606–2612.

5 Estner HL, Hessling G, Ndrepepa G, et al. Electrogram-guided substrate ablation with or without pulmonary vein isolation in patients with persistent atrial fibrillation. Europace. 2008;10:1281–1287.

6 Verma A, Mantovan R, Macle L, et al. Substrate and Trigger Ablation for Reduction of Atrial Fibrillation (STARAF): a randomized, multicentre, international trial. Eur Heart J. 2010;31:1344–1356.

7 Deisenhofer I, Estner H, Reents T, et al. Does electrogram guided substrate ablation add to the success of pulmonary vein isolation in patients with paroxysmal atrial fibrillation? A prospective, randomized study. J Cardiovasc Electrophysiol. 2009;20:514–521.

8 Di Biase L, Elayi CS, Fahmy TS, et al. Atrial fibrillation ablation strategies for paroxysmal patients: randomized comparison between different techniques. Circ Arrhythm Electrophysiol. 2009;2:113–119.

9 Verma A, Patel D, Famy T, et al. Efficacy of adjuvant anterior left atrial ablation during intracardiac echocardiography-guided pulmonary vein antrum isolation for atrial fibrillation. J Cardiovasc Electrophysiol. 2007;18:151–156.

10 Elayi CS, Verma A, Di Biase L, et al. Ablation for long-standing permanent atrial fibrillation: results from a randomized study comparing three different strategies. Heart Rhythm. 2008;5:1658–1664.

11 Haissaguerre M, Hocini M, Sanders P, et al. Catheter ablation of long-lasting persistent atrial fibrillation: clinical outcome and mechanisms of subsequent arrhythmias. J Cardiovasc Electrophysiol. 2005;16:1138–1147.

12 Oral H, Chugh A, Yoshida K, et al. A randomized assessment of the incremental role of ablation of complex fractionated atrial electrograms after antral pulmonary vein isolation for long-lasting persistent atrial fibrillation. J Am Coll Cardiol. 2009;53:782–789.

13 Dixit S, Marchlinski FE, Lin D, et al. Randomized ablation strategies for the treatment of persistent atrial fibrillation: RASTA study. Circ Arrhythm Electrophysiol. 2012;5: 287–294.

14 Li WJ, Bai YY, Zhang HY, et al. Additional ablation of complex fractionated atrial electrograms after pulmonary vein isolation in patients with atrial fibrillation: a meta-analysis. Circ Arrhythm Electrophysiol. 2011;4:143–148.

15 Hayward RM, Upadhyay GA, Mela T, et al. Pulmonary vein isolation with complex fractionated atrial electrogram ablation for paroxysmal and nonparoxysmal atrial fibrillation: a meta-analysis. Heart Rhythm. 2011; 8:994–1000.

16 Kalifa J, Tanaka K, Zaitsev AV, et al. Mechanisms of wave fractionation at boundaries of high-frequency excitation in the posterior left atrium of the isolated sheep heart during atrial fibrillation. Circulation. 2006;113:626–633.

17 Lee G, Roberts-Thomson K, Madry A, et al. Relationship among complex signals, short cycle length activity, and dominant frequency in patients with long-lasting persistent AF: a high-density epicardial mapping study in humans. Heart Rhythm. 2011;8:1714–1719.

18 Verma A, Novak P, Macle L, et al. A prospective, multi-center evaluation of ablating complex fractionated electrograms (CFEs) during atrial fibrillation (AF) identified by an automated mapping algorithm: acute effects on AF and efficacy as an adjuvant strategy. Heart Rhythm. 2008;5:198–205.

19 Porter M, Spear W, Akar JG, et al. Prospective study of atrial fibrillation termination during ablation guided by automated detection of fractionated electrograms. J Cardiovasc Electrophysiol. 2008;19:613–620.

20 Kabra R, Singh JP. Catheter ablation targeting complex fractionated atrial electrograms for the control of atrial fibrillation. Curr Opin Cardiol. 2012;27:49–54.

21 Konings KT, Smeets JL, Penn OC, et al. Configuration of unipolar atrial electrograms during electrically induced atrial fibrillation in humans. Circulation. 1997;95: 1231–1241.

22 Zlochiver S, Yamazaki M, Kalifa J, et al. Rotor meandering contributes to irregularity in electrograms during atrial fibrillation. Heart Rhythm. 2008;5:846–854.

23 Lin J, Scherlag BJ, Zhou J, et al. Autonomic mechanism to explain complex fractionated atrial electrograms (CFAE). J Cardiovasc Electrophysiol. 2007;18:1197–1205.

24 Narayan SM, Wright M, Derval N, et al. Classifying fractionated electrograms in human atrial fibrillation using monophasic action potentials and activation mapping: evidence for localized drivers, rate acceleration, and non-local signal etiologies. Heart Rhythm. 2011;8:244–253.

25 Tada H, Yoshida K, Chugh A, et al. Prevalence and characteristics of continuous electrical activity in patients with paroxysmal and persistent atrial fibrillation. J Cardiovasc Electrophysiol. 2008;19:606–612.

26 Takahashi Y, O'Neill MD, Hocini M, et al. Characterization of electrograms associated with termination of chronic atrial fibrillation by catheter ablation. J Am Coll Cardiol. 2008;51:1003–1010.

27 Hunter RJ, Diab I, Tayebjee M, et al. Characterization of fractionated atrial electrograms critical for maintenance of atrial fibrillation: a randomized, controlled trial of ablation strategies (the CFAEAF trial). Circ Arrhythm Electrophysiol. 2011;4:622–629.

28 Roux JF, Gojraty S, Bala R, et al. Effect of pulmonary vein isolation on the distribution of complex fractionated electrograms in humans. Heart Rhythm. 2009;6:156–160.

29 Oral H, Chugh A, Good E, et al. Randomized evaluation of right atrial ablation after left atrial ablation of complex fractionated atrial electrograms for long-lasting persistent atrial fibrillation. Circ Arrhythm Electrophysiol. 2008; 1:6–13.

30 Haissaguerre M, Sanders P, Hocini M, et al. Catheter ablation of long-lasting persistent atrial fibrillation: critical structures for termination. J Cardiovasc Electrophysiol. 2005;16:1125–1137.

31 Singh SM, D'Avila A, Kim SJ, et al. Intraprocedural use of ibutilide to organize and guide ablation of complex fractionated atrial electrograms: preliminary assessment of a modified step-wise approach to ablation of persistent atrial fibrillation. J Cardiovasc Electrophysiol. 2010;21:608–616.

32 Narayan SM, Krummen DE, Shivkumar K, et al. Treatment of atrial fibrillation by the ablation of localized sources: CONFIRM (Conventional Ablation for Atrial Fibrillation With or Without Focal Impulse and Rotor Modulation) Trial. J Am Coll Cardiol. 2012;60:628–636.

33 Narayan SM, Krummen DE, Clopton P, et al. Direct or coincidental elimination of stable rotors or focal sources may explain successful atrial fibrillation ablation: on-treatment analysis of the CONFIRM trial (Conventional Ablation for AF With or Without Focal Impulse and Rotor Modulation). J Am Coll Cardiol. 2013;62:138–147.

CHAPTER 15

Left atrial linear lesions

Stephan Zellerhoff, Han S. Lim, & Pierre Jaïs

CHU de Bordeaux, Hopital Cardiologique Haut Leveque, Pessac, France
Université de Bordeaux, IHU LIRYC, Bordeaux, France

Introduction

Left atrial linear lesions are an indispensable part of an electrophysiologists' armory of ablation strategies, especially in the treatment of persistent atrial fibrillation (AF) and associated macroreentries. Various ablation techniques have been developed over the recent years, although the mechanisms of atrial fibrillation are still incompletely understood [1]. In the context of AF ablation, catheter-based application of linear lesions mimics the surgical Cox maze procedure. It has been shown that linear ablation at the mitral isthmus or the roof of the left atrium contributes to the increase of AF cycle length approximately as much as the isolation of the pulmonary veins, favoring the termination of AF either directly to sinus rhythm or to atrial tachycardia [1–3]. Moreover, linear lesions are needed in the treatment of *de novo* left atrial macroreentrant tachycardia or, more frequently, in post-AF ablation tachycardias. The latter consist of about 50% of macroreentrant ATs requiring linear lesions [4]. Nevertheless, the proarrhythmic effect of incomplete linear lesions, the prerequisite to accurately prove bidirectional block and technical difficulties need to be taken into account while considering the application of linear lesions [5–7].

Techniques

Materials and ablation settings

Creating a contiguous transmural line of radiofrequency (RF) lesions is challenging in the complex

anatomy of the left atrium. Therefore, the use of long sheaths (e.g., Daig SL0 from St. Jude Medical, St. Paul, MN, USA) or Preface (Biosense Webster, Diamond Bar, CA, USA) to stabilize the ablation catheter is helpful. Irrigated tip catheters are the preferred RF ablation catheters, because they provide highest efficacy with a reasonable safety margin. In our institution, the power used for ablation depends on the site of ablation: for the left atrial roof, usually a power setting of 25–30 W is sufficient, whereas at the mitral isthmus higher power settings of 30–37 W are needed to achieve complete lesions. To limit damage to collateral structures and avoid complications, ablation in the coronary sinus (frequently required) is performed with a lower power of 20–25 W. Temperature is limited to 43–45 °C. In general, the irrigation rate is adjusted manually between 7 and 60 ml/min to achieve the desired power and temperature. By this, "overrigation" (reflected as electrode temperature <40 °C), which may reduce lesion size, and "underirrigation," which may prevent obtainment of the desired power, is prevented. Moreover, by limiting the temperature to 43–45 °C, charring and thrombus formation at the catheter tip is reduced.

Confirmation of complete bidirectional block by differential pacing

The principle of differential pacing for proving complete bidirectional conduction block is applied to left atrial linear lesions in the same manner as initially described for the right atrial isthmus ablation [8].

Three essential points are observed during differential pacing next to an ablation line:
1 Pacing on either side of the line results in two activation fronts, each propagating toward one side of the ablation line.

Practical Guide to Catheter Ablation of Atrial Fibrillation, Second Edition. Edited by Jonathan S. Steinberg, Pierre Jaïs and Hugh Calkins.
© 2016 John Wiley & Sons, Ltd. Published 2016 by John Wiley & Sons, Ltd.

2 This results in the presence of widely separated local double potentials along the length of the ablation line, without bridging fragmented potentials. The activation delay associated with complete block depends on individual tissue conduction velocity. Therefore, absolute values of conduction delay are an unreliable predictor of complete block, although a delay of 100 ms is almost always observed in the presence of complete block.

3 While pacing further away from the ablation line, the distance to the opposite side decreases, and the interval should shorten accordingly.

The Detection of very slow conduction is nevertheless challenging. Due to edema acutely caused by RF ablation, the detection of low amplitude, fractionated electrograms at the site of a conduction gap is sometimes prohibited during the initial ablation procedure. Moreover, tissue swelling may result in increased thickness preventing transmural ablation. Therefore, the closure of the conduction gap and achievement of complete block may be possible only during repeat procedures in some cases – after complete lesion formation and reduction of tissue edema. Pitfalls in assessing conduction block will be discussed in the context of the respective linear lesion.

Left atrial linear lesions

Mitral isthmus ablation

The mitral isthmus is defined as the distance between the lateral mitral annulus and the ostium of the left pulmonary vein usually the inferior one. Between these two structures, a linear lesion is applied using RF energy [9]. To achieve this, a multipolar diagnostic catheter is placed in the coronary sinus with the distal pole placed immediately proximal to the planned line of ablation. Bearing in mind the frequent need of epicardial ablation within the coronary sinus to accomplish

conduction block, mitral isthmus ablation should not be performed if the distal coronary sinus cannot be reached with the ablation catheter, to avoid an incomplete, potentially proarrhythmic line [6,7,10].

The ablation catheter is introduced via a long sheath into the left atrium. Ablation is started at the ventricular aspect of the mitral annulus with an atrioventricular ratio of 1:1 or 2:1. The ablation catheter can be positioned at an angle of 90–180° to the lateral mitral annulus. The parallel position often provides good contact, but higher irrigation rates may be required because of occlusion of the irrigation holes with this orientation. In contrast to this, the perpendicular orientation at 90° provides less problems with irrigation, but frequently also less good contact. The sheath and catheter are rotated clockwise to extend the lesion posteriorly to the ostium of the left PVs (Figure 1).

Radiofrequency energy is delivered for 1–2 min at each site in a dragging fashion. Intermittent fluoroscopy and careful electrogram inspection during RF application are mandatory to avoid inadvertent dislodgement of the catheter into the left pulmonary vein or the left atrial appendage, which could result in pulmonary vein stenosis and/or cardiac perforation. Assessment of the impact of ablation and the development of conduction block is facilitated by distal CS pacing during ablation. The observation of local split signals suggests a sufficient local lesion. Gaps in the ablation line can be identified by a short delay (<100 ms) between pacing artifact and the second atrial electrogram on the other side of the ablation line. Although narrow splitting and fractionation may be a sign of persistent slow conduction across the line, a single potential might also be the site of conduction gap.

If a complete conduction block cannot be achieved, an extension of the ablation line at the base of the appendage is sometimes necessary. This higher position usually results in a connection to the left superior

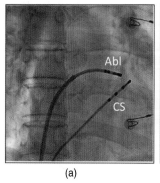 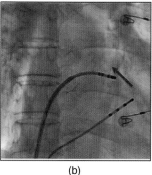 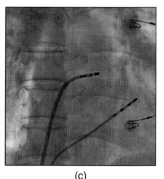

(a)   (b)   (c)

Figure 1 Ablation of the lateral mitral isthmus: starting RF application at the ventricular margin, the catheter is pulled back progressively while the sheath is rotated clockwise to extend the lesions to the ostium of the LIPV.

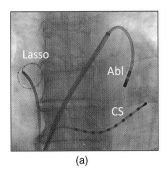
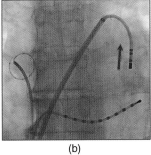
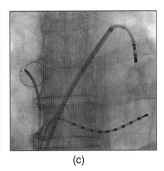

(a)   (b)   (c)

Figure 2 Improving contact: the sheath is placed close to the LAA and the catheter is aligned in a 180° angle to the mitral isthmus. Careful assessment of catheter position and electrograms is necessary to avoid dislodgment of the catheter. Starting from the ventricular aspect (a), the catheter is pulled back during ablation (b) until close to the LSPV (c).

PV. To obtain good contact in this position, the long sheath can be placed at the os of the LAA while the ablation catheter is curved in order to achieve a parallel orientation to the tissue (Figure 2).

Despite extensive endocardial ablation, ablation within the coronary sinus *en face* the endocardial line is frequently required. In this case, the ablation catheter tip should be oriented toward the atrial endocardium to minimize injury of the circumflex artery or free wall of the CS [11,12]. The use of low power and high irrigation rates is also mandatory.

End point and validation
The end point of ablation is achievement of bidirectional block, which is assessed by differential pacing using the following criteria [8,9] (Figure 3):
1 Pacing lateral (higher) to the line in the left atrial appendage results in a proximal-to-distal activation sequence along the coronary sinus.
2 Pacing on the septal side of the line (below the line) via the coronary sinus results in late activation on the opposite side.
3 While pacing the coronary sinus further septal (proximal), the conduction time to the opposite side should shorten.
4 Widely separated local double potentials along the length of the ablation line are invariably observed.

Trouble shooting
Insufficient lesion creation is, in part, due to too low contact force at the site of ablation. There is increasing evidence that the use of a deflectable sheath (e.g., Agilis from St Jude Medical, St. Paul, MN, USA)) for the ablation catheter can enhance the contact force and thereby increase the rate of complete block in the mitral isthmus even without ablating epicardially [5]. Moreover, the histo-anatomical architecture of the tissue in the mitral isthmus possesses special features

that prevent the creation of transmural lesions: apart from the tissue thickness and myocardial sleeves around the coronary sinus, both the local arterial and the venous vessels can act as a "heat sink" and thereby impede sufficient lesion creation [13–16]. This effect can be partially overcome by temporally occluding the coronary sinus and thus reducing the need for epicardial ablation [17,18]. Individual anatomic features and potential obstacles can be identified preprocedurally and taken into account while planning linear ablation at the mitral isthmus [19].

The assessment of the ablation's end point poses several pitfalls: the complete bidirectional block and the persistent conduction can both be diagnosed by mistake [20]. Attention should be paid to carefully differentiate between left atrial and local coronary sinus electrograms in order to assess endo- and epicardial conduction accurately and thereby localize potential conduction gaps. Besides, appropriate adjustments in catheter position and pacing outputs are necessary to ensure correct capture of atrial tissue in relation to the deployed ablation line.

Roof line ablation
This ablation line connects the superior part of both superior pulmonary veins through the roof of the left atrium [21]. Usually, pulmonary vein isolation has already been performed, facilitating the anchoring of this ablation line to the electrically inexcitable pulmonary veins. The use of a long sheath to improve stability is again recommended. Starting ablation from the left superior pulmonary vein and extending the line to the right superior pulmonary vein in a dragging fashion is one technique. The catheter tip is most of the time perpendicular to the left atrial roof during the maneuver, which carries a higher risk of "popping" necessitating a power reduction. Alternatively, ablation can start from the right pulmonary

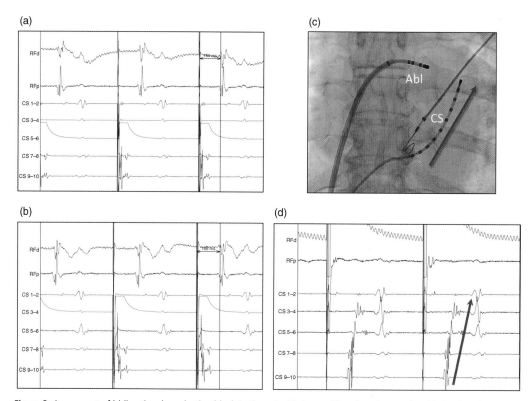

Figure 3 Assessment of bidirectional conduction block in the mitral isthmus: CS pacing close to the ablation line (bipole 3–4) displays a delay of 188 ms measured in the ablation catheter, placed lateral to the ablation line (a). Pacing more septally (bipole 5–6) displays a shorter delay of 154 ms, indicating unidirectional block (b). Pacing lateral to the ablation line with the ablation catheter is associated with proximal to distal activation in the CS, proving bidirectional block (c and d).

vein with the catheter curved toward this vein. Both sheath and catheter are then pushed toward the left superior pulmonary vein (Figure 4). With this method, a more parallel orientation of the catheter tip is achieved, reducing the risk of "popping" and perforation. Looping the ablation catheter within the left atrium and applying a roof line by simply pulling back the catheter from the left superior to the right

superior pulmonary vein is the third alternative. (Figure 5) A posterior line should be avoided to reduce the risk of esophageal injury [22].

End point and validation

1 The activation sequence of the posterior left atrial wall between the pulmonary vein should be low to high in the presence of a completely blocked roof line.

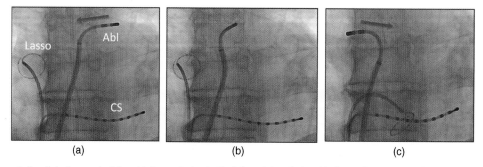

Figure 4 Parallel alignment of the ablation catheter to the left atrial roof: the ablation catheter is curved toward the LSPV (a) and RSPV (c), respectively. The assembly of sheath and catheter is then pushed and rotated to the contralateral superior pulmonary vein.

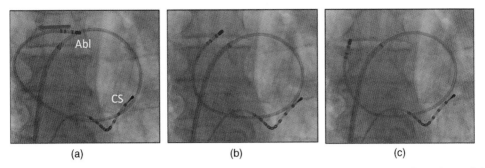

(a)	(b)	(c)

Figure 5 Looping the ablation catheter in the LA: the roof line ablation is started while the loop is still complete and the catheter tip is placed close to the LSPV (a). Ablation is continued while slowly dragging back the catheter toward the RSPV (b) and stopped when reaching it (c).

This can be assessed by sequentially mapping the posterior wall with the ablation catheter either during LAA pacing or during sinus rhythm [21,23] (Figure 6). 2 Widely separated double potentials should be registered along the length of the ablation.

If a mitral line has already been applied, activation of the posterior left atrium is not only low to high but also right to left due to the conduction block in the lateral mitral isthmus. Low amplitude, fractionated electrograms at the site of a conduction gap can sometimes be localized only during repeat after abatement of tissue edema (Figure 7).

Trouble shooting
Tissue thickness at the left atrial roof is usually less than at the mitral isthmus. However, if conduction block cannot be achieved using one ablation technique, another of the described methods should be considered. Similar to mitral isthmus ablation, branches of coronary arteries acting as a "heat sink" may prevent achievement of complete conduction block [13,24]. Other sites within the circuit of the roof-dependent flutter may then have to be targeted.

Anterior mitral isthmus ablation
A potential alternative to the previously described ablation line located at the lateral mitral isthmus is an ablation line in the anterior left atrium, connecting the anterior mitral annulus with either the right superior pulmonary vein or a previously established roof line [25]. In some patients, a diffusely diseased

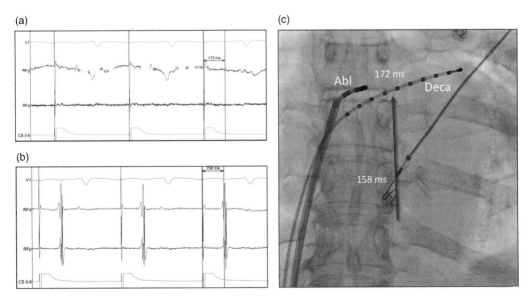

Figure 6 Assessment of conduction block in the roof line: the tip of the decapolar catheter is placed in the LAA; the proximal electrode is located at the septum. The ablation catheter is used to map the high posterior LA, where a delay of 172 ms is registered (a) during pacing in the anterior LA (bipole 5–6). In the low posterior LA, further away from the roof line, a 158 ms delay is recorded (b), demonstrating a low to high activation of the posterior LA.

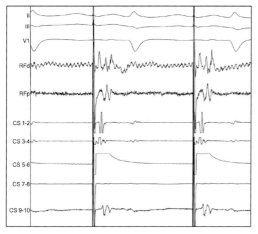
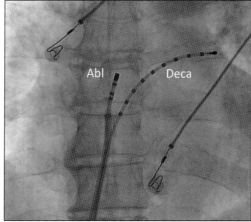

Figure 7 Localization of conduction gaps: during pacing of the anterior LA, a low amplitude, fractionated potential is detected in the roof line suggestive of slow conduction at the site of a gap.

left atrial myocardium with profound reduced voltage is encountered in the anterior left atrium, which may facilitate the achievement of conduction block [26]. In these patients, if a mitral isthmus line has to be performed, the anterior location may be considered as first line given the already altered conduction of this region.

Achieving good contact may be especially difficult, even with the help of a long sheath, due to catheter instability. Catheter ablation is started at the mitral annulus. The ablation catheter is progressively withdrawn while the sheath is rotated counterclockwise to increase contact with the anterior and anteroseptal wall of the left atrium. The ablation catheter is progressively dragged to the right superior pulmonary vein or to the roof line (Figure 8). Alternatively, a modified anterior mitral line can be used to connect the anterior/anterolateral mitral annulus to the left superior pulmonary vein [27].

End point and validation

Bidirectional block is assessed by means of differential pacing [8,25]:

1 Pacing at the anterior left atrium immediately lateral to the ablation line results in activation propagating laterally and posteriorly around the mitral annulus to reach the septal left atrium and the opposite side of the line.

2 As the anterior pacing site is moved further lateral from the ablation line, the conduction time to the opposite side should correspondingly shorten.

3 Widely separated local double potentials along the length of the ablation line are invariably observed.

Trouble shooting

Employing this line may substantially delay the activation of the lateral left atrium and the left atrial appendage, particularly in patients who have undergone extensive left atrial ablation including a lateral

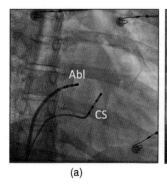
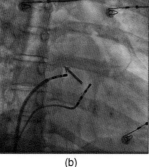
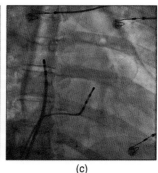

(a)   (b)   (c)

Figure 8 The anterior mitral line: ablation is started at the ventricular margin of the mitral annulus (a). The assembly of ablation catheter and sheath is increasingly rotated counterclockwise toward the septum (b) and to the lesion encircling the right pulmonary veins or to the roof line (c).

mitral isthmus line. Ultimately, this may result in considerable delay or even isolation of the left atrial appendage, potentially increasing the thrombembolic risk and necessitating long-term oral anticoagulation in these patients. The hemodynamic consequences of the LAA isolation or contraction after mitral valve closure are largely unknown and this should probably be avoided.

Conclusions

The application of linear lesions in the LA is frequently necessary in the setting of catheter ablation of persistent AF. The prerequisite of proving complete conduction block to avoid incomplete proarrhythmic lines, potential difficulties, and pitfalls in performing the described linear lesions need to be taken into account before starting each procedure. Technical tools such as deflectable sheaths might be considered in difficult cases.

References

1 Schotten U, Verheule S, Kirchhof P, Goette A. Pathophysiological mechanisms of atrial fibrillation: a translational appraisal. Physiol Rev. 2011;91(1):265–325.

2 Haïssaguerre M, Sanders P, Hocini M, Takahashi Y, Rotter M, Sacher F, et al. Catheter ablation of long-lasting persistent atrial fibrillation: critical structures for termination. J Cardiovasc Electrophysiol. 2005;16(11): 1125–1137.

3 Knecht S, Hocini M, Wright M, Lellouche N, O'neill MD, Matsuo S, et al. Left atrial linear lesions are required for successful treatment of persistent atrial fibrillation. Eur Heart J. 2008;29(19):2359–2366.

4 Haïssaguerre M, Hocini M, Sanders P, Sacher F, Rotter M, Takahashi Y, et al. Catheter ablation of long-lasting persistent atrial fibrillation: clinical outcome and mechanisms of subsequent arrhythmias. J Cardiovasc Electrophysiol. 2005;16(11):1138–1147.

5 Matsuo S, Yamane T, Date T, Hioki M, Narui R, Ito K, et al. Completion of mitral isthmus ablation using a steerable sheath: prospective randomized comparison with a nonsteerable sheath. J Cardiovasc Electrophysiol. 2011;22(12):1331–1338.

6 Anousheh R, Sawhney N, Panutich M, Tate C, Chen W-C, Feld GK. Effect of mitral isthmus block on development of atrial tachycardia following ablation for atrial fibrillation. Pacing Clin Electrophysiol. 2010;33(4): 460–468.

7 Sawhney N, Anand K, Robertson CE, Wurdeman T, Anousheh R, Feld GK. Recovery of mitral isthmus conduction leads to the development of macro-reentrant tachycardia after left atrial linear ablation for atrial fibrillation. Circ Arrhythm Electrophysiol. 2011;4 (6):832–837.

8 Shah D, Haïssaguerre M, Takahashi A, Jaïs P, Hocini M, Clémenty J. Differential pacing for distinguishing block from persistent conduction through an ablation line. Circulation. 2000;102(13):1517–1522.

9 Jaïs P, Hocini M, Hsu L-F, Sanders P, Scavee C, Weerasooriya R, et al. Technique and results of linear ablation at the mitral isthmus. Circulation. 2004;110(19):2996–3002.

10 Matsuo S, Wright M, Knecht S, Nault I, Lellouche N, Lim K-T, et al. Peri-mitral atrial flutter in patients with atrial fibrillation ablation. Heart Rhythm. 2010;7(1):2–8.

11 Takahashi Y, Jais P, Hocini M, Sanders P, Rotter M, Rostock T, et al. Acute occlusion of the left circumflex coronary artery during mitral isthmus linear ablation. J Cardiovasc Electrophysiol. 2005;16(10):1104–1107.

12 Wong KCK, Lim C, Sadarmin PP, Jones M, Qureshi N, De Bono J, et al. High incidence of acute sub-clinical circumflex artery "injury" following mitral isthmus ablation. Eur Heart J. 2011;32(15):1881–1890.

13 Pardo Meo J, Scanavacca M, Sosa E, Correia A, Hachul D, Darrieux F, et al. Atrial coronary arteries in areas involved in atrial fibrillation catheter ablation. Circ Arrhythm Electrophysiol. 2010;3(6):600–605.

14 Wittkampf FHM, van Oosterhout MF, Loh P, Derksen R, Vonken E-J, Slootweg PJ, et al. Where to draw the mitral isthmus line in catheter ablation of atrial fibrillation: histological analysis. Eur Heart J. 2005;26(7):689–695.

15 Kurotobi T, Shimada Y, Kino N, Iwakura K, Inoue K, Kimura R, et al. Local coronary flow is associated with an unsuccessful complete block line at the mitral isthmus in patients with atrial fibrillation. Circ Arrhythm Electrophysiol. 2011;4(6):838–843.

16 Wong KCK, Jones M, Sadarmin PP, De Bono J, Qureshi N, Rajappan K, et al. Larger coronary sinus diameter predicts the need for epicardial delivery during mitral isthmus ablation. Europace. 2011;13(4):555–561.

17 Wong KCK, Jones M, Qureshi N, Sadarmin PP, De Bono J, Rajappan K, et al. Balloon occlusion of the distal coronary sinus facilitates mitral isthmus ablation. Heart Rhythm. 2011;8(6):833–839.

18 Hocini M, Shah AJ, Nault I, Rivard L, Linton N, Narayan S, et al. Mitral isthmus ablation with and without temporary spot occlusion of the coronary sinus: a randomized clinical comparison of acute outcomes. J Cardiovasc Electrophysiol. 2012;23(5):489–496.

19 Yokokawa M, Sundaram B, Garg A, Stojanovska J, Oral H, Morady F, et al. Impact of mitral isthmus anatomy on the likelihood of achieving linear block in patients undergoing catheter ablation of persistent atrial fibrillation. Heart Rhythm. 2011;8(9):1404–1410.

20 Shah AJ, Pascale P, Miyazaki S, Liu X, Roten L, Derval N, et al. Prevalence and types of pitfall in the assessment of mitral isthmus linear conduction block. Circ Arrhythm Electrophysiol. 2012;5(5):957–967.

21 Hocini M, Jaïs P, Sanders P, Takahashi Y, Rotter M, Rostock T, et al. Techniques, evaluation, and consequences of linear block at the left atrial roof in paroxysmal atrial fibrillation: a prospective randomized study. Circulation. 2005;112(24):3688–3696.

22 Zellerhoff S, Ullerich H, Lenze F, Meister T, Wasmer K, Mönnig G, et al. Damage to the esophagus after atrial fibrillation ablation: just the tip of the iceberg? High

prevalence of mediastinal changes diagnosed by endosonography. Circ Arrhythm Electrophysiol. 2010;3(2):155–159.

23 Sang C, Jiang C, Dong J, Liu X, Yu R, Long D, et al. A new method to evaluate linear block at the left atrial roof: is it reliable without pacing? J Cardiovasc Electrophysiol. 2010;21(7):741–746.

24 Yokokawa M, Sundaram B, Oral H, Morady F, Chugh A. The course of the sinus node artery and its impact on achieving linear block at the left atrial roof in patients with persistent atrial fibrillation. Heart Rhythm. 2012; 9(9):1395–1402.

25 Sanders P, Jaïs P, Hocini M, Hsu L-F, Scavée C, Sacher F, et al. Electrophysiologic and clinical consequences of linear catheter ablation to transect the anterior left atrium in patients with atrial fibrillation. Heart Rhythm. 2004;1 (2):176–184.

26 Pak H-N, Oh Y-S, Lim HE, Kim Y-H, Hwang C. Comparison of voltage map-guided left atrial anterior wall ablation versus left lateral mitral isthmus ablation in patients with persistent atrial fibrillation. Heart Rhythm. 2011;8(2):199–206.

27 Tzeis S, Luik A, Jilek C, Schmitt C, Estner HL, Wu J, et al. The modified anterior line: an alternative linear lesion in perimitral flutter. J Cardiovasc Electrophysiol. 2010;21(6): 665–670.

CHAPTER 16

Ablation of autonomic ganglia

Evgeny Pokushalov[1] & Jonathan S. Steinberg[2]

[1]State Research Institute of Circulation Pathology, Novosibirsk, Russia
[2]Arrhythmia Institute, The Valley Health System, University of Rochester School of Medicine & Dentistry, New York, NY and Ridgewood, NJ, USA

Introduction

It is known that the intrinsic cardiac autonomic nervous system (ANS) in the form of a neural network is a key element in the initiation and maintenance of atrial fibrillation (AF) [1,2]. This is supported by the marked reduction of AF inducibility after denervation of the cardiac ANS in animal models [3,4]. The clinical effectiveness of catheter ablation of the ANS, ganglionated plexi (GP) ablation, in patients with AF remains controversial mainly because of the lack of a sensitive and specific means to localize the GP in patients [5–8].

The most commonly used method to localize the major atrial GP is to apply high-frequency stimulation (HFS) to the presumed GP sites to elicit AV block. There are several major drawbacks of this approach. First, the specificity of HFS is not clear. One cannot distinguish stimulation of the autonomic nerves from the stimulation of GP; the latter contains hundreds of autonomic neurons and has been proposed to be the "integration centers" of the intrinsic cardiac ANS and, therefore, serves as a better target than the former [9]. Second, it has not been verified if HFS applied endocardially can effectively elicit a vagal response from the GP that are embedded in epicardial fat pads. Thus, there have been concerns that using HFS as the sole approach to guide GP ablation may not be either specific or sensitive [10].

Recently, it was revealed that one of the major mechanisms underlying the formation of the complex fractionated atrial electrograms (CFAE) is the hyperactive state of the intrinsic cardiac ANS. In addition to the original report by Nadamanee et al. showing that the distribution of the CFAE appeared to coincide with the presumed locations of the major atrial GP, several clinical studies also demonstrated that the distribution of CFAE often encompass those of the GP [10,11]. Some researchers had already suggested that additional identification of CFAE around the areas with a positive reaction to HFS might improve the accuracy of GP's boundary location, enhancing the success rate of ablation [10–12].

Role of the autonomic nervous system in initiation and maintenance of AF: justification for ablation of GP

Widespread clinical interest in the interventional treatment of AF emerged after the publication of data by Haissaguerre et al. showing for the first time that AF can emerge spontaneously as a result of triggering activity originating from the pulmonary vein ostia [13]. Further experimental and clinical data have provided strong evidence for an important role of the ANS in the genesis of AF. It is well known that vagal stimulation and acetylcholine administration induce considerable changes in cardiac electrophysiology. Vagal stimulation shortens the atrial refractoriness and facilitates the induction of atrial fibrillation [14]. Schauerte et al. showed that high-frequency electrical stimulation of ganglionated plexi may induce triggering activity in pulmonary veins and induce atrial fibrillation [15]. Later, Scherlag et al. showed that stimulation of epicardial fat pads that contain clusters of ganglionated plexi may cause atrial fibrillation after an atrial premature stimulus [16]. Nakagawa et al. showed that radiofrequency ablation of these ganglionated plexi reversed the refractory period change and abolished the ability of the right superior pulmonary vein (RSPV) and the left superior

Practical Guide to Catheter Ablation of Atrial Fibrillation, Second Edition. Edited by Jonathan S. Steinberg, Pierre Jaïs and Hugh Calkins.
© 2016 John Wiley & Sons, Ltd. Published 2016 by John Wiley & Sons, Ltd.

pulmonary vein (LSPV) premature stimuli to induce atrial fibrillation [17]. The electrophysiological basis for these findings was addressed in a recent study by Patterson et al. who recorded intracellular action potentials from the sleeve of myocardium from an excised and superfused pulmonary vein–atrial preparation [18]. They showed the synergistic actions of both the sympathetic and the parasympathetic neurotransmitters required to initiate rapid pulmonary vein discharges. Chevalier et al. described the gradients of nerve density in an anatomical study of human hearts [19]. Their research showed that the highest concentration of neural inputs occurs at the pulmonary vein–left atrial junction, fanning out toward the distal pulmonary vein and anterior wall of the left atrium. These reports have recently formed the basis of novel therapeutic strategies for catheter ablation of atrial fibrillation.

Pappone et al. found that patients with documented autonomic denervation had fewer recurrences of atrial fibrillation after catheter ablation [20]. Furthermore, additional radiofrequency applications to sites that elicited a vagal response considerably increased the effectiveness of the procedure in patients with paroxysmal atrial fibrillation. An interesting finding by Scherlag et al. was that ablation of ganglionated plexi before pulmonary vein isolation abolished pulmonary vein triggering activity in 95% of cases [1].

In a recent study, Tan et al. showed that adrenergic and cholinergic nerve densities were highest in the left atrium within 5 mm from the pulmonary vein–left atrial junction, higher in the superior aspect of the left superior pulmonary vein, the anterosuperior aspect of right superior pulmonary vein, and the inferior aspects of both inferior pulmonary veins than diametrically opposite, and higher in the epicardial than endocardial half of the tissue [21]. These data showed that the areas most suitable for ANS modification procedures are located in the immediate vicinity of the pulmonary vein–left atrial junction. Radiofrequency ablation of these sites will destroy either adrenergic or cholinergic nerves because both nerve types are highly colocated in these regions.

In another study, Zhou et al. showed that stimulation of the right anterior ganglionated plexi converts isolated premature depolarization from the right superior pulmonary vein into atrial fibrillation inducing premature depolarizations [22]. This results in progressive changes in the refractory period and window of vulnerability with increasing levels of ganglionated plexi stimulation, thereby indicating a strong link between ganglionated plexi activity and atrial fibrillation inducibility.

More than 85% of the total population is born with pulmonary vein structures whose electrical properties and muscle structure facilitate the formation of triggering activity and reentry circuit sites, but only 3–5% develop atrial fibrillation [21]. This means that other changes are needed to induce atrial fibrillation. Experimental studies have provided compelling evidence that these changes occur as a result of some changes in the ANS [1,14–19,23]. There is strong evidence of the involvement of autonomic nerves in the initiation and maintenance of atrial fibrillation [14–18]. This is related to changes occurring in the ANS, that is, ANS hyperactivity with the uncontrolled release of excess amounts of neurotransmitters. It is known that these neurotransmitters shorten the refractoriness in the atrium [6]. The highest levels of neurotransmitter release would be in the vicinity of the autonomic ganglia concentrated at the ganglionated plexi interfacing with both the atria and the pulmonary vein. Taken together, these neurotransmitters, particularly in locally excessive concentrations, could induce rapid ectopic firing and thereby serve as the "drivers" for initiating atrial fibrillation [22]. In addition to shortened atrial refractoriness, a gradient of atrial refractoriness (electrical dispersion) is a necessary factor of atrial fibrillation. Experimental data have shown that electrical dispersion is caused not only by the ANS innervation gradient but probably also by a gradient of distribution of compromised ganglionated plexi in the atrial myocardium [19,22].

If all the conditions of the development of atrial fibrillation are related to changes occurring in the ANS, then one could ask why the "fight" against cardiomyocytes by means of ostial pulmonary vein ablation or left atrial ablation when we need to reverse the changes in their innervation? Electrical isolation of pulmonary veins does not address the problem of ANS hyperactivity, and this results in new triggering activity located in another area and involving adjacent cardiomyocytes, which causes a recurrence of atrial fibrillation. All this recalls the tilting at windmills.

A new trend in radiofrequency atrial fibrillation ablation is targeted at reversing ANS hyperactivity, that is, eliminating compromised ganglionated plexi that produce excess amounts of neurotransmitters. The first steps have already been taken; however, the results are still far from perfect [5–8]. Unfortunately, a considerable difference remains between the results of experimental and clinical studies. Experimental data provide compelling evidence that atrial fibrillation cannot be initiated and maintained after autonomic denervation of the left atrial myocardium. This means that the clinical goal must be to eliminate the maximum amount of compromised ganglionated plexi.

Localization of left atrial GP

The cardiac ANS can be divided into the extrinsic and intrinsic components. The extrinsic cardiac ANS consists of the soma in brain nuclei and chains of ganglia along the spinal cord and the axons that course en route to the heart. The intrinsic cardiac ANS is composed of a neural network formed by axons and autonomic ganglia concentrated at the GP embedded within epicardial fat pads and the ligament of Marshall [24]. Armour et al. provided a comprehensive anatomic study of the intrinsic ANS in the human heart by delineating the locations of the major GP, their axonal fields and peripheral ganglia (Figure 1) [24]. Further elaboration of the anatomy of intrinsic ANS has been published by Pauza et al. [25]. Four major GPs lie adjacent to the PVs and have been reported to contain 200 or more neuronal cell bodies.

In patients undergoing surgical ablation of AF, the left atrial epicardial fad pads are visualized directly (Figure 2) [10]. GP can also be identified and localized using endocardial HFS in patients undergoing catheter ablation of AF [6,8,11,12]. The sites with a positive vagal response is localized in five major areas are superior left GP, inferior left GP, Marshall tract, inferior right GP, and anterior right GP (Figure 3).

GP ablation for AF: strategies not involving PVI

An effect of PVI may be explained by the hyperactive GP. Some investigators have concluded that complete electrical isolation of the PVs is not a requirement for a successful outcome after PVI [8,20,26–28]. The GP, or the axons traversing the atrial–PV junction, could be destroyed during ablation, which might explain how a PV isolation procedure works. The interruption of axons from these hyperactive GP to PVs may have also contributed to PV focal firing.

Although nowadays GP ablation is not considered as a stand-alone procedure, it still serves as an adjunct therapy to pulmonary vein isolation [29].

GP ablation technique: selective approach

Theoretically, high-frequency stimulation is useful in defining the areas of vagal innervation sites during electrophysiologic procedures. Stimulation of GP associated with a vagal response caused by release of acetylcholine results in reduced atrial action potential duration and development of AF with continued stimulation [1,2]. However, the response to high-frequency stimulation depends on the coupling between the neural elements stimulated and the AV node. High-frequency stimulation at a particular site might elicit the parasympathetic response by stimulating not the autonomic ganglia but the autonomic nerves in the neural network of the intrinsic cardiac autonomic nervous system. In addition, despite detailed endocardial localization of GP sites, we could not usually show a vagal response during ablation. It is probable that during high-frequency stimulation, the afferent link reaction is expressed more fully and the areas with vagal response to high-frequency stimulation may not necessarily correspond to the anatomic regions of GP concentration. In keeping with the observations of Pappone et al., we observed RF-induced vagal reaction only in one-third of the patients, although all of them showed a degree of vagal denervation [20].

The technique of selective GP ablation has been proposed by the Oklahoma group [11,30]. In brief, mapping and ablation are performed under general anesthesia. Atrial ablation target sites are identified as the places where vagal reflexes were evoked by transcatheter HFS (Figure 4). Rectangular electrical stimuli is delivered at a frequency of 20–50 Hz, actual output amplitude 15 V, and pulse duration of 10 ms for 5 s [6]. High-frequency stimulation is performed in five major GP areas: *superior left GP area* (left atrial area interfacing LSPV, left atrial roof), *inferior left GP area* (left atrial area interfacing left inferior pulmonary vein (LIPV), left atrial inferoposterior area), *Marshall tract GP* (along the left atrial appendage ridge), *inferior right GP area* (left atrial area interfacing RIPV, coronary sinus ostium area), and *anterior right GP area* (left atrial area interfacing RSPV, superior vena cava, right atrial septum). When high-frequency stimulation is applied during sinus rhythm, AF generally occurs and then terminates within the next minute. Repeated stimulation usually results in sustained AF, at least in patients with a clinical history of AF. The predominant vagal response to high-frequency stimulation usually is observed during AF, manifested by obvious AV block and hypotension. This response is elicited within 10 s of application of high-frequency stimulation; if no response occurs, the catheter is positioned at adjacent sites. A predominantly efferent sympathetic response to high-frequency stimulation is an increase in blood pressure.

Radiofrequency energy is applied to each site exhibiting a positive vagal response to HFS and continued over the CFAE area. It is preferred to stimulate and ablate the GP in the following order: (1) SLGP, (2) ILGP, (3) ARGP, and (4) IRGP [11]. This practice is based on animal studies from our laboratory showing that IRGP (and the GP in the fat pad in the crux of the heart) appears to serve as the "gateway" for the

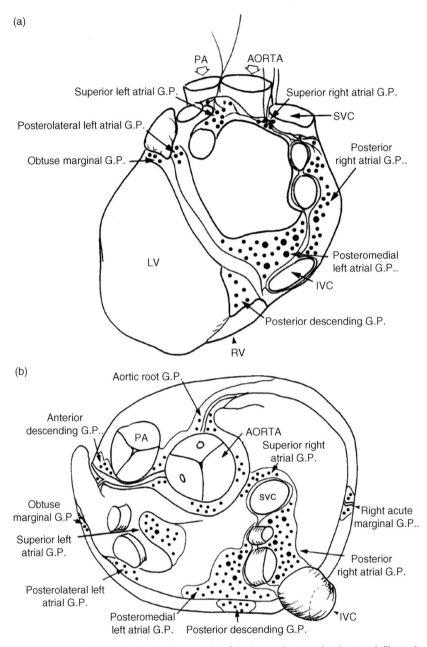

Figure 1 Drawing of a posterior view (a) and superior view (b) of the human heart and major vessels illustrating the locations of posterior atrial and ventricular GP. Note the mediastinal nerves coursing adjacent to the aortic root and joining the two superior atrial GP. SVC, superior vena cava; IVC, inferior vena cava; RV, right ventricle; LV, left ventricle. *Source:* Armour et al., 1997 [24]. Reproduced with permission of Wiley.

autonomic innervation to the AV node. HFS at ARGP, ILGP, or SLGP failed to elicit a parasympathetic response in dogs if IRGP was ablated first [9]. Post-ablation HFS is performed directly after the end of ablation by precise catheter reposition over the ganglionated plexus sites. If a vagal response is still present, radiofrequency energy is reapplied until the vagal response is eliminated. The end point of ablation is the failure to reproduce vagal reflexes with repeated high-frequency stimulation and elimination

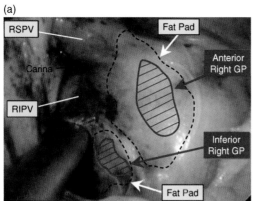 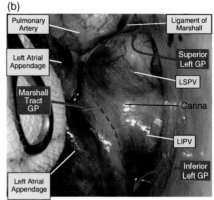

Figure 2 Locations of the five major left atrial autonomic ganglionated plexi in patients undergoing surgical ablation of atrial fibrillation. (a) Thoracoscopic photograph of the right side of the chest during minimally invasive surgical ablation in a patient with persistent AF. An epicardial left atrial fat pad is located anterior to the right superior pulmonary vein and another epicardial fat pad is located inferoposterior to the right inferior pulmonary vein. High-frequency stimulation was delivered within the entire area of the fat pads and in the PVs. However, the sites exhibiting a vagal response were limited to the red crossed hatch areas, corresponding to the anterior right GP and the inferior right GP. (b) Thoracoscopic photograph of the left side of the chest in the same patient showing the LSPV, LIPV, and pulmonary artery. The left atrial appendage was retracted beneath the gauze. The fat pad is located between the left PVs and the left atrial appendage. HFS along this fat pad resulted in a vagal response, corresponding to the Marshall tract GP. Note the ligament of Marshall courses between the LSPV and the pulmonary artery and inserts into the pericardium. The superior left GP is located deep within the pocket beneath the ligament of Marshall, confirmed by a vagal response to HFS. The inferior left GP is located within the fat pad below the LIPV, confirmed by a vagal response to HFS. *Source:* Nakagawa et al., 2009 [10]. Reproduced with permission of Elsevier.

of electrical activity (peak-to-peak bipolar electrogram <0.1 mV) in the CFAE areas (Figure 5).

In the study by Pokushalov et al., the selective ablation of GP identified by high-frequency stimulation showed low clinical efficacy, and within 12 months of observation, AF relapsed among more than 50% of the patients (Figure 6) [8]. Similar results were published in a prior study by Lemery et al. and Scanavacca et al. with even lower efficiency: after 8 months only 29% of the patients did not have AF relapse [5,6].

Unfortunately, the described technique cannot estimate the extent of the full GP area. Autonomic ganglia are located mainly epicardially and the sensitivity of endocardial HFS to localize the GP may not be optimal. The coupling between the stimulated GP and the AV node determines the parasympathetic response elicited by HFS. If this coupling is weak, the precise location of GP area is impossible.

Conventional PVI often involves ablation of the axons of the autonomic nerves, part of the ARGP, SLGP, and ligament of Marshall. However, after the PV antrum isolation the ILGP and IRGP remain intact.

Some researchers had already suggested that additional identification of CFAE around the areas with a positive reaction to HFS might improve the accuracy of GPs boundaries' location and then

enhancing the success rate of ablation [10–12]. At the electrophysiologic laboratory of the University of Oklahoma, the first step of AF ablation is CFAE mapping during AF [31]. This CFAE map then serves as the basis for localization of the major atrial GP. High-frequency stimulation (20 Hz) delivered to these sites invariably elicited a prominent vagal response (AV block). A consistent observation is that the distribution of CFAE encompasses the sites where a vagal response is achieved (the presumed GP sites). The findings of Pokushalov et al. study was that the ablation of areas with positive vagal response by HFS and enhanced ablation of areas with CFAE around the areas where vagal reflexes were evoked is effective (71% patients were free from AF at 12 months) for PAF without PV isolation (Figure 7) [32].

GP ablation technique: anatomical approach

We are of the strong opinion that the location of ganglionated plexi clusters is a key factor for obtaining a good clinical result. Clinical studies have shown that HFS may be used to locate sites of vagal innervation during electrophysiological examination [1,5,6]. This method has a very low sensitivity; however, only

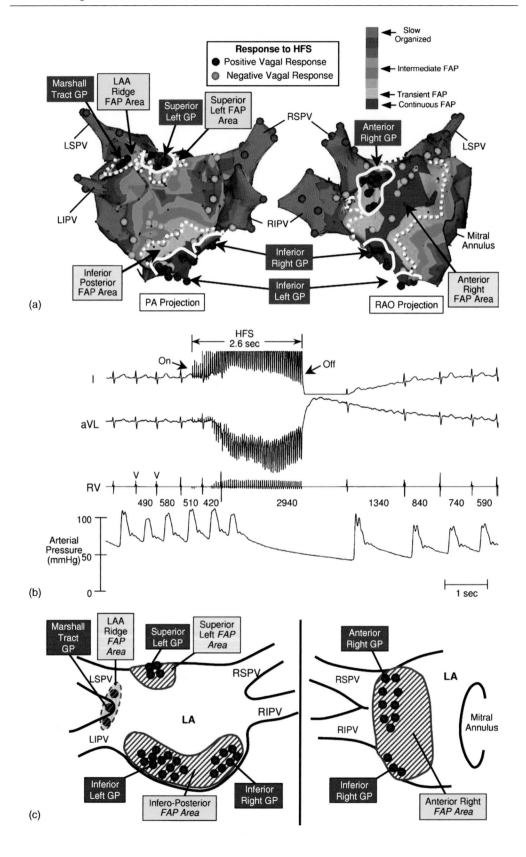

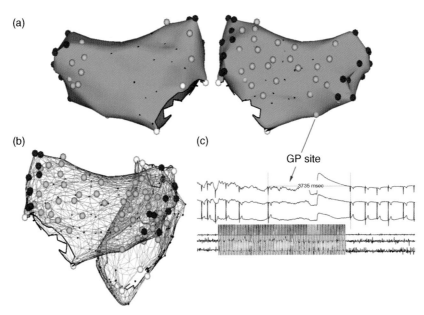

Figure 4 Electroanatomic maps showing high-frequency stimulation in patient 21. (a) Anteroposterior and posteroanterior view of the left atrium. (b) Posteroanterior view of the right atrium and left atrium in a mesh representation to see through the image in the same patient. In both maps, the rose 2-mm dots represent pulmonary vein ostia, the gray 2-mm dots represent high-frequency stimulation negative sites, and the yellow 2-mm dots represent high-frequency stimulation positive sites. See text for details about high-frequency stimulation. (c) Vagal response (pause, 3.7 s) elicited during endocardial high-frequency stimulation (20 Hz, amplitude 15 V, pulse duration 10 ms) in the crux region. *Source:* Pokushalov et al., 2013 [8]. Reproduced with permission of Elsevier.

28–71% of sites with a well-developed ANS responded to HFS [5]. As a result of this, despite the detailed mapping of endocardial and epicardial surfaces, the effectiveness of this procedure needs improvement.

The only possible way to explain such a low effectiveness of HFS is to assume that the stimulated sites that emit vagal responses do not anatomically correspond to actual ganglionated plexi clusters. Zhou et al. clearly demonstrated the possibility that the appropriate stimulation of the axons of the intrinsic cardiac ANS can retrogradely activate the ganglionated plexi at a distance from the site of stimulation and initiate

◀────────────────────────────────────

Figure 3 Correlation between the locations of fractionated atrial potentials (FAP) and the ganglionated plexi in patients undergoing catheter ablation of atrial fibrillation. (a) Electroanatomic map of FAP in a patient with paroxysmal AF. Electrograms were recorded for 2.5 s at each site. Sites exhibiting FAP for the entire 2.5 s were classified as *continuous FAP* and are colored *red*. Sites with FAP for 0.5 s but with organized atrial potentials for the remainder of the 2.5 s were classified as *transient FAP* and are colored *orange*. Sites exhibiting periods of irregular amplitude, polarity, and cycle length but not rapid were classified as "intermediate FAP" and are colored *green* and *light blue*. Sites exhibiting large-amplitude discrete atrial potentials with an average cycle length 180 ms were classified as "slow organized atrial potentials" and are colored *purple*. An *FAP area* was defined as a contiguous area of fractionated atrial potentials (continuous or transient FAP). Four FAP areas were identified: LAA ridge FAP area, superior left FAP area, inferior posterior FAP area, and anterior right FAP area. Sites where endocardial high-frequency stimulation produced a vagal response (see b) are marked by *brown tags*, corresponding the five major GP areas: (1) Marshall tract GP, (2) superior left GP, (3) inferior left GP, (4) inferior right GP, and (5) anterior right GP. HFS failed to produce a vagal response at the sites marked by *orange tags*. Note that all five GP are located within the four FAP areas (see c). (b) Tracings shown from top to bottom are ECG leads I and aVL, electrogram from the right ventricle (RV), and arterial pressure. During AF, endocardial HFS (cycle length 50 ms, pulse width 10 ms) in the posterior left atrium, 2.5 cm inferior to the ostium of the LIPV, results in transient complete AV block (R–R interval 2940 ms) and hypotension (vagal response), identifying the inferior left GP. (c) Schematic representation of the relationship between the FAP areas and the GP locations. *Brown tags* indicate sites with a positive HFS response. Red crossed hatch areas indicate FAP areas. LAA ridge FAP area and Marshall tract GP are located anterior to the left pulmonary veins. All five GP are located within one of the four FAP areas. LSPV, left superior pulmonary vein; PA, posteroanterior; RAO, right anterior oblique; RIPV, right inferior pulmonary vein; RSPV, right superior pulmonary vein.

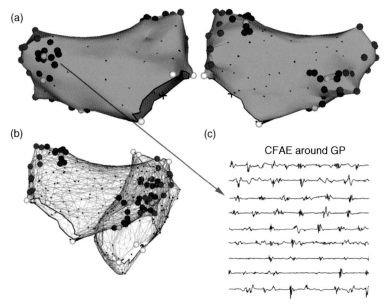

Figure 5 Electroanatomic maps showing RF ablation. (a) Anteroposterior and posteroanterior view of the left atrium. (b) Posteroanterior view of the right atrium and left atrium in a mesh representation to see through the image in the same patients. In both maps, the rose 2-mm dots represent pulmonary vein ostia, the yellow 2-mm dots represent RF applications to high-frequency stimulation positive sites, and the maroon 2-mm dots represent RF applications to complex fractionated atrial electrograms sites. (c) Nine sets of recordings of complex fractionated atrial electrograms from adjacent sites around the ganglionated plexus were obtained. *Source:* Pokushalov et al., 2009 [8]. Reproduced with permission of Elsevier.

atrial fibrillation, possibly by the local release of excessive amounts of neurotransmitters [22]. They proposed a model of highly integrated atrial neural network in which a hyperactive state of the ganglionated plexi may release a gradient of locally excessive concentrations of neurotransmitters and subsequently initiate atrial fibrillation, whereas the activation of the axons may "retrogradely" excite

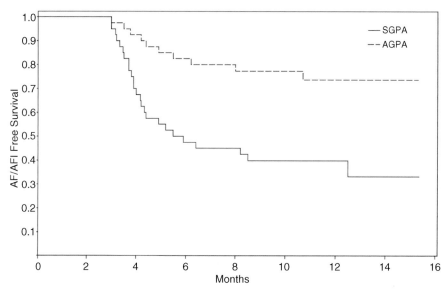

Figure 6 Freedom from recurrent AF or flutter after selective ganglionated plexi ablation (solid line) and anatomic ablation (dashed line). *Source:* Pokushalov et al., 2009 [8]. Reproduced with permission of Elsevier.

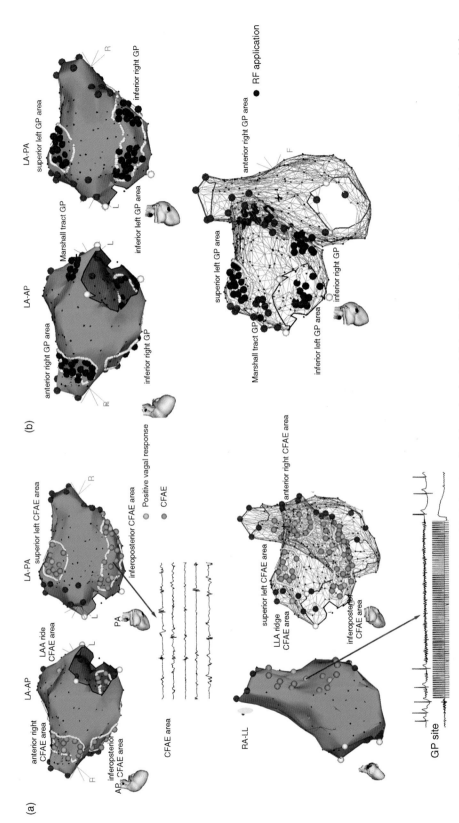

Figure 7 (a) Anteroposterior (AP) and posteroanterior (PA) view of the left atrium; the right atrium in the left lateral (LL) projection; posteroanterior view of the right atrium and left atrium in a mesh representation to see through the image in the same patient. In all maps, the rose 2-mm dots represent pulmonary vein ostia, the yellow 2-mm dots represent high-frequency stimulation positive sites, whereas the blue 2-mm dots represent complex fractionated atrial electrograms from adjacent sites around the positive vagal response. The boundary of the design line passes through the most remote blue dots (demonstrating the fractional activity) on the field vagal response highlighting the GP area. These CFAE areas display the location and boundaries of ganglionic plexus. The pink 2-mm dots represent PV ostia, the maroon red 2-mm dots represent applications of RF energy and the design line represents boundaries of ganglionic plexus. (b) Electroanatomic maps showing RF ablation in the same patient with the same projections. The pink 2-mm dots represent PV ostia, the maroon red 2-mm dots represent applications of RF energy, and the design line represents boundaries of ganglionic plexus. *Source:* Pokushalov et al., 2012 [32]. Reproduced with permission of Wiley.

the ganglionated plexi at a distance to cause the release of neurotransmitters to induce atrial fibrillation.

In analogy, the intrinsic cardiac ANS may behave like an octopus. Activation of the head (ganglionated plexi) may trigger the release of neurotransmitter and initiate atrial fibrillation, whereas stimulation of the tentacles (axons) can retrogradely activate the ganglionated plexi at a distance and trigger the release of neurotransmitters, thus initiating atrial fibrillation in the vicinity of the ganglionated plexi. The octopus theory can provide a logical explanation for the discrepancy between the sites of vagal response (which are also the sites of radiofrequency ablation) and the actual ganglionated plexi sites.

Most current studies focus on the possibility of inducing vagal efferent denervation by means of radiofrequency procedures. Chen et al. suggested that HFS mainly reveals the response of the afferent link of the ANS [23]. Only the stimulation of its afferent link can account for reflex bradycardia and vasodilation upon HFS. These data suggest that sites eliciting vagal responses do not coincide with sites where ganglionated plexi clusters and efferent autonomic nerves are located.

Radiofrequency ablation probably destroys efferent autonomic nerves, which causes a massive release of acetylcholine. Because of this, radiofrequency mapping can be considered a more accurate tool for locating sites of efferent innervation, that is, ganglionated plexi clusters. Radiofrequency mapping is not, however, an absolutely precise tool either, and its sensitivity is also rather low because only one-third of patients had a vagal response to radiofrequency applications, although autonomic denervation was achieved in all patients [20].

As a result of this, the validity of existing methods for the selective location of ganglionated plexi clusters is in question. Unfortunately at present, we have no acceptable method for their location other than HFS. Pokushalov et al. suggested using an anatomical approach to the ablation of ganglionated plexi, that is, performing extended radiofrequency ablation of the sites of their highest density found in anatomical studies [33]. In 1997, Armour et al. provided a detailed description of the localization of all the major ganglionated plexi clusters in the human heart (Figure 8a) [24]. The authors described the exact locations of the five main ganglionated plexi clusters in the wall of the left atrium. In our study, we used these anatomical localization data and performed radiofrequency ablation of these areas until their atrial potentials were completely suppressed to the isoelectric line and the vagal response to their radiofrequency applications disappeared. The first

clinical results of this anatomical approach were encouraging [33].

This technique has been previously described in detail [33]. In brief, the method considers the sites of GP clustering as they are established from anatomic and experimental studies in the human and animal hearts (Figure 8a) [5,21,24,25]. Anatomic GP ablation is not technically challenging because the locations of the four major atrial GP vary minimally among patients. Presumed GP clusters are identified near the pulmonary vein–left atrial junctions at the following sites: left superolateral area (left superior GP), right superoanterior area (right anterior GP of the left atrium and anterior right GP of the right atrium), left inferoposterior area (left inferior GP), and right inferoposterior area (right inferior GP of the left atrium and inferior right GP of the right atrium) (Figure 8b and c).

RF energy is delivered to describe the locations of assumed GP clustering. The quantity of RF energy varied depending on the left atrial volume. Ablation lesions is delivered at the following areas, as seen in the left anterior oblique projection: left superolateral area around the circumference of the pulmonary vein ostium from 11 to 1 o'clock, inferoposterior area from 5 to 9 o'clock, right superoanterior area from 7 to 12 o'clock, right inferoposterior area 5 to 8 o'clock, and between the left and the right inferior pulmonary vein (RIPV) at the crux area (Figure 8c and d). Because the exact anatomic borders of GP clusters are unknown and their location can vary slightly in different patients, an expanded number of RF applications forming a cloud-like shape, and not a line, are delivered. A higher number of applications was delivered in the right side, as both left and right atrial GP clusters are contained in these areas, and there is evidence that the right GP are more arrhythmogenic than the left [2,24]. The end point of the ablation procedure is elimination of electrical activity (peak-to-peak bipolar electrogram 0.1 mV) in the specified areas, and abolition of any vagal effects during RF energy delivery.

The results of selective versus anatomical approach indicate that selective GP ablation directed by high-frequency stimulation is inferior to extensive regional ablation at the presumed anatomic sites of the plexi (Figure 6) [8].

GP ablation for AF: PVI plus GP ablation

The prevailing procedure for catheter ablation now consists of some or all of the following steps: (1) circumferential lesions for PV isolation of the four

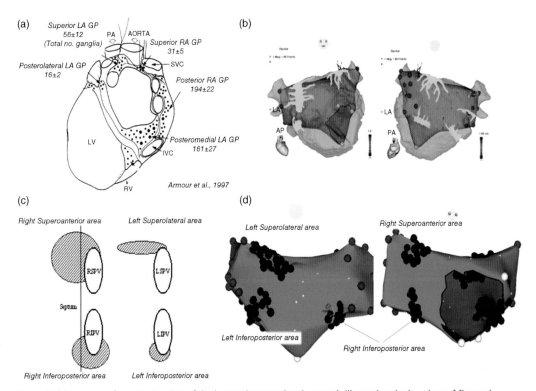

Figure 8 (a) Drawing of a posterior view of the human heart and major vessels illustrating the locations of five major atrial ganglionated plexi. (b) Integration of the computed tomography image and electroanatomic map of the left atrium. (c) Schematic image of the sites of contact of areas of ganglionated plexi ablation with the pulmonary vein–left atrial junction. (d) Imaging of four areas of RF ablation. In both maps, the pink 2-mm dots represent pulmonary vein ostia and the maroon red 2-mm dots represent applications of RF energy. *Source:* Pokushalov et al., 2009 [8]. Reproduced with permission of Elsevier.

PVs from the left atrium, (2) a lesion line connecting the circumferential lines at the atrial roof, (3) mitral isthmus ablation, (4) ablation of CFAE/GP. Lesion sets 2 and 3 are instituted to treat iatrogenically induced macroreentrant tachycardias. Notwithstanding these modifications, the pulmonary vein isolation procedure remains the foundation of the strategy for the treatment of drug-resistant AF.

Since 2004, several reports have indicated a relatively high success rate when PVI was combined with the ablation of ganglionated plexi adjacent to the PV [1,20,34,35]. Recently published studies of 83 patients with paroxysmal and persistent AF who were subjected to this combined procedure were followed for a period of 22 months. The number of patients free of AF or atrial tachycardia after a single ablation procedure was 80% at 12 months and 86% at 22 months [11]. In another study, 67 patients with paroxysmal AF were followed for 12 months; recurrence of AF was documented in 18 (54.5%) patients in the group of PVI alone, whereas recurrence was documented in nine (26.5%) patients in the GP + PVI

group [35]. Overall, 20 (60.6%) patients in the PVI group and 29 (85.3%) patients in the GP + PVI group remained AF free. It should be pointed out that the two groups of studies are not temporally comparable and that the PVI + GP data may show similar results as the PVI group over a longer period of follow-up.

This technique of the PVI + GP has been previously described in detail [34,35]. After the four left atrial GP are ablated, pulmonary vein antrum isolation is performed. The end point of PV antrum isolation is the elimination of potentials within the isolated antral area. As antrum isolation typically transects the ARGP and SLGP areas, we use the ARGP and SLGP ablation sites as the starting points for right and left antrum isolation, respectively. Antrum isolation is not extended to the IRGP and ILGP because of the significant distance between these two GP and the inferior edge of the usual antral isolation area.

The additional benefit of PVI + GP ablation may result from a combination of destroying and/or isolating the triggers of PV firing by PVI and more complete autonomic denervation by GP ablation combined with PVI. Another possibility is that ablation at the GP area resulted in the elimination of the complex electrical activity located at these parts of the left atrium. Katritsis et al. have previously shown that fractionated electrograms are usually found at the areas of GP [36,37]. Choi et al. have also identified intrinsic cardiac nerve activity as a source of electrogram fractionation and trigger of paroxysmal atrial tachyarrhythmias including AF, consistent with the possibility that GP ablation may target both autonomic neural elements and fractionated electrograms [38].

The PVI + GP approach did not confer a higher risk of ablation-induced proarrhythmia despite more RF applications delivered and longer ablation time. Selective GP modification added to PVI has been reported to carry a higher risk of iatrogenic left atrial tachycardias than PVI [11]. Selective anatomic or HFS-mediated GP ablation was complicated by atrial macroreentry in 2–10% of patients after ablation, but did not always require a repeat procedure, since these tachycardias may spontaneously resolve with time [7,8,35,39]. In the present study, GP ablation sites were either on the circumferential PVI lines or were extended to connect with the circumferential lines to avoid creating arrhythmogenic channels. This precaution may account for the lower incidence of left atrial tachycardias that potentially can be introduced by adding GP ablation to PVI.

Efficacy of cardiac autonomic denervation for atrial fibrillation

In recent years, adjunctive CFAE or GP ablation have been proposed as new strategies to increase the rate of elimination of AF. Several studies demonstrated that adjuvant CFAEs ablation in addition to PVI increased the rate of long-term sinus rhythm maintenance in nonparoxysmal AF after a single procedure with or without antiarrhythmic drugs, but did not provide additional benefit to sinus rhythm maintenance in PAF patients [40–42].

Meta-analysis performed by Zhang et al. suggested the benefit of combined CFAE/GP ablation and PVI for the maintenance of sinus rhythm ($n = 887$; OR 1.85; 95% CI: 1.33–2.59; Figure 9) [43]. A previous meta-analysis by Li et al. showed that adjuvant CFAEs ablation in addition to standard PVI increased the rate of long-term sinus rhythm maintenance in nonparoxysmal PAF patients but not in PAF [41]. However, results of Zhang et al. suggested that CFAEs/GP ablation in addition to standard PVI increased the rate of long-term sinus rhythm maintenance not only in nonparoxysmal PAF patients ($n = 360$; OR 2.11; 95% CI: 1.14–3.90) but also in PAF patients ($n = 457$; OR 1.69; 95% CI: 1.09–2.62) [43].

In another subgroup analysis, both adjunctive CFAE and GP ablations significantly increased the freedom from AF (CAFE + PVI subgroup: $n = 820$; OR 1.75; 95% CI: 1.24–2.47; GP + PVI subgroup: $n = 67$; OR 3.33; 95% CI: 1.20–9.29), and no significant differences were found between the subgroups.

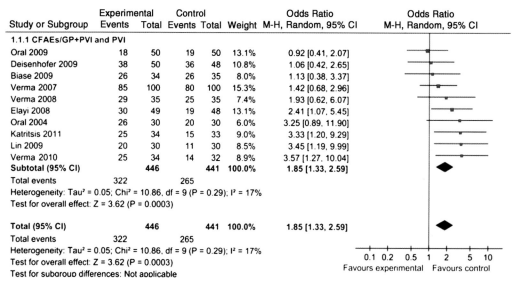

Figure 9 The benefit of CFAE/GP plus PVI compared with PVI. CFAE, complex fractionated atrial electrogram ablation; GP, ganglionated plexi ablation; PVI, pulmonary vein isolation. *Source:* Zhang et al., 2012 [43]. Reproduced with permission of Wiley.

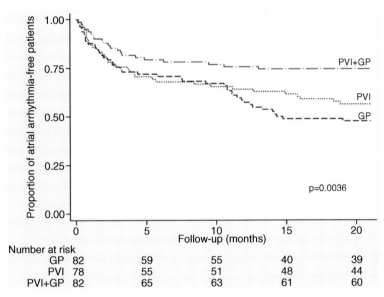

Figure 10 Atrial fibrillation or other sustained atrial arrhythmia recurrence across the three different ablation strategies. Kaplan–Meier estimates were used to calculate the 2-year event rates and comparison was performed with the use of the log-rank test stratified by study site. A blanking period of 3-months after the ablation procedure was adopted. Abbreviations: GP, ganglionated plexi; PVI, pulmonary vein isolation. *Source:* Katritsis et al., 2013 [34]. Reproduced with permission of Elsevier.

It is possible that autonomic denervation by GP ablation plays a central role in the efficacy of PVI, but there remain several questions: (1) Is GP ablation alone as effective as PVI? (2) Does addition of GP ablation to PVI increase the success rate of AF ablation in patients with PAF without an increase in the procedural risks and complication rates? Katritsis et al. provided data to address these questions [34]. Two hundred forty-two patients with symptomatic PAF were recruited and randomized as follows: (1) circumferential PVI, (2) anatomic ablation of the main right and left atrial GP, or (3) circumferential PVI followed by anatomic ablation of the four major atrial GP. Freedom from AF or AT was achieved in 44 (56%), 39 (48%), and 61 (74%) patients in the PVI, GP, and PVI + GP groups, respectively (Figure 10). These results indicate that addition of anatomic GP ablation to conventional PVI improves clinical outcome in patients with PAF. Notably, the success rate of GP ablation alone was not significantly different from that of conventional PVI in which the lesion sets of both approaches have significant overlap.

Katritsis et al. study included only patients with PAF. Although a recent meta-analysis suggested that autonomic denervation plus PVI significantly increases the freedom from recurrence of AF both in paroxysmal and in nonparoxysmal patients, the value of additional ablation (e.g., lines or fractionated electrograms) to PVI in persistent AF continues to be

questioned [43]. As a stand-alone therapy, GP ablation is not enough to confer a favourable outcome on patients with long-standing persistent AF [39]. However, GP ablation alone was still effective in maintaining sinus rhythm in 38.2% (at 24 ± 3 months) patients with long-standing persistent AF, indicating that the autonomic nervous system still contributes to the maintenance of AF in more advanced stages of AF [39].

References

1 Scherlag B, Nakagawa H, Jackman W, Yamanashi WS, Patterson E, Po S, Lazzara R. Electrical stimulation to identify neural elements on the heart: their role in atrial fibrillation. J Cardiovasc Electrophysiol. 2005;13: 37–42.

2 Hou Y, Scherlag BJ, Lin J, Zhang Y, Lu Z, Truong K, Patterson E, Lazzara R, Jackman WM, Po SS. Ganglionated plexi modulate extrinsic cardiac autonomic nerve input: effects on sinus rate, atrioventricular conduction, refractoriness, and inducibility of atrial fibrillation. J Am Coll Cardiol. 2007;50:61–68.

3 Schauerte P, Scherlag BJ, Pitha J, Scherlag MA, Reynolds D, Lazzara R, Jackman WM. Catheter ablation of cardiac autonomic nerves for prevention of vagal atrial fibrillation. Circulation. 2000;102:2774–2780.

4 Lemola K, Chartier D, Yeh YH, Dubuc M, Cartier R, Armour A, Ting M, Sakabe M, Shiroshita-Takeshita A, Comtois P, Nattel S. Pulmonary vein region ablation in experimental vagal atrial fibrillation: role of pulmonary

veins versus autonomic ganglia. Circulation. 2008;117:470–477.

5 Scanavacca M, Pisani C, Hachul D, Lara S, Hardy C, Darrieux F, Trombetta I, Negrão CE, Sosa E. Selective atrial vagal denervation guided by evoked vagal reflex to treat patients with paroxysmal atrial fibrillation. Circulation. 2006;114:876–885.

6 Lemery R, Birnie D, Tang A, Green M, Gollob M. Feasibility study of endocardial mapping of ganglionated plexuses during catheter ablation of atrial fibrillation. Heart Rhythm. 2006;3:387–396.

7 Katritsis D, Giazitzoglou E, Sougiannis D, Goumas N, Paxinos G, Camm AJ. Anatomic approach for ganglionic plexi ablation in patients with paroxysmal atrial fibrillation. Am J Cardiol. 2008;102:330–334.

8 Pokushalov E, Romanov A, Shugayev P, Artyomenko S, Shirokova N, Turov A, Katritsis DG. Selective ganglionated plexi ablation for paroxysmal atrial fibrillation. Heart Rhythm. 2009;6:1257–1264.

9 Hou YL, Scherlag BJ, Lin J, Zhou J, Song J, Zhang Y, Patterson E, Lazzara R, Jackman WM, Po SS. Interactive atrial neural network: determining the connection between ganglionated plexi. Heart Rhythm. 2007;4:56–63.

10 Nakagawa H, Scherlag B, Patterson E, Ikeda A, Lockwood D, Jackman W. Pathophysiologic basis of autonomic ganglionated plexus ablation in patients with atrial fibrillation. Heart Rhythm. 2009;6:S26–S34.

11 Po S, Nakagawa H, Jackman W. Localization of left atrial ganglionated plexi in patients with atrial fibrillation. J Cardiovasc Electrophysiol. 2009. 20:1186–1189.

12 Lemery R. How to perform ablation of the parasympathetic ganglia of the left atrium. Heart Rhythm. 2006;3:1237–1239.

13 Haissaguerre M, Jais P, Shah DC, et al. Spontaneous initiation of atrial fibrillation by ectopic beats originating in the pulmonary veins. N Engl J Med. 1998;339:659–666.

14 Hirose M, Leatmanoratn Z, Laurita KR, et al. Partial vagal denervation increases vulnerability to vagally induced atrial fibrillation. J Cardiovasc Electrophysiol. 2002;13:1272–1279.

15 Schauerte P, Scherlag BJ, Patterson E, et al. Focal atrial fibrillation: experimental evidence for a pathophysiologic role of the autonomic nervous system. J Cardiovasc Electrophysiol. 2001;12:592–599.

16 Scherlag BJ, Yamanashi WS, Patel U, et al. Autonomically induced conversion of pulmonary vein focal firing into atrial fibrillation. J Am Coll Cardiol. 2005;45:1878–1886.

17 Nakagawa H, Scherlag BJ, Aoyama H, et al. Catheter ablation of cardiac autonomic nerves for prevention of atrial fibrillation in a caninemodel [Abstract]. Heart Rhythm. 2004;1:S10.

18 Patterson E, Po S, Scherlag BJ, Lazzara R. Triggered firing in pulmonary veins initiated by in vitro autonomic nerve stimulation. Heart Rhythm. 2005;2:624–631.

19 Chevalier P, Tabib A, Meyronnet D, et al. Quantitative study of nerves of the human left atrium. Heart Rhythm. 2005;2:518–522.

20 Pappone C, Santinelli V, Manguso F, et al. Pulmonary vein denervation enhances long-term benefit after circumferential ablation for paroxysmal atrial fibrillation. Circulation. 2004;109:327–334.

21 Tan AY, Li H, Wachsmann-Hogiu S, et al. Autonomic innervation and segmental muscular disconnections at the human pulmonary vein–atrial junction: implications for catheter ablation of atrial–pulmonary vein junction. J Am Coll Cardiol. 2006;48:132–143.

22 Zhou J, Scherlag B, Ewards J, et al. Gradients of atrial refractoriness and inducibility of atrial fibrillation due to stimulation of ganglionated plexi. J Cardiovasc Electrophysiol. 2007;18:83–90.

23 Chen J, Wasmund S, Hamdan M, et al. Back to the future: the role of the autonomic nervous system in atrial fibrillation. PACE. 2006;29:413–421.

24 Armour JA, Yuan BX, Macdonald S, et al. Gross and microscopic anatomy of the human intrinsic cardiac nervous system. Anat Rec. 1997;247:289–298.

25 Pauza DH, Skripka V, Pauziene N, et al. Morphology, distribution, and variability of the epicardiac neural ganglionated subplexuses in the human heart. Anat Rec. 2000;259:353–382.

26 Stabile G, Turco P, LaRocca V, Nocerio P, Stabile E, DeSimeone A. Is pulmonary vein isolation necessary for curing atrial fibrillation. Circulation. 2003;108:657–660.

27 Lemola K, Oral H, Chugh A, Hall B, Cheung P, Han J, et al. Pulmonary vein isolation as an end point for left atrial circumferential ablation of atrial fibrillation. J Am Coll Cardiol. 2005;46:1060–1066.

28 Pratola C, Baldo E, Notarstefano P, Toselli T, Ferrari R. Radiofrequency ablation of atrial fibrillation. Circulation. 2008;117:136–143.

29 Calkins H, Kuck KH, Cappato R, C et al. Heart Rhythm, 2012;9(4):632–696.e21. HRS/EHRA/ECAS expert consensus statement on catheter and surgical ablation of atrial fibrillation: recommendations for patient selection, procedural techniques, patient management and follow-up, definitions, endpoints, and research trial design: a report of the Heart Rhythm Society (HRS) Task Force on Catheter and Surgical Ablation of Atrial Fibrillation. Developed in partnership with the European Heart Rhythm Association (EHRA), a registered branch of the European Society of Cardiology (ESC) and the European Cardiac Arrhythmia Society (ECAS); and in collaboration with the American College of Cardiology (ACC), American Heart Association (AHA), the Asia Pacific Heart Rhythm Society (APHRS), and the Society of Thoracic Surgeons (STS). Endorsed by the governing bodies of the American College of Cardiology Foundation, the American Heart Association, the European Cardiac Arrhythmia Society, the European Heart Rhythm Association, the Society of Thoracic Surgeons, the Asia Pacific Heart Rhythm Society, and the Heart Rhythm Society.

30 Nakagawa H, Scherlag BJ, Wu R. Addition of selective ablation of autonomic ganglia to pulmonary vein antrum isolation for treatment of paroxysmal and persistent atrial fibrillation [Abstract]. Circulation. 2004;110:III-543.

31 Po SS, Scherlag BJ. CFAE: "I know it when I see it!" But what does it mean? J Cardiovasc Electrophysiol. 2012; 23(1):34–35.

32 Pokushalov E, Romanov A, Artyomenko S, Shirokova N, Turov A, Karaskov A, Katritsis DG, Po SS. Ganglionated plexi ablation directed by high-frequency stimulation and complex fractionated atrial electrograms for paroxysmal atrial fibrillation. Pacing Clin Electrophysiol. 2012;35(7): 776–784.

33 Pokushalov E, Turov A, Shugayev P, Artyomenko S, Romanov A, Shirokova N. Catheter ablation of left atrial ganglionated plexi for atrial fibrillation. Asian Cardiovasc Thorac Ann. 2008;16(3):194–201.

34 Katritsis D, Pokushalov E, Romanov A, Giazitzoglou E, Siontis G, Po S, Camm J, Ioannidis J. Autonomic denervation added to pulmonary vein isolation for paroxysmal atrial fibrillation: a randomized clinical trial. JACC, J Am Coll Cardiol. 2013;62(24):2318–25.

35 Kastritsis DG, Giazitzoglou E, Zografos T, Pokushalov E, Po SS, Camm AJ. Rapid pulmonary vein isolation combined with autonomic ganglia modification: a randomized study. Heart Rhythm. 2011;8:672–678.

36 Katritsis D, Giazitzoglou E, Sougiannis D, Voridis E, Po SS. Complex fractionated atrial electrograms at anatomic sites of ganglionated plexi in atrial fibrillation. Europace. 2009;11:308–315.

37 Katritsis D, Sougiannis D, Batsikas K, et al. Autonomic modulation of complex fractionated atrial electrograms in patients with paroxysmal atrial fibrillation. J Interv Card Electrophysiol. 2011;31:217–223.

38 Choi EK, Shen MJ, Han S, et al. Intrinsic cardiac nerve activity and paroxysmal atrial tachyarrhythmia in ambulatory dogs. Circulation. 2010;121:2615–2623.

39 Pokushalov E, Romanov A, Artyomenko S, et al. Ganglionated plexi ablation for longstanding persistent atrial fibrillation. Europace. 2010;12:342–346.

40 Kong MH, Piccini JP, Bahnson TD. Efficacy of adjunctive ablation of complex fractionated atrial electrograms and pulmonary vein isolation for the treatment of atrial fibrillation: a meta-analysis of randomized controlled trials. Europace. 2011;13:193–204.

41 Li WJ, Bai YY, Zhang HY, Tang RB, Miao CL, Sang CH, Yin XD, Dong JZ, Ma CS. Additional ablation of complex fractionated atrial electrograms (CFAEs) after pulmonary vein isolation (PVAI) in patients with atrial fibrillation: a meta-analysis. Circ Arrhythm Electrophysiol. 2011;4:143–148.

42 Hayward RM, Upadhyay GA, Mela T, Ellinor PT, Barrett CD, Heist EK, Verma A, Choudhry NK, Singh JP. Pulmonary vein isolation with complex fractionated atrial electrogram ablation for paroxysmal and nonparoxysmal atrial fibrillation: a meta-analysis. Heart Rhythm. 2011;8:994–1000.

43 Zhang Y, Wang Z, Zhang Y, Wang W, Wang J, Gao M, Hou Y. Efficacy of cardiac autonomic denervation for atrial fibrillation: a meta-analysis. J Cardiovasc Electrophysiol. 2012;23(6):592–600.

CHAPTER 17

Trigger mapping

Pasquale Santangeli & Francis E. Marchlinski

Cardiovascular Division, Hospital of the University of Pennsylvania, Philadelphia, PA, USA

Introduction

The goal of current catheter-based ablation approaches for the treatment of atrial fibrillation (AF) is to achieve long-term maintenance of sinus rhythm through the elimination of all the possible arrhythmia triggers with the least amount of ablation necessary. Once all the arrhythmia triggers have been eliminated, the incremental value of additional substrate modification with linear ablation and/or ablation of complex fractionated atrial electrograms (CFAE) remains unproven [1–3]. The role of novel substrate-based ablation approaches targeting putative localized sources of AF (e.g., rotors) identified by means of computational mapping techniques is also unclear, as they have never been compared with trigger ablation in an adequately designed randomized trial [4].

The importance of focal triggers initiating AF in humans was first highlighted in 1998 by Haissaguerre et al. [5]. The authors demonstrated that focal discharges from the pulmonary veins (PVs) are able to trigger AF paroxysms [5], and that ablation of such arrhythmogenic foci results in AF suppression. Over the past 15 years, different catheter-based techniques to target PV triggers have been developed and tested in clinical studies. The initial experience with PV trigger ablation targeted solely the arrhythmogenic PV(s) responsible for precipitating AF. The major drawback of such approach was that up to 30% of cases presented no sufficient ectopies to allow accurate mapping, and multiple periprocedural cardioversions were required as sustained episodes of AF were frequently induced. In addition, the clinical outcome of focal PV trigger ablation was suboptimal and the risk of PV stenosis

considerable [5–9]. Subsequent evolution of PV trigger ablation involved empirical isolation of all the PVs, as it became clear that the majority of AF patients have multiple arrhythmogenic PVs, and moving downstream in the atrium to minimize the risk of PV stenosis and target triggers localized in the more proximal antral region of the PVs [9–11]. In the current AF ablation era, an accurate mapping of triggers arising from the PVs has lost some of its original value, since the PVs are empirically isolated regardless of their proven arrhythmogenic activity [12]. Of note, targeting arrhythmogenic veins early in the process of isolating the PVs may still have merit to give them the greatest chance for intraprocedure recovery. Moreover, PV trigger mapping is still extremely useful in patients presenting with isolated focal atrial tachycardia, in whom isolation of only the arrhythmogenic vein is associated with excellent arrhythmia-free survival. A correct understanding of the typical mapping features of PV ectopic activities is also crucial for the differential diagnosis with other non-PV trigger sites during AF ablation procedures, in order to adequately extend ablation beyond the PVs.

Non-PV ectopic activities triggering AF can be elicited in up to 20% of unselected cohorts referred for AF ablation [1,3,13], and are typically clustered in discrete regions such as the inferior mitral annulus (MA), the posterior left atrium (LA), the interatrial septum particularly at the fossa ovalis/limbus region, the Eustachian ridge, the coronary sinus (CS), the crista terminalis (CT) region, and the superior vena cava (SVC) [3,14]. Other sites implicated in AF initiation include the left atrial appendage (LAA) [15], the left superior vena cava (LSVC) [16,17], and its remnant – the ligament of Marshall (LOM) [18,19].

Finally, a minority of subjects, particularly younger patients with lone paroxysmal AF, may have other mechanisms for AF induction (e.g., atrioventricular reentrant tachycardia (AVRT) or atrioventricular nodal reentrant tachycardia (AVNRT) inducing AF). If such

Practical Guide to Catheter Ablation of Atrial Fibrillation,
Second Edition. Edited by Jonathan S. Steinberg, Pierre Jaïs and Hugh Calkins.
© 2016 John Wiley & Sons, Ltd. Published 2016 by John Wiley & Sons, Ltd.

triggers are suspected, the primary target would be the elimination of the inciting arrhythmia [20].

This chapter will describe a systematic approach to elicit and localize AF triggers using standard stimulation protocols, and integrating ECG criteria with intracardiac recordings from multipolar catheters positioned at specific locations.

Preprocedural drug therapy considerations for patients undergoing trigger mapping

In patients undergoing trigger-based AF ablation, preprocedural discontinuation of antiarrhythmic drug therapy plays an essential role. All antiarrhythmics should be discontinued for at least five half-lives in order to avoid interference with trigger inducibility, and possibly reduce the effectiveness of catheter ablation procedures. While adequate drug washout can be achieved in reasonable time before the procedure (i.e., 4–7 days) in most patients treated with conventional antiarrhythmic agents, subjects receiving chronic treatment with amiodarone represent a particular challenge due to the long elimination half-life of the drug (i.e., 58 days on average) [21]. Recent evidence, however, supports an incremental benefit of preprocedural amiodarone washout [22]. In the setting of long-standing persistent AF ablation, preliminary data suggest that amiodarone discontinuation 4–6 months before the procedure increases the chance of disclosing latent non-PV trigger sites, which translates into better long-term arrhythmia-free survival [22].

Although no data are available from clinical studies, there is a strong rationale supporting the benefit of beta-blocker discontinuation before AF trigger ablation. Beta-blockers might interfere with arrhythmia inducibility, negatively affect the blood pressure response during sustained arrhythmias, and significantly blunt the effect of drugs commonly used to elicit triggers, such as isoproterenol. In particular, isoproterenol testing in patients under chronic therapy with cardioselective beta-blockers might induce significant hypotension, due to the need for increasing dosages to overcome the beta-1 blockade, coupled with the unrestricted stimulation of beta-2 adrenergic receptors in vascular smooth muscle cells leading to systemic vasodilation.

In patients with concomitant AF and heart failure due to rapid ventricular rates, however, beta-blocker discontinuation is not recommended without adequate rate control provided by alternative agents [23]. Similarly, patients with risk factors for ischemic heart disease or those with established ischemic heart disease may also benefit from periprocedural continuation of beta-blockers [24].

Stimulation protocols to elicit AF triggers

A reliable induction of triggers represents a key step of the ablation procedure, since the majority of subjects referred for AF ablation do not present recurrent spontaneous firings. At the University of Pennsylvania, we adopt a rigorous and reproducible stimulation protocol that includes both pacing maneuvers and pharmacological challenges [13,14]. At the beginning of the procedure, programmed atrial stimulation is performed to exclude the presence of triggers approachable from the right atrium, such as AVNRT or right atrial tachycardias; these triggers can be elicited in up to 9% of cases [25]. As mentioned, AVNRT might also represent the only trigger of AF, particularly in young subjects with lone paroxysmal AF [20], and slow pathway ablation results in excellent long-term freedom from AF in these patients. The presence of other PV and non-PV triggers is elicited with the following standardized protocol [13,14]: (1) isoproterenol infusion (starting at 3 μg and incrementing every 3–5 min to 6, 12, and 20 μg) and (2) cardioversion of AF induced by left or right atrial pacing (15-beat drive train at an amplitude of 10 mA and pulse width of 2 ms; decrementing by 10 ms from 250 ms to 180 ms and failure to capture with 5 s pause between drives). This protocol has been extensively validated in multiple studies [1,3,13,14,25] and has been demonstrated to be able to elicit arrhythmogenic PV and/or non-PV firing in over 90% of patients referred for AF ablation.

Catheter positioning for trigger mapping

In order to identify triggers based on intracardiac activation, a correct positioning of multipolar catheters is crucial. The CS catheter should be positioned with the most proximal electrode at the CS ostium; this might be validated either fluoroscopically, visualizing the proximal electrode just anteriorly to the epicardial fat in the posteroseptal space – as assessed in the right anterior oblique (RAO) view – or with intracardiac echocardiography (ICE), directly imaging the CS ostium with a gentle clockwise torque of the ICE catheter from the "home view" in the mid right atrium (RA) (Figure 1).

Importantly, CS catheters from different manufacturers may have different electrode sizes and inter-electrode distances; such differences might be relevant when analyzing the CS activation patterns. In humans, the length of the CS varies between 3 and 5.5 cm, and depends upon the site of the drainage of the postero-lateral vein, often marked by the insertion of the valve

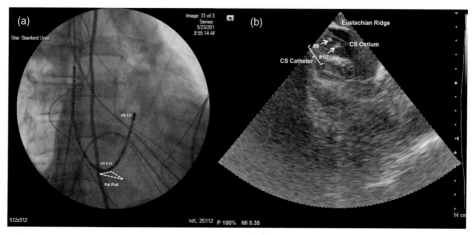

Figure 1 Example of catheter position in the CS for trigger mapping. The proximal electrode pair (9,10) is positioned at the CS ostium. This can be validated with fluoroscopy, visualizing the proximal electrode pair just anteriorly to the epicardial fat pad in the RAO view (a), and with ICE, directly imaging the proximal electrode pair in the CS ostium (b).

of Vieussens [26]. The wall of the CS up to the insertion of the valve of Vieussens (3–5.5 cm from the CS ostium) is made of striated myocardium [27], which may serve either as a trigger for AF, or as a part of a reentrant circuit [27,28]. The vein of Marshall that terminates in the ligament of Marshall and represents the anatomic remnant of the left superior vena cava also inserts into the CS at the level of the valve of Vieussens [29].

When a decapolar catheter with 5-mm electrodes and 2-mm interelectrode distance is used to record the CS activation, it can be anticipated that with the proximal electrode at the CS ostium, the first 3–4 pairs of electrodes will be positioned before the insertion of the valve of Vieussens and the last 1–2 pairs will be beyond the valve of Vieussens. Therefore, both the near-field activation of the CS musculature and the far-field activation of the LA are usually recorded by the first 3–4 electrode pairs, whereas only far-field LA signals are recorded by the distal 1–2 electrode pairs (Figure 2). When mapping a focal trigger with the earliest activation recorded at the proximal 3–4 electrode pairs of the CS catheter, particular attention should be paid to distinguish a true CS trigger from a trigger originating from a left atrial structure. When the earliest activation is recorded approximately at the level of the valve of Vieussens (first or second electrode pair), a trigger from the LOM should also be ruled out. When the earliest activation is recorded at the distal electrode pair, attention should be directed primarily to left atrial structures, since at that level no myocardium is usually present within the CS (see Section Coronary Sinus Triggers) [26,27].

Most laboratories couple the multipolar CS catheter with a multipolar (10- or 20-poles) catheter positioned in the posteromedial RA, along the CT and extending up to the SVC. The distal electrode pair of this catheter should be positioned in the SVC, just above the junction with the RA. Ideally, this should be validated with ICE imaging; the distal electrode pair should be positioned at the lower border of the right pulmonary artery (Figure 3). When correctly positioned, the distal electrode pair of the RA catheter will typically record a far-field RA potential followed by a discrete near-field SVC potential (see also Section Superior Vena Cava Triggers). The SVC muscle sleeve typically extends for several centimeters to the level of the azygous vein.

As an alternative to a catheter placed into the SVC, the proximal 10-poles of a spaced duo-decapolar catheter can replace the multipolar RA catheter, although anatomical variations between patients, such as different RA sizes, might influence the location of the proximal 10 poles.

Once the CS and RA catheters have been positioned, analysis of their pattern of activation during normal sinus rhythm might provide important information regarding the presence and relative contribution of different routes of interatrial activation. During normal sinus rhythm, atrial activation begins from the high right atrium (typically second bipolar pair of the RA catheter when the most distal pair is in the SVC), spreads toward the low right atrium and then to the left atrium. The activation of the left atrium during normal sinus rhythm may occur through three different routes: (1) cranially through the Bachmann's bundle (up to 70% of patients), (2) at the level of

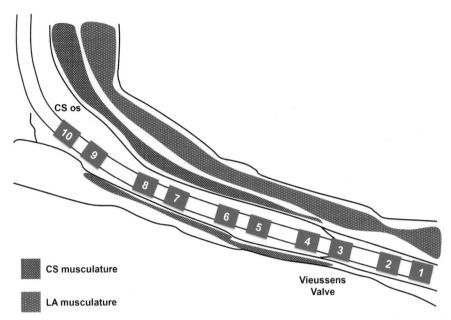

Figure 2 Longitudinal section of the CS with a multielectrode catheter positioned within the vessel. The CS musculature extends from the CS ostium to the valve of Vieussens. The CS musculature is distinguishable from left atrial myocardium. Using a standard decapolar catheter with 5-mm electrodes and 2-mm interelectrode distance, it can be anticipated that the first three–four pairs of electrodes will be positioned before the insertion of the valve of Vieussens, and the last one–two pairs will be beyond the valve of Vieussens (see text for details).

the fossa ovalis, and (3) caudally at the region of the triangle of Koch. Predominant left atrial activation through the Bachmann's bundle can be demonstrated by distal coronary sinus activation (superior and lateral) preceding mid-coronary sinus activation (inferior and septal). On the other hand, predominant left atrial activation through the fossa ovalis/caudal right atrium is suggested by a proximal-to-distal activation of the coronary sinus.

As will be highlighted later in the chapter, a correct understanding of the relative contribution of different routes of interatrial activation plays a crucial role in identifying the site of origin during trigger mapping.

Finally, some laboratories integrate the information collected by the CS and RA catheters with recordings from the circular mapping catheter and from the ablation catheter positioned in specific locations, in order to increase the mapping resolution. For

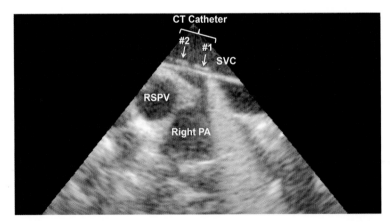

Figure 3 Correct catheter positioning in the crista terminalis/SVC for trigger mapping. The distal electrode pair (1,2) is at the level of the lower border of the right pulmonary artery, confirming its position in the SVC. RSPV, right superior pulmonary vein; CT, crista terminalis.

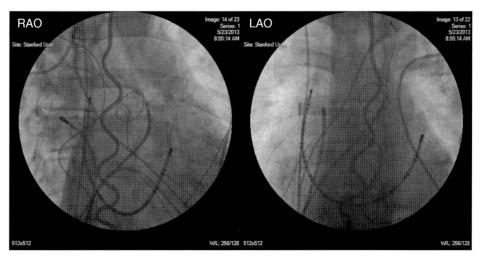

Figure 4 Catheter positioning for trigger mapping: apart from the CS and crista terminalis catheters, additional left atrial recordings are obtained from the ablation catheter positioned in the right superior PV and from the circular mapping catheter positioned within the left superior PV recording far-field signals from the LAA. Far-field LAA potentials will be typically recorded on the electrodes facing the anterior segments of the left superior PV (i.e., poles 1–5 of the circular mapping catheter).

instance, the approach of the Austin group during the Isoproterenol test at the end of PV antrum Isolation includes positioning the circular mapping catheter within the left superior PV recording far-field potentials from the LAA, and the ablation catheter within the right superior PV (Figure 4). When positioning the circular mapping catheter within the left superior PV, far-field LAA potentials will be typically recorded on the electrodes facing the anterior segments of the PV, which are typically the poles 1–5 of a decapolar circular mapping catheter (Figure 4), or poles 1–10 of a duodecapolar circular mapping catheter.

Mapping of triggers: a systematic approach

Ideally, a detailed activation mapping would be the gold standard to detect the origin of AF triggers. Unfortunately, it is very rare to be able to obtain a detailed activation mapping of AF triggers, given their transient nature and/or rapid degeneration into AF. In the majority of the cases, however, triggers can be localized integrating the information from 12-lead ECG and the intracardiac activation timings/patterns at the multipolar CS and RA catheters. In the following section, we will describe a systematic approach to AF triggers mapping, which includes (1) analysis of the P wave morphology on the 12-lead ECG, (2) analysis of the earliest endocardial site of activation at the multipolar CS and crista terminalis catheters referenced to the P-wave onset, and (3) analysis of the

activation patterns at the multipolar CS and crista terminalis catheters.

When analyzing intracardiac activation timings/patterns, it is important to keep in mind the possible confounding effect of atrial scarring and/or previous ablation(s), which might generate bizarre ECG and intracardiac activation patterns. In these cases, creating a "template" of the P-wave morphology and intracardiac activation pattern(s) at the beginning of the procedure with pacing from common AF triggers sites might be particularly helpful. As a general rule, if the P wave in sinus rhythm cannot be clearly recognized as originating from the sinus node region, then one cannot use the P wave during the atrial rhythm as an index of the origin.

Mapping of pulmonary vein triggers

The PVs constitute the major part of the so-called venous component of the left atrium, which is the most posterior structure in the heart. Typical PV anatomy with the presence of four distinct PVs and PV ostia is present in up to 60% of subjects, with the most common variant being a common left trunk, and one or more than one right middle PVs [30,31]. A correct understanding of the PV anatomy by means of preprocedural imaging techniques (e.g., cardiac CT or MRI) and/or intraprocedurally with ICE is crucial when mapping PV triggers.

Owing to their posterior location in the left atrium, triggers from the PVs are characterized by positive P waves across the precordium (leads V1–V6) and a negative P wave in lead aVR. In addition, since the left PVs are localized laterally and more superiorly than the right PVs, the duration of the P wave for the left PV triggers is typically longer than for the right PV triggers (usually a notched P wave is present in V1–V6 for left PV triggers), with more positive forces in lead III than lead II (Figure 5).

Intracardiac activation at the level of the CS and RA catheters is extremely useful to distinguish right versus left PV triggers [32]. In a study by our group on 15 patients with either spontaneous or reproduced PV triggers (with pace mapping), activation at the crista terminalis always preceded CS activation by at least 15 ms (range −15 to −58 ms) in right PVs, while for the left-sided PVs, CS activation was simultaneous or preceded the crista terminalis activation (earliest CS to crista terminalis activation ranging from −14 to + 54 ms) (Figure 6). The direction of CS activation was also a peculiar feature, with left PVs always demonstrating a distal-to-proximal direction of activation, while the right PVs had a proximal-to-distal direction of activation (Figure 7). Such results have been replicated in other studies [33,34]. For instance, Deen et al. analyzed the CS activation sequence while pacing from each of the four PVs and found 100% accuracy for distinguishing right PVs (i.e., proximal-to-distal CS activation) versus left PVs (distal-to-proximal CS activation) [33]. In a subsequent study, Lee et al. validated the CS activation sequence in a prospective series of 38 patients undergoing trigger-based AF ablation. A proximal-to-distal CS activation sequence had 100% specificity in distinguishing right versus left PV triggers. Overall, these results would support the notion that triggers from the right and left PVs are characterized by very different routes of atrial activation, with a predominant transseptal activation over either the Bachmann's bundle or the fossa ovalis for right PVs ectopies, and a predominant activation of the inferolateral LA with an interatrial activation through the CS musculature (distal-to-proximal) for left PVs triggers.

It is important to emphasize that the patterns of CS activation described above do not take into account possible anatomical variants that might produce bizarre patterns of CS activation. For instance, when the left superior PV is displaced superiorly, or right inferior PVs are displaced posteriorly, multiple poles of the CS catheter might be activated simultaneously. Intraprocedural imaging of the PVs with ICE is particularly useful to recognize such typical anatomic variants.

Particular caution should be exercised in the presence of an apparent trigger from the anterior aspect of the left superior PV ostium, especially when there is an

early breakthrough at the mid-CS. In these cases, a trigger from the LOM might be operative (see Section Ligament of Marshall Triggers). Furthermore, the CS activation sequence is not able to differentiate PV triggers from those arising from nearby structures. For instance, a proximal-to-distal pattern of CS activation can be observed also for RA triggers (superior vena cava, crista terminalis), for triggers from the CS os, as well as for LA triggers with a rapid transseptal conduction through the Bachmann's bundle. On the other side of the left atrium, a distal-to-proximal pattern of CS activation is present also for triggers arising from the inferolateral mitral annulus, from the body of the CS, and for lateral LA structures like the left atrial appendage. Establishing the site of origin between PV triggers and other non-PV trigger sites sharing the same patterns of CS activation can be achieved by analyzing the pattern of activation at the crista terminalis catheter, the P-wave morphology on 12-lead ECG, and the earliest site of activation at CS and crista terminalis catheters referenced to the P-wave onset (see Section Mapping of Non-Pulmonary Vein Triggers: General Considerations). In this regard, since neither the CS nor the crista terminalis catheters are recording signals directly from the PVs, the earliest site of activation at these catheters is not expected to precede the P-wave onset on the surface ECG for PVs triggers. Conversely, when a trigger arises from a site directly recorded by the crista terminalis/CS catheters (e.g., SVC, crista terminalis, and CS), the earliest site of activation at the crista terminalis/CS catheters will always precede the P-wave onset on the surface ECG.

The differential diagnosis between a superior and inferior PV site of origin based on the activation timings and patterns recorded from the CS and crista terminalis catheters is more difficult, although some criteria have been suggested [32–34]. In the study by Deen et al., there was a clear separation between the relative timings of activation of the CS and crista terminalis catheters for superior versus inferior PVs. In particular, the activation at the crista terminalis was typically earlier than the CS activation for right superior PVs (CS to crista terminalis activation −36 ± 11.3 ms), while it was almost simultaneous (with an early breakthrough in the middle-lower crista teminalis) for right inferior PVs [33]. For the left PVs, the authors reported a nearly simultaneous crista terminalis and CS activation for left superior PVs (CS to crista terminalis activation 9.4 ± 7.2 ms), and always an earlier CS activation for left inferior PVs (CS to crista terminalis activation 53.9 ± 17.6 ms) [33].

Overall, these results were in line with those reported by our group [32], although we were not able to find a consistent separation in activation

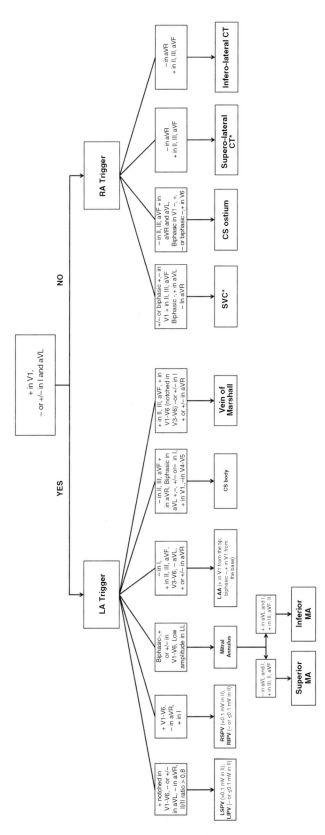

Figure 5 Algorithm for the localization of AF triggers based on the P wave morphology at the 12-lead ECG. LA, left atrial; RA, right atrial; LSPV, left superior pulmonary vein; LIPV, left inferior pulmonary vein; RSPV, right superior pulmonary vein; RIPV, right inferior pulmonary vein; MA, mitral annulus; LAA, left atrial appendage; CS, coronary sinus; SVC, superior vena cava; CT, crista terminalis. *Substantial overlap with RSPV has been described.

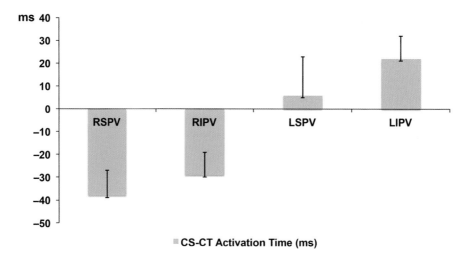

CS-CT Activation Time (ms)

Figure 6 Mean and standard deviation of the earliest coronary sinus to earliest the crista terminalis activation times for the right superior pulmonary vein (RSPV), right inferior pulmonary vein (RIPV), left superior pulmonary vein (LSPV), and left inferior pulmonary vein (LIPV). (See text for details). *Source:* Ashar et al., 2000 [32]. Reproduced with permission of Wiley.

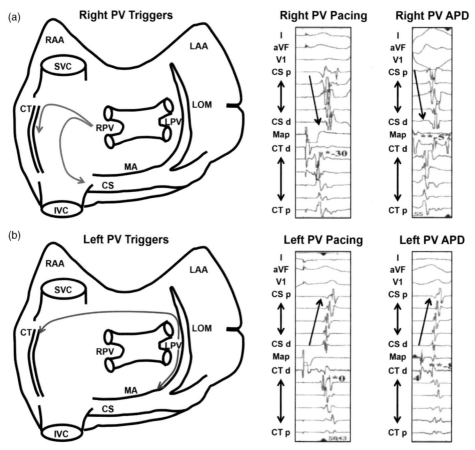

Figure 7 Surface ECG leads I, aVF, and V1, and intracardiac activation sequence at the CS and crista terminalis catheters. The intracardiac activation sequence during either spontaneous or paced right and left PV ectopy is shown. The ablation catheter (Map) is positioned at the lateral right atrium.

timings of the CS/crista terminalis in superior versus inferior PVs. Therefore, the analysis of the activation timing and pattern at the CS and crista terminalis might be used only as a general guide to anticipate the superior versus inferior site of origin of a PV trigger, although considerable overlap exists. Different sites within the same PVs (ostial versus deep within the vein; superior versus inferior border of the vein) and different coupling intervals might also influence the activation patterns and relative timings between the CS and the RA catheters [35–37]. Pace-mapping studies from our group have demonstrated a change in crista terminalis and CS activation timings by >10 ms in up to 21% of PVs when pacing at the ostium compared to pacing deep inside the vein [35], and by >25 ms in 7% of the PVs when pacing from the upper versus the lower border of a PV [36]. Finally, different coupling intervals might account for substantial differences in intracardiac activation timings. Beshai et al. evaluated the effect of coupling interval on the activation sequence at the CS–crista terminalis catheters by delivering a single synchronized atrial premature beat from the PVs and decreasing the coupling intervals from 550 ms until refractoriness [37]. Remarkably, a significant activation change with more premature stimuli was observed in 18% of cases and, occasionally, a complete reversal in the CS activation pattern was observed. These findings likely reflect regional differences in atrial refractory periods, with development of functional areas of block with shorter coupling intervals [38,39].

In addition to the information acquired by the 12-lead ECG and by the intracardiac recordings at the crista terminalis and CS catheters, additional recordings from the LA can further improve the mapping resolution for both PV and non-PV triggers. In a preliminary study, Schweikert et al. evaluated the incremental diagnostic value of direct left atrial recording with a bipolar esophageal catheter in addition to a spaced 16-electrode CS–crista terminalis catheter in 29 patients with drug-refractory AF [40]. The authors showed that the activation sequence and relative timing of the recordings obtained with such catheter configuration were highly predictive not only of right and left atrial origin but also of right and left PV triggers [40].

As mentioned, the approach to trigger mapping currently implemented by the Austin group involves positioning the circular mapping catheter in the left superior PV recording far-field potentials from the LAA, and the ablation catheter in the right superior PV (Figure 4). This approach is systematically adopted after empirical PV antrum isolation during the isoproterenol test and allows a rapid

differentiation between PV and non-PV triggers with similar patterns of CS activation [15].

Mapping of nonpulmonary vein triggers: general considerations

Non-PV triggers account for up to 20–30% of AF initiators [1,3,13,41], and extending ablation to target such sites improves the long-term arrhythmia-free survival [1,3,41–43]. Most non-PV ectopic beats initiating AF are clustered in specific anatomical areas, with varying prevalence across different studies; this likely reflects different patient populations, heterogeneous trigger stimulation protocols, and different definitions for AF triggers (Table 1) [15,41,44–49].

Eliciting non-PV triggers is a key step of AF ablation procedures; lack of a thorough search for such trigger sites is a leading cause for recurrent arrhythmia after successful PV isolation. Recent evidences from studies with ablation technologies targeting solely the PVs have shown that AF might recur in up to 30% of patients with paroxysmal AF despite permanent PV isolation [50], a finding attributable to the presence of non-PV triggers that were not addressed at the time of the index procedure [50]. Although there is no reliable way to predict which patient will present non-PV triggers, several clinical characteristics have been associated with the presence of extra-PV sites of firing [48,51]. In a consecutive series of 293 patients with paroxysmal drug-refractory AF, Lee et al. analyzed the prevalence and clinical characteristics of patients with non-PV ectopies initiating AF [51]. The authors reported an overall prevalence of non-PV triggers of 32%, with 12% of cases having only non-PV firing as a trigger for AF paroxysms. Multivariable analysis showed that female gender and left atrial enlargement were the only independent predictors of non-PV triggers [51]. More recently, Santangeli et al. have investigated the predictors of non-PV triggers in a group of 226 patients with lone paroxysmal AF [48]. In this particular study, non-PV triggers were defined as any consistent non-PV ectopic activity ($\geq$10 premature atrial beats/min and/or atrial tachycardia/fibrillation/flutter). Non-PV triggers were detected in 63 (28%) patients. Patients with non-PV triggers were older (64 ± 11 versus 56 ± 11 years, $P < 0.001$), more frequently females (44% versus 24%, $P = 0.004$), with higher prevalence of associated comorbidities (diabetes: 14% versus 4%, $P = 0.008$; hypertension: 51% versus 29%, $P = 0.002$; high body mass index: 30 ± 7 versus 27 ± 5 kg/m^2, $P = 0.005$), and had longer duration (>10 h) of AF paroxysms ($P = 0.006$). The results of this study, albeit preliminary, would indicate that non-PV triggers can be

Table 1 Prevalence and distribution of non-PV triggers inducing AF in selected studies.

Study name	Year	No. of Patents	Non-PV Triggers, n (%)	Age, years	Females, n (%)	Mapping method	Areas of Non-PV triggers, n (%)
Lin et al. [47]	2003	240	68 (28)	61 ± 13[b]	25 (37)[b]	Conventional, Basket	SVC: 27 (39.7) CT: 10 (14.7) CS: 1 (1.5) IAS: 1 (1.5) LOM: 6 (8.8) LAPW: 28 (41.2)
Shah et al. [41][a]	2003	160	36 (23)	53 ± 11	30 (19)	Conventional	SVC: 3 (8.3) RA: 5 (13.9) CS: 4 (11.1) LAPW: 30 (83.3)
Beldner et al. [44]	2004	401	68 (17)	NR	NR	Conventional, CARTO®	SVC: 4 (5.9) CT: 11 (16.2) TA: 4 (5.9) ER: 13 (19.1) CS: 3 (4.4) IAS: 4 (5.9) LAPW: 15 (22.1) MA: 7 (10.3) Others (AVNRT/AVRT): 20 (29.4)
Suzuki et al. [101]	2004	127	18 (14)	53 ± 11	21 (17)	Conventional	SVC: 5 (27.7) CT: 4 (22.2) CS: 1 (5.6) IAS: 7 (38.9) LOM: 1 (5.6)
Kurotobi et al. [46]	2006	97	63 (65)	59 ± 11	26 (27)	Conventional	SVC: 28 (44.4) CT: 3 (4.8) CS: 10 (15.9) LOM: 11 (17.5)
Yamada et al. [102]	2007	147	31 (21)	NR	NR	Basket	SVC: 12 (38.7) CT: 5 (16.1) CS: 2 (6.5) IAS: 5 (16.1) Other: 5 (16.1)[c]
Valles et al. [49]	2008	45	63[d]	56 ± 9	10 (22)	Conventional	SVC: 2 (3.2)[d] CT: 2 (3.2)[d] CS: 1 (1.6)[d] LAPW: 1 (1.6)[d]
Bhargava et al. [117]	2009	1404	PAF: 2.9% PerAF: 8.2% LPAF: 19.1%	56 ± 11	338 (24)	Conventional, CARTO®/NavX®	NR

Abbreviations: NR, not reported; PAF, paroxysmal AF; PerAF, persistent AF; LPAF, longstanding persistent AF; SVC, superior vena cava; CT, crista terminalis; RA, right atrium; IAS, interatrial septum; LOM, ligament of Marshall; LAPW, left atrial posterior wall; MA, mitral annulus; AVNRT, atrioventricular nodal reentrant tachycardia; AVRT, atrioventricular reentrant tachycardia.
[a] Unknown origin of the trigger in 16 cases.
[b] Data are referred to patients with non-PV triggers.
[c] Possible epicardial triggers in these cases.
[d] Data represent number of triggers.

predicted by simple baseline clinical characteristics, such as advanced age, female gender, presence of associated comorbidities, and longer duration of AF episodes.

Coronary sinus triggers

The CS wall is composed by striated muscle, with macroscopic architecture and histological structure resembling that of the left atrium [27,28]. Similar to the left atrial myocardium, the CS musculature is capable of spontaneous firing [52,53], and has been consistently reported as a trigger site for AF [47,54–57]. Triggers arising from the CS are invariably characterized by negative P waves in the inferior leads (II, III, and aVF). Analysis of the P-wave morphology in the precordial leads is useful to anticipate whether a CS trigger arises from the ostium (biphasic P wave in V1, negative P wave in V6) or from the body of the vessel (positive P wave in V1, negative P wave in V4–V5), although considerable overlap exists (Figure 5).

In the presence of CS triggers, the CS catheter will record the earliest activity preceding the P-wave onset on the surface ECG (Figure 8). On the other hand, caution should be exercised to distinguish between CS triggers and triggers from nearby structures with similar early CS activation.

As mentioned, with conventional decapolar catheters it can be anticipated that the distal pair of electrodes (i.e., 1–2) are positioned beyond the valve of Vieussens, where no CS musculature is present (see Section Catheter Positioning for Trigger Mapping) [27,28]. At this level, the CS catheter will record only far-field signals arising from either the inferolateral MA or from the posterolateral aspect of the LAA that can occasionally be displaced posteriorly. Therefore, when the earliest endocardial activity is recorded at the distal CS catheter, attention should be directed primarily to left atrial structures (Figure 8).

When the earliest endocardial activity is recorded between the CS ostium and the valve of Vieussens (e.g., electrode pair 9–10 to 3–4), attention should be directed to distinguish between a CS trigger and a trigger arising from the nearby structures (i.e., inferior MA or LOM). In addition to the information derived from the P-wave analysis and timing between the earliest CS signal and the onset of the P wave on surface ECG, a careful analysis of the morphology of CS electrograms during sinus rhythm and during the ectopic beat might provide important information. Between the CS ostium and the valve of Vieussens, two atrial components can be recorded, namely, a sharp near-field electrogram due to depolarization of the CS musculature and a blunt far-field electrogram generated by the depolarization of the inferior MA myocardium. The differentiation between the two components is not always straightforward and can be facilitated by introducing atrial extrastimuli at the posterior mitral valve annulus [58]. Such maneuver should be able to selectively bring in the far-field left atrial component and allow the recognition of the near-field CS electrogram. The adoption of CS

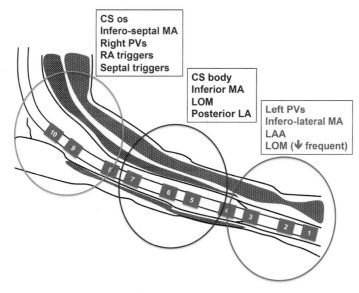

Figure 8 Diagram representing the possible sites of origin of AF triggers according to the earliest activity at the CS catheter.

catheters with closely spaced electrodes improves the mapping resolution and the ability to differentiate between near-field and far-field electrograms.

In the presence of a trigger with the earliest activation between the CS ostium and the valve of Vieussens, the near-field sharp CS electrograms will be earlier than the far-field electrogram for true CS triggers, while the opposite will be true for MA triggers. It is important to emphasize that triggers from the LOM can also display and early activation of the mid-CS musculature (i.e., near-field CS electrogram), owing to the direct anatomical connection between the LOM and the mid-CS [18,46]. Of note, triggers from the LOM typically present multiple early breakthroughs along left atrial posterior wall and left PVs (see Section Ligament of Marshall Triggers). The latter is never observed for pure CS triggers.

Once a CS trigger has been identified, complete CS isolation is the procedural end point (Table 2) [54,55,58]. In a recent multicenter study, Di Biase et al. evaluated the impact of CS isolation versus focal ablation in a series of 225 patients undergoing catheter ablation of AF and showing CS triggers. A total of 140 patients underwent CS isolation, while focal CS ablation was performed in 85 patients. Over a mean follow-up of 21 ± 7 months, freedom from recurrent arrhythmia was achieved in 74% of patients who received CS isolation versus 51% of those receiving focal CS ablation [54].

The most common approach to achieve CS isolation is to target both the endocardial (from the LA) and the epicardial (from within the CS) aspect of the vessel, with the end point of disappearance of CS potentials [54,55]. An alternative approach would be to selectively target the sites of electrical connection between the CS and the LA, as described by Oral et al. [58]. Sites of electrical connection can be identified analyzing the earliest near-field unipolar recordings at the CS catheter while pacing the posterior mitral valve annulus. In a group of 22 patients, Oral et al. described an average of 3 ± 1 electrical connections between the CS and the left atrium, and focal ablation at those sites resulted in CS electrical disconnection [58]. The technique described by Oral et al. has the theoretical advantage of achieving CS isolation with minimal amount of ablation only from the LA aspect, thus minimizing the risk of CS perforation or collateral injury to the coronary arteries. On the other hand, focal ablation of CS–LA connections requires careful mapping and might be time-consuming, and whether it is equivalent to endo-epicardial CS ablation in terms of long-term arrhythmia-free survival requires further investigation.

Mitral annular triggers

The left atrial myocardium around the MA represents another common non-PV trigger site [1,3]. Triggers from the MA can arise from both the superior and the inferior aspect of the annulus. Typically, lateral MA triggers are characterized by biphasic notched P waves in the precordial leads and by low-amplitude P waves in limb leads (Figure 5). In addition, superior MA triggers are characterized by a positive P wave in the inferior leads (II, III, and aVF) and a negative P wave in aVL and lead I, whereas the opposite is valid for triggers arising from the inferior MA. The P wave from the medial mitral annulus will typically be narrow and when originating superiorly may have a negative component in V2.

Table 2 Summary of studies on catheter ablation of AF initiated by triggers from the coronary sinus.

Study name	Year	No. of Patents	Age, years	Sex, M/F	Mapping method	Ablation technique	F/U, mos	Success	Complications[a]
Jais et al. [57]	1997	1	37	F	Conventional	Focal ablation	17	100%	0%
Lin et al. [47]	2003	1	67	M	Conventional	Focal ablation	NA	100% acute	0%
Rotter et al. [55]	2004	1	59	M	Conventional	Isolation	NA	100% acute	0%
Sanders et al. [56]	2004	1	53	M	Conventional	Isolation	2	100%	0%
Knecht et al. [103]	2007	4	51 ± 7	4 M	Conventional	Isolation	NR	100%	1 case of CS narrowing
Di Biase et al. [54]	2011	225	65 ± 10	142 M/ 83 F	Conventional, CARTO®	Focal ablation (38%); isolation (62%)	21 ± 7	51% focal abl.; 74% isolation	0%

Abbreviations: NR, not reported; NA, not available; CS, coronary sinus; abl., ablation.
[a] Complications related to CS ablation/isolation.

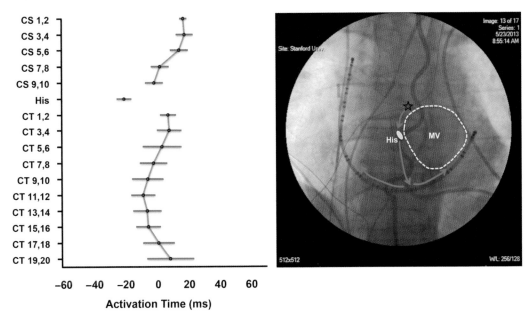

Figure 9 Activation patterns at the crista terminalis, CS and His catheters for superior mitral annular triggers. (Data from Kistler et al. [59].)

The intracardiac activation sequence of triggers from the superior medial MA often shows a proximal-to-distal pattern of CS activation, with the earliest CS activation always following the onset of the P wave on the surface ECG. In addition, the earliest CS activation will occur almost simultaneously to the earliest activation at the crista terminalis catheter [59]. Direct recording from the His bundle region is particularly valuable in these cases, since superior MA triggers typically display an early activity in the right para-Hisian region (Figure 9) [59]. Nevertheless, when a superior MA trigger is suspected, direct recording in the area is crucial in order to distinguish a true MA trigger from a trigger arising from a nearby structure, such as the LAA.

Owing to the anatomical proximity to the CS, inferior MA triggers are always characterized by an early CS activation, which precedes the onset of the P wave on the surface ECG. In addition, CS activation is always earlier than the crista terminalis activation. Since virtually any location along the inferior MA can be a trigger site for AF, the earliest CS activation can span from the distal CS electrode pair (inferolateral MA), to mid-CS (mid-inferior MA), or more proximal CS electrodes (inferoseptal MA). As mentioned, since no CS musculature is expected at the level of the distal CS electrode pairs (i.e., beyond the valve of Vieussens), inferolateral MA triggers can be easily diagnosed, provided that a trigger from a posteriorly displaced LAA has been adequately ruled out. This can be achieved by positioning a circular mapping catheter in the left superior PV recording far-field activation from the LAA or by direct recordings from the LAA (see Section Left Atrial Appendage Triggers).

When the earliest CS activation is in the mid-CS, particular caution should be exercised to differentiate a true mid-inferior MA trigger from a trigger from the CS body or from the LOM. The differential diagnosis between a trigger from the CS body and a MA trigger has been covered previously (see Section Mitral Annular Triggers). Triggers from the LOM typically present early activation of the mid-distal CS often simultaneously to other areas along the left atrial posterior wall and left PVs, due to the presence of muscular connections between the LOM and the posterior left atrial structures (see Section Ligament of Marshall Triggers). When an MA trigger is identified, focal ablation is recommended to eliminate the trigger [1,3,59]. Detailed mapping of the noncoronary cusp in the root of the aorta may be required to successfully eliminate an atrial focus with earliest endocardial activation along the superior medial mitral annulus.

Superior vena cava triggers

The SVC contains embryonic sinus venous tissue capable of spontaneous depolarization [60], and has been consistently demonstrated as one of the most important sites of origin for non-PV triggers (Table 3) [41,45,60–67]. Due to the close proximity between the SVC and other structures, such as the

Table 3 Summary of studies on catheter ablation of AF initiated by triggers from the superior vena cava.

Study name	Year	No. of Patents	Age, years	Sex, M/F	Mapping Method	Ablation technique	F/U, mos	Success	Complications[b]
Ino et al. [45]	2000	1	34	M	Conventional	Focal ablation	15	100%	0%
Tsai et al. [67]	2000	8	55 ± 12	4/4	Conventional	Focal ablation	9 ± 3	100%	0%
Chang et al. [62]	2001	2	50 M/57 F	1/1	Conventional	Focal ablation	3–6	100%	NR
Ooie et al. [66]	2002	1	42	F	Conventional	Isolation	7	100%	0%
Goya et al. [64][a]	2002	16	59 ± 5	14/2	Conventional, CARTO®	Isolation	13 ± 1	81%	0%
Shah et al. [41]	2003	1	NR	NR	Conventional	Isolation	12	100%	NR
Liu et al. [104]	2003	2	73 M/57 F	1/1	EnSite®	Isolation	2	100%	0%
Lin et al. [47]	2003	27	57 ± 12	NR	Conventional	Focal ablation (74%); isolation (26%)	NR	89%	0%
Weiss et al. [105]	2003	1	54	M	EnSite®	Isolation	4	100%	NR
Jayam et al. [65]	2004	1	39	M	Conventional	Isolation	NR	NR	NR
Arruda et al. [61]	2007	24	NR	NR	Conventional	Isolation	15 ± 6	100%	0%
Pastor et al. [106]	2007	3	50 ± 11	1 M/2 F	Conventional	Focal ablation (67%); isolation (33%)	29 ± 17	100%	NR
Wang et al. [107][a]	2008	52	65 ± 9	30 M/22 F	Conventional, CARTO®	Isolation	4 ± 2	81%	0%
Steven et al. [108]	2009	1	49	M	Conventional	Isolation	NA	100% acute	0%
Miyazaki et al. [96]	2010	1	63	F	Conventional	Isolation	12	100%	0%
Kato et al. [109]	2010	1	19	M	Conventional	Isolation	36	100%	0%
Higuchi et al. [110]	2010	12	60 ± 10	8 M/4 F	Conventional	Isolation	12	83%	1 transient PN palsy
Corrado et al. [63][a]	2010	134	55 ± 10	99 M/35 F	Conventional	Isolation	12	81%	0%
Chang et al. [111]	2011	1	62	F	Conventional, CARTO®	Isolation	NA	100% acute	0%
Fukumoto et al. [112]	2011	1	52	M	Conventional, CARTO®	Isolation	10	100%	0%
Miyazaki et al. [113]	2012	1	54	F	Conventional	Isolation	NA	100% acute	0%
Chang et al. [114]	2012	68	56 ± 12	32 M/36 F	Conventional, EnSite®	Focal ablation (47%); isolation (53%)	88 ± 50	65%	1 SN injury (after the third proc.)
Miyazaki et al. [115][a]	2013	76	65 ± 9	59 M/17 F	Conventional, CARTO®	Isolation	NA	NA	4 transient PN palsy
Miyazaki et al. [98]	2013	46	59 ± 11	34 M/12 F	Conventional, CARTO®	Isolation	NA	NA	1 transient PN palsy

Abbreviations: NR, not reported; NA, not available; PN, phrenic nerve; SN, sinus node.

[a] Goya et al. [64] included also patents without SVC ectopy; Wang et al. [107] and Corrado et al. [63] were randomized controlled trials evaluating empirical SVC isolation plus PV isolation versus PV isolation only; Miyazaki et al. [115] performed empirical SVC isolation in addition to PV isolation.

[b] Complications related to SVC ablation/isolation.

right superior PV and the superior crista terminalis, the differential diagnosis between SVC triggers and triggers from the nearby structures based on 12-lead ECG might be challenging (Figure 5) [68]. Typically, the P wave from the SVC will have a larger negative component in V1 compared to a right PV focus. To this purpose, the analysis of intracardiac activation patterns at the crista terminalis and CS catheters is crucial. When the two distal bipoles of the crista terminalis catheter are correctly positioned in the SVC, an early activation of the distal crista terminalis poles will always be recorded for SVC triggers, with a clear distal-to-proximal crista terminalis and CS activation sequence. Conversely, triggers from the right superior PV and those from the upper crista terminalis will show an early activation at more proximal poles of the crista terminalis catheter (Figure 10). The intracardiac recordings from the bipolar electrodes in the SVC will typically show two distinct components: a near-field sharp SVC potential and a far-field blunt potential. The latter might represent either far-field electrogram from the superior RA or a far-field recording from the right superior PV. During sinus rhythm, the far-field activation of the superior RA will always precede the near-field SVC potential, whereas the opposite is true if the far-field recording is due to the right superior PV depolarization.

During SVC ectopy, the activation sequence of the double potentials will be reversed when the far-field electrogram is due to the superior RA depolarization, and will be the same as during sinus rhythm when the far-field electrogram reflects right superior PV activation.

Activation timing to the right para-Hisian region can be also used to differentiate SVC/superior crista terminalis triggers from triggers arising from the right superior PV [34]. Lee et al. developed a simple algorithm with high positive and negative predictive values to distinguish between SVC/superior crista terminalis and right superior PV triggers [34]. Specifically, the authors assessed the difference in time intervals between the activation at the high right atrium and that at the His bundle for sinus beats versus atrial premature beats and found that the difference was <0 ms when the foci arose from the SVC and ≥0 for right superior PV triggers.

In the presence of a SVC trigger, complete SVC isolation is the procedural end point (Table 2) [45,61–65,67]. Isolation is often achieved with a segmental approach targeting the area just proximal to the arrhythmogenic focus [61,63]. The junction between the SVC and the RA can be easily imaged with ICE, and a circular mapping catheter is placed just above the junction between SVC and RA at the level of the lower border of the right pulmonary artery. Radiofrequency

energy is delivered with a segmental approach until SVC isolation is achieved [64]. When the circular mapping catheter is properly placed and radiofrequency energy is applied just proximally to the circular mapping catheter, collateral injury to the sinus node is extremely rare. When delivering RF energy to the anterolateral SVC ostium, caution should still be applied. Increase in sinus node automaticity may be a warning of impending injury to the sinus node. Ablation should not be performed during isoproterenol infusion to avoid masking sinus node injury. Particular caution should be exercised when applying radiofrequency energy at the posterolateral aspect of the SVC, due to6 the risk of collateral injury to the phrenic nerve. Pacing at high output (>20 mA) should be performed before radiofrequency delivery at the posterolateral aspect of the SVC, and ablation should be avoided if phrenic nerve capture with pacing is observed.

Crista terminalis triggers

Ectopy originating from the superior portion of the crista terminalis presents P-wave morphologies and intracardiac activation sequences very similar to SVC or right superior PV triggers (Figures 5 and 10). However, unlike SVC triggers, ectopies from the superior crista terminalis very rarely display the earliest endocardial activation at the distal poles of the crista terminalis catheter (i.e., SVC poles). In addition, the activation sequence of the double potentials in the SVC region is never reversed (see Section Superior Vena Cava Triggers).

The differential diagnosis between a superior crista terminalis trigger and ectopy from the right superior PV can be achieved either by analyzing the difference in time intervals between the activation at the high RA and at the His bundle (as described above) [34] or by direct recording from the right superior PV. Furthermore, the local activation at the crista terminalis catheter rarely precedes the P-wave onset when the trigger arises from the right superior PV, while it always precedes the P-wave onset for superior crista terminalis ectopy.

Triggers from the inferior portion of the crista terminalis are relatively straightforward to diagnose, owing to the peculiar P-wave morphology (Figure 5) together with the earliest endocardial activation at the more proximal poles of the crista terminalis catheter. The intracardiac activation for inferior crista terminalis triggers spreads centrifugally from the more proximal poles of the crista terminalis catheter to the rest of the RA and CS poles, in a proximal-to-distal sequence. Crista terminalis triggers can be eliminated with focal ablation at the earliest activation site [69]; ICE imaging is particularly useful to identify

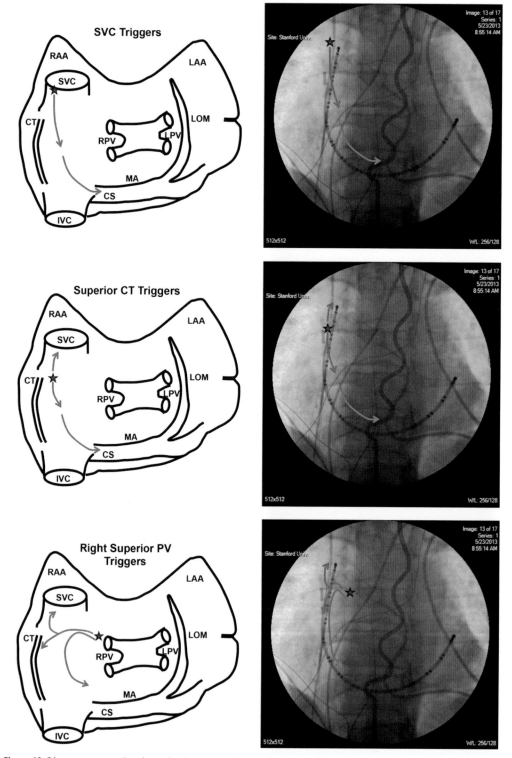

Figure 10 Diagram representing the activation patterns for superior vena cava, superior crista terminalis, and right superior pulmonary vein triggers. During ectopy from the SVC, the distal CT catheter bipole (1,2) is activated earliest, with clear distal to proximal activation, and the CT catheter is activated well in advance of the CS catheter. During RSPV or CT ectopy, the CT catheter is activated earlier at poles 3,4 than at 1,2.

the crista terminalis and assist catheter positioning and radiofrequency delivery.

Septal triggers

The interatrial septum, particularly at the level of the fossa ovalis/limbus, is another well-documented trigger site for AF (Table 1) [1,3,70,71]. Several ECG characteristics have been reported to predict a septal origin of the ectopy, namely, (1) a P-wave duration shorter than that during sinus rhythm [71], (2) a biphasic P wave in V1 (predominantly positive for left posteroseptal and predominantly negative for right anteroseptal) [70,71], (3) a negative P wave in the inferior leads for posteroseptal triggers versus a biphasic or positive P wave for anteroseptal triggers [70,71]. The intracardiac activation pattern in septal triggers is not specific if CS and posterior RA triggers are used to record atrial activation. A posteroseptal CS breakthrough is often observed. Direct recording from the interatrial septum is crucial to identify the site of origin, and focal ablation is commonly adopted to eliminate the trigger.

Left atrial appendage triggers

The LAA originates from the primordial atrial tissue, which is formed by the adsorption of the primordial PVs and their branches. This peculiar embryological origin suggests that the LAA may initiate AF like the PVs [15,72]. In a recent study, Di Biase et al. reported the prevalence of AF triggers from the LAA in a consecutive series of 987 patients (71% nonparoxysmal AF) referred for repeat catheter ablation [15]. LAA firing was assessed only after all the potential sites of reconnection, including the PVs, the posterior wall, and the septum were checked and targeted if reconnected. Overall, 266 (27%) patients showed firing from the LAA at baseline or after administration of

isoproterenol, and in 8.7% of patients the LAA was found to be the only source of arrhythmia. In this study, LAA firing was defined as consistent atrial premature contractions with the earliest activation in the LAA or as AF/atrial tachyarrhythmia originating from the LAA.

Several ECG criteria have been associated with LAA ectopy (Figure 5). The P wave is positive in the inferior leads (III greater than II and aVF), negative in lead I and aVL, and biphasic or frankly positive in V1 [73]. Nonetheless, direct recording from the LAA is mandatory to correctly identify a trigger from this structure. To avoid mechanical ectopy due to direct catheter placement within the LAA, the circular mapping catheter should be positioned in the left superior PV recording far-field potentials from the LAA (Figure 4). In the absence of direct recording from the LAA, analysis of the intracardiac activation at the crista terminalis and CS catheters might be misleading. Indeed, the earliest CS activation (often distal CS) occurs almost simultaneously to the superior crista terminalis activation, due to the rapid transseptal activation through the Bachmann's bundle, which is directly connected to the LAA (Figure 11).

Triggers from the LAA might originate from the LAA ostium (either posteriorly in the region of the ridge separating the LAA from the left superior PV that harbors the ligament of Marshall or from the anterior aspect) or from the LAA body including the LAA tip [15,72–77]. Once the earliest endocardial activity has been recorded in the LAA, it is useful to reposition the circular mapping catheter at the ostium of the LAA (as assessed with ICE) for further mapping [15]. When positioning the circular mapping catheter at the ostium of the LAA, the electrodes recording activity from the posterior aspect of the ostium will often be the poles 1–5 (decapolar catheter)

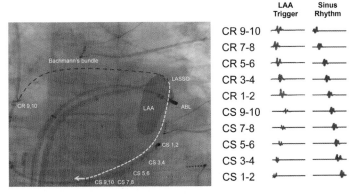

Figure 11 Characteristic activation pattern of triggers from the left atrial appendage (LAA). Note that the earliest CS activation occurs almost simultaneously to the superior crista terminalis activation, due to the rapid transseptal activation through the Bachmann's bundle (see text for details).

or poles 1–10 (duodecapolar catheter). While triggers from the anterior aspect of the LAA ostium or from the LAA body always represent true LAA triggers, particular caution should be exercised when recording ectopies with the earliest endocardial activation in the posterior aspect of the LAA ostium (i.e., ridge region), which might represent triggers from the LOM. However, due to the direct connection between the LOM and the CS, triggers from the LOM are also characterized by an early breakthrough at the mid-CS (see Section Ligament of Marshall Triggers), which is almost never observed in true LAA triggers. Furthermore, LOM triggers often display multiple early breakthroughs along the posterior left atrium, which is also never observed with LAA triggers.

When a LAA trigger has been identified, isolation of the LAA is maybe the optimal procedural end point because precise localization of the trigger may be difficult. In the study by Di Biase et al., out of the 266 patients presenting with LAA firing, 43 (16%) were not ablated, 56 (24%) received a focal ablation, and 167 (63%) underwent LAA isolation. After a mean follow-up of 1 year, AF recurred in 74% of patients who did not receive any LAA ablation, compared to 68% of those treated with focal LAA ablation and 15% of those treated with LAA isolation ($P < 0.001$ for multiple comparison) [15]. The technique employed for LAA isolation is similar to that adopted for PV isolation, although the procedure requires more ablation time. Moreover, since some areas of the LAA have a very thin wall and may be prone to perforation, particular caution should be exercised when isolating this structure. Further studies are necessary to disclose the clinical relevance of LAA isolation and its consequences with respect to potential complications. LAA isolation should be done only when long-term anticoagulation can be instituted or left atrial occlusion is being considered.

Ligament of Marshall triggers

According to the initial description by Marshall [78], the LOM is a vestigial structure containing portions of the embryonic sinus venosus and left cardinal vein. It contains striated muscular bundles that connect to the mid-CS, usually at the level of the valve of Vieussens [29], and to the posterolateral left atrium extending to the epicardial aspect of the muscular ridge between the LAA and the left superior PV. The relevance of the LOM in arrhythmogenesis was first hypothesized by Scherlag et al. in a seminal preclinical study [79] and subsequently confirmed in multiple clinical studies [19,47,80–84]. LOM triggers are extraordinarily sensitive to isoproterenol infusion; patients with classical LOM-dependent AF often report exercise or other hypercatecholaminergic states as a trigger for AF paroxysms [85].

The most reliable method to detect a trigger from the LOM is via direct cannulation from the CS with a small multipolar catheter [19,83,86]. Theoretically, pericardial access might be also useful to obtain direct recordings from the LOM, although such an approach is unpractical.

Hwang et al. first described the technique of direct cannulation of the LOM via the CS in humans [86]. The authors performed balloon occlusion angiograms of the CS to identify the vein of Marshall in 28 consecutive patients with drug-refractory paroxysmal AF. A 1.5-Fr quadripolar catheter was inserted in the vein of Marshall to acquire bipolar recordings. Overall, the vein of Marshall was visualized in 19/28 (68%) patients, and successful cannulation was achieved in 17/19 (89%) cases. Discrete near-field LOM potentials (following the far-field blunt left atrial potential) were recorded in 8/17 (47%) patients between the CS and the left PVs [86]. The reasons for the lack of discrete LOM potentials in about half the cases were investigated in a subsequent study using a canine model [87]. The authors found that direct muscular connections between the posterolateral left atrium and the LOM, which were present in about 50% of dogs, accounted for simultaneous activation of the left atrium and the LOM. On the other hand, in the absence of a direct connection between the posterior left atrium and the LOM, two different potentials in the LOM could be recorded, due to the far-field activation of the left atrium and the near-field activation of the LOM musculature occurring at different times [87].

In the absence of direct recordings from the LOM, a trigger from this structure might be suspected in the presence of (1) early activation in the mid-CS (especially at the approximate level of the valve of Vieussens, that is, 3–5.5 cm from the CS ostium), (2) multiple regions of early endocardial activation in the posterolateral left atrium between the endocardial aspect of the mid-CS and the left inferior PV, and (3) an early endocardial activation in the ridge between the LAA and the left superior PV (Figure 12). Owing to the different conduction patterns between the LOM and the left atrium, analysis of the P-wave morphology is unable to predict a LOM trigger with adequate reliability, although some ECG criteria have been suggested (Figure 5) [80].

In the presence of a LOM trigger, complete electrical isolation of the LOM is the optimal ablation end point. This could be achieved endocardially targeting the areas of muscular connection with the posterolateral left atrium and CS, which are clustered in the ridge between the LAA and the left superior PV, and

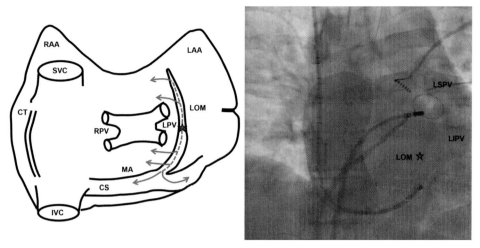

Figure 12 Diagram illustrating the intracardiac activation pattern of triggers originating from the ligament of Marshall. Note the multiple areas of early breakthrough between the mid-CS and the left PVs.

between the mid-CS and the left inferior PV [86]. Rarely, direct catheterization from within the coronary sinus is required to complete LOM isolation. More recently, Valderrabano et al. described a novel technique for LOM ablation using direct ethanol injection in the LOM through an angioplasty wire and balloon. This strategy has been demonstrated to achieve effective ablation of this structure throughout its course between the CS and the left superior PV without significant complications (Table 4) [19,83].

Other triggers

Failure of involution of the left cardinal vein during embryogenesis results in a persistent LSVC [88], which represents the embryologic counterpart of the LOM. The LSVC is also a well-documented trigger site for AF [16,17,89], and many authors suggest to empirically target the LSVC when present regardless of its demonstrated arrhythmogenic activity [17]. The LSVC travels across the posterolateral left atrium between the LAA and the left PVs, and is often directly connected to the mid-CS. In this instance, the CS is significantly dilated and the LSVC can be easily accessed via the CS with a retrograde approach, provided that the CS ostium is patent. Similar to LOM triggers, triggers from the LSVC present multiple early endocardial breakthroughs along the posterolateral left atrium and mid-CS. Complete LSVC isolation is the procedural end point [17,90]. This could be achieved with a retrograde approach via the dilated CS under ICE guidance. In brief, the circular mapping catheter is advanced retrogradely through the enlarged CS into the LSVC for mapping, and

ablation lesions can be delivered along the entire course of the LSVC, proceeding from its most distal aspect (at the level of the left superior PV) to its proximal connection to the CS [17,90].

The inferior vena cava (IVC) has been rarely implicated in the initiation of AF in few case reports [91–93]. This is not surprising given the fact that the atrial muscle sleeve uncommonly extends for any distance into the IVC. Triggers from the IVC presents P-wave morphology and intracardiac activation sequence similar to inferolateral CT ectopies; therefore, direct recording from the IVC is crucial to establish the definitive site of origin. In published studies, patients with IVC triggers have been successfully treated with focal ablation [91–93].

A small minority of patients, particularly young subjects with lone paroxysmal AF, might present with AVNRT or AVRT as a triggering mechanism for AF paroxysms. In these cases, elimination of the triggering arrhythmia is the optimal approach to achieve lasting AF-free survival [20].

Areas of uncertainty and future directions

Current approaches to trigger induction include a combination of pacing maneuvers and pharmacological challenges [13,14]. Intravenous infusion of high doses of isoproterenol is the pharmacological challenge most commonly utilized to elicit triggers. The value of other types of pharmacological challenges, such as intravenous adenosine or other agents (e.g., cholinergic drugs), remains to be proven. Intravenous adenosine has been demonstrated to unmask

Table 4 Summary of studies on catheter ablation of AF initiated by triggers from the ligament of Marshall.

Study name	Year	No. of Patents	Age, years	Sex, M/F	Mapping method	Ablation technique	F/U, mos	Success	Complications[d]
Katritsis et al. [81]	2001	10	54 ± 9	NR	Conventional	Focal ablation (LA, 40%; CS, 10%; LA/CS, 50%)	11 ± 5	70% acute, long-term NR	1 cardiac tamponade
Polymeropoulos et al. [82]	2002	1	66	F	Conventional, CARTO®	Focal ablation (LA)	3	100%	0%
Lin et al. [47]	2003	6	66 ± 13	NR	Conventional	Focal ablation (LA)	NA	50% acute	0%
Hwang et al. [86]	2004	21	43 ± 9	16 M/5 F	Conventional (LOM cannulation)	Focal ablation (CS)	19 ± 10	89%	0%
Kurotobi et al. [46]	2006	73	NR	NR	Conventional	Focal ablation in 11 cases (LA)	10	64%	NA
Valderrabano et al. [19][a]	2009	7	NR	NR	Conventional, CARTO®	Ethanol injection in the LOM	NR	86%	1 CS dissection
Valderrabano et al. [83][b]	2009	10	57.1	9 M/1 F	Conventional, CARTO®	Ethanol injection in the LOM	7 ± 2	80%	0%
Dave et al. [84][c]	2012	54	63 ± 9	41 M/13 F	Conventional, CARTO®, NavX®	Ethanol injection in the LOM	14 (1–30)	85%	1 late cardiac tamponade
Varma and Abi-Saleh [116]	2012	1	52	M	NavX®	Focal ablation (LA)	>12	100% after second proc.	0%

Abbreviations: NR, not reported; NA, not available; LA, left atrium; CS, coronary sinus; proc., procedures.
[a] Initial feasibility study, demonstration of LOM triggers not required.
[b] Demonstration of LOM triggers not required.
[c] LOM triggers were demonstrated only in one patient.
[d] Complications possibly related to LOM ablation.

dormant PV conduction [94,95] and to induce firing from non-PV structures [96–98]. However, adenosine does not seem to provide additional benefit compared to isoproterenol alone [99].

The majority of the published studies have focused on triggers that result in sustained atrial tachyarrhythmias (AF/AT). Nonsustained triggers are also frequently observed during ablation procedures; whether or not an aggressive treatment of nonsustained triggers results in improved arrhythmia-free survival is still unclear and warrants further investigation.

Thus far, there is no reliable way to predict which patient will present with non-PV triggers. A correct identification of such patients before the ablation procedure would have a profound therapeutic impact. Preliminary studies have shown that baseline clinical characteristics such as female gender and

comorbidities are associated with a higher rate of non-PV triggers [48]; these factors might account for a higher degree of left atrial electrical/structural remodeling, which could be detected with noninvasive imaging tools [100]. Genetic factors might also play a role and should be investigated in properly designed case–control studies.

Conclusions

Trigger mapping is a crucial step of current catheter ablation approaches for the treatment of AF. While the majority of AF triggers arise from the PVs, non-PV ectopic activities account for up to 20% of AF initiators and are typically clustered in discrete anatomical regions. These include the MA, the posterior LA, the interatrial septum, the CS, the CT, the SVC, the LAA, and the LOM. A systematic mapping approach based on the analysis of the P-wave morphology and of the earliest activation site and activation pattern at the multipolar CS and crista terminalis catheters allows for a rapid and reliable distinction between different AF trigger sites.

References

1 Dixit S, Lin D, Frankel DS, Marchlinski FE. Catheter ablation for persistent atrial fibrillation: antral pulmonary vein isolation and elimination of nonpulmonary vein triggers are sufficient. Circ Arrhythm Electrophysiol. 2012;5:1216–1223; discussion 1223.

2 Bai R, Di Biase L, Mohanty P, Dello Russo A, Casella M, Pelargonio G, Themistoclakis S, Mohanty S, Elayi CS, Sanchez J, Burkhardt JD, Horton R, Gallinghouse GJ, Bailey SM, Bonso A, Beheiry S, Hongo RH, Raviele A, Tondo C, Natale A. Ablation of perimitral flutter following catheter ablation of atrial fibrillation: impact on outcomes from a randomized study (PROPOSE). J Cardiovasc Electrophysiol. 2012;23:137–144.

3 Dixit S, Marchlinski FE, Lin D, Callans DJ, Bala R, Riley MP, Garcia FC, Hutchinson MD, Ratcliffe SJ, Cooper JM, Verdino RJ, Patel VV, Zado ES, Cash NR, Killian T, Tomson TT, Gerstenfeld EP. Randomized ablation strategies for the treatment of persistent atrial fibrillation: RASTA study. Circ Arrhythm Electrophysiol. 2012;5:287–294.

4 Narayan SM, Krummen DE, Shivkumar K, Clopton P, Rappel WJ, Miller JM. Treatment of atrial fibrillation by the ablation of localized sources: CONFIRM (Conventional Ablation for Atrial Fibrillation With or Without Focal Impulse and Rotor Modulation) Trial. J Am Coll Cardiol. 2012;60:628–636.

5 Haissaguerre M, Jais P, Shah DC, Takahashi A, Hocini M, Quiniou G, Garrigue S, Le Mouroux A, Le Metayer P, Clementy J. Spontaneous initiation of atrial fibrillation by ectopic beats originating in the pulmonary veins. N Engl J Med. 1998;339:659–666.

6 Chen SA, Hsieh MH, Tai CT, Tsai CF, Prakash VS, Yu WC, Hsu TL, Ding YA, Chang MS. Initiation of atrial fibrillation by ectopic beats originating from the pulmonary veins: electrophysiological characteristics, pharmacological responses, and effects of radiofrequency ablation. Circulation. 1999;100:1879–1886.

7 Gerstenfeld EP, Guerra P, Sparks PB, Hattori K, Lesh MD. Clinical outcome after radiofrequency catheter ablation of focal atrial fibrillation triggers. J Cardiovasc Electrophysiol. 2001;12:900–908.

8 Saad EB, Marrouche NF, Natale A. Ablation of atrial fibrillation. Curr Cardiol Rep. 2002;4:379–387.

9 Kanagaratnam L, Tomassoni G, Schweikert R, Pavia S, Bash D, Beheiry S, Lesh M, Niebauer M, Saliba W, Chung M, Tchou P, Natale A. Empirical pulmonary vein isolation in patients with chronic atrial fibrillation using a three-dimensional nonfluoroscopic mapping system: long-term follow-up. Pacing Clin Electrophysiol. 2001;24:1774–1779.

10 Marrouche NF, Dresing T, Cole C, Bash D, Saad E, Balaban K, Pavia SV, Schweikert R, Saliba W, Abdul-Karim A, Pisano E, Fanelli R, Tchou P, Natale A. Circular mapping and ablation of the pulmonary vein for treatment of atrial fibrillation: impact of different catheter technologies. J Am Coll Cardiol. 2002;40: 464–474.

11 Pappone C, Santinelli V, Manguso F, Vicedomini G, Gugliotta F, Augello G, Mazzone P, Tortoriello V, Landoni G, Zangrillo A, Lang C, Tomita T, Mesas C, Mastella E, Alfieri O. Pulmonary vein denervation enhances long-term benefit after circumferential ablation for paroxysmal atrial fibrillation. Circulation. 2004;109:327–334.

12 Calkins H, Kuck KH, Cappato R, Brugada J, Camm AJ, Chen SA, Crijns HJ, Damiano RJ, Jr., Davies DW, DiMarco J, Edgerton J, Ellenbogen K, Ezekowitz MD, Haines DE, Haissaguerre M, Hindricks G, Iesaka Y, Jackman W, Jalife J, Jais P, Kalman J, Keane D, Kim YH, Kirchhof P, Klein G, Kottkamp H, Kumagai K, Lindsay BD, Mansour M, Marchlinski FE, McCarthy PM, Mont JL, Morady F, Nademanee K, Nakagawa H, Natale A, Nattel S, Packer DL, Pappone C, Prystowsky E, Raviele A, Reddy V, Ruskin JN, Shemin RJ, Tsao HM, Wilber D, Heart Rhythm Society Task Force on C, Surgical Ablation of Atrial F. 2012 HRS/EHRA/ECAS Expert Consensus Statement on Catheter and Surgical Ablation of Atrial Fibrillation: recommendations for patient selection, procedural techniques, patient management and follow-up, definitions, endpoints, and research trial design: a report of the Heart Rhythm Society (HRS) Task Force on Catheter and Surgical Ablation of Atrial Fibrillation. Developed in partnership with the European Heart Rhythm Association (EHRA), a registered branch of the European Society of Cardiology (ESC) and the European Cardiac Arrhythmia Society (ECAS); and in collaboration with the American College of Cardiology (ACC), American Heart Association (AHA), the Asia Pacific Heart Rhythm Society (APHRS), and the Society of Thoracic Surgeons (STS). Endorsed by the governing bodies of the American College of Cardiology Foundation, the American Heart Association, the European Cardiac Arrhythmia Society, the European Heart Rhythm Association, the Society of Thoracic Surgeons, the Asia Pacific Heart Rhythm Society, and the Heart Rhythm Society. Heart Rhythm. 2012;9:632–696 e621.

13 Lin D, Poku JW, Beshai JF, Lewkowiez L, Gerstenfeld EP, Dixit S, Nayak H, Zado ES, Calovic Z, Alonso C, Callans DJ, Marchlinski FE. High dose isoproterenol is tolerated and effective in potentiating triggers and assessing the efficacy of atrial fibrillation ablation. Pacing Clin Electrophysiol. 2003;26:1001.

14 Dixit S, Gerstenfeld EP, Ratcliffe SJ, Cooper JM, Russo AM, Kimmel SE, Callans DJ, Lin D, Verdino RJ, Patel VV, Zado E, Marchlinski FE. Single procedure efficacy of isolating all versus arrhythmogenic pulmonary veins on long-term control of atrial fibrillation: a prospective randomized study. Heart Rhythm. 2008;5:174–181.

15 Di Biase L, Burkhardt JD, Mohanty P, Sanchez J, Mohanty S, Horton R, Gallinghouse GJ, Bailey SM, Zagrodzky JD, Santangeli P, Hao S, Hongo R, Beheiry S, Themistoclakis S, Bonso A, Rossillo A, Corrado A, Raviele A, Al-Ahmad A, Wang P, Cummings JE, Schweikert RA, Pelargonio G, Dello Russo A, Casella M, Santarelli P, Lewis WR, Natale A. Left atrial appendage: an underrecognized trigger site of atrial fibrillation. Circulation. 2010;122:109–118.

16 Hsu LF, Jais P, Keane D, Wharton JM, Deisenhofer I, Hocini M, Shah DC, Sanders P, Scavee C, Weerasooriya R, Clementy J, Haissaguerre M. Atrial fibrillation originating from persistent left superior vena cava. Circulation. 2004;109:828–832.

17 Elayi CS, Fahmy TS, Wazni OM, Patel D, Saliba W, Natale A. Left superior vena cava isolation in patients undergoing pulmonary vein antrum isolation: impact on atrial fibrillation recurrence. Heart Rhythm. 2006;3:1019–1023.

18 Han S, Joung B, Scanavacca M, Sosa E, Chen PS, Hwang C. Electrophysiological characteristics of the Marshall bundle in humans. Heart Rhythm. 2010;7:786–793.

19 Valderrabano M, Chen HR, Sidhu J, Rao L, Ling Y, Khoury DS. Retrograde ethanol infusion in the vein of Marshall: regional left atrial ablation, vagal denervation and feasibility in humans. Circ Arrhythm Electrophysiol. 2009;2:50–56.

20 Sauer WH, Alonso C, Zado E, Cooper JM, Lin D, Dixit S, Russo A, Verdino R, Ji S, Gerstenfeld EP, Callans DJ, Marchlinski FE. Atrioventricular nodal reentrant tachycardia in patients referred for atrial fibrillation ablation: response to ablation that incorporates slow-pathway modification. Circulation. 2006;114:191–195.

21 Santangeli P, Di Biase L, Burkhardt JD, Bai R, Mohanty P, Pump A, Natale A. Examining the safety of amiodarone. Expert Opin Drug Safety 2012;11:191–214.

22 Di Biase L, Santangeli P, Mohanty P, Burkhardt D, Sanchez J, Massaro R, Potenza D, Pelargonio G, Lakkireddy D, Reddy M, Forleo G, Bai R, Mohanty S, Pump A, Elayi CS, Rossillo A, Themistoclakis S, Raviele A, Beheiry S, Hongo R, Gibson D, Casella M, Dello Russo A, Tondo C, Natale A. Amiodarone increases the AF termination during ablation but reduces the long term success rate of patients undergoing ablation of long-standing persistent atrial fibrillation: preliminary results from the SPECULATE study. Heart Rhythm. 2012;9:S37.

23 Fonarow GC, Abraham WT, Albert NM, Stough WG, Gheorghiade M, Greenberg BH, O'Connor CM, Sun JL, Yancy CW, Young JB, Investigators O-H, Coordinators. Influence of beta-blocker continuation or withdrawal on outcomes in patients hospitalized with heart failure: findings from the OPTIMIZE-HF program. J Am Coll Cardiol. 2008;52:190–199.

24 Bangalore S, Wetterslev J, Pranesh S, Sawhney S, Gluud C, Messerli FH. Perioperative beta blockers in patients having non-cardiac surgery: a meta-analysis. Lancet. 2008;372:1962–1976.

25 Marchlinski FE, Callans D, Dixit S, Gerstenfeld EP, Rho R, Ren JF, Zado E. Efficacy and safety of targeted focal ablation versus PV isolation assisted by magnetic

electroanatomic mapping. J Cardiovasc Electrophysiol. 2003;14:358–365.

26 von Ludinghausen M. Clinical anatomy of cardiac veins, Vv. cardiacae. Surg Radiol Anat. 1987;9:159–168.

27 von Ludinghausen M, Ohmachi N, Boot C. Myocardial coverage of the coronary sinus and related veins. Clin Anat. 1992;5:1–15.

28 Chauvin M, Shah DC, Haissaguerre M, Marcellin L, Brechenmacher C. The anatomic basis of connections between the coronary sinus musculature and the left atrium in humans. Circulation. 2000;101:647–652.

29 Cendrowska-Pinkosz M, Urbanowicz Z. Analysis of the course and the ostium of the oblique vein of the left atrium. Folia Morphol (Warsz). 2000;59:163–166.

30 Mlcochova H, Tintera J, Porod V, Peichl P, Cihak R, Kautzner J. Magnetic resonance angiography of pulmonary veins: implications for catheter ablation of atrial fibrillation. Pacing Clin Electrophysiol. 2005;28:1073–1080.

31 Kato R, Lickfett L, Meininger G, Dickfeld T, Wu R, Juang G, Angkeow P, LaCorte J, Bluemke D, Berger R, Halperin HR, Calkins H. Pulmonary vein anatomy in patients undergoing catheter ablation of atrial fibrillation: lessons learned by use of magnetic resonance imaging. Circulation. 2003;107:2004–2010.

32 Ashar MS, Pennington J, Callans DJ, Marchlinski FE. Localization of arrhythmogenic triggers of atrial fibrillation. J Cardiovasc Electrophysiol. 2000;11:1300–1305.

33 Deen VR, Morton JB, Vohra JK, Kalman JM. Pulmonary vein paced activation sequence mapping: comparison with activation sequences during onset of focal atrial fibrillation. J Cardiovasc Electrophysiol. 2002;13:101–107.

34 Lee SH, Tai CT, Lin WS, Tsai CF, Hsieh MH, Yu WC, Lin YK, Chen CC, Ding YA, Chang MS, Chen SA. Predicting the arrhythmogenic foci of atrial fibrillation before atrial transseptal procedure: implication for catheter ablation. J Cardiovasc Electrophysiol. 2000;11:750–757.

35 Ashar MS, Callans D, Zado E, Marchlinski FE. Influence of pacing sites in an individual pulmonary vein on intracardiac electrograms in coronary sinus and posteromedial right atrium for pace-mapping triggers of atrial fibrillation originating in pulmonary veins. J Am Coll Cardiol. 2001;37:97A.

36 Dixit S, Gerstenfeld EP, Rho RW, Patel V, Callans DJ, Marchlinski FE. Change in distant atrial activation patterns during circumferential pacemapping of pulmonic vein ostium: implications for localizing triggers for atrial fibrillation. J Interv Card Electrophysiol. 2003;8:187–194.

37 Beshai JF, Marchlinski FE, Gerstenfeld EP, Rho R, Dixit S, Patel VV, Poku JW, Callans D, Zado E, Lin D. Effect of prematurity from pulmonary veins on activation of coronary sinus and posterior right atrium: implications for mapping triggers for atrial fibrillation. Pacing Clin Electrophysiol. 2002;25:708.

38 Fareh S, Villemaire C, Nattel S. Importance of refractoriness heterogeneity in the enhanced vulnerability to atrial fibrillation induction caused by tachycardia-induced atrial electrical remodeling. Circulation. 1998;98:2202–2209.

39 Wang J, Liu L, Feng J, Nattel S. Regional and functional factors determining induction and maintenance of atrial fibrillation in dogs. Am J Physiol. 1996;271:H148–158.

40 Schweikert RA, Perez Lugones A, Kanagaratnam L, Tomassoni G, Beheiry S, Bash D, Pisano E, Saliba W, Tchou PJ, Natale A. A simple method of mapping atrial premature depolarizations triggering atrial fibrillation. Pacing Clin Electrophysiol. 2001;24:22–27.

41 Shah D, Haissaguerre M, Jais P, Hocini M. Nonpulmonary vein foci: do they exist? Pacing Clin Electrophysiol. 2003;26:1631–1635.

42 Santangeli P, Di Biase L, Mohanty P, Burkhardt JD, Horton R, Bai R, Mohanty S, Pump A, Gibson D, Couts L, Hongo R, Beheiry S, Natale A. Catheter ablation of atrial fibrillation in octogenarians: safety and outcomes. J Cardiovasc Electrophysiol. 2012;23:687–693.

43 Mohanty S, Mohanty P, Di Biase L, Bai R, Pump A, Santangeli P, Burkhardt D, Gallinghouse JG, Horton R, Sanchez JE, Bailey S, Zagrodzky J, Natale A. Impact of metabolic syndrome on procedural outcomes in patients with atrial fibrillation undergoing catheter ablation. J Am Coll Cardiol. 2012;59:1295–1301.

44 Beldner SJ, Zado E, Lin D, Callans D, Gerstenfeld EP, Marchlinski FE. Anatomic targets for non-pulmonary vein triggers: identification with intracardiac echo and magnetic mapping. Heart Rhythm. 2004;1:S237.

45 Ino T, Miyamoto S, Ohno T, Tadera T. Exit block of focal repetitive activity in the superior vena cava masquerading as a high right atrial tachycardia. J Cardiovasc Electrophysiol. 2000;11:480–483.

46 Kurotobi T, Ito H, Inoue K, Iwakura K, Kawano S, Okamura A, Date M, Fujii K. Marshall vein as arrhythmogenic source in patients with atrial fibrillation: correlation between its anatomy and electrophysiological findings. J Cardiovasc Electrophysiol. 2006;17:1062–1067.

47 Lin WS, Tai CT, Hsieh MH, Tsai CF, Lin YK, Tsao HM, Huang JL, Yu WC, Yang SP, Ding YA, Chang MS, Chen SA. Catheter ablation of paroxysmal atrial fibrillation initiated by non-pulmonary vein ectopy. Circulation. 2003;107:3176–3183.

48 Santangeli P, Di Biase L, Horton R, Burkhardt D, Gallinghouse GJ, Bailey SM, Sanchez J, Zagrodzky JD, Bai R, Mohanty P, Pump A, Mohanty S, Yan R, Beheiry S, Hongo R, Natale A. Non-pulmonary vein triggers in lone paroxysmal atrial fibrillation: prevalence, clinical profile and ablation outcomes. Heart Rhythm. 2012;9:S342.

49 Valles E, Fan R, Roux JF, Liu CF, Harding JD, Dhruvakumar S, Hutchinson MD, Riley M, Bala R, Garcia FC, Lin D, Dixit S, Callans DJ, Gerstenfeld EP, Marchlinski FE. Localization of atrial fibrillation triggers in patients undergoing pulmonary vein isolation: importance of the carina region. J Am Coll Cardiol. 2008;52:1413–1420.

50 Dukkipati SR, Neuzil P, Kautzner J, Petru J, Wichterle D, Skoda J, Cihak R, Peichl P, Dello Russo A, Pelargonio G, Tondo C, Natale A, Reddy VY. The durability of pulmonary vein isolation using the visually guided laser balloon catheter: multicenter results of pulmonary vein remapping studies. Heart Rhythm. 2012;9:919–925.

51 Lee SH, Tai CT, Hsieh MH, Tsao HM, Lin YJ, Chang SL, Huang JL, Lee KT, Chen YJ, Cheng JJ, Chen SA. Predictors of non-pulmonary vein ectopic beats initiating paroxysmal atrial fibrillation: implication for catheter ablation. J Am Coll Cardiol. 2005;46:1054–1059.

52 Eckardt L. Automaticity in the coronary sinus. J Cardiovasc Electrophysiol. 2002;13:288–289.

53 Volkmer M, Antz M, Hebe J, Kuck KH. Focal atrial tachycardia originating from the musculature of the coronary sinus. J Cardiovasc Electrophysiol. 2002;13: 68–71.

54 Di Biase L, Bai R, Mohanty P, Sanchez J, Mohanty S, Burkhardt D, Horton R, Bailey SM, Zagrodzky JD, Gallinghouse GJ, Santangeli P, Dello Russo A, Casella M, Pelargonio G, Riva S, Fassini G, Hongo R, Beheiry S, Lakkireddy D, Vanga SR, Schweikert R, Gibson D, Lewis WR, Tondo C, Natale A. Atrial fibrillation triggers from the coronary sinus: comparison between isolation versus focal ablation. Heart Rhythm. 2011;8:S78.

55 Rotter M, Sanders P, Takahashi Y, Hsu LF, Sacher F, Hocini M, Jais P, Haissaguerre M. Images in cardiovascular medicine. Coronary sinus tachycardia driving atrial fibrillation. Circulation. 2004;110:e59–e60.

56 Sanders P, Jais P, Hocini M, Haissaguerre M. Electrical disconnection of the coronary sinus by radiofrequency catheter ablation to isolate a trigger of atrial fibrillation. J Cardiovasc Electrophysiol. 2004;15:364–368.

57 Jais P, Haissaguerre M, Shah DC, Chouairi S, Gencel L, Hocini M, Clementy J. A focal source of atrial fibrillation treated by discrete radiofrequency ablation. Circulation. 1997;95:572–576.

58 Oral H, Ozaydin M, Chugh A, Scharf C, Tada H, Hall B, Cheung P, Pelosi F, Knight BP, Morady F. Role of the coronary sinus in maintenance of atrial fibrillation. J Cardiovasc Electrophysiol. 2003;14:1329–1336.

59 Kistler PM, Sanders P, Hussin A, Morton JB, Vohra JK, Sparks PB, Kalman JM. Focal atrial tachycardia arising from the mitral annulus: electrocardiographic and electrophysiologic characterization. J Am Coll Cardiol. 2003;41:2212–2219.

60 Yeh HI, Lai YJ, Lee SH, Lee YN, Ko YS, Chen SA, Severs NJ, Tsai CH. Heterogeneity of myocardial sleeve morphology and gap junctions in canine superior vena cava. Circulation. 2001;104:3152–3157.

61 Arruda M, Mlcochova H, Prasad SK, Kilicaslan F, Saliba W, Patel D, Fahmy T, Morales LS, Schweikert R, Martin D, Burkhardt D, Cummings J, Bhargava M, Dresing T, Wazni O, Kanj M, Natale A. Electrical isolation of the superior vena cava: an adjunctive strategy to pulmonary vein antrum isolation improving the outcome of AF ablation. J Cardiovasc Electrophysiol. 2007;18:1261–1266.

62 Chang KC, Lin YC, Chen JY, Chou HT, Hung JS. Electrophysiological characteristics and radiofrequency ablation of focal atrial tachycardia originating from the superior vena cava. Jpn Circ J. 2001;65:1034–1040.

63 Corrado A, Bonso A, Madalosso M, Rossillo A, Themistoclakis S, Di Biase L, Natale A, Raviele A. Impact of systematic isolation of superior vena cava in addition to pulmonary vein antrum isolation on the outcome of

paroxysmal, persistent, and permanent atrial fibrillation ablation: results from a randomized study. J Cardiovasc Electrophysiol. 2010;21:1–5.

64 Goya M, Ouyang F, Ernst S, Volkmer M, Antz M, Kuck KH. Electroanatomic mapping and catheter ablation of breakthroughs from the right atrium to the superior vena cava in patients with atrial fibrillation. Circulation. 2002;106:1317–1320.

65 Jayam VK, Vasamreddy C, Berger R, Calkins H. Electrical disconnection of the superior vena cava from the right atrium. J Cardiovasc Electrophysiol. 2004;15:614.

66 Ooie T, Tsuchiya T, Ashikaga K, Takahashi N. Electrical connection between the right atrium and the superior vena cava, and the extent of myocardial sleeve in a patient with atrial fibrillation originating from the superior vena cava. J Cardiovasc Electrophysiol. 2002;13:482–485.

67 Tsai CF, Tai CT, Hsieh MH, Lin WS, Yu WC, Ueng KC, Ding YA, Chang MS, Chen SA. Initiation of atrial fibrillation by ectopic beats originating from the superior vena cava: electrophysiological characteristics and results of radiofrequency ablation. Circulation. 2000;102:67–74.

68 Kuo JY, Tai CT, Tsao HM, Hsieh MH, Tsai CF, Lin WS, Lin YK, Ding YA, Hou CJ, Tsai CH, Chen SA. P wave polarities of an arrhythmogenic focus in patients with paroxysmal atrial fibrillation originating from superior vena cava or right superior pulmonary vein. J Cardiovasc Electrophysiol. 2003;14:350–357.

69 Lin YJ, Tai CT, Liu TY, Higa S, Lee PC, Huang JL, Yuniadi Y, Huang BH, Lee KT, Lee SH, Ueng KC, Hsieh MH, Ding YA, Chen SA. Electrophysiological mechanisms and catheter ablation of complex atrial arrhythmias from crista terminalis. Pacing Clin Electrophysiol. 2004;27:1231–1239.

70 Chen CC, Tai CT, Chiang CE, Yu WC, Lee SH, Chen YJ, Hsieh MH, Tsai CF, Lee KW, Ding YA, Chang MS, Chen SA. Atrial tachycardias originating from the atrial septum: electrophysiologic characteristics and radiofrequency ablation. J Cardiovasc Electrophysiol. 2000;11:744–749.

71 Marrouche NF, SippensGroenewegen A, Yang Y, Dibs S, Scheinman MM. Clinical and electrophysiologic characteristics of left septal atrial tachycardia. J Am Coll Cardiol. 2002;40:1133–1139.

72 Takahashi Y, Sanders P, Rotter M, Haissaguerre M. Disconnection of the left atrial appendage for elimination of foci maintaining atrial fibrillation. J Cardiovasc Electrophysiol. 2005;16:917–919.

73 Wang YL, Li XB, Quan X, Ma JX, Zhang P, Xu Y, Zhang HC, Guo JH. Focal atrial tachycardia originating from the left atrial appendage: electrocardiographic and electrophysiologic characterization and long-term outcomes of radiofrequency ablation. J Cardiovasc Electrophysiol. 2007;18:459–464.

74 Kato M, Adachi M, Yano A, Inoue Y, Ogura K, Iitsuka K, Igawa O. Radiofrequency catheter ablation for atrial tachycardia originating from the left atrial appendage. J Interv Card Electrophysiol. 2007;19:45–48.

75 Miyazaki S, Nault I, Jais P, Haissaguerre M. Atrial tachycardia confined within the left atrial appendage. J Cardiovasc Electrophysiol. 2010;21:933–935.

76 Yamada T, Murakami Y, Yoshida Y, Okada T, Yoshida N, Toyama J, Tsuboi N, Inden Y, Hirai M, Murohara T, McElderry HT, Epstein AE, Plumb VJ, Kay GN. Electrophysiologic and electrocardiographic characteristics and radiofrequency catheter ablation of focal atrial tachycardia originating from the left atrial appendage. Heart Rhythm. 2007;4:1284–1291.

77 Yang Q, Ma J, Zhang S, Hu JQ, Liao ZL. Focal atrial tachycardia originating from the distal portion of the left atrial appendage: characteristics and long-term outcomes of radiofrequency ablation. Europace. 2012;14:254–260.

78 Marshall J. On the development of the great anterior veins in man and mammalia: including an account of certain remnants of foetal structure found in the adult, a comparative view of these great veins in the different mammalia, and an analysis of their occasional peculiarities in the human subject. Phil Trans R Soc Lond. 1850;140:133–169.

79 Scherlag BJ, Yeh BK, Robinson MJ. Inferior interatrial pathway in the dog. Circ Res. 1972;31:18–35.

80 Huang C, Chen PS. Clinical electrophysiology and catheter ablation of atrial fibrillation from the ligament of Marshall. In: Chen SA, Haissaguerre M, Zipes DP (eds), Thoracic Vein Arrhythmias: Mechanisms and Treatment, Blackwell Futura: Malden, MA, 2004, pp. 226–284.

81 Katritsis D, Ioannidis JP, Anagnostopoulos CE, Sarris GE, Giazitzoglou E, Korovesis S, Camm AJ. Identification and catheter ablation of extracardiac and intracardiac components of ligament of Marshall tissue for treatment of paroxysmal atrial fibrillation. J Cardiovasc Electrophysiol. 2001;12:750–758.

82 Polymeropoulos KP, Rodriguez LM, Timmermans C, Wellens HJ. Images in cardiovascular medicine. Radiofrequency ablation of a focal atrial tachycardia originating from the Marshall ligament as a trigger for atrial fibrillation. Circulation. 2002;105:2112–2113.

83 Valderrabano M, Liu X, Sasaridis C, Sidhu J, Little S, Khoury DS. Ethanol infusion in the vein of Marshall: adjunctive effects during ablation of atrial fibrillation. Heart Rhythm. 2009;6:1552–1558.

84 Dave AS, Baez-Escudero JL, Sasaridis C, Hong TE, Rami T, Valderrabano M. Role of the vein of Marshall in atrial fibrillation recurrences after catheter ablation: therapeutic effect of ethanol infusion. J Cardiovasc Electrophysiol. 2012;23:583–591.

85 Coumel P. Autonomic influences in atrial tachyarrhythmias. J Cardiovasc Electrophysiol. 1996;7:999–1007.

86 Hwang C, Wu TJ, Doshi RN, Peter CT, Chen PS. Vein of Marshall cannulation for the analysis of electrical activity in patients with focal atrial fibrillation. Circulation. 2000;101:1503–1505.

87 Omichi C, Chou CC, Lee MH, Chang CM, Lai AC, Hayashi H, Zhou S, Miyauchi Y, Okuyama Y, Hamabe A, Hwang C, Fishbein MC, Lin SF, Karagueuzian HS, Chen PS. Demonstration of electrical and anatomic connections between Marshall bundles and left atrium in dogs: implications on the generation of P waves on surface electrocardiogram. J Cardiovasc Electrophysiol. 2002;13:1283–1291.

88 Steinberg I, Dubilier W, Jr., Lukas DS. Persistence of left superior vena cava. Dis Chest. 1953;24:479–488.

89 Tsutsui K, Ajiki K, Fujiu K, Imai Y, Hayami N, Murakawa Y. Successful catheter ablation of atrial tachycardia and atrial fibrillation in persistent left superior vena cava. Int Heart J. 2010;51:72–74.

90 Santangeli P, Di Biase L, Burkhardt JD, Horton R, Sanchez J, Bailey S, Zagrodzky JD, Lakkireddy D, Bai R, Mohanty P, Beheiry S, Hongo R, Natale A. Transseptal access and atrial fibrillation ablation guided by intracardiac echocardiography in patients with atrial septal closure devices. Heart Rhythm. 2011;8: 1669–1675.

91 Mansour M, Ruskin J, Keane D. Initiation of atrial fibrillation by ectopic beats originating from the ostium of the inferior vena cava. J Cardiovasc Electrophysiol. 2002;13:1292–1295.

92 Scavee C, Jais P, Weerasooriya R, Haissaguerre M. The inferior vena cava: an exceptional source of atrial fibrillation. J Cardiovasc Electrophysiol. 2003;14:659–662.

93 Mizobuchi M, Enjoji Y, Shibata K, Funatsu A, Yokouchi I, Kambayashi D, Kobayashi T, Nakamura S. Case report: focal ablation for atrial fibrillation originating from the inferior vena cava and the posterior left atrium. J Interv Card Electrophysiol. 2006;16:131–134.

94 Datino T, Macle L, Qi XY, Maguy A, Comtois P, Chartier D, Guerra PG, Arenal A, Fernandez-Aviles F, Nattel S. Mechanisms by which adenosine restores conduction in dormant canine pulmonary veins. Circulation. 2010;121:963–972.

95 Matsuo S, Yamane T, Date T, Lellouche N, Tokutake K, Hioki M, Ito K, Narui R, Tanigawa S, Nakane T, Tokuda M, Yamashita S, Aramaki Y, Inada K, Shibayama K, Miyanaga S, Yoshida H, Miyazaki H, Abe K, Sugimoto K, Taniguchi I, Yoshimura M. Dormant pulmonary vein conduction induced by adenosine in patients with atrial fibrillation who underwent catheter ablation. Am Heart J. 2011;161:188–196.

96 Miyazaki S, Kobori A, Kuwahara T, Takahashi A. Adenosine triphosphate exposes dormant superior vena cava conduction responsible for recurrent atrial fibrillation. J Cardiovasc Electrophysiol. 2010;21:464–465.

97 Miyazaki S, Takahashi Y, Fujii A, Takahashi A. Adenosine triphosphate exposes multiple extra pulmonary vein foci of atrial fibrillation. Int J Cardiol. 2011;148:249–250.

98 Miyazaki S, Taniguchi H, Komatsu Y, Uchiyama T, Kusa S, Nakamura H, Hachiya H, Hirao K, Iesaka Y. Clinical impact of adenosine triphosphate injection on arrhythmogenic superior vena cava in the context of atrial fibrillation ablation. Circ Arrhythm Electrophysiol. 2013;6:497–503.

99 Elayi CS, Di Biase L, Bai R, Burkhardt D, Mohanty P, Sanchez J, Santangeli P, Hongo R, Gallinghouse GJ, Horton R, Bailey SM, Beheiry S, Natale A. Administration of isoproterenol and adenosine to guide supplemental ablation after pulmonary vein antrum isolation. Heart Rhythm. 2011;8:S333.

100 Oakes RS, Badger TJ, Kholmovski EG, Akoum N, Burgon NS, Fish EN, Blauer JJ, Rao SN, DiBella EV, Segerson NM, Daccarett M, Windfelder J, McGann CJ, Parker D, MacLeod RS, Marrouche NF. Detection and quantification of left atrial structural remodeling with delayed-enhancement magnetic resonance imaging in patients with atrial fibrillation. Circulation. 2009;119: 1758–1767.

101 Suzuki K, Nagata Y, Goya M, Takahashi Y, Takahashi A, Fujiwara H, Hiraoka M, Iesaka Y. Impact of non-pulmonary vein focus on early recurrence of atrial fibrillation after pulmonary vein isolation. Heart Rhythm. 2004;1:S203–S204.

102 Yamada T, Murakami Y, Okada T, Yoshida N, Ninomiya Y, Toyama J, Yoshida Y, Tsuboi N, Inden Y, Hirai M, Murohara T, McElderry HT, Epstein AE, Plumb VJ, Kay GN. Non-pulmonary vein epicardial foci of atrial fibrillation identified in the left atrium after pulmonary vein isolation. Pacing Clin Electrophysiol. 2007;30:1323–1330.

103 Knecht S, O'Neill MD, Matsuo S, Lim KT, Arantes L, Derval N, Klein GJ, Hocini M, Jais P, Clementy J, Haissaguerre M. Focal arrhythmia confined within the coronary sinus and maintaining atrial fibrillation. J Cardiovasc Electrophysiol. 2007;18:1140–1146.

104 Liu TY, Tai CT, Lee PC, Hsieh MH, Higa S, Ding YA, Chen SA. Novel concept of atrial tachyarrhythmias originating from the superior vena cava: insight from noncontact mapping. J Cardiovasc Electrophysiol. 2003;14:533–539.

105 Weiss C, Willems S, Rostock T, Risius T, Ventura R, Meinertz T. Electrical disconnection of an arrhythmogenic superior vena cava with discrete radiofrequency current lesions guided by noncontact mapping. Pacing Clin Electrophysiol. 2003;26:1758–1761.

106 Pastor A, Nunez A, Magalhaes A, Awamleh P, Garcia-Cosio F. The superior vena cava as a site of ectopic foci in atrial fibrillation. Rev Esp Cardiol. 2007;60:68–71.

107 Wang XH, Liu X, Sun YM, Shi HF, Zhou L, Gu JN. Pulmonary vein isolation combined with superior vena cava isolation for atrial fibrillation ablation: a prospective randomized study. Europace. 2008;10:600–605.

108 Steven D, Roberts-Thomson KC, Seiler J, Michaud GF, John RM, Stevenson WG. Fibrillation in the superior vena cava mimicking atrial tachycardia. Circ Arrhythm Electrophysiol. 2009;2:e4–e7.

109 Kato Y, Horigome H, Takahashi-Igari M, Yoshida K, Aonuma K. Isolation of pulmonary vein and superior vena cava for paroxysmal atrial fibrillation in a young adult with left ventricular non-compaction. Europace. 2010;12:1040–1041.

110 Higuchi K, Yamauchi Y, Hirao K, Sasaki T, Hachiya H, Sekiguchi Y, Nitta J, Isobe M. Superior vena cava as initiator of atrial fibrillation: factors related to its arrhythmogenicity. Heart Rhythm. 2010;7:1186–1191.

111 Chang HY, Chang SL, Feng AN, Chen SA. Atrial fibrillation originating from superior vena cava mimics typical atrial flutter. J Cardiovasc Electrophysiol. 2011;22:1398.

112 Fukumoto K, Takatsuki S, Endo A. Arrhythmogenic superior vena cava caused by partial anomalous pulmonary venous return. Heart. 2011;97:437.

113 Miyazaki S, Kuwahara T, Takahashi A. Confined driver of atrial fibrillation in the superior vena cava. J Cardiovasc Electrophysiol. 2012;23:440.

114 Chang HY, Lo LW, Lin YJ, Chang SL, Hu YF, Feng AN, Yin WH, Li CH, Chao TF, Hartono B, Chung FP, Cheng CC, Lin WS, Tsao HM, Chen SA. Long-term outcome of catheter ablation in patients with atrial fibrillation originating from the superior vena cava. J Cardiovasc Electrophysiol. 2012;23:955–961.

115 Miyazaki S, Taniguchi H, Kusa S, Uchiyama T, Hirao K, Iesaka Y. Conduction recovery after electrical isolation of superior vena cava; prevalence and electrophysiological properties. Circ J. 2013;77:352–358.

116 Varma N, Abi-Saleh B. Electrical isolation of both left pulmonary veins by a single left atrial endocardial radiofrequency energy application: ablation of Marshall bundle bypass. Pacing Clin Electrophysiol. 2012;35: e325–329.

117 Bhargava et al. Heart Rhythm. 2009;Oct6(10): 1403–1412.

CHAPTER 18

Mapping and ablation of electrical rotor and focal sources for atrial fibrillation: a patient-tailored mechanistic approach

Junaid A. B. Zaman,[3] Siva K. Mulpuru,[1] David E. Krummen,[2] & Sanjiv M. Narayan[3]

[1]Division of Cardiovascular Diseases, Mayo Clinic, Rochester, MN, USA
[2]Division of Cardiovascular Medicine, Department of Medicine, University of California at San Diego, San Diego, CA, USA
[3]Cardiovascular Medicine, Stanford University, Stanford, CA, USA

Introduction

Despite great strides in our understanding of atrial fibrillation (AF), therapy using pharmacological, percutaneous, and surgical interventional approaches remains suboptimal [1]. A major limitation of therapy is our lack of mechanistic understanding for AF [2]. While advances have been made in ablating pulmonary vein (PV) AF triggers, durable PV isolation remains elusive [1], and triggers commonly arise outside the PVs [3,4] while, in other arrhythmias, ablation targets central substrates (sustaining mechanisms) [2] that circumvent the need to identify or ablate potentially diverse triggers. The future of personalized therapy will likely require the mapping of AF substrates in each patient, as has been the cornerstone of successful diagnosis and therapy for essentially all other arrhythmias.

Prior mapping for human AF

We hypothesized that a novel physiologically based mapping approach may produce patient-specific

Practical Guide to Catheter Ablation of Atrial Fibrillation,
Second Edition. Edited by Jonathan S. Steinberg, Pierre Jaïs and Hugh Calkins.
© 2016 John Wiley & Sons, Ltd. Published 2016 by John Wiley & Sons, Ltd.

dynamic spatiotemporal maps of AF at the precise time of electrophysiology study, to enable patient-tailored therapy. Notably, traditional mapping for AF is challenging, since clinical signals may not faithfully represent local activation [5], while "virtual" electrograms from noncontact methods may distort information in AF [6].

Substantial data support *localized sources for AF*, first postulated by Mines and Lewis, then reported in seminal studies by Schuessler, Cox and Boineau [7,8] who showed that AF may be sustained by stable drivers and by Jalife et al. [9,10] who demonstrated *electrical spiral waves (rotors)* that perpetuate fibrillation in various models. Indeed, ablation at AF rotors was recently shown to suppress AF in a canine model [11]. Indirectly, stable sources for human AF explain localized regions of stable high dominant frequency [12–15] and consistent activation vectors over time [16].

Conversely, the *multiple wavelet model of AF*, shown in early computer models [17], posits that AF is driven by meandering wavelets that collide and extinguish. While shown in some mapping studies of small atrial regions, this model has recently been challenged [18] and does not easily explain either the clinical observations of AF termination by limited ablation at PVs [19,20] or other sites [21,22] or the above evidence for spatiotemporal stability in AF.

Development of focal impulse and rotor mapping

The CONFIRM trial [21] set out to identify potential deterministic mechanisms for human AF by developing and testing novel computational mapping (focal impulse and rotor mapping, FIRM), with ablation to establish whether identified mechanisms were etiological or bystander. We recruited 92 subjects undergoing 107 consecutive ablation procedures for drug-refractory AF, referred for ablation to the Veterans Affairs and University of California Medical Centers in San Diego, under an IRB approved protocol. The trial is summarized below, and its results have since been validated in more than 200 patients at more than 10 centers [23,24].

Consecutive cases prospectively received FIRM mapping of AF, as described below, and were enrolled in a 2-arm 1:2 case cohort design. FIRM-guided patients received ablation targeted at identified mechanisms, while FIRM-blinded patients underwent conventional ablation blinded to the results of FIRM mapping. We included patients with paroxysmal and persistent AF. By design, we included patients at their first ablation as well as a minority with AF after unsuccessful conventional ablation. The goal of broad inclusion was to test if patients with and without prior attempted ablation, who are often clinically indistinguishable, have similar or different AF mechanisms. The only patient exclusions were an unwillness or inability to provide informed consent.

Table 1 displays the clinical characteristics of the patient group. Persistent AF was present in 81% of the FIRM-guided group, and in 66% of the FIRM-blinded group.

Electrophysiological mapping (focal impulse and rotor mapping)

Native AF was mapped when possible but, when required, induced by pacing from the coronary sinus using a continuous incremental pacing protocol from cycle lengths (CL) 500 ms, continuously decrementing to 450 ms, 400 ms, 350 ms, 300 ms, then in 10 ms steps to AF. If required, isoproterenol was infused and pacing was repeated.

Simultaneous contact recordings of the atria were taken using 64-pole catheters (Constellation, Boston Scientific, MA) advanced transseptally to the left atrium in all patients, and the right atrium in 73 patients. AF electrograms were recorded for minutes and then exported for analysis using Rhythmview (Topera, Palo Alto, CA). Electrode locations within each patient's atrium were identified from fluoroscopy and electroanatomic mapping if desired [21].

Analysis and interpretation of computational maps of AF

Figure 1c illustrates the nomenclature of FIRM maps, in which the left atrium is opened at its "equator" and the right atrium is opened along a meridian. Mapping analyzes contact electrograms, which are the reference standard for signal fidelity, using recently reported human rate-response properties of atrial repolarization and regional conduction [25–28].

Clinically, rotors (stable rotational activation) or focal sources from FIRM mapping are diagnosed only if stable for >50 cycles in patient-specific movies, and typically thousands of cycles, depicted in this chapter as static images of representative cycles. This

Table 1 Clinical characteristics of patients in the CONFIRM trial.

Characteristic	Conventional ablation (n = 71)	FIRM-guided ablation (n = 36)	P
AF presentation			0.12
Paroxysmal	24 (34%)	7 (19%)	
Persistent	47 (66%)	29 (81%)	
Age (years)	61 ± 8	63 ± 9	0.34
Gender (male/female)	68/3	34/2	1.00
Nonwhite race	9 (13%)	6 (17%)	0.57
History of AF (months)	45 (18–79)	52 (38–110)	0.04
Left atrial diameter (mm)	43 ± 6	48 ± 7	0.001
LVEF (%)	55 ± 12	53 ± 15	0.59
CHADS2 score			
0 or 1	38 (54%)	13 (36%)	0.09
2 or more	33 (46%)	23 (64%)	
Previously failed >1 AAD	16 (23%)	16 (44%)	<0.05

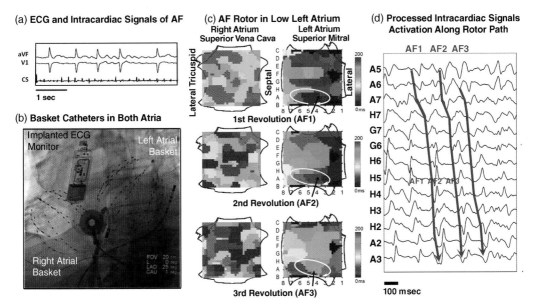

Figure 1 FIRM mapping for AF. (a) Electrocardiogram (ECG) and intracardiac signals in an 85-year-old man during paroxysmal AF. (b) Fluoroscopy shows a 64-pole catheter in each atrium, an implanted continuous electrocardiography monitor, diagnostic catheters in the coronary sinus and left atrium, and an esophageal temperature probe at the inferior left atrium. (c) Left atrial AF rotor, showing clockwise revolution (red to blue) around a precessing center for three cycles. The right atrium depicts the superior and inferior vena cavae above and below and lateral and medial tricuspid annuli at left and right. The left atrium depicts superior and inferior mitral annuli above and below, and pulmonary vein pairs. Electrodes are labeled A to H1 to 8, respectively. (d) Computationally processed and filtered intracardiac signals show sequential activation over the rotor path for cycles AF1 to AF3 (arrowed). FIRM-guided ablation at this rotor terminated AF to sinus rhythm in ≤1 min, prior to any other intervention.

definition excludes transient or migratory activity more consistent with fibrillatory conduction [29]. We have shown that identifying spiral waves in human AF requires a contact electrode separation of $< \approx 1$ cm [30], although precise defininition of the rotor core requires higher resolution. This spatial resolution analysis is illustrated in Figure 2. Figure 3 presents several examples.

Direct ablation at sources (FIRM) and postprocedure management

In FIRM-guided subjects, ablation commenced with the elimination of AF rotors or focal sources using various radiofrequency sources (and in a recent multicenter experience, cryoablation [23]). In each case, the catheter is maneuvered to tissue subtending each source identified by basket splines. The typical approach is to apply a 15–30 s lesion, then move the catheter within the source precession area. In detailed phase analyses in AF patients [30,31], rotors and sources precess in areas of 1.7–2.5 cm^2, requiring 5–10 min ablation per source. If AF terminated,

vigorous attempts were made to reinitiate AF. FIRM ablation was repeated for ≤3 sources and then conventional ablation was performed.

Conventional ablation, performed after FIRM ablation in the FIRM-guided group, and as sole therapy in the FIRM-blinded group, comprised wide area circumferential ablation to isolate the left and right pulmonary veins in pairs, with verification of pulmonary vein isolation. In cases of persistent AF, a left atrial roof line was also applied. Atrial tachycardia or flutters were ablated appropriately, but no other ablation was performed.

Study end points

The prespecified acute end point was ≤10 min ablation per source, recording AF termination or ≥10% AF slowing (previously, 3% slowing was significant [32]). Within a 3-month blanking period postablation, antiarrhythmic medications were continued and arrhythmias were managed as indicated but repeat ablation was not permitted. The prespecified primary chronic efficacy end point was freedom from AF after a single procedure using continuous implanted ECG (88% of patients) or intermittent

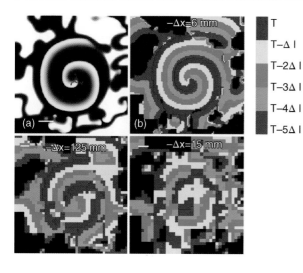

Figure 2 Spatial resolution analysis of human AF rotors, showing rotor detection until spatial resolution falls under ≈1 cm. (a) A 15 × 15 cm computational domain, with spatial resolution $\Delta x = 0.5$ mm, contains a stable rotor, clearly evident organized domain with a meandering spiral tip path (red) and peripheral disorganization. Scale bar = 2 cm. (b) Isochronal map using a spatial resolution of $\Delta x = 6$ mm, as indicated by the scale bar, using the data from (a). (c) Snapshot of an isochronal map on a 12 × 12 grid. The scale bar represents the spatial resolution ($\Delta x = 12.5$ mm). (d) Snapshot of an isochronal map on a 15 × 15 grid from an animated sequence (enhanced online). All isochronal maps used an isochronal interval of $\Delta I = 20$ ms.

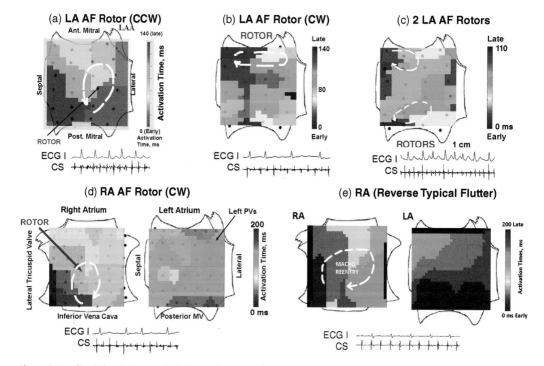

Figure 3 Localized electrical rotors (spiral waves) revealed by computational mapping. (a) Counterclockwise rotor in persistent AF in the high posterior LA (rotor, arrow) near the left superior PV (color-coded from red to blue). (b) CCW rotor in persistent AF in the lateral LA. (c) CW rotor in persistent AF in the anterior LA. (d) Two concurrent rotors during paroxysmal AF in the anterior LA (CW) and inferior LA (CCW). (e) Right atrial rotor (CW) during paroxysmal AF in the midposterior wall, with fibrillatory conduction to the LA. AF, atrial fibrillation; LA, left atrium; LAA, left atrial appendage; MV, mitral valve; PV, pulmonary vein. *Source:* Narayan et al., 2012. [21]. Reproduced with permission of Wiley.

Table 2 Acute results of ablation at localized AF sources.

Characteristic	Conventional ablation	FIRM-guided ablation	P
Cases with intraprocedural sustained AF	65/71 (92%)	36/36 (100%)	0.10
Subjects with AF sources	63/65 (97%)	35/36 (97%)	1.00
Acute end point achieved	13/65 (20%)	31/36 (86%)	<0.001
AF termination end point	6/65 (9%)	20/36 (56%)	<0.001
AF CL prolongation end point, n (%)	7/65 (11%)	11/36 (31%)	0.01
Total procedural ablation (all cases), min	52.1 ± 17.8	57.8 ± 22.8	0.16
Complications (all cases)	6 (8%)	2 (6%)	0.72

Values are number (%), mean ± SD, or median (interquartile range).

monitors. The safety end point was a comparison of adverse events between groups.

Results: localized sources were highly prevalent in human AF

Stable AF sources were present in 98 of 101 cases with sustained AF (97%), each subject demonstrating 2.1 ± 1.0 sources (median 2, IQR: 1–3) of which 70% were rotors and 30% focal impulses (Table 2). AF sources controlled local activation during AF on directionality analyses [31], with secondary disorganization as predicted [9,10]. The number of concurrent AF sources was higher in patients with persistent than paroxysmal AF (2.2 ± 1.0 versus 1.7 ± 0.9; median 2.0 versus 1.0; $p = 0.03$) but, in these patients with troublesome symptomatic drug-refractory AF, was unrelated to whether ablation has not or had been attempted before (2.1 ± 1.1 versus 2.0 ± 0.8; median 2.0 versus 2.0; $p = 0.71$). Recent multicenter validations showed remarkably similar results in >200 patients at 11 independent centers [23,24].

Demonstration of electrical rotors during human AF

Figure 3 illustrates electrical rotors in human AF and differences from atrial flutter on FIRM mapping. Figure 3a shows a solitary rotor in the midposterior LA with counterclockwise (CCW) activation with surrounding fibrillatory conduction. Figure 3b illustrates a CCW rotor during persistent AF, and Figure 3c shows a clockwise (CW) rotor during persistent AF in the anterior LA. Finally, Figure 3d shows a right atrial AF rotor, with fibrillatory breakdown in the left atrium while, conversely, Figure 3e shows clockwise (reverse typical) right atrial flutter with no fibrillatory breakdown. Figure 4a shows a focal AF source with breakdown to AF peripherally in right and left atrium. Conversely, Figure 4b shows focal atrial tachycardia on FIRM mapping with no peripheral disorganization.

Acute results of FIRM-guided ablation

FIRM-guided ablation alone in the CONFIRM trial achieved AF termination with noninducibility or AF slowing (including terminations with subsequently reinducible AF) in 31 of 36 (86%) patients. Cases in whom FIRM ablation slowed rather than terminated AF had larger LA diameters (53 ± 8 mm versus 46 ± 6 mm; $p = 0.01$). Total FIRM-guided ablation time (all sources) was 16.1 ± 9.8 min (median 18.5 min, IQR: 7.9–24.5 min) (Table 2). By comparison, in the FIRM-blinded group, the acute end point was achieved in 13 of 65 cases (20%) after 43.4 ± 28.0 min (median 31.8 min, IQR: 22.1–71.5 min) ablation ($p = 0.001$ for both comparisons).

Location of rotors and focal sources in the CONFIRM trial

Stable AF sources lay at diverse patient-specific locations with ≈40–50% near PVs (22.8%) and left atrial roof (16%), 28% elsewhere in the left atrium, and 33% in right atrium, and were more widely distributed in persistent than paroxysmal AF. Figure 5 indicates these locations [33].

Relationship between localized sources and CFAE sites

Notably, sites of localized sources did not show a specific electrogram fingerprint [31]. Even in cases where rotors overlay CFAE, additional sites of CFAE were frequently noted at distant locations. This corresponds to clinical experience in which ablation of CFAE is sometimes dramatically effective and other times does not appear to have acute impact.

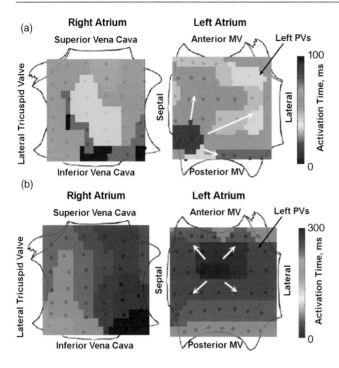

Figure 4 Localized focal beats in a 50-year-old man with persistent AF and LA diameter 52 mm revealed by FIRM. (a) Low septal LA focal beat in paroxysmal AF, with centrifugal activation to the remaining LA and activation to RA over Bachmann's bundle (CL: 100 ms). In contrast, (b) focal atrial tachycardia from the high posterior LA, differing from AF by showing discrete activation centrifugally to the ipsilateral and then contralateral atria (CL: 300 ms). AF, atrial fibrillation; LA, left atrium; RA, right atrium; CL, cycle length; MV, mitral valve; PV, pulmonary vein. *Source:* Narayan et al., 2012. [21]. Reproduced with permission of Wiley.

Long-term efficacy of FIRM-guided ablation versus conventional ablation

Two subjects per group were lost to follow-up. By intention-to-treat analysis, single procedure freedom from AF was higher for FIRM-guided (FIRM + PVI) than conventional ablation (Figure 6; 82.4% versus 44.9%; $p = 0.001$) after median 273 days (IQR: 132–681 days). FIRM ablation could not be completed in 4 of 36 cases. The benefits of FIRM-guided therapy were maintained for the first and all ablation cases ($p = 0.001$). Substudy analysis recently showed that patients with traditionally adverse comorbidities such as obstructive sleep apnea and obesity had more sources, often away from pulmonary veins [34]. However, the benefits of FIRM-guided ablation was maintained in these patients. FIRM-guided patients also had higher freedom from any atrial tachyarrhythmia than FIRM-blinded cases (70.6%, including three typical flutter, one atrial macroreentry, versus 39.1%, two typical flutter, one atrial macroreentry; $p = 0.001$). Neither the total duration of ablation, the aggregate number, nor the type of adverse events differed between groups. Multicenter experiences of FIRM ablation in >10 independent laboratories have now confirmed the acute results of FIRM and benefits of FIRM-guided over conventional ablation [23,24].

Relationship of patient-specific sources to ablation lesions

We set out to study how ablation impacted rotors in both limbs of CONFIRM [33]. In Figure 7, two left atrial rotors were ablated by FIRM. Conventional ablation, subsequently performed per protocol, would clearly have eliminated the superior rotor but not the inferior rotor. A preplanned on-treatment analysis set out to investigate whether ablation of rotors by any strategy impacted the outcome, performed by all investigators blinded to the outcome. In patients in whom ablation passed through AF sources (directly by FIRM or coincidentally by anatomical ablation), freedom from AF was 80.3%, while when ablation missed all sources, success was 18.8% (Figure 8). Freedom from AF was highest when all sources were eliminated, intermediate when some were eliminated, and lowest when all were missed.

Discussion: computational mapping compared with prior mapping of human AF

The demonstration of stable rotors in human AF actually reconciles several otherwise disparate clinical observations. First, despite its complexity, AF can be terminated by targeted interventions [20,22] that

(a)   **AF Source Locations - CONFIRM Paroxysmal AF**

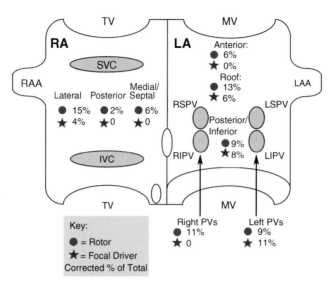

AF Source Locations - CONFIRM Persistent AF

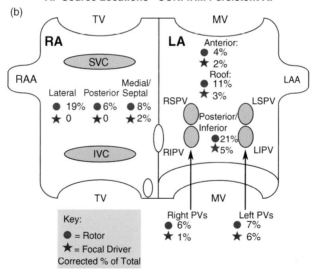

Figure 5 Location of focal sources and rotors in patients enrolled in the CONFIRM trial.

support localized mechanisms at least in some patients. Second, human AF may show stable high dominant frequency sites in diverse biatrial locations [12–15] and stable activation vectors in given subjects [16], which are difficult to explain by meandering wavelets but consistent with stable sources in patient-specific locations. The on-treatment analysis of CONFIRM further supports this hypothesis [33], and the notion that sources sometimes are

and other times are not ablated by anatomical lesion sets. Recent data on the efficacy of FIRM-only ablation (without trigger ablation) in patients with paroxysmal AF [35] further supports this concept. In persistent AF, the improved efficacy of extensive ablation, but success of localized ablation in some patients, is explained by more diverse AF sources' locations [33]. This also explains our findings in AF patients with comorbidities. Third, the inconsistent relationship of

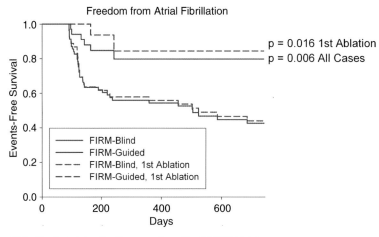

Figure 6 Kaplan–Meier Survival plots of both groups from the CONFIRM trial.

FIRM Sites (LA PosteroInferolateral Rotors) Near L WACA

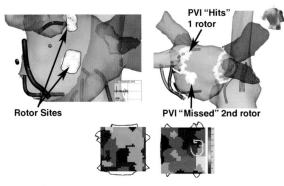

Figure 7 Electroanatomic maps of the left atrium with rotor annotations as revealed by computational mapping. Conventional WACA ablation would pass through one source but not the other.

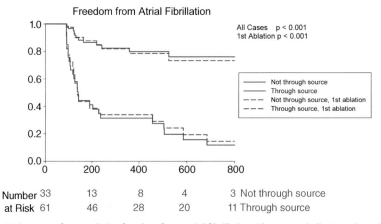

Figure 8 Kaplan–Meier curves for cumulative freedom from atrial fibrillation. Blue curves indicate patients in whom WACA passed through areas identified as rotors or focal sources by computational mapping.

AF rotors to CFAE [31] explains the sporadic but sometimes dramatic success of ablating at CFAE areas.

Differing results from other human mapping studies likely reflect technical factors. Elegant work by Allessie et al. mapped small atrial areas (10 cm² plaques in persistent AF patients [36], yet left atrial areas [37] are 100–130 cm²), and may have missed sources. However, their descriptions of epicardial–endocardial dissociation may provide insights into the processes governing fibrillatory conduction. Recent work from Ganesan et al. [29] used "Shannon entropy" on bipolar electograms to localize rotors in animal and clinical AF. The inverse solution has also been used to identify AF rotors using virtual electrograms constructed from the body surface in 26 patients [38], and such rotors were ablated in a preliminary study of 3 patients [39]. These studies add to a growing body of literature on the identification and ablation of patient-specific sources.

Limitations

CONFIRM and recent confirmatory multicenter studies of FIRM were not randomized, although subjects were enrolled and treated prospectively for prespecified end points. In CONFIRM, the FIRM-guided group had more subjects with persistent AF, higher comorbidity, and more intense monitoring than FIRM-blinded subjects, thus potentially underestimating the benefit of FIRM-guided ablation. Second, current baskets map the atria suboptimally, and it is possible that improved designs may reduce this significant technical limitation. Third, as with any new technology, interpreting FIRM maps requires a learning curve, although this was relatively short in the recent multicenter experience [23].

Clinical implications and directions for future studies

Targeted FIRM ablation has already been shown to substantially improve upon the success of conventional AF ablation. The recent PRECISE (*Precise Rotor Elimination without Concomitant pulmonary vein Isolation for the Successful Elimination of Paroxysmal AF*) trial [35] supports the elimination of precisely defined sustaining mechanisms (substrates) alone for AF, as is currently being tested at multiple institutions and compared against trigger-elimination. Future studies should also define the role of FIRM-based ablation in patients with long-standing persistent AF, and should focus on optical mapping studies of human AF which have recently revealed stable rotors on the endocardium that can be ablated

to eliminate arrhythmia (40), yet which produced transient fibrillatory disorganization on the epicardium which correlate with other methods (39).

Conclusions

A rapidly growing body of literature shows that using FIRM mapping based on human atrial physiology, clinical AF is sustained by stable electrical rotors and repetitive focal sources. In multicenter studies, sources were stable for unexpectedly long durations and were found in nearly all AF patients in diverse patient-specific locations in both atria. Targeted elimination of stable sources, combined with conventional ablation, substantially increased ablation success after a single procedure compared to conventional ablation alone. On-treatment analysis shows that ablation was more effective when AF sources were eliminated, directly by FIRM or coincidentally by anatomical lesions, than when they were not. Preliminary data show that targeted FIRM-only ablation may be an effective therapy for AF without the need for trigger elimination. These mechanistic findings open the real and immediate possibility of patient-tailored therapy for AF.

Acknowledgments

This work was supported by grants to S.M. Narayan from the NIH (HL70529, HL83359, HL103800) and the Doris Duke Charitable Foundation, and by a Career Development grant from the Department of Medicine, Mayo Clinic, Rochester, MN to S.K. Mulpuru.

References

1 Calkins H, Kuck KH, Cappato R, Brugada J, Camm AJ, et al. 2012 HRS/EHRA/ECAS Expert Consensus Statement on Catheter and Surgical Ablation of Atrial Fibrillation: Recommendations for Patient Selection, Procedural Techniques, Patient Management and Follow-up, Definitions, Endpoints, and Research Trial Design: a report of the Heart Rhythm Society (HRS) Task Force on Catheter and Surgical Ablation of Atrial Fibrillation. Developed in partnership with the European Heart Rhythm Association (EHRA), a registered branch of the European Society of Cardiology (ESC) and the European Cardiac Arrhythmia Society (ECAS); and in collaboration with the American College of Cardiology (ACC), American Heart Association (AHA), the Asia Pacific Heart Rhythm Society (APHRS), and the Society of Thoracic Surgeons (STS). Endorsed by the governing bodies of the American College of Cardiology Foundation, the American Heart Association, the European Cardiac Arrhythmia Society, the European Heart Rhythm

Association, the Society of Thoracic Surgeons, the Asia Pacific Heart Rhythm Society, and the Heart Rhythm Society. Heart Rhythm. 2012;9:632–696. e621.

2 Nattel S. New ideas about atrial fibrillation 50 years on. Nature. 2002;415:219–226.

3 Elayi CS, Di Biase L, Barrett C, Ching CK, al Aly M, et al. Atrial fibrillation termination as a procedural endpoint during ablation in long-standing persistent atrial fibrillation. Heart Rhythm. 2010;7:1216–1223.

4 Schmitt C, Ndrepepa G, Weber S, Schmieder S, Weyerbrock S, et al. Biatrial multisite mapping of atrial premature complexes triggering onset of atrial fibrillation. Am J Cardiol. 2002;89:1381–1387.

5 Narayan SM, Wright M, Derval N, Jadidi A, Forclaz A, et al. Classifying fractionated electrograms in human atrial fibrillation using monophasic action potentials and activation mapping: evidence for localized drivers, rate acceleration and non-local signal etiologies. Heart Rhythm. 2011a;8:244–253.

6 Earley M, Abrams D, Sporton S, Schilling R. Validation of the non-contact mapping system in the left atrium during permanent atrial fibrillation and sinus rhythm. J Am Coll Cardiol. 2006;48:485–491.

7 Cox JL, Canavan TE, Schuessler RB, Cain ME, Lindsay BD, et al. The surgical treatment of atrial fibrillation. II. Intraoperative electrophysiologic mapping and description of the electrophysiologic basis of atrial flutter and atrial fibrillation. J Thorac Cardiovasc Surg. 1991;101:406–426.

8 Schuessler RB, Grayson TM, Bromberg BI, Cox JL, Boineau JP. Cholinergically mediated tachyarrhythmias induced by a single extrastimulus in the isolated canine right atrium. Circ Res. 1992;71:1254–1267.

9 Davidenko JM, Pertsov AV, Salomonsz R, Baxter W, Jalife J. Stationary and drifting spiral waves of excitation in isolated cardiac muscle. Nature. 1992;355:349–351.

10 Pandit SV, Jalife J. Rotors and the dynamics of cardiac fibrillation. Circ Res. 2013;112:849–862.

11 Chou CC, Chang PC, Wen MS, Lee HL, Chen TC, et al. Epicardial ablation of rotors suppresses inducibility of acetylcholine-induced atrial fibrillation in left pulmonary vein-left atrium preparations in a beagle heart failure model. J Am Coll Cardiol. 2011;58:158–166.

12 Wu T-J, Doshi RN, Huang H-LA, Blanche C, Kass RM, et al. Simultaneous biatrial computerized mapping during permanent atrial fibrillation in patients with organic heart disease. J Cardiovasc Electrophysiol. 2002;13:571–577.

13 Lazar S, Dixit S, Marchlinski FE, Callans DJ, Gerstenfeld EP. Presence of left-to-right atrial frequency gradient in paroxysmal but not persistent atrial fibrillation in humans. Circulation. 2004;110:3181–3186.

14 Sahadevan J, Ryu K, Peltz L, Khrestian CM, Stewart RW, et al. Epicardial mapping of chronic atrial fibrillation in patients: preliminary observations. Circulation. 2004;110:3293–3299.

15 Sanders P, Berenfeld O, Hocini M, Jais P, Vaidyanathan R, et al. Spectral analysis identifies sites of high-frequency activity maintaining atrial fibrillation in humans. Circulation. 2005;112:789–797.

16 Gerstenfeld E, Sahakian A, Swiryn S. Evidence for transient linking of atrial excitation during atrial fibrillation in humans. Circulation. 1992;86:375–382.

17 Moe GK, Rheinboldt W, Abildskov J. A computer model of atrial fibrillation. Am Heart J. 1964;67:200–220.

18 Lee S, Sahadevan J, Khrestian CM, Durand DM, Waldo AL. High density mapping of atrial fibrillation during vagal nerve stimulation in the canine heart: restudying the Moe hypothesis. J Cardiovasc Electrophysiol. 2013;24:328–335.

19 Haissaguerre M, Sanders P, Hocini M, Takahashi Y, Rotter M, et al. Catheter ablation of long-lasting persistent atrial fibrillation: critical structures for termination. J Cardiovasc Electrophysiol. 2005a;16:1125–1137.

20 Herweg B, Kowalski M, Steinberg JS. Termination of persistent atrial fibrillation resistant to cardioversion by a single radiofrequency application. Pacing Clin Electrophysiol. 2003;26:1420–1423.

21 Narayan SM, Krummen DE, Shivkumar K, Clopton P, Rappel W-J, et al. Treatment of Atrial Fibrillation by the Ablation of Localized Sources: The Conventional Ablation for Atrial Fibrillation With or Without Focal Impulse and Rotor Modulation (CONFIRM) Trial. J Am Coll Cardiol. 2012d;60:628–636.

22 Tzou WS, Saghy L, Lin D. Termination of persistent atrial fibrillation during left atrial mapping. J Cardiovasc Electrophysiol. 2011;22:1171–1173.

23 Kowal RC, Daubert J, Day J, Ellenbogen K, Hummel J, et al. Results of focal impulse and rotor modulation (FIRM) for atrial fibrillation are equivalent between patients treated in san diego compared with sites new to FIRM ablation: an extended multi-center experience [Abstract]. Heart Rhythm. 2013;10:S479.

24 Shivkumar K, Ellenbogen KA, Hummel JD, Miller JM, Steinberg JS. Acute termination of human atrial fibrillation by identification and catheter ablation of localized rotors and sources: first multicenter experience of focal impulse and rotor modulation (FIRM) ablation. J Cardiovasc Electrophysiol. 2012;23:1277–1285.

25 Klos M, Calvo D, Yamazaki M, Zlochiver S, Mironov S, et al. Atrial septopulmonary bundle of the posterior left atrium provides a substrate for atrial fibrillation initiation in a model of vagally mediated pulmonary vein tachycardia of the structurally normal heart. Circ Arrhythm Electrophysiol. 2008;1:175–183.

26 Narayan SM, Franz MR, Clopton P, Pruvot EJ, Krummen DE. Repolarization alternans reveals vulnerability to human atrial fibrillation. Circulation. 2011b;123:2922–2930.

27 Narayan SM, Kazi D, Krummen DE, Rappel W-J. Repolarization and activation restitution near human pulmonary veins and atrial fibrillation initiation: a mechanism for the initiation of atrial fibrillation by premature beats. J Am Coll Cardiol. 2008c;52:1222–1230.

28 Lalani G, Gibson M, Schricker A, Rostamanian A, Krummen DE, et al. Dynamic conduction slowing precedes human atrial fibrillation initiation: insights from biatrial basket mapping during burst pacing. J Am Coll Cardiol. 2011b.

29 Ganesan AN, Kuklik P, Lau DH, Brooks AG, Baumert M, et al. Bipolar electrogram Shannon entropy at sites of rotational activation: implications for ablation of atrial fibrillation. Circ Arrhythmia Electrophysiol. 2013;6: 48–57.

30 Rappel W-J, Narayan SM. Theoretical Considerations for Mapping Activation in Human Cardiac Fibrillation. Chaos. 2013;23 (2): 023113

31 Narayan SM, Shivkumar K, Krummen DE, Miller JM, Rappel W-J. Panoramic electrophysiological mapping but not individual electrogram morphology identifies sustaining sites for human atrial fibrillation (af rotors and focal sources relate poorly to fractionated electrograms). Circ Arrhythm Electrophysiol. 2013;6:58–67.

32 Takahashi Y, O'Neill MD, Hocini M, Dubois R, Matsuo S, et al. Characterization of electrograms associated with termination of chronic atrial fibrillation by catheter ablation. J Am Coll Cardiol. 2008;51: 1003–1010.

33 Narayan SM, Krummen DE, Clopton P, Shivkumar K, Miller JM. Direct or coincidental elimination of stable rotors or focal sources may explain successful atrial fibrillation ablation: on-treatment analysis of the CONFIRM (CONventional ablation for AF with or without Focal Impulse and Rotor Modulation) trial. J Am Coll Cardiol. 2013.

34 Baykaner T, Clopton P, Schricker AA, Lalani G, Krummen DE, et al. Targeted ablation at stable atrial fibrillation sources improves success over conventional ablation in high risk patients: a substudy of the CONFIRM Trial [Abstract]. Heart Rhythm. 2013; 29 (10): 1218–1226.

35 Narayan SM, Krummen DE, Donsky A, Swarup V, Miller JM. Precise rotor elimination without concomitant pulmonary vein isolation for the successful elimination of paroxysmal atrial fibrillation. Precise PAF. Heart Rhythm. 2013;10:LBCT4.

36 de Groot NM, Houben RP, Smeets JL, Boersma E, Schotten U, et al. Electropathological substrate of long-standing persistent atrial fibrillation in patients with structural heart disease: epicardial breakthrough. Circulation. 2010;122:1674–1682.

37 Jadidi AS, Cochet H, Shah AJ, Kim SJ, Duncan E, et al. Inverse relationship between fractionated electrograms and atrial fibrosis in persistent atrial fibrillation: a combined MRI and high density mapping. J Am Coll Cardiol. 2013;62 (9): 802–812

38 Cuculich PS, Wang Y, Lindsay BD, Faddis MN, Schuessler RB, et al. Noninvasive characterization of epicardial activation in humans with diverse atrial fibrillation patterns. Circulation. 2010;122:1364–1372.

39 Haissaguerre M, Hocini M, Shah AJ, Derval N, Sacher F, et al. Noninvasive panoramic mapping of human atrial fibrillation mechanisms: a feasibility report. J Cardiovasc Electrophysiol.. 2012.

40 Hansen BJ, Zhao J, Csepe TA, Moore BT, Li N, et al. Atrial fibrillation driven by micro-anatomic intramural re-entry revealed by simultaneous sub-epicardial and sub-endocardial optical mapping in explanted human hearts. Eur Heart J. 2015; in press.

CHAPTER 19

Renal artery denervation: modulation of the autonomic nervous system to treat atrial fibrillation

Evgeny Pokushalov[1] & Jonathan S. Steinberg[2]

[1]State Research Institute of Circulation Pathology, Novosibirsk, Russia
[2]Arrhythmia Institute, The Valley Health System University of Rochester School of Medicine & Dentistry New York, NY and Ridgewood, NJ, USA

An integral role in the modulation of normal cardiac electrophysiology is played by the autonomic nervous system (ANS). Nevertheless, with the increasing recognition of anatomic and functional relationships between the nervous system and the heart, also comes a litany of new questions. Particularly, studies, to date, have not so much clarified these relationships in so much as they have revealed a multiplicity of complexity [1–11].

Renal artery denervation (RDN) has emerged as an important invasive remedy for drug-resistant hypertension (HTN). As HTN is perhaps the most common cardiovascular condition that complicates arrhythmic conditions, especially atrial fibrillation (AF), it would seem logical to explore the potential value of RDN as an antiarrhythmic tool. Moreover, because RDN likely initiates a complex series of sympatholytic phenomena, there is even greater need to understand these relationships.

Practical Guide to Catheter Ablation of Atrial Fibrillation, Second Edition. Edited by Jonathan S. Steinberg, Pierre Jaïs and Hugh Calkins.
© 2016 John Wiley & Sons, Ltd. Published 2016 by John Wiley & Sons, Ltd.

The autonomic nervous system and the substrate for atrial fibrillation

Much published literature demonstrates the ANS as a prime contributor to AF with the sympathetic and the parasympathetic nervous systems playing an integral role. It has been shown that the onset of AF was preceded by a primary increase in the sympathetic drive, followed by marked modulation toward vagal predominance [12,13]. There is presently strong evidence for the implication of autonomic nerves in the initiation and maintenance of AF [14–17]. Hyperactivity of ANS with the uncontrolled release of excess amounts of neurotransmitters underlies these changes, which in turn shorten the refractoriness in the atrium [14]. The highest levels of neurotransmitter release would be in the vicinity of the autonomic ganglia concentrated at the ganglionated plexi (GP) interfacing with both the atria and the pulmonary veins. Accordingly, these neurotransmitters, especially in locally excessive concentrations, could induce rapid ectopic firing and thereby serve as the "drivers" for initiating atrial fibrillation [18]. Shortened atrial refractoriness with gradients across the atria serves to facilitate the development of AF. Experimental data have shown that electrical dispersion (gradient of atrial refractoriness) is caused not only by the ANS innervation gradient [19,20] but possibly also by a gradient of allocation of compromised GP in the atrial myocardium.

Sources of pathological activity influencing the ANS in AF include afferent signals arising from extrinsic and intrinsic nervous systems (kidney, baroreceptors, carotid bodies, and intracardiac GP), efferent signals from extrinsic nervous system, epicardial GP or/and myocardial GP, and groups of intrinsic ganglia-complex neural network modulate the interactions between the extrinsic and the intrinsic nervous systems. Modulation of the autonomic nervous system might be a promising strategy to protect the myocardium from proarrhythmic autonomic influences and the development of electrical, autonomic, and structural atrial remodeling [21]. Nowadays we have several strategies to modulate the complex interaction between the ANS and the heart. However, different approaches target the problem differently making the prediction of arrhythmogenic and/or antiarrhythmic effects difficult. These strategies are based on renal sympathetic denervation, GP ablation, ganglion stellatum ablation, high thoracic epidural anesthesia, low-level vagal nerve stimulation, and baroreflex stimulation.

Renal sympathetic denervation is a new method that may be effective for control of resistant hypertension [22]. Apart from its antihypertensive effects, renal denervation may also exert antiarrhythmic effects, with reports suggesting a potential role for both AF [23] and ventricular tachyarrhythmias [24]. Hypertension is an established risk factor for AF [25,26], and many cases of apparently "lone" AF can be attributed to latent hypertension [27]. The sympathetic nervous system also appears to play an important role in the initiation and maintenance of AF [28,29]. Increases in sympathetic tone frequently precede the onset of AF [30] and excessive sympathetic activation can predict recurrences of AF after catheter ablation [31]. Autonomic denervation, which inevitably affects both the parasympathetic and the sympathetic components of the autonomic innervation of the atria, has also been found beneficial in patients subjected to PVI for AF [32,33].

The renal nerves and renal denervation

The kidney has an extensive network of afferent unmyelinated fibers that transmit important sensory information to the central nervous system. Afferent fibers from the kidney travel along with the sympathetic nerves and enter the dorsal roots and project to neurons at both spinal and supraspinal levels. The renal afferent nerves carry information to the CNS from renal chemo- and mechanoreceptors. Most of the brainstem regions involved in cardiovascular

control including the hypothalamus receive inputs from the renal afferents [34–36]. Renal afferent nerve activity then directly influences sympathetic outflow to the kidneys and other highly innervated organs involved in cardiovascular control such as the heart and the vascular system.

Renal sympathetic efferent nerves stimulate neuroeffectors throughout the kidney. Sympathetic nerve activation of juxtaglomerular cells results in increased renin secretion and reduced urinary sodium excretion and renal vasoconstriction. The results are diverse, but they include decreased renal blood flow and glomerular filtration rate via vascular smooth muscle cell contraction of the resistance vessels and preferential preglomerular vasoconstriction of the microvessels, renin secretion and activation of the renin–angiotensin–aldosterone system (RAAS), and sodium retention.

There are important interactions between the kidney and the heart in various cardiac conditions, which are mediated by the autonomic nervous system. These include upregulation of the sympathetic nerve system, activation of the RAAS, and vasopressin secretion. For example, compromised hemodynamics during AF leads to an increase in catecholamines and sympathetic tone with parasympathetic withdrawal [37]. The activation of sympathetic nervous system is, in part, related to the effects of circulating renin released from the kidneys. The kidney receives a dense innervation of sympathetic and sensory fibers and can be both a target of sympathetic activity and a source of signals that drive sympathetic tone.

Electrical and structural remodeling are fundamental contributors to the AF substrate, and their progression perpetuates the development and maintenance of AF. The RAAS may be involved in this progression, particularly via the actions of angiotensin II and aldosterone. It is well known that renal sympathetic stimulation induces renin release; conversely, angiotensin II appears to have important actions in modulating sympathetic nerve activity. The RAAS is involved in myocardial fibrosis and increased angiotensin II production causes marked atrial dilation with focal fibrosis and AF [38]. Inhibition of the RAAS might have a protective effect on remodeling and deleterious influences on AF occurrence and progression. For example, the inhibition of endogenous angiotensin II interfered with the expected electrical remodeling responses during rapid atrial pacing [39]. During continuous AF, the presence of persistent elevated sympathetic and RAAS activity may be mutually reinforcing.

There is some evidence that inhibition of RAAS in patients may reduce the likelihood of AF. For example, renin–angiotensin system blockers protected against AF recurrences after PVI in patients with low-burden paroxysmal AF and hypertension. Published meta-analyses suggest decreased AF incidence in patients with hypertension treated with ACEI or ARBs [40]. More recent prospective data, however, has not confirmed the potential value of RAAS inhibition to prevent AF [41].

Further evidence to support the importance of cardiorenal interactions has been observed in the presence of left ventricular hypertrophy and even more pronounced in heart failure [42–44]. Renal sympathetic activation has been shown to predict all-cause mortality and need for heart transplantation in patients with heart failure [45].

If sympathetic activity potentiates conditions that promote AF, modulation of the autonomic nervous system has been shown to favorably influence neural remodeling during AF. Thoracic epidural anesthesia reduced afferent and efferent sympathetic nerve impulse traffic and prevented sustained AF created by rapid atrial pacing. This was associated with inhibition of atrial nerve sprouting [46]. Interestingly, local ablation of sympathovagal nerves did not achieve the same effect in a similar model [47]. These data suggest that a blockade of afferent and efferent sympathetic fibers is more effective than elimination of cardiac efferent nerve fibers. In this regard, it is critically important to emphasize that ablation of the afferent and efferent renal sympathetic nerves by RDN has been shown to reduce renal and whole-body sympathetic activity [48]. Radiotracer dilution methodologies were used to assess the overflow of norepinephrine from the kidneys into the circulation before and after RDN. These analyses revealed a substantial reduction in norepinephrine spillover, in addition to decreased renin secretion and increased renal blood flow [49].

Some experimental work suggests that the most effective autonomic manipulation to limit triggering of AF is via combined antisympathetic and antiparasympathetic intervention. Patterson et al. used isolated pulmonary vein muscle sleeves to demonstrate the synergistic value of AF triggering by combined sympathetic and parasympathetic stimulation [50]. Conversely, the suppression of Ca transients and inhibition of forward Na/Ca exchange reduced arrhythmogenicity. If combined autonomic blockade is necessary for optimal AF suppression, a local cardiac denervation approach would be a logical treatment effort. If so, then RDN may be most efficacious only when HTN control is part of the response, that is, lowering the elevated blood pressure imparts an antiarrhythmic response. On the other hand, if more thorough sympathetic denervation is achieved by RDN than alternative methods (e.g., beta-blockers, ablation of autonomic cardiac ganglia), this could potentially contribute mightily to an antiarrhythmic response if accompanying parasympathetic blockade is not a therapeutic requirement.

Experimental work in arrhythmia models

Poorly controlled HTN is likely a negative contributor to the outcome after ablation of AF. Lau et al. showed in a sheep model of AF that a hypertensive group developed a progressive increase in mean arterial pressure, longer mean effective atrial refractory periods, progressive biatrial hypertrophy, left atrial dysfunction and greater AF inducibility (with increased inflammation after 5 weeks of HTN) [51].

In a pig model of rapid atrial pacing, RDN exhibited inhibition of cardiac sympathetic tone with negative chronotropic and dromotropic effects, prolongation of AV node effective refractory period and antegrade Wenckebach cycle length, and improved rate control during induced AF [52]. Interestingly, the duration of induced AF episodes was shortened after RDN compared to control experiments; however, inducibility was not changed. The latter may be due to the observation that RDN had no effect on atrial pacing-induced atrial effective refractory period shortening or intraatrial conduction. The findings in this study raise the possibility that RDN may be useful for rate control in AF.

Zhao et al. used a dog model of rapid atrial pacing and demonstrated that the number of episodes and duration of AF were decreased by RDN, associated with decreased activity of RAAS [53].

In a pig model of obstructive sleep apnea, RDN inhibited shortening of atrial refractory periods and the anticipated increased AF susceptibility [54].

After RDN, the efferent nerves experienced functional reinnervation of the renal vasculature with complete return of neural function by 8 weeks [55]. It is, therefore, possible that some efferent sympathetic reinnervation may occur in patients after RDN, although the magnitude and time course of this potential response is unknown. Interestingly, in contrast to efferent nerves, the afferent nerves do not appear to have the capacity to regenerate [56].

Clinical experience

Hypertension is an important risk factor for developing AF. The incidence of AF also increases with left ventricular hypertrophy, coronary heart disease, and heart failure, all consequences of poorly controlled hypertension. We have previously shown in a randomized controlled pilot study that RDN provided incremental AF suppression after PVI in patients with symptomatic and refractory AF in the setting of drug-resistant hypertension [23]. The mechanisms by which RDN could help were believed to fall into 2 nonmutually exclusive possibilities: by improving blood pressure control and by reducing central sympathetic cardiac stimulation. The implication of the latter is very important, that is, this technique has potential value in nonhypertensives.

We enrolled 27 patients (14 randomized to PVI only and 13 randomized to PVI with RDN), all of whom were followed for 12 months after ablation. All had a history of PAF, but 18 (67%) also had a history of PersAF. HTN was uncontrolled in all patients despite multidrug therapy. At the 12-month follow-up examination, 9 (69%) of the 13 PVI with renal artery ablation group patients were AF free. In contrast, in the PVI-only group, only 4 (29%) of the 14 patients were AF free on no antiarrhythmic drugs ($p = 0.033$) (Figure 1). Patients who underwent PVI only did not show any significant variation in systolic or diastolic blood pressures (Figure 2). By contrast, patients treated with RDN displayed a significant decrease in systolic and diastolic blood pressures at each of the visits at 3, 6, 9, and 12 months. At 12 months, the reductions in systolic and diastolic blood pressures were successfully and

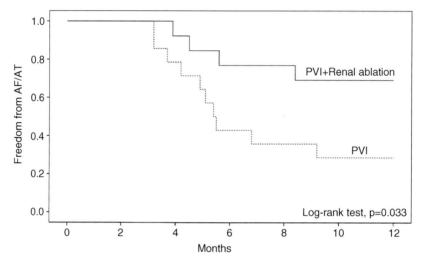

Figure 1 Incidence of AF recurrences in patients with and without renal artery denervation.

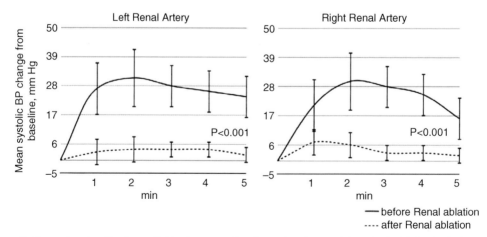

Figure 2 Change from baseline in systolic blood pressures (continuous invasive arterial monitoring) following high-frequency stimulation (20 Hz, 15 V, 10 ms, for 10 s) of the right and left renal arteries during the ablation procedure.

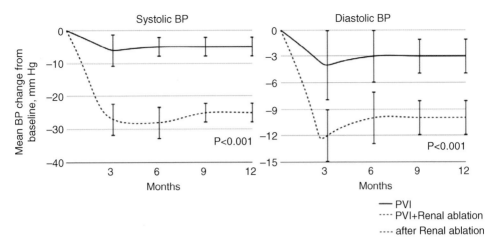

Figure 3 Change from baseline in systolic and diastolic blood pressures throughout follow-up.

significantly maintained ($P < 0.001$ versus PVI only) resulting in a fall from baseline of 25 ± 5 mm Hg and 10 ± 2 mm Hg, respectively (Figure 3). Mean LV mass was reduced in the PVI with renal artery ablation group during follow-up by approximately 10%.

Recent analysis from two prospective double-blind randomized studies confirm our earlier findings but in a larger and more diverse cohort of patients, that is, RDN reduces the likelihood of AF when performed with PVI in hypertensive patients [57]. The benefit was most dramatic in patients with severe drug-resistant hypertension and those with PersAF, although nonsignificant trends were also seen in patients with moderate hypertension and those with PAF (Figure 4). Perhaps, we could speculate that the limited number of patients enrolled did not allow this trend to reach statistical significance. The use of RDN in moderate hypertension and the effect on PAF deserve further investigation.

Whether the benefit of RDN results from reduced vascular tone and atrial unloading or diminished sympathetic activity, or both, cannot be deduced by our study. Hypertension is the most common cause of AF encountered in clinical practice [58,59], and its control should be valuable for patients undergoing a primary AF ablation procedure using PVI, the fundamental interventional technique in contemporary use.

PersAF, a disease attributed to a remodeled substrate in addition to PV firing, also seems to be affected by the addition of RDN. This benefit, despite the detection of a trend toward improvement, was not statistically significant in patients with PAF. It might be that in patients with paroxysmal AF, elimination of the sympathetic hyperactivity and/or reduced atrial loading through treatment of hypertension may not be sufficient to translate into clear and dramatic clinical outcomes or that PVI works well enough that it is more difficult to substantiate its incremental benefit. The observed trend toward improvement, however, suggests further evaluation is needed in future trials.

In our study, RDN delivered a significant reduction in systolic and diastolic blood pressures. These results are compatible with those reported by the Symplicity HTN-1, 2 and Ott et al. trials [60] for moderate resistant hypertension. The Symplicity HTN-3 was recently stopped due to inadequate therapeutic effect [61]. Although we do not have full data of this trial for comparison, there are two important differences between the methodology of our study and that of the Symplicity HTN-3. First, we have used high-frequency stimulation (HFS) that was not used by the Symplicity HTN-3 trial. We believe this is a critical procedural online measure of success of this procedure. We found that HFS delivered at the ostium of the targeted renal artery caused a sudden increase of blood pressure by a mean of 30 mm Hg and could be used to confirm the completion of RDN. Our observations confirm the anatomic finding of Norvell et al. in that the aortorenal ganglia are located near the ostia of the renal arteries and the aorta [62]. Second, we used office measurements, according to the Standard Joint National Committee VII, European Society of Cardiology, and European Society of Hypertension recommendations [63,64]. If we would have used 24-h monitoring, results may have been different. Another limitation of this study is the relatively small number of patients. In addition, 60 out of 146 patients were excluded due to their declining to participate or ineligible renal artery anatomy. Thus, our results certainly require validation in additional and larger trials.

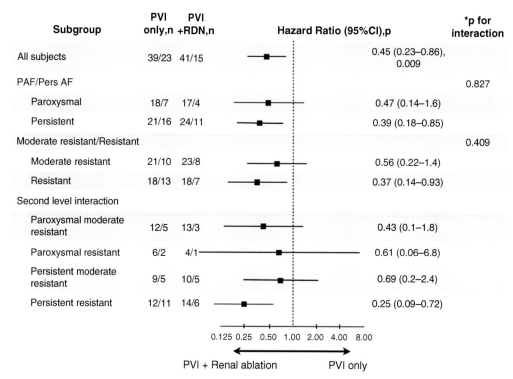

Subgroup	PVI only,n	PVI +RDN,n	Hazard Ratio (95%CI),p	*p for interaction
All subjects	39/23	41/15	0.45 (0.23–0.86), 0.009	
PAF/Pers AF				0.827
Paroxysmal	18/7	17/4	0.47 (0.14–1.6)	
Persistent	21/16	24/11	0.39 (0.18–0.85)	
Moderate resistant/Resistant				0.409
Moderate resistant	21/10	23/8	0.56 (0.22–1.4)	
Resistant	18/13	18/7	0.37 (0.14–0.93)	
Second level interaction				
Paroxysmal moderate resistant	12/5	13/3	0.43 (0.1–1.8)	
Paroxysmal resistant	6/2	4/1	0.61 (0.06–6.8)	
Persistent moderate resistant	9/5	10/5	0.69 (0.2–2.4)	
Persistent resistant	12/11	14/6	0.25 (0.09–0.72)	

0.125 0.25 0.50 1.00 2.00 4.00 8.00

PVI + Renal ablation ← → PVI only

Figure 4 Hazard ratio for AF recurrence. The main effect models are calculated using proportional hazard regression with adjustment for study and type of AF. *p for interaction was calculated using the interaction term treatment*type of AF and treatment*study for each interaction, respectively.

The technique of renal artery denervation

Our patients underwent bilateral renal denervation directly after PVI during the same procedure. The renal artery ablation procedure has been defined in detail previously [23,57,65]. Renal arteries were assessed for suitability of ablation by renal angiography. In some patients, real-time three-dimensional aorta–renal artery maps were reconstructed with the use of the same navigation system, CARTO XP, and the NaviStar ThermoCool ablation catheter, used for PVI (Biosense-Webster Inc., Diamond Bar, CA) via femoral artery access (Figure 5). Other patients underwent renal ablation with the use of Simplicity™ renal denervation system (Medtronic Inc, Mountain View, CA). There is no great advantage to one system over another, and operators can use catheters/systems with which they are comfortable, including expense considerations. Both mapping and ablation were performed under modified sedation using a propofol infusion. RF ablations of 8–12 watts (impedance drop >10%) were applied discretely from the first distal main renal artery bifurcation all the way back to the ostium. The duration of each RF delivery was 60–120 s, and up to six lesions (separated by >5 mm) were performed both longitudinally and rotationally within each renal artery.

To confirm renal denervation, we used HFS before the initial and after each RF delivery within the renal artery. Rectangular electrical stimuli were delivered at the ostium of the targeted renal artery at a frequency of 20 Hz, with an amplitude of 15 V and pulse duration of 10 ms (Stimulator B-53, Biotok Inc, Russia) for 10 s. Renal sympathetic denervation was considered to have been achieved when the sudden increase of blood pressure (>15 mm Hg from invasive arterial monitoring) was eliminated in the presence of HFS (Figure 3).

Conclusions

Available data indicate that autonomic influences contribute to the development of AF. Therefore, modulation of the autonomic nervous system is a promising strategy for antiarrhythmic treatment. Randomized trials are required to investigate the definite effect of the different strategies on atrial arrhythmogenesis.

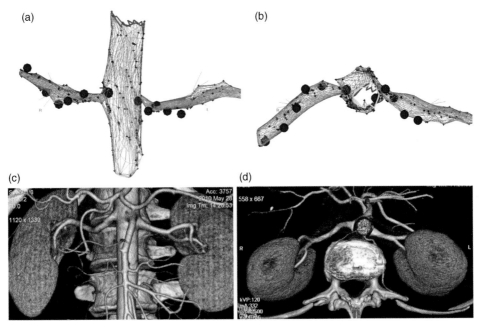

Figure 5 (a) and (b) are 3D reconstructions with sites of RF ablation represented in dark gray. (c) and (d) are MRI scans performed 6 months after ablation that demonstrate no evidence of renal artery stenosis.

References

1 Kapa S, Venkatachalam KL, Samuel J. Asirvatham, The Autonomic Nervous System in Cardiac Electrophysiology. Cardiol Rev. 2010;18(6):275–284.

2 Armour JA, Murphy DA, Yuan BX, et al. Gross and microscopic anatomy of the human intrinsic cardiac nervous system. Anat Rec. 1997;247:289–298.

3 Davies F, Francis ET, King TS. Neurological studies of the cardiac ventricles of mammals. J Anat. 1952;86:130–143.

4 Kuntz A. The Autonomic Nervous System. Philadelphia, PA: Lea & Febiger, 1934.

5 Janes RD, Brandys JC, Hopkins DA, et al. Anatomy of human extrinsic cardiac nerves and ganglia. Am J Cardiol. 1986;57:299–309.

6 Lloyd TC, Jr. Control of systemic vascular resistance by pulmonary and left heart baroreflexes. Am J Physiol. 1972;222:1511–1517.

7 Lloyd TC, Jr, Fried JJ. Effect of a left atrium–pulmonary vein baroreflex on peripheral vascular beds. Am J Physiol. 1977;233:H587–H591.

8 Edis AJ. Aortic baroreflex function in the dog. Am J Physiol. 1971;221:1352–1357.

9 Mitchell RA. Location and function of medullary respiratory neurons. Am Rev Respir Dis. 1977;115:209–216.

10 Thoren PN. Characteristics of left ventricular receptors with nonmedullated vagal afferents in cats. Circ Res. 1977;40:415–421.

11 Tan AY, Verrier RL. The role of the autonomic nervous system in cardiac arrhythmias. Handb Clin Neurol. 2013;117:135–145.

12 Shen MJ, Choi EK, Tan AY, Lin SF, Fishben MC, Chen LS, Chen PS. Neural mechanisms of atria arrhythmias. Nat Rev Cardiol. 2012;9:30–39.

13 Chou CC, Chen PS. New concepts in atrial fibrillation: neural mechanisms and calcium dynamics. Cardiol Clin. 2009.

14 Schauerte P, Scherlag BJ, Patterson E, et al. Focal atrial fibrillation: experimental evidence for a pathophysiologic role of the autonomic nervous system. J Cardiovasc Electrophysiol. 2001;12:592–599.

15 Scherlag BJ, Yamanashi WS, Patel U, et al. Autonomically induced conversion of pulmonary vein focal firing into atrial fibrillation. J Am Coll Cardiol. 2005;45:1878–1886.

16 Nakagawa H, Scherlag BJ, Aoyama H, et al. Catheter ablation of cardiac autonomic nerves for prevention of atrial fibrillation in a caninemodel. [Abstract] Heart Rhythm. 2004;1:S10.

17 Patterson E, Po S, Scherlag BJ, Lazzara R. Triggered firing in pulmonary veins initiated by *in vitro* autonomic nerve stimulation. Heart Rhythm. 2005;2:624–631.

18 Zhou J, Scherlag B, Ewards J, et al. Gradients of atrial refractoriness and inducibility of atrial fibrillation due to stimulation of ganglionated plexi. J Cardiovasc Electrophysiol. 2007;18:83–90.

19 Chevalier P, Tabib A, Meyronnet D, et al. Quantitative study of nerves of the human left atrium. Heart Rhythm. 2005;2:518–522.

20 Zhou J, Scherlag B, Ewards J, et al. Gradients of atrial refractoriness and inducibility of atrial fibrillation due to stimulation of ganglionated plexi. J Cardiovasc Electrophysiol. 2007;18:83–90.

21 Linz D, Ukena C, Mahfoud F, Neuberger H, Böhm M. Atrial autonomic innervation a target for interventional antiarrhythmic therapy? J Am Coll Cardiol. 2014;63(3):215–224.

22 Schlaich MP, Schmieder RE, Bakris G, et al. International Expert Consensus Statement: percutneous transluminal renal denervation for the treatment of resistant hypertension. J Am Coll ardiol. 2013;62(22):2031–2045.

23 Pokushalov E, Romanov A, Corbucci G, Artyomenko S, Baranova V, Turov A, Shirokova N, Karaskov A, Mittal S, Steinberg JS. A randomized comparison of pulmonary vein isolation with versus without concomitant renal artery denervation in patients with refractory symptomatic atrial fibrillation and resistant hypertension. J Am Coll Cardiol. 2012;60:1163–1170.

24 Remo BF, Preminger M, Bradfield J, Mittal S, Boyle N, Gupta A, Shivkumar K, Steinberg JS, Dickfeld T. Safety and efficacy of renal denervation as a novel treatment of ventricular tachycardia storm in patients with cardiomyopathy. Heart Rhythm. 2014;11:541–546.

25 Huxley RR, Lopez FL, Folsom AR, et al. Absolute and attributable risks of atrial fibrillation in relation to optimal and borderline risk factors: the Atherosclerosis Risk in Communities (ARIC) Study. Circulation. 2011;123:1501–1508.

26 Fuster V, Ryden LE, Cannom DS, et al. 2011 ACCF/AHA/HRS focused updates incorporated into the ACC/AHA/ESC 2006 guidelines for the management of patients with atrial fibrillation: a report of the American College of Cardiology Foundation/American Heart Association Task Force on Practice Guidelines. Circulation. 2011;123:e269–e367.

27 Katritsis DG, Toumpoulis IK, Giazitzoglou E, Korovesis S, Karabinos I, Paxinos G, Zambartas C, Anagnostopoulos CE. Latent arterial hypertension in apparently lone atrial fibrillation. J Interv Card Electrophysiol. 2005;13:203–207.

28 Schotten U, Verheule S, Kirchhof P, Goette A. Pathophysiological mechanisms of atrial fibrillation: a translational appraisal. Physiol Rev. 2011;91:265–325.

29 Lau D, Mackenzie L, Kelly D, et al. Hypertension and atrial fibrillation: evidence of progressive atrial remodeling with electrostructural correlate in a conscious chronically instrumented ovine model. Heart Rhythm. 2010;7:1282–1290.

30 Bettoni M, Zimmermann M. Autonomic tone variations before the onset of paroxysmal atrial fibrillation. Circulation. 2002;105:2753–2759.

31 Arimoto T, Tada H, Igarashi M, Sekiguchi Y, Sato A, Koyama T, Yamasaki H, Machino T, Kuroki K, Kuga K, Aonuma K. High washout rate of iodine-123-metaiodobenzylguanidine imaging predicts the outcome of catheter ablation of atrial fibrillation. J Cardiovasc Electrophysiol. 2011;22:1297–1304.

32 Katritsis DG, Pokushalov E, Romanov A, Giazitzoglou E, Siontis GC, Po SS, Camm AJ, Ioannidis JP. Autonomic denervation added to pulmonary vein isolation for paroxysmal atrial fibrillation: a randomized clinical trial. J Am Coll Cardiol. 2013; 735–1097.

33 Pokushalov E. The role of autonomic denervation during catheter ablation of atrial fibrillation. Curr Opin Cardiol. 2008;23(1):55–9.

34 Stella A, Zanchetti A. Functional role of renal afferents. Physiol Rev. 1991;71:659–682.

35 DiBona GF, Kopp UC. Neural control of renal function. Physiol Rev. 1997;77:75–197.

36 Ye S, Ozgur B, Campese VM. Renal afferent impulses, the posterior hypothalamus, and hypertension in rats with chronic renal failure. Kidney Int. 1997;51:722–727.

37 Kumagai K, Nakashima H, Urata H, et al. Effects of angiotensin II type 1 receptor antagonist on electrical and structural remodeling in atrial fibrillation. J Am Coll Cardiol. 2003;41:2197–2204.

38 Nakashima H, Kumagai K, Urata H, et al. Angiotensin II antagonist prevents electrical remodeling in atrial fibrillation. Circulation. 2000;101:2612–2617.

39 Berkowitsch A, Neumann T, Kuniss M, et al. Therapy with renin-angiotensin system blockers after pulmonary vein isolation in patients with atrial fibrillation: who is a responder? PACE. 2010;33:1101–1111.

40 Healy JS, Baranchuk A, Crystal E, et al. Prevention of atrial fibrillation with angiotensin-converting enzyme inhibitors and angiotensin receptor blockers: a meta-analysis. J Am Coll Cardiol. 2005;45:1832–1839.

41 GISSI-AF Investigators. Valsartan for prevention of recurrent atrial fibrillation. N Eng J Med. 2009;360:1606–1617.

42 Schlaich MP, Kaye DM, Lambert E, et al. Relation between cardiac sympathetic activity and hypertensive left ventricular hypertrophy. Circulation. 2003;108:560–565.

43 Burns J, Sivananthan MU, Ball SG, et al. Relationship between central sympathetic drive and magnetic resonance imaging-determined left ventricular mass in essential hypertension. Circulation. 2007;115:1999–2005.

44 Kaye DM, Lambert GW, Lefkovits J, et al. Neurochemical evidence of cardiac sympathetic activation and increased central nervous system norepinephrine turnover in severe congestive heart failure. J Am Coll Cardiol. 1994;23:570–578.

45 Kaye DM, Lefkovits J, Jennings GL, et al. Adverse consequences of high sympathetic nervous activity in the failing human heart. J Am Coll Cardiol. 1995;26:1257–1263.

46 Yang SS, Han W, Cao Y, et al. Effects of high thoracic epidural anesthesia on atrial electrophysiological characteristics and sympathetic nerve sprouting in a canine model of atrial fibrillation. Basic Res Cardiol. 2011;106:495–506.

47 Tan AY, Zhou S, Ogawa M, et al. Neural mechanisms of paroxysmal atrial fibrillation and paroxysmal atrial tachycardia in ambulatory canines. Circulation. 2008;118:916–925.

48 Sobotka PA, Mahfoud F, Schlaich MP, et al. Sympathorenal axis in chronic disease. Clin Res Cardiol. 2011;100:1049–1057.

49 Schlaich MP, Sobotka PA, Krum H, Lambert E, Esler MD. Renal sympathetic-nerve ablation for uncontrolled hypertension. N Eng J Med. 2009;361:932–934.

50 Patterson E, Po SS, Scherlag BJ, Lazzara R. Triggered firing of pulmonary veins by *in vitro* autonomic nerve stimulation. Heart Rhythm. 2005;2:624–631.

51 Lau DH, Mackenzie L, Kelly DJ, et al. Hypertension and atrial fibrillation: evidence of progressive atrial remodeling with electrostructural correlate in a conscious chronically instrumented ovine model. Heart Rhythm. 2010;7: 1282–1290.

52 Linz D, Mahfoud F, Schotten U, et al. Renal sympathetic denervation provide ventricular rate control but does not prevent atrial electrical remodeling during atrial fibrillation. Hypertension. 2013;61:225–231.

53 Zhao Q, Yu S, Zou M, et al. Effects of renal sympathetic denervation on the inducibility of atrial fibrillation during rapid atrial pacing. JICE. 2012;35:119–125.

54 Linz D, Mahfoud F, Schotten U, et al. Renal sympathetic denervation suppresses postapneic blood pressure rises and atrial fibrillation in a model for sleep apnea. Hypertension. 2012;60:172–178.

55 Kline RL, Mercer PF. Functional reinnervation and development of supersensitivity to NE after renal denervation in rats. Am J Physiol. 1980;238:R353–R358.

56 Arrowood JA, Goureau JA, Minisi AJ, Davis AB, Mohanty PK. Evidence against reinnervation of cardiac vagal afferents after human orthotopic cardiac transplantation. Circulation. 1995;92:402–408.

57 Pokushalov E, Romanov A, Katritsis DG, Artyomenko S, Bayramova S, Losik D, Baranova V, Karaskov A, Steinberg JS. Renal denervation for improving outcomes of catheter ablation in patients with atrial fibrillation and hypertension: early experience. Heart Rhythm. 2014; 11(7):1131–1138.

58 Huxley RR, Lopez FL, Folsom AR, et al. Absolute and attributable risks of atrial fibrillation in relation to optimal and borderline risk factors: the Atherosclerosis Risk in Communities (ARIC) Study. Circulation. 2011; 123:1501–1508.

59 Fuster V, Ryden LE, Cannom DS, et al. 2011 ACCF/ AHA/HRS focused updates incorporated into the ACC/ AHA/ESC 2006 guidelines for the management of patients with atrial fibrillation: a report of the American College of Cardiology Foundation/American Heart Association Task Force on Practice Guidelines. Circulation. 2011;123:e269–e367.

60 Ott C, Mahfoud F, Schmid A, Ditting T, Sobotka PA, Veelken R, Spies A, Ukena C, Laufs U, Uder M, Böhm M, Schmieder RE. Renal denervation in moderate treatment resistant hypertension. J Am Coll Cardiol. 2013;62(20): 1880–1886.

61 Bhatt DL, Kandzari DE, O'Neill WW, D'Agostino R, Flack JM, Katzen BT, Leon MB, Liu M, Mauri L, Negoita M, Cohen SA, Oparil S, Rocha-Singh K, Townsend RR, Bakris GL, SYMPLICITY HTN-3 Investigators. A controlled trial of renal denervation for resistant hypertension. N Engl J Med. 2014;370(15):1393–1401.

62 Norvell JE. The aorticorenal ganglion and its role in renal innervation. J Comp Neur. 1968;133:101–112.

63 Chobanian AV, Bakris GL, Black HR, et al. The Seventh Report of the Joint National Committee on Prevention, Detection, Evaluation, and Treatment of High Blood Pressure: the JNC 7 Report. JAMA. 2003;289: 2560–2572.

64 Mancia G, De Backer G, Dominiczak A, et al. 2007 Guidelines for the Management of Arterial Hypertension: The Task Force for the Management of Arterial Hypertension of the European Society of Hypertension (ESH) and of the European Society of Cardiology (ESC). J Hypertens. 2007;25:1105–1187.

65 Krum H, Schlaich M, Whitbourn R, Sobotka PA, Sadowski J, Bartus K, Kapelak B, Walton A, Sievert H, Thambar S, Abraham WT, Esler M. Catheter-based renal sympathetic denervation for resistant hypertension: a multicentre safety and proof-of-principle cohort study. Lancet. 2009;11 373 (9671):1275–1281.

CHAPTER 20

The stepwise ablation approach for persistent atrial fibrillation

Han S. Lim, Stephan Zellerhoff, & Pierre Jaïs

CHU de Bordeaux, Hopital Cardiologique Haut Leveque, Pessac, France
Université de Bordeaux, IHU LIRYC, Bordeaux, France

Introduction

Persistent atrial fibrillation (AF) ablation remains a challenge with variable clinical success reported. The lack of efficacy of pulmonary vein isolation (PVI) alone in treating persistent AF compared with paroxysmal AF suggests the further involvement of atrial substrate in these patients [1,2]. Several techniques have been proposed to provide incremental benefit to PVI, including ablation of complex fractionated electrograms (CFE), linear ablation, and ablation of localized sources maintaining AF [3–7]. The stepwise ablation approach combines the abovementioned techniques – PVI, electrogram-based ablation, and linear lesions – to achieve a cumulative effect with the procedural end point of AF termination [8,9]. This chapter summarizes the technique, clinical outcomes, recovery of cardiac function, recurrence of atrial tachycardias (ATs), and current limitations of the stepwise ablation strategy in persistent AF.

Rationale for the stepwise ablation approach

Although pulmonary vein isolation (PVI) is efficacious in the treatment of paroxysmal AF, its limited success in persistent AF suggests more diffuse involvement of the biatrial substrate and the need to perform further substrate modification [2,4]. Various techniques have demonstrated incremental benefit in

Practical Guide to Catheter Ablation of Atrial Fibrillation, Second Edition. Edited by Jonathan S. Steinberg, Pierre Jaïs and Hugh Calkins.

addition to PVI, including ablation of complex fractionated electrograms (CFE) [3,6,10], ablation of localized sources maintaining AF [5], and linear ablation [4,7]. The stepwise ablation strategy combines the above techniques for persistent AF ablation in a sequential fashion, with the end point of AF termination. This strategy aims to target all sources and foci contributing to the initiation and maintenance of AF, until AF is no longer sustained.

Technique of stepwise ablation

Step 1: Thoracic/pulmonary vein isolation

Isolation of the pulmonary veins remains the cornerstone of most AF ablation procedures. Circumferential PVI is performed at least about 1 cm proximal to the PV ostia to avoid the risk of PV stenosis whenever possible. Pulmonary vein potentials can be mapped with the use of a circular multielectrode catheter. Pacing maneuvers, such as pacing from the coronary sinus and left atrial appendage, help distinguish overlapping far-field signals from PV potentials. The delay, sequence, and polarity reversal of PV potentials provide information on progressive conduction delay between the LA and the PV and on sites of breakthrough. Isolation of the PVs results in termination of AF in a minority of patients and frequently further steps are required in persistent AF. The superior vena cava may also be targeted as a non-PV trigger in this step when proved arrhythmogenic. Following AF termination at the end of the procedure, isolation of the PVs is confirmed and further consolidative ablation performed as necessary in sinus rhythm (SR).

Step 2: Electrogram-based ablation

The next step following PVI is electrogram-based ablation. Sites of continuous electrical activity, complex fractionated electrograms, rapid local cycle lengths, and significant gradient of activation between adjacent and surrounding electrodes are targeted [11,12]. These regions vary with the individual patient. However, often important sites for cycle length slowing include the base of the left atrial appendage and the inferior LA–coronary sinus interface, in addition to the PV–LA junction [12]. Additional ablation within the coronary sinus or at the coronary sinus ostium may also be needed to eliminate residual sharp potentials or to dissociate the proximal coronary sinus musculature from the atria. Other areas of interest include the interatrial septum and parts of the posterior and anterior LA wall. In the setting of disparate progression of AF cycle length between the right and the left atria, right atrial drivers of AF are suspected, indicating the need for right atrial ablation [13].

Step 3: Linear ablation

If AF persists following the first two steps, ablation proceeds to linear ablation, in the form of roof line ablation, mitral isthmus line ablation, and cavotricuspid isthmus ablation. Linear ablation prevents the formation of macroreentrant circuits and further debulks the atrium. The roof line forms a continuous linear lesion between the isolated left and the right superior pulmonary veins. The mitral isthmus line extends from the ventricular aspect of the mitral annulus to the ostium of the left inferior pulmonary vein, and is reserved for patients with persisting AF despite prior ablation steps and patients with perimitral macroreentrant AT. Bidirectional block across

these linear lesions is imperative, as patients with incomplete linear conduction block are noted to have a much higher rate of AT recurrence [14]. Following AF termination, bidirectional linear conduction block across the linear lesions is confirmed by differential pacing, evidence of activation detour, and demonstration of wide double potentials along the line. Consolidative ablation is performed in SR to achieve linear conduction block as required.

Monitoring of AF cycle length

The AF cycle length is an indicator of procedural (AF termination) and long-term success. Longer baseline AF cycle length predicts AF termination and mid-to-long-term freedom from arrhythmia recurrence. The AF cycle length is assessed at baseline and at each step of the procedure, shown in Figure 1. The AF cycle length can be reliably and simultaneously recorded from the left and right atrial appendages, where discrete potentials can be measured. During the procedure, progressive prolongation of AF cycle length precedes AF termination. A cumulative effect is observed with each step of the ablation approach [9].

Right atrial ablation

In a series of patients with chronic AF who underwent stepwise ablation, termination of AF occurred during ablation in the LA in 55% of patients, right atrium in 26%, and coronary sinus in 19% [15]. By monitoring AF cycle length, in about 20% of persistent AF cases, a divergent pattern of AF cycle length prolongation is observed during the procedure, with a shorter right atrial AF cycle length compared to LA AF cycle length [13]. Right atrial ablation in these cases resulted in AF termination in 55% [14].

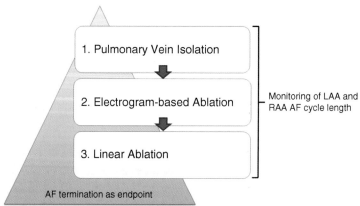

Figure 1 Assessment of AF cycle length.

Termination of AF as the procedural end point

The procedural end point for stepwise ablation is termination of AF, either directly to SR or to an intermediate AT. Termination of AF during ablation has been demonstrated to be an independent predictor of single procedure success, success after the last procedure, and overall clinical success with multiple procedures [16–19]. In the setting of AF termination into an intermediate AT, the importance of successful ablation of these ATs is demonstrated in several studies where outcomes were significantly better in patients with intermediate ATs terminated by ablation compared to cardioversion [20,21]. A systematic approach may be taken to map and ablate these intermediate ATs [22]. This involves first excluding a macroreentrant tachycardia and then diagnosing a focal arrhythmia from activation and entrainment mapping.

Each component of the stepwise ablation approach provides a cumulative effect toward prolongation of the AF cycle length and eventual AF termination [9,23]. In the study by O'Neill et al., AF termination was achieved during PVI in 11%, electrogram-based ablation in 68% and linear ablation in 21% [16].

Clinical outcomes

In the initial study of 60 patients with persistent AF who underwent ablation utilizing a stepwise approach, AF was successfully terminated in 87% of patients during ablation and maintenance of SR was achieved in 95% of patients with repeat ablation [8]. Termination of AF can be achieved in about 66–90% of patients from the majority of studies with the stepwise approach [8,15–17,19,24]. Patients may represent following the index procedure with recurrent AT (up to 45% in a study), and repeat procedures are required for long-term maintenance of SR [16]. Studies utilizing the stepwise ablation approach have reported freedom from atrial arrhythmias with multiple procedures between 79 and 98% with the use of AADs [8,13,15–17,24–26]. The clinical outcome of studies utilizing stepwise ablation for persistent AF is summarized in Table 1.

Predictors of successful clinical outcome

Several studies have examined factors associated with successful clinical outcome following the stepwise ablation approach. Two of the strongest predictors of mid-to-long-term clinical success are longer baseline AF cycle length and procedural AF termination [17–19,27]. Termination of AF during

the index procedure was associated with patients with shorter duration of persistent AF, longer baseline AF cycle length, and smaller LA dimension [16]. An AF cycle length >142 ms and duration of persistent AF <21 months was predictive of procedural AF termination [28]. Duration of persistent AF was also predictive of clinical outcome, whereby duration of persistent AF >6 months was predictive of arrhythmia recurrences after the index procedure [17]. In another study, in patients with continuous AF duration ≥3 years, the clinical success was comparable regardless of whether AF termination was achieved or not [29].

Other factors associated with poorer clinical outcome include female gender, older age, and the presence of structural heart disease or congestive heart failure [17–19]. A larger LA diameter, the presence of LA spontaneous echocardiographic contrast, and a CHADS2 score of ≥3 have also been shown to be significant predictors of arrhythmic recurrences and poor clinical outcome [30,31]. Recent advancements in magnetic resonance imaging (MRI) techniques have provided a noninvasive method for the quantification and assessment of LA structural remodeling and fibrosis [32]. Delayed enhancement MRI in the LA may predict outcomes following ablation and provides a metric for disease progression in patients with AF [32]. Finally, studies have demonstrated that restoration of sinus rhythm (with either pharmacological or electrical cardioversion) prior to persistent AF ablation is associated with less extensive ablation and similar high clinical success [33].

Cardiac function following stepwise ablation

One consideration with the extent of ablation to achieve SR is whether atrial mechanical function is impaired. Despite extensive ablation, in the initial reported series, 97% of patients had evidence of atrial transport assessed by Doppler echocardiography by 6 months, and all patients in SR demonstrated improved exercise capacity [8]. The effects of stepwise ablation of chronic AF on atrial electrical and mechanical properties were studied by Takahashi et al. in 40 patients after a mean of 4 ± 3 months [24]. Atrial electrical activity in the LA was significantly affected with a wide range of conduction times. However, recovery of LA mechanical function was observed and LA diameter decreased significantly [24]. Utilizing cardiac MRI, reversibility of LA and right atrial dysfunction were demonstrated after 6-month follow-up following ablation and maintenance of SR [34] (Table 2).

Table 1 Clinical outcome of stepwise ablation for persistent and long-standing persistent AF.

Study	Year	No. of patients	Follow-up duration (months)	Acute AF termination rate	Freedom from AF/AT from single procedure	Freedom from AF/AT with multiple procedures	Freedom from AF/AT with multiple procedures and AADs
Haissaguerre et al. [8]	2005	60	11 ± 6	87	–	88	95
Takahashi et al. [24]	2007	40	9 ± 5	90	–	88	98
Rostock et al. [15]	2008	88	20 ± 4	77	38	–	81
O'Neill et al. [16]	2009	153	32 ± 11	85	–	–	89
Matsuo et al. [28]	2009	90	28 ± 4	84	31	84	–
Hocini et al. [13]	2010	148	22 ± 9	86	–	–	87
Rostock et al. [17]	2011	395	27 ± 7	66	27	–	79
Chao et al. [30]	2012	88	37^a	30	28	51	–
Park et al. [19]	2012	140	19 ± 8	68	47	–	–
Sacher et al. [25]	2008	43	18 ± 5	70	–	–	84
Lin et al. [41]	2009	30^b	19 ± 11	47	70	77	83
Bortone et al. [35]	2013	34	26 ± 9	44	65	100^c	–
Li et al. [42]	2008	92	12 ± 11	35	58	–	–
Fiala et al. [26]	2008	135	31 ± 14	83^d; 38^e	–	80^d; 66^e	89^d; 87^e
Ning et al. [43]	2010	86	17 ± 4	85	44	–	–

[a] Median.
[b] Duration of persistent AF.
[c] Group with PVI, linear, and CFE ablation.
[d] $17.6 \pm$ months after the last procedure.
[e] Short-lasting persistent, defined as AF lasting for 7 days to 6 months.
[f] Long-lasting persistent, defined as AF lasting >6 months.

In selected patients with depressed cardiac function and persistent AF unresponsive to DC cardioversion, catheter ablation with the stepwise strategy was shown to improve left ventricular ejection fraction and New York Heart Association class after 3–6 months of SR [35]. In patients with a baseline left ventricular ejection fraction ≤45%, left ventricular ejection fraction was also shown to significantly improve from baseline on follow-up [24]. Levels of ANP and BNP (atrial and brain naturipeptides) also decreased significantly at 3 months with restoration of SR, following stepwise ablation in patients with persistent and long-standing persistent AF [25]. Listed in Table 3 are studies examining atrial and ventricular functions following stepwise ablation.

Atrial tachycardia following stepwise ablation

Patients undergoing stepwise ablation may experience recurrence of atrial tachycardia (AT) after the first procedure, necessitating further procedures. Recurrence with AT is not uncommon after the index procedure and was reported to be as high as 45% in one study [16]. A significant proportion of recurrent arrhythmias in these patients is due to AT rather

Table 2 Cardiac mechanical function poststepwise ablation.

Study	Year	Time of reassessment of cardiac function	Findings
Haissaguerre et al. [8]	2005	6 months	Evidence of atrial transport (mitral A-wave velocity) by Doppler echocardiography. Improved exercise capacity in patients with SR
Sacher et al. [25]	2008	3 months	Decreased LA diameter, improved presence of A waves, improved LVEF
			Decreased ANP and BNP with SR restoration
Takahashi et al. [24]	2010	4 ± 3 months	Atrial electrical conduction diversely affected with wide range of LA conduction times. Decreased LA diameter, recovery of LA mechanical function
			Improvement of LVEF in patients with baseline LVEF ≤45%
Muellerleile et al. [34]	2013	6 months	Reversibility of LA, LA appendage, and RA dysfunction
			Resorption of periatrial edema (cardiac MRI) with SR
Bortone et al. [35]	2013	3–6 months (of SR)	Improved LVEF and NYHA class in selected patients with depressed LVEF and persistent AF with maintenance of SR

Abbreviations: ANP, atrial natriuretic peptide; BNP, brain natriuretic peptide; LVEF, left ventricular ejection fraction; NYHA, New York Heart Association; SR, sinus rhythm.

Table 3 Factors associated with successful clinical outcome for the stepwise ablation approach.

Study	Year	Factors associated with better clinical outcome	Factors associated with poorer clinical outcome
O'Neill et al. [16]	2009	Procedural AF termination	
		Longer AF cycle length	
Drewitz et al. [27]	2010	Longer baseline AF cycle length	
Rostock et al. [17]	2011	Longer baseline AF cycle length	Female gender
		Procedural AF termination	Long duration of persistent AF
			Congestive heart failure
Heist et al. [18]	2012	AF termination by ablation	
		Younger age	
		Male gender	
		Shorter duration of radiofrequency energy	
Rivard et al. [33]	2012	Restoration of sinus rhythm prior to ablation (decreased the extent of ablation with similar clinical success rates)	
Park et al. [19]	2012	AF termination by ablation	Structural heart disease
Chao et al. [30]	2012		CHADS2 score ≥3
			Larger left atrial diameter
Komatsu et al. [29]	2012		Continuous AF duration ≥3 years (clinical success was comparable regardless of whether AF termination was achieved or not)
Hartono et al. [31]	2012		LASEC noted at baseline
Combes et al. [44]	2013	High left atrial appendage flow velocity >0.3 m/s	

Abbreviations: CHADS2 score, congestive heart failure, hypertension, age ≥75 years, diabetes mellitus, and prior stroke or transient ischemic attack (doubled); LASEC, left atrial spontaneous echocardiographic contrast.

than AF. A study observed that patients with AF termination had predominantly ATs as the representing arrhythmia (83%), whereas those without termination mainly represented with recurrent AF (85%) [15]. Studies have documented that the majority of recurrent atrial arrhythmias were due to conduction recovery from previous linear lesions and PVI [8,17,24,30].

Among the recurrent ATs, in about 50% the AT mechanism is macroreentrant. This includes macroreentry around the left atrial roof, the mitral annulus, and the cavotricuspid isthmus [8,15,16,24]. The remaining comprises focal ATs and localized reentry, with a centrifugal activation pattern from a localized area. Focal ATs can originate from sites such as the left atrial appendage, coronary sinus, recovered pulmonary veins, inferior LA, fossa ovalis, or right atrium [8,12,36]. In cases of localized reentry, almost the entire cycle length may be recorded in a localized area of several centimeters. Lozalized reentry may originate from sites such as the left atrial appendage, septum, coronary sinus, or left atrial wall [16,36,37]. Interestingly, these sites were similar to those at which the greatest impact was observed on the atrial fibrillatory process during the initial ablation procedure [8,12]. Furthermore, one study noted that in almost all redo procedures due to AT, at least 1 AT encountered during the repeat procedure had been documented previously [15].

The majority of these recurrent ATs can be successfully ablated with good long-term outcome. Rostock et al. reported 61 out of 320 patients who presented with recurrent ATs following *de novo* ablation for chronic AF. Out of 124 ATs, 93% were successfully ablated. After a mean follow-up of 21 ± 4 months and following a single redo procedure, 82% of these patients were free of any recurrent arrhythmia [36]. The type of arrhythmia recurrence following ablation of persistent AF was shown to predict clinical outcome at the repeat procedure, whereby the occurrence of AT was associated with significantly better outcomes compared to recurrent persistent AF [38]. With the evidence that AF termination is associated with better long-term outcomes and the high success rate of AT ablation, ablating these ATs can be considered as a step toward restoring SR [8,16,36,38].

Current limitations

Current limitations of the stepwise ablation strategy include extensive ablation and long procedure times, recurrent ATs necessitating repeat procedures, the inability to achieve linear conduction block in all patients, and the nonspecificity of CFE in guiding ablation. In the stepwise approach, linear ablation is reserved in the setting of a macroreentrant AT or when isolation of the thoracic veins and ablation of fractionated electrograms fail to terminate AF. Although linear ablation is performed only when necessary, failure to achieve conduction block may result in further recurrence of AT [14]. The mechanism underlying complex fractionated atrial electrograms is multifactorial. The CFE signals can be influenced by local areas of anisotropic or slow conduction, contiguity of different structures, the autonomic nervous system, and the temporal overlap and direction of multiple wave fronts. This may account for the relatively low specificity of CFEs in defining areas of localized sources and drivers in AF.

Newer mapping techniques such as computational mapping with a multielectrode basket catheter and noninvasive mapping facilitate identification of active rotors and focal discharges driving persistent AF [39,40]. The use of these newer technologies may help decrease procedural time and minimize the extent of ablation.

Conclusions

The stepwise approach offers an ablation strategy combining different techniques with high AF termination rates and clinical success for persistent AF. However, the incidence of recurrent ATs after the index procedure is not uncommon and multiple procedures are often required for long-term maintenance of SR. Newer mapping technologies will further facilitate the process of localizing drivers and foci maintaining AF, potentially decreasing the extent of ablation and procedural time.

References

1 Calkins H, Kuck KH, Cappato R, Brugada J, Camm AJ, Chen SA, Crijns HJ, Damiano RJ, Jr., Davies DW, DiMarco J, Edgerton J, Ellenbogen K, Ezekowitz MD, Haines DE, Haissaguerre M, Hindricks G, Iesaka Y, Jackman W, Jalife J, Jais P, Kalman J, Keane D, Kim YH, Kirchhof P, Klein G, Kottkamp H, Kumagai K, Lindsay BD, Mansour M, Marchlinski FE, McCarthy PM, Mont JL, Morady F, Nademanee K, Nakagawa H, Natale A, Nattel S, Packer DL, Pappone C, Prystowsky E, Raviele A, Reddy V, Ruskin JN, Shemin RJ, Tsao HM, Wilber D. Heart Rhythm Society Task Force on C, Surgical Ablation of Atrial F. 2012 HRS/EHRA/ECAS Expert Consensus Statement on Catheter and Surgical Ablation of Atrial Fibrillation: recommendations for patient selection, procedural techniques, patient management and follow-up, definitions, endpoints, and research trial design: a report of the Heart Rhythm Society (HRS)

Task Force on Catheter and Surgical Ablation of Atrial Fibrillation. Developed in partnership with the European Heart Rhythm Association (EHRA), a registered branch of the European Society of Cardiology (ESC) and the European Cardiac Arrhythmia Society (ECAS); and in collaboration with the American College of Cardiology (ACC), American Heart Association (AHA), the Asia Pacific Heart Rhythm Society (APHRS), and the Society of Thoracic Surgeons (STS). Endorsed by the governing bodies of the American College of Cardiology Foundation, the American Heart Association, the European Cardiac Arrhythmia Society, the European Heart Rhythm Association, the Society of Thoracic Surgeons, the Asia Pacific Heart Rhythm Society, and the Heart Rhythm Society. Heart Rhythm. 2012;9:632–696 e621.

2 Brooks AG, Stiles MK, Laborderie J, Lau DH, Kuklik P, Shipp NJ, Hsu LF, Sanders P. Outcomes of long-standing persistent atrial fibrillation ablation: a systematic review. Heart Rhythm. 2010;7:835–846.

3 Nademanee K, McKenzie J, Kosar E, Schwab M, Sunsaneewitayakul B, Vasavakul T, Khunnawat C, Ngarmukos T. A new approach for catheter ablation of atrial fibrillation: mapping of the electrophysiologic substrate. J Am Coll Cardiol. 2004;43:2044–2053.

4 Willems S, Klemm H, Rostock T, Brandstrup B, Ventura R, Steven D, Risius T, Lutomsky B, Meinertz T. Substrate modification combined with pulmonary vein isolation improves outcome of catheter ablation in patients with persistent atrial fibrillation: a prospective randomized comparison. Eur Heart J. 2006;27:2871–2878.

5 Haissaguerre M, Hocini M, Sanders P, Takahashi Y, Rotter M, Sacher F, Rostock T, Hsu LF, Jonsson A, O'Neill MD, Bordachar P, Reuter S, Roudaut R, Clementy J, Jais P. Localized sources maintaining atrial fibrillation organized by prior ablation. Circulation. 2006;113: 616–625.

6 Elayi CS, Verma A, Di Biase L, Ching CK, Patel D, Barrett C, Martin D, Rong B, Fahmy TS, Khaykin Y, Hongo R, Hao S, Pelargonio G, Dello Russo A, Casella M, Santarelli P, Potenza D, Fanelli R, Massaro R, Arruda M, Schweikert RA, Natale A. Ablation for longstanding permanent atrial fibrillation: results from a randomized study comparing three different strategies. Heart Rhythm. 2008;5: 1658–1664.

7 O'Neill MD, Jais P, Hocini M, Sacher F, Klein GJ, Clementy J, Haissaguerre M. Catheter ablation for atrial fibrillation. Circulation. 2007;116:1515–1523.

8 Haissaguerre M, Hocini M, Sanders P, Sacher F, Rotter M, Takahashi Y, Rostock T, Hsu LF, Bordachar P, Reuter S, Roudaut R, Clementy J, Jais P. Catheter ablation of long-lasting persistent atrial fibrillation: clinical outcome and mechanisms of subsequent arrhythmias. J Cardiovasc Electrophysiol. 2005;16:1138–1147.

9 O'Neill MD, Jais P, Takahashi Y, Jonsson A, Sacher F, Hocini M, Sanders P, Rostock T, Rotter M, Pernat A, Clementy J, Haissaguerre M. The stepwise ablation approach for chronic atrial fibrillation: evidence for a cumulative effect. J Interv Card Electrophysiol. 2006;16: 153–167.

10 Verma A, Novak P, Macle L, Whaley B, Beardsall M, Wulffhart Z, Khaykin Y. A prospective, multicenter evaluation of ablating complex fractionated electrograms (CFES) during atrial fibrillation (AF) identified by an automated mapping algorithm: acute effects on AF and efficacy as an adjuvant strategy. Heart Rhythm. 2008;5:198–205.

11 Takahashi Y, O'Neill MD, Hocini M, Dubois R, Matsuo S, Knecht S, Mahapatra S, Lim KT, Jais P, Jonsson A, Sacher F, Sanders P, Rostock T, Bordachar P, Clementy J, Klein GJ, Haissaguerre M. Characterization of electrograms associated with termination of chronic atrial fibrillation by catheter ablation. J Am Coll Cardiol. 2008;51: 1003–1010.

12 Haissaguerre M, Sanders P, Hocini M, Takahashi Y, Rotter M, Sacher F, Rostock T, Hsu LF, Bordachar P, Reuter S, Roudaut R, Clementy J, Jais P. Catheter ablation of long-lasting persistent atrial fibrillation: critical structures for termination. J Cardiovasc Electrophysiol. 2005;16:1125–1137.

13 Hocini M, Nault I, Wright M, Veenhuyzen G, Narayan SM, Jais P, Lim KT, Knecht S, Matsuo S, Forclaz A, Miyazaki S, Jadidi A, O'Neill MD, Sacher F, Clementy J, Haissaguerre M. Disparate evolution of right and left atrial rate during ablation of long-lasting persistent atrial fibrillation. J Am Coll Cardiol. 2010;55:1007–1016.

14 Knecht S, Hocini M, Wright M, Lellouche N, O'Neill MD, Matsuo S, Nault I, Chauhan VS, Makati KJ, Bevilacqua M, Lim KT, Sacher F, Deplagne A, Derval N, Bordachar P, Jais P, Clementy J, Haissaguerre M. Left atrial linear lesions are required for successful treatment of persistent atrial fibrillation. Eur Heart J. 2008;29:2359–2366.

15 Rostock T, Steven D, Hoffmann B, Servatius H, Drewitz I, Sydow K, Mullerleile K, Ventura R, Wegscheider K, Meinertz T, Willems S. Chronic atrial fibrillation is a biatrial arrhythmia: data from catheter ablation of chronic atrial fibrillation aiming arrhythmia termination using a sequential ablation approach. Circ Arrhythmia Electrophysiol. 2008;1:344–353.

16 O'Neill MD, Wright M, Knecht S, Jais P, Hocini M, Takahashi Y, Jonsson A, Sacher F, Matsuo S, Lim KT, Arantes L, Derval N, Lellouche N, Nault I, Bordachar P, Clementy J, Haissaguerre M. Long-term follow-up of persistent atrial fibrillation ablation using termination as a procedural endpoint. Eur Heart J. 2009;30: 1105–1112.

17 Rostock T, Salukhe TV, Steven D, Drewitz I, Hoffmann BA, Bock K, Servatius H, Mullerleile K, Sultan A, Gosau N, Meinertz T, Wegscheider K, Willems S. Long-term single- and multiple-procedure outcome and predictors of success after catheter ablation for persistent atrial fibrillation. Heart Rhythm. 2011;8:1391–1397.

18 Heist EK, Chalhoub F, Barrett C, Danik S, Ruskin JN, Mansour M. Predictors of atrial fibrillation termination and clinical success of catheter ablation of persistent atrial fibrillation. Am J Cardiol. 2012;110:545–551.

19 Park YM, Choi JI, Lim HE, Park SW, Kim YH. Is pursuit of termination of atrial fibrillation during catheter ablation of great value in patients with longstanding

persistent atrial fibrillation? J Cardiovasc Electrophysiol. 2012;23:1051–1058.

20 Ammar S, Hessling G, Reents T, Paulik M, Fichtner S, Schon P, Dillier R, Kathan S, Jilek C, Kolb C, Haller B, Deisenhofer I. Importance of sinus rhythm as endpoint of persistent atrial fibrillation ablation. J Cardiovasc Electrophysiol. 2013;24:388–395.

21 Zhou G, Chen S, Chen G, Zhang F, Meng W, Yan Y, Lu X, Wei Y, Liu S. Procedural arrhythmia termination and long-term single-procedure clinical outcome in patients with non-paroxysmal atrial fibrillation. J Cardiovasc Electrophysiol. 2013.

22 Jais P, Matsuo S, Knecht S, Weerasooriya R, Hocini M, Sacher F, Wright M, Nault I, Lellouche N, Klein G, Clementy J, Haissaguerre M. A deductive mapping strategy for atrial tachycardia following atrial fibrillation ablation: importance of localized reentry. J Cardiovasc Electrophysiol. 2009;20:480–491.

23 Haissaguerre M, Sanders P, Hocini M, Hsu LF, Shah DC, Scavee C, Takahashi Y, Rotter M, Pasquie JL, Garrigue S, Clementy J, Jais P. Changes in atrial fibrillation cycle length and inducibility during catheter ablation and their relation to outcome. Circulation. 2004;109:3007–3013.

24 Takahashi Y, O'Neill MD, Hocini M, Reant P, Jonsson A, Jais P, Sanders P, Rostock T, Rotter M, Sacher F, Laffite S, Roudaut R, Clementy J, Haissaguerre M. Effects of stepwise ablation of chronic atrial fibrillation on atrial electrical and mechanical properties. J Am Coll Cardiol.. 2007;49:1306–1314.

25 Sacher F, Corcuff JB, Schraub P, Le Bouffos V, Georges A, Jones SO, Lafitte S, Bordachar P, Hocini M, Clementy J, Haissaguerre M, Bordenave L, Roudaut R, Jais P. Chronic atrial fibrillation ablation impact on endocrine and mechanical cardiac functions. Eur Heart J. 2008;29:1290–1295.

26 Fiala M, Chovancik J, Nevralova R, Neuwirth R, Jiravsky O, Januska J, Branny M. Termination of long-lasting persistent versus short-lasting persistent and paroxysmal atrial fibrillation by ablation. Pacing Clin Electrophysiol. 2008;31:985–997.

27 Drewitz I, Willems S, Salukhe TV, Steven D, Hoffmann BA, Servatius H, Bock K, Aydin MA, Wegscheider K, Meinertz T, Rostock T. Atrial fibrillation cycle length is a sole independent predictor of a substrate for consecutive arrhythmias in patients with persistent atrial fibrillation. Circ Arrhythmia Electrophysiol. 2010;3:351–360.

28 Matsuo S, Lellouche N, Wright M, Bevilacqua M, Knecht S, Nault I, Lim KT, Arantes L, O'Neill MD, Platonov PG, Carlson J, Sacher F, Hocini M, Jais P, Haissaguerre M. Clinical predictors of termination and clinical outcome of catheter ablation for persistent atrial fibrillation. J Am Coll Cardiol. 2009;54:788–795.

29 Komatsu Y, Taniguchi H, Miyazaki S, Nakamura H, Kusa S, Uchiyama T, Kakita K, Kakuta T, Hachiya H, Iesaka Y. Impact of atrial fibrillation termination on clinical outcome after ablation in relation to the duration of persistent atrial fibrillation. Pacing Clin Electrophysiol. 2012;35:1436–1443.

30 Chao TF, Tsao HM, Lin YJ, Tsai CF, Lin WS, Chang SL, Lo LW, Hu YF, Tuan TC, Suenari K, Li CH, Hartono B, Chang HY, Ambrose K, Wu TJ, Chen SA. Clinical outcome of catheter ablation in patients with nonparoxysmal atrial fibrillation: results of 3-year follow-up. Circ Arrhythmia Electrophysiol. 2012;5:514–520.

31 Hartono B, Lo LW, Cheng CC, Lin YJ, Chang SL, Hu YF, Suenari K, Li CH, Chao TF, Liu SH, Niu YL, Chang HY, Ambrose K, Yu WC, Hsu TL, Chen SA. A novel finding of the atrial substrate properties and long-term results of catheter ablation in chronic atrial fibrillation patients with left atrial spontaneous echo contrast. J Cardiovasc Electrophysiol. 2012;23:239–246.

32 Oakes RS, Badger TJ, Kholmovski EG, Akoum N, Burgon NS, Fish EN, Blauer JJ, Rao SN, DiBella EV, Segerson NM, Daccarett M, Windfelder J, McGann CJ, Parker D, MacLeod RS, Marrouche NF. Detection and quantification of left atrial structural remodeling with delayed-enhancement magnetic resonance imaging in patients with atrial fibrillation. Circulation. 2009;119:1758–1767.

33 Rivard L, Hocini M, Rostock T, Cauchemez B, Forclaz A, Jadidi AS, Linton N, Nault I, Miyazaki S, Liu X, Xhaet O, Shah A, Sacher F, Derval N, Jais P, Khairy P, Macle L, Nattel S, Willems S, Haissaguerre M. Improved outcome following restoration of sinus rhythm prior to catheter ablation of persistent atrial fibrillation: a comparative multicenter study. Heart Rhythm. 2012;9:1025–1030.

34 Muellerleile K, Groth M, Steven D, Hoffmann BA, Saring D, Radunski UK, Lund GK, Adam G, Rostock T, Willems S. Cardiovascular magnetic resonance demonstrates reversible atrial dysfunction after catheter ablation of persistent atrial fibrillation. J Cardiovasc Electrophysiol. 2013.

35 Bortone A, Pujadas-Berthault P, Karam N, Maupas E, Boulenc JM, Rioux P, Durrleman N, Ciobotaru V, Marijon E. Catheter ablation in selected patients with depressed left ventricular ejection fraction and persistent atrial fibrillation unresponsive to current cardioversion. Europace. 2013.

36 Rostock T, Drewitz I, Steven D, Hoffmann BA, Salukhe TV, Bock K, Servatius H, Aydin MA, Meinertz T, Willems S. Characterization, mapping, and catheter ablation of recurrent atrial tachycardias after stepwise ablation of long-lasting persistent atrial fibrillation. Circ Arrhythmia Electrophysiol. 2010;3:160–169.

37 Hocini M, Shah AJ, Nault I, Sanders P, Wright M, Narayan SM, Takahashi Y, Jais P, Matsuo S, Knecht S, Sacher F, Lim KT, Clementy J, Haissaguerre M. Localized reentry within the left atrial appendage: arrhythmogenic role in patients undergoing ablation of persistent atrial fibrillation. Heart Rhythm Soc. 2011;8:1853–1861.

38 Ammar S, Hessling G, Reents T, Fichtner S, Wu J, Zhu P, Kathan S, Estner HL, Jilek C, Kolb C, Haller B, Deisenhofer I. Arrhythmia type after persistent atrial fibrillation ablation predicts success of the repeat procedure. Circ Arrhythmia Electrophysiol. 2011;4:609–614.

39 Narayan SM, Krummen DE, Rappel WJ. Clinical mapping approach to diagnose electrical rotors and focal

impulse sources for human atrial fibrillation. J Cardiovasc Electrophysiol. 2012;23:447–454.

40 Haissaguerre M, Hocini M, Shah AJ, Derval N, Sacher F, Jais P, Dubois R. Noninvasive panoramic mapping of human atrial fibrillation mechanisms: A feasibility report. J Cardiovasc Electrophysiol. 2013;24:711–717.

41 Lin YJ, Tai CT, Chang SL, Lo LW, Tuan TC, Wongchar-oen W, Udyavar AR, Hu YF, Chang CJ, Tsai WC, Kao T, Higa S, Chen SA. Efficacy of additional ablation of complex fractionated atrial electrograms for catheter ablation of nonparoxysmal atrial fibrillation. J Cardiovasc Electrophysiol. 2009;20:607–615.

42 Li XP, Dong JZ, Liu XP, Long de Y, Yu RH, Tian Y, Tang RB, Zheng B, Hu FL, Shi LS, He H, Ma CS. Predictive value of early recurrence and delayed cure after catheter ablation for patients with chronic atrial fibrillation. Circulation. 2008;72:1125–1129.

43 Ning M, Dong JZ, Liu XP, Yu RH, Long DY, Tang RB, Sang CH, Ma CS. Mechanisms of organized atrial tachycardia during catheter ablation of chronic atrial fibrillation by stepwise approach. Chin Med J. 2010;123:852–856.

44 Combes S, Jacob S, Combes N, Karam N, Chaumeil A, Guy-Moyat B, Treguer F, Deplagne A, Boveda S, Marijon E, Albenque JP. Predicting favourable outcomes in the setting of radiofrequency catheter ablation of long-standing persistent atrial fibrillation: a pilot study assessing the value of left atrial appendage peak flow velocity. Arch Cardiovasc Dis. 2013;106:36–43.

CHAPTER 21

Limited ablation for persistent atrial fibrillation using preprocedure reverse remodeling

David J. Slotwiner[1] & Jonathan S. Steinberg[2]

[1]Department of Medicine and School of Health Policy and Research, Weill Cornell Medical College, New York, NY

[2]Arrhythmia Institute, The Valley Health System University of Rochester School of Medicine & Dentistry New York, NY and Ridgewood, NJ, USA

Background

Pulmonary vein isolation (PVI) has been demonstrated to be a highly effective treatment option for patients with paroxysmal atrial fibrillation (AF), but less effective for patients with persistent AF. The lower efficacy of PVI alone has been attributed to adverse atrial electrical and structural remodeling in the setting of AF.

Strategies to improve efficacy of catheter ablation for persistent AF alter these pathophysiological characteristics of atrial tissue remodeling. These techniques largely depend upon creation of linear lesions, ablation of complex fractionated electrograms (CFAEs), ablation of autonomic ganglia, and/or mapping of rotors that drive persistent AF.

Based upon the known physiology of electrical remodeling and evidence that it can be reversed by restoration of sinus rhythm (SR), two studies have revealed that pretreatment of patients with persistent AF with antiarrhythmic drug therapy (AAD) can be utilized to improve the efficacy of PVI alone for patients with persistent AF. This strategy provides the advantage of a shorter ablation procedure, lower risks of time-dependent intraprocedural complications, fewer ablation lesions, and less possibility of

Practical Guide to Catheter Ablation of Atrial Fibrillation, Second Edition. Edited by Jonathan S. Steinberg, Pierre Jaïs and Hugh Calkins.
© 2016 John Wiley & Sons, Ltd. Published 2016 by John Wiley & Sons, Ltd.

postablation atrial tachycardias that result from incomplete linear ablation lesions.

This chapter will review atrial remodeling observed with AF and evidence that the electrical component of remodeling is reversible by restoration of sinus rhythm, and we will discuss how this physiologic property of atrial tissue can be used to reduce the amount of atrial tissue that needs to be ablated to successfully treat patients with persistent AF. Finally, the relative advantages and limitations of this technique will be compared with other ablation strategies for treatment of patients with persistent AF.

Electrical remodeling

Evidence supporting atrial remodeling

The term atrial remodeling is used to describe the physiological changes of atrial tissue observed in persistent AF. The concept was first introduced in 1995 simultaneously by Wijffels et al. [1] and Morillo et al. [2] who demonstrated that once sustained AF was induced in goats, or rapid atrial pacing was performed in dogs, physiological changes occurred that favored the maintenance of AF [3]. This has led to the concept that "AF begets AF."

Atrial tissue remodeling is characterized by the following structural, electrical, and mechanical changes:

1 Structural remodeling: Rapid atrial pacing models used to simulate AF in animals consistently result in biatrial enlargement. This correlates with humans, in whom the burden and duration of AF has been

correlated with left atrial volume. Interstitial fibrosis, which usually accompanies atrial enlargement, has been demonstrated in humans to be an independent predictor of AF ablation success [4]. While chamber enlargement may be an adaptive response of the heart to reduced contractility, the end result is increased atrial size, the ability of the atria to accommodate reentrant circuits, and an increase in AF burden.

2 Electrical remodeling: Several aspects of the cellular and ion channel function changes that occur during persistent AF have been defined. These include:

a Reduced inward I_{CaL} by up to 70%, reducing action potential duration (APD) and effective refractory period (ERP) [5,6].

b Downregulation of I_{CaL} occurs to prevent Ca^{2+} overload during rapid atrial rates [7].

c Upregulation of acetylcholine-dependent potassium current (I_{KACh}) that may contribute to shortening of the atrial ERP.

d Dysregulated connexin function, which plays an important role in electrical propagation, during persistent AF [3,8].

The rapid rates of atrial fibrillation induce shortening of both the atrial ERP and APD [2]. Shortening of the ERP has been attributed to downregulation of the L-type Ca^{2+} current (I_{CaL}) caused by Ca^{2+} accumulation within atrial myocytes [3,7]. Spatial heterogeneity of ERP and conduction velocity also contribute to the proarrhythmic electrical changes observed in AF [9]. The effects of atrial remodeling have been correlated with measurement of the P-wave duration on surface ECG recordings [10,11]. The shortened ERP reduces the wavelength of atrial impulses that promotes wavebreak and multiple wavelet reentry.

3 Mechanical remodeling: The structural and electrical changes of atrial tissue observed in chronic AF result in up to 75% reduction in contractile force of the right atrial appendage [12,13].

Together, the effect of structural, mechanical, and electrical remodeling increases the frequency of ectopic and reentrant arrhythmias and provides atrial tissue substrate that favors sustained reentrant arrhythmias [7,14].

Evidence for reverse remodeling
The electrical components of atrial remodeling have been demonstrated to be reversible. Soon after studies revealed that AF begets AF, a study from Wijffels et al. recorded complete recovery of atrial ERP a week after cardioversion (goat model, AF duration 24 h prior to cardioversion) [1,15].

Surface ECG measurements of P-wave duration, including the maximum P-wave duration, P-wave dispersion, and high-resolution signal-averaged P wave (SAPW) have proven to be accurate noninvasive measures of atrial electrical remodeling [10,11,16–19].

Several studies have demonstrated that reverse electrical remodeling occurs in humans once sinus rhythm is restored. Using SAPW postcardioversion, two studies revealed significant reduction in SAPW duration at 1 and 3 months postcardioversion, but no reduction for patients who experienced recurrent AF [16,20]. Another study demonstrated that patients who maintain sinus rhythm 6 months postcardioversion have shorter P-wave duration compared to those with AF recurrence [21]. Two studies evaluated invasive measures of electrical remodeling (ERP) 4 days and 1 week postcardioversion [22,23]. The studies revealed significant decreased duration of SAPW, and prolongation of atrial ERP, elegantly proving both the physiological phenomenon of atrial electrical reverse-remodeling and the fact that surface P-wave characteristics can be used as a noninvasive measure of atrial electrical remodeling. While the precise duration of time in sinus rhythm required for complete electrical remodeling to occur has not been defined, several studies have indicated that 3 months is probably sufficient [16,23–27].

Evidence supporting preprocedure atrial remodeling

Based upon the physiologic ability to promote reverse atrial electrical remodeling by restoring sinus rhythm, we and others have hypothesized that successful atrial remodeling by either cardioversion alone or with the assistance of temporary AAD therapy would facilitate the performance of PVI as the primary ablation strategy for patients with persistent AF [28,29].

Clinical study using preablation antiarrhythmic drug therapy
One study focused on consecutive patients with symptomatic, drug-refractory, persistent AF. To be included, patients had to be (1) in a persistent pattern of AF (≥ 7 days and ≤ 1 year) despite prior efforts at control using at least one class I or class III AAD and (2) be free of contraindications to use dofetilide. Patients underwent pretreatment with dofetilide 3 months prior to ablation (with electrical cardioversion after six doses if required), and the drug was continued 1–3 months post-PVI ablation. Electrical remodeling was evaluated by measuring P-wave duration immediately postelectrical cardioversion, and again at the time of presentation for PVI. If AF had recurred by the

time the patient presented for ablation, P-wave duration was measured immediately after cardioversion to normal sinus rhythm. P-wave duration was measured in limb lead II, with ECGs in random order, by an observer blinded to the clinical outcome. The difference in P-wave duration (ΔP) between the ECG at the time of cardioversion and at the time of PVI was used as a measure of reverse remodeling.

The technique used for pulmonary vein catheter ablation isolation is described in detail in the original manuscript [28]. Briefly, real-time three-dimensional left atrial maps were constructed using a nonfluoroscopic navigation system (Carto, Biosense-Webster Inc., Diamond Bar CA, USA). A 20-pole catheter with distal ring configuration (LASSO Catheter; Biosense-Webster) was positioned within the ostium of each PV. Radiofrequency catheter ablation was performed until all left atrial pulmonary vein connections were severed, as verified by the circumferential mapping catheter. All pulmonary vein connections were severed in each study patient. No patient underwent non-PV ablation including linear lesions or targeting of CFAEs.

A control cohort of patients with symptomatic, paroxysmal AF who were referred for ablation and did not have prior pretreatment of AF with AAD functioned as a control group for comparison purposes. P-wave durations at comparable points in time preablation and at ablation were recorded. The treated persistent AF group was largely converted by AAD with dofetilide to paroxysmal AF. The control group was matched for age, gender, duration of AF, concomitant cardiovascular conditions, left atrial size and left ventricular function. Paroxysmal AF was defined as lasting less than 7 days in duration and terminating spontaneously. Control patients underwent identical ablation protocol. A sinus rhythm ECG recorded 3 months prior to ablation was compared with that recorded at ablation.

Patients were seen at 1, 3, 6, and 12 months or more frequently following PVI to assess for recurrence of AF. AF burden was evaluated using patient symptoms, 12-lead ECG, 24 h Holter monitoring, and mobile cardiac outpatient telemetry. Specifically, after hospital discharge, each patient underwent a minimum of 4 weeks of mobile outpatient telemetry. At each office visit an ECG was recorded and an extended autotrigger transtelephonic monitor and/or 24–48 h Holter recording was performed as needed to document asymptomatic AF episodes or to clarify symptoms. Antiarrhythmic drug treatment was discontinued 3 months postablation when complete freedom of AF was achieved.

Seventy-one consecutive patients with persistent AF were included. The median duration of the persistent AF episodes was 6 months. Overall, the group had mild LA dilatation and preserved left ventricular function. A median of 1 AAD had been ineffective in preventing recurrences of AF before initiation of dofetilide and the ablation procedure. Of the 71 study patients, 15% required an early second PVI procedure. ECG analysis of the P-wave duration was performed on all patients at a median of 85 days prior to PVI and again at the time of PVI. Baseline characteristics for the 35 patients in the control cohort were not significantly different from the study group.

Efficacy of dofetilide

All 71 patients in the treatment group tolerated AAD therapy with dofetilide (768 ± 291 mcg/day) preablation for a median of 85 days. During dofetilide initiation, all patients were converted to sinus rhythm. Sixty-nine (97%) successfully transformed from persistent AF to paroxysmal AF (56 patients, 81%) or the AF was completely suppressed (13 patients, 19%). The remaining two patients (3%) remained in persistent AF.

Response to PVI

All patients in both the treatment and the control groups underwent successful catheter ablation isolation of all pulmonary vein connections. In the study patients with persistent AF, 76% were completely free of AF recurrence on no drug therapy at 6 months post-PVI, while 70% were completely free of AF at 12 months post-PVI (responders). At 6 and 12 months, 24% and 30%, respectively, continued to have AF and required continued medical therapy or repeat ablation (nonresponders).

Among the control patients with paroxysmal AF, 80% had complete response to PVI at 6 months and 75% at 12 months. There was no significant difference in the 6-and 12-month PVI response in the study group versus the control group (Figure 1). During the postablation period, there was a single case of sustained left-sided atrial tachycardia, which occurred in the control paroxysmal AF group.

Of the 13 patients whose AF was completely suppressed with dofetilide pretreatment, 12 (92%) had complete response to PVI at 6 months. Neither of the two patients who remained in persistent AF despite dofetilide pretreatment responded to PVI. Seventy-five percent of the patients with persistent AF who responded to pretreatment with dofetilide responded to PVI at 6 months.

Change in P-wave duration

P-wave duration at baseline was significantly longer in the persistent AF group compared with the

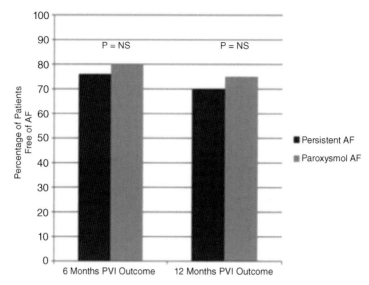

Figure 1 Six and twelve-month outcome postpulmonary vein isolation. Patients with persistent atrial fibrillation were pretreated with dofetilide and then underwent pulmonary vein isolation had a similar outcome at 6 and 12 months as patients with paroxysmal AF (76% versus 80% and 70% versus 75%, respectively; P=NS). AF, atrial fibrillation; PVI, pulmonary vein isolation. *Source:* Khan et al., 2011 [28]. Reproduced with permission of Wiley.

paroxysmal AF group ($p < 0.001$). Patients in the treatment group with persistent AF treated with dofetilide demonstrated a statistically significant reduction in the mean P-wave duration by the time they returned for PVI 3 months later (Figure 2). In contrast, the cohort patients with paroxysmal AF who were not treated with AAD during the 3 months prior to PVI experienced no significant change in P-wave duration (Figure 2). Patients with persistent AF who responded to PVI after pretreatment with dofetilide had a significantly greater

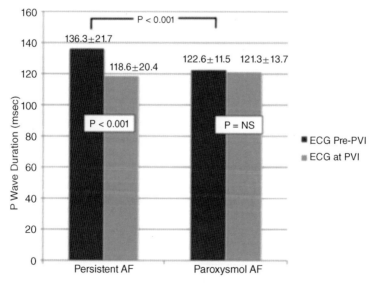

Figure 2 Comparison of P-wave duration changes over time in study and control patients. In patients with persistent AF, dofetilide treatment was associated with a significant reduction in P-wave duration; in contrast, the P-wave duration remained unchanged in control patients with paroxysmal AF. At baseline, the P-wave duration was significantly longer in the study group compared to the control group. AF, atrial fibrillation; PVI, pulmonary vein isolation. *Source:* Khan et al., 2011 [28]. Reproduced with permission of Wiley.

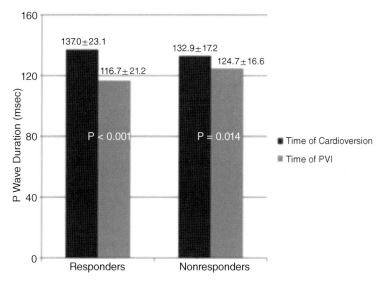

Figure 3 Comparison of change in P-wave duration between responders and nonresponders. In patients with persistent atrial fibrillation, dofetilide therapy was associated with a significant reduction in P-wave duration in both responders and nonresponders. PVI, pulmonary vein isolation. *Source:* Khan et al., 2011 [28]. Reproduced with permission of Wiley.

decrease in P-wave duration in response to dofetilide (137.0 ± 23.1 to 116.7 ± 21.2 ms (20.3 ± 16.9 ms or 15% decrease), $P < 0.001$) compared to nonresponders (132.9 ± 17.2 ms to 124.7 ± 16.6 ms (8.2 ± 12.4 ms or 6% decrease), $P = 0.014$) (Figures 3 and 4).

Predictors of freedom from recurrent atrial fibrillation following ablation

Age, gender, hypertension, left atrial size, duration of persistent AF episodes, duration of AF history, dose of dofetilide, and clinical response (suppression versus

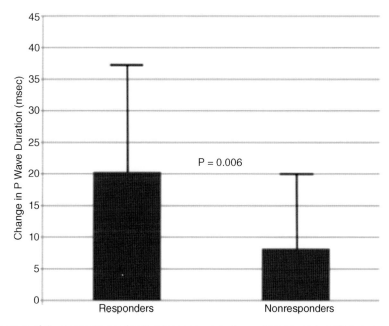

Figure 4 Comparison of changes in P-wave duration between responders and nonresponders. Clinical response was assessed following pulmonary vein isolation in patients with persistent atrial fibrillation who were treated with dofetilide. Responders demonstrated a significantly greater decrease in P-wave duration compared to nonresponders (20.3 ± 16.9 ms versus 8.2 ± 12.4 ms; $P = 0.006$). *Source:* Khan et al., 2011 [28]. Reproduced with permission of Wiley.

paroxysmal AF) to dofetilide all failed to predict a complete clinical response to PVI. A decrease in P-wave duration was the only significant predictor of clinical response to PVI (HR = 0.94; CI = 0.90–0.98; $P = 0.009$ on univariate analysis. For each decrease in P-wave duration of 1 ms from baseline to ablation, there was a 6% increase in the likelihood of a complete response to PVI. Similarly, on multivariate analysis a decrease in P-wave duration was again the only significant predictor of clinical response to PVI (HR = 0.092; CI = 0.86–0.98; $P = 0.007$).

Clinical study using cardioversion preablation

A similar study, based upon the same hypothesis of reverse atrial electrical remodeling as a potential tool to limit the extent of catheter ablation required for successful treatment of persistent AF, was published by Rivard et al. in 2012 [29].

This two-group cohort study was conducted from 2007 through 2009 and included patients undergoing a first catheter ablation procedure for persistent and long-standing persistent AF. The study group consisted of 40 consecutive patients from 3 European centers who underwent electrical cardioversion 1 month prior to ablation. Patients who did not remain in sinus rhythm were excluded from the study, and all patients were required to have LA diameters ≤55 mm. These patients were retrospectively matched 1:1 with contemporary controls (matched for age, gender, and duration of AF) with persistent AF in whom no attempt to restore sinus rhythm was made prior to ablation.

Radiofrequency catheter ablation was performed 1 month after cardioversion (for the study group), and after 4 weeks of therapeutic anticoagulation for both study arms. Antiarrhythmic drug therapy was discontinued five half-lives before the ablation procedure, with the exception of amiodarone. Ablation was performed during AF in all patients according to a sequential stepwise approach previously described in detail [30]. AF was induced by burst atrial pacing for patients who presented in sinus rhythm due to previous cardioversion. Briefly, left atrial antral PVI was performed using a 3.5-mm irrigated tip catheter (ThermoCool, Diamond Bar, CA) and guided by a circular mapping catheter (LASSO; Biosense Webster, Inc, Diamond Bar, CA). Next, electrogram-based ablation was performed at right atrial and/or LA sites demonstrating features of continuous electrical activity, complex rapid and fractionated electrograms, and a gradient of activation. If AF persisted after this step, linear ablation lesions were created across the LA roof between the superior PVs and then from the left inferior PV to the mitral annulus. The end point was termination of AF during ablation. However, if AF persisted beyond these ablation lesions, electrical cardioversion was performed.

Patients were evaluated at 1, 3, 6, and 12 months postablation with 48 h Holter monitoring performed at each visit. Success was defined as the absence of AF or atrial tachycardia lasting 30 s or longer off antiarrhythmic drug therapy.

Eighty patients were included in the study (forty in each arm). Both groups were similar with the exception of a slightly lower ejection fraction among patients in the control arm (63.9 ± 11.7 versus 55.7 ± 14.9; $P < 0.05$).

AF cycle length was greater among patients who presented for ablation in sinus rhythm (i.e., induced AF in the treatment arm). Termination of AF occurred more frequently during ablation of patients in the treatment arm, with less extensive application of ablation and with less fluoroscopic exposure (Table 1).

Table 1 Characteristics of the first procedure.

	SR group (n = 40)	Control group (n = 40)	P
Amiodarone within the preceding 3 months, n (%)	17 (42.5)	19 (47.5)	.59
Atrial fibrillation cycle length (ms), mean ± SD	183 ± 32	166 ± 20	.06
Procedural duration (min), mean ± SD	199.8 ± 69.8	283.5 ± 72.3	***
Fluoroscopy time (min), mean ± SD	51.0 ± 24.9	96.3 ± 32.1	***
Radiofrequency duration (min), mean ± SD	47.5 ± 18.9	97.0 ± 30.6	***
Left line, n (%)	17 (42.5)	33 (82.5)	***
Roof line, n (%)	14 (35.0)	33 (82.5)	***
Mitral line, n (%)	7 (17.5)	30 (75.0)	***
CFAE ablation, n (%)	16 (40.0)	35 (87.5)	***
Ablation in the coronary sinus, n (%)	5 (12.5)	28 (70.0)	***
Termination of AF by ablation, n (%)	38 (95.0)	31 (77.5)	*

Source: Rivard et al., 2012 [29]. Reproduced with permission of Elsevier.
Abbreviations: AF, atrial fibrillation; CFAE, complex fractionated atrial electrogram; SD, standard deviation; SR, sinus rhythm.
*$P < 0.05$; ***$P < 0.001$.

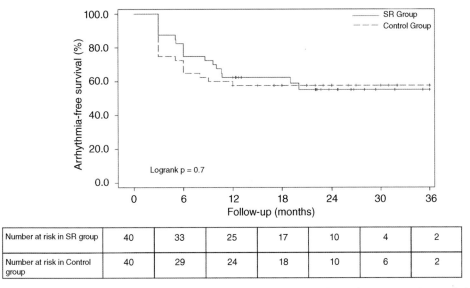

Figure 5 Arrhythmia-free survival after a single catheter ablation intervention. Kaplan–Meier recurrence-free survival rates are shown for patients having undergone a single catheter ablation procedure in the sinus rhythm and control groups.

Clinical success without the use of antiarrhythmic drug therapy was similar in both groups up to 36 months following ablation (Figure 5). The need for repeat ablation was similar in both groups, and after the last procedure success rates off antiarrhythmic drug therapy were 80% in the treatment arm versus 70% in the control group ($P = 0.47$).

The authors concluded that cardioversion and maintenance of sinus rhythm 1 month prior to ablation decreased the extent of ablation required to restore and maintain sinus rhythm without compromising efficacy.

Discussion

Together, these studies confirm that (1) electrical remodeling plays a role in the maintenance of persistent AF, (2) restoration of sinus rhythm allows electrical remodeling to occur, (3) electrical modeling is a time-dependent phenomenon, and (4) catheter ablation for patients with persistent AF may at least be less complicated if electrical remodeling is allowed to occur first, and it may even be more effective. The reduction in fluoroscopy exposure and procedure duration are also advantageous.

The physiological evidence for reverse remodeling is demonstrated by the shortening of the P-wave duration and the longer AF cycle length among patients converted first to sinus rhythm. One potential explanation for the difference between these studies is the difference in the duration of sinus rhythm prior to

AF ablation. It is possible that 1 month is insufficient time to allow for full electrical remodeling. Whether 3 months is adequate remains unanswered.

Limitations

Both studies presented are nonrandomized and relatively small. It is possible that by identifying patients who could remain in sinus rhythm (with dofetilide or after cardioversion alone), a cohort of patients more likely to respond favorably to ablation was selected [31]. A larger, multicenter trial is needed to confirm these findings and the long-term benefits of this approach. And finally, a randomized clinical trial is needed to definitively establish the value of the clinical strategy described in these manuscripts with alternative ablation techniques for persistent AF.

Selecting ablation strategies for persistent AF

Several catheter ablation techniques have been developed to treat persistent or long-standing persistent AF for symptomatic patients who have failed or are unable to take antiarrhythmic drug therapy. Pulmonary vein isolation remains the cornerstone for all of these strategies, isolating the most common source of triggers of AF. Additional lesions sets are then created to target known physiological conditions that favor continued propagation of chaotic reentrant wavelets.

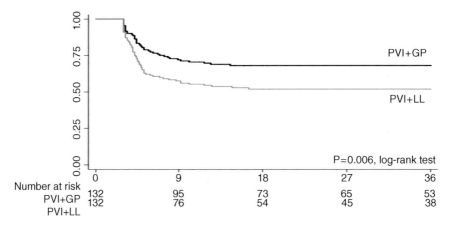

Figure 6 The long-term overall success rate including repeat ablation procedure, if needed. GP, ganglionated plexus; LL, linear lesion; PVI, pulmonary vein isolation. *Source:* Pokushalov et al., 2013 [36]. Reproduced with permission of Elsevier.

Linear lesions

Among the more common techniques employed for ablation of persistent AF is the creation of linear ablation lesions. A combination of a left atrial roof line, posterior wall line, and mitral isthmus line reduces the area of atrial substrate required to support the reentrant wave fronts of AF and thereby increase the efficacy of catheter ablation above PVI alone. Results from the surgical MAZE procedure have demonstrated that this concept, when executed with consistent, transmural lesions, is valid and highly effective. Results from the electrophysiology laboratory have been limited by the technical challenges of achieving long-lasting transmural bidirectional conduction block particularly across the mitral isthmus, and the subsequent occurrence of proarrhythmic left atrial flutters.

Autonomic ganglia

Cellular electrophysiological properties of left atrial tissue are profoundly influenced by autonomic ganglionated plexi (GP) located in epicardial fat pads and the ligament of Marshall [32]. These GP contain afferent neurons from the atrial myocardium and central autonomic nervous system, efferent cholinergic and adrenergic neurons, and interconnecting neurons between GPs. The initiation and maintenance of AF is enhanced by parasympathetic stimulation (which markedly shortens the atrial and pulmonary vein myocardium refractory periods) and sympathetic stimulation (intracellular calcium loading resulting in delayed after depolarizations and abnormal triggered activity from the pulmonary vein myocardium) [33]. The addition of GP ablation to PVI has been demonstrated to increase AF-free survival in patients with paroxysmal as well as long-standing persistent AF without conferring the risk of proarrhythmic left atrial flutters commonly associated with linear ablation lesions [34–36]. Our experience (single center, prospective randomized controlled trial) indicated that for patients with persistent or long-standing persistent AF, PVI + GP ablation conferred significantly superior outcomes over a PVI + linear lesion approach (Figure 6) [36].

Complex fractionated atrial electrograms

The pathophysiology of atrial triggers as initiatorsl of atrial fibrillation has been well defined, with pulmonary vein muscle sleeves known to be the most common but not the exclusive origin. Reentrant propagation of wavelets around structural and functionally refractory barriers allows AF to sustain, assisted by the electrical and structural remodeling discussed earlier in this chapter. Given the limited success of catheter ablation techniques to treat persistent AF by preventing triggers alone, identification and ablation of the reentrant wavelets driving sustained AF has attracted great attention. Complex fractionated atrial electrograms (CFAE), low-voltage signals with fractionated electrograms with continuous deflections and/or very short cycle lengths ($\leq$120 ms) appear to represent a complex interplay between the epicardial GP and the atrial tissue and they may represent critical pivot points or rotors that are responsible for the maintenance of AF [2,37]. These sites also appear to represent regions of hyperactive autonomic activity within the LA [38]. Catheter ablation targeting CFAE have been shown to slow AF, often resulting in regularization of the reentrant circuit and/or termination of AF. These acute changes have been correlated with long-term freedom from AF recurrence [39,40]. CFAE ablation has become an established component of catheter ablation protocols at many centers for patients with paroxysmal or persistent AF refractory to pulmonary vein isolation alone. A prospective, multicenter, randomized trial (Selective CFAE Targeting for Atrial Fibrillation Study (SELECT AF)) is underway to better define the techniques and efficacy of this approach for treatment of patients with persistent AF [40].

Rotor Mapping & Ablation

There are two prevailing hypotheses describing how AF sustains once an ectopic trigger beat emanates from the pulmonary veins or other site starts the process. The multiwavelet hypothesis proposes that continuously meandering electoral waves cause AF [41]. An alternative explanation based upon experimental models proposes that local organized reentrant circuits (rotors) or focal impulse generators drive AF [42]. Electrical wavelets of AF appear disorganized unless the central driving rotor is identified. Narayan and colleagues have developed algorithms to create computational AF maps obtained by recording endocardial left atrial activation at 64 sites during AF. These focal impulse and rotor modulation (FIRM) maps are reviewed off-line to identify sites at the center of rotation corresponding to the hypothesized focal impulse origins of AF.

Results from the CONFIRM Trial are provocative. The investigators prospectively enrolled 92 consecutive subjects with symptomatic paroxysmal, persistent, or long-standing persistent AF, as well as patients with AF that failed to respond to prior conventional ablation. Patients were randomized in a 2-arm 1: 2 case cohort design to receive either (1) FIRM-guided ablation followed by conventional ablation versus (2) conventional ablation alone. During a median of 273 days follow-up after a single procedure, FIRM-guided cases had a remarkably higher freedom from AF (84.2% versus 44.9%; $P < 0.001$) [42]. These remarkable results are presently being evaluated in a multicenter prospective randomized controlled trial.

Practical application of the reverse remodeling concept

Catheter ablation for patients with symptomatic atrial fibrillation (paroxysmal or persistent) remains a long-term management strategy. Cardioversion with or without subsequent antiarrhythmic drug therapy is often required acutely to alleviate severe symptoms and achieve adequate ventricular rate control, while a more definitive long-term treatment strategy is

identified and then performed. Even for patients with persistent AF who have only mild to moderate symptoms, elective cardioversion with or without antiarrhythmic drug therapy as a temporizing intervention until a more definitive intervention such as catheter ablation may be viewed favorably by both the patient and the physician. In addition to the benefits of atrial electrical remodeling, this period of time allows the patient time to consider the complex treatment options for persistent atrial fibrillation and confirm the symptom that was associated with AF. It also allows time for scheduling the catheter ablation that is resource-intensive and often must be scheduled weeks to months in advance.

Therefore, from a practical standpoint, many patients are already undergoing a period of reverse atrial electrical remodeling prior to catheter ablation of persistent atrial fibrillation. The optimal period of time in sinus rhythm is not clearly defined. Evidence suggests that between 1 and 3 months is probably adequate.

While our study utilized dofetilide to assist in maintenance of sinus rhythm prior to ablation of persistent AF, sinus rhythm is the essential component that allows electrical remodeling to occur, not the antiarrhythmic drug [1,3,15,29]. If dofetilide is not available or not appropriate for an individual patient, evidence suggests that the same benefit of preprocedural electrical remodeling would be achieved with any antiarrhythmic agent that effectively maintains sinus rhythm.

For these reasons, the application of atrial reverse electrical remodeling may be considered a complementary tool to AF ablation strategies. For some patients, electrical remodeling effectively limits ablation requirements to PVI alone. For others, more extensive mechanical remodeling and structural heart disease may dictate the need for additional ablation strategies such as ablation of autonomic ganglia, CFAE and/or rotor mapping and ablation, or even creation of linear ablation lesions. But even for these patients, the benefit of atrial electrical remodeling exists, potentially reducing the quantity of substrate modification required to achieve maintenance of sinus rhythm.

Conclusions

Atrial fibrillation, the most common heart rhythm disturbance, represents the end result of complex structural, electrical, and mechanical changes of the atrial tissue. Early in the disease process, elimination of pulmonary vein triggers has been demonstrated to be an effective therapy for many patients. However, as the disease process progresses, electrical and structural remodeling create conditions that favor continuation of AF. The effectiveness of catheter ablation techniques to treat the more advanced stages of AF once it has become persistent remains suboptimal.

Most ablation techniques for persistent AF are founded upon the theory that atrial tissue substrate modification, in addition to elimination of AF triggers, is required to improve ablation efficacy. Ablation of autonomic ganglia, complex fractionated electrograms and rotor mapping/ablation all extend the amount of tissue ablated. These techniques, in their present form, therefore lengthen the ablation procedure and increase the risk of time-dependent complications associated with AF ablation. Creation of LA linear lesions is the most common technique employed for ablation of persistent AF, but it remains associated with a high rate of postablation left atrial flutters, and creation of the mitral annular lesion is challenging and time-consuming, with success rates of only 75–85% in the most experienced laboratories.

In contrast, preprocedure electrical remodeling by restoration and maintenance of sinus rhythm 1 to 3 months prior to ablation for persistent AF offers the only strategy to improve ablation efficacy without extending the procedure duration and without exposing patients to the associated risks of prolonged procedures and extensive ablation lesions.

Randomized, controlled multicenter studies are needed to further characterize the effectiveness of preprocedure electrical remodeling prior to ablation of persistent AF, to clearly define the optimal duration of sinus rhythm required for electrical remodeling to complete, and to compare this technique to the alternative strategies described in this chapter. Given the complex physiology and pathophysiology that exists in AF, it is likely that no single ablation approach will be a magic bullet. Rather, a combination of elimination of triggers (PVI) along with electrical remodeling, GP ablation, rotor mapping, and as a last resort linear lesion ablation may prove most effective.

References

1 Wijffels M, Kirchhof C, Dorland R, Allessie MA. Atrial fibrillation begets atrial fibrillation: a study in awake chronically instrumented goats. Circulation. 1995;92(7): 1954–1968.

2 Morillo CA, Klein GJ, Jones DL, Guiraudon CM. Chronic rapid atrial pacing: structural, functional, and electrophysiological characteristics of a new model of sustained atrial fibrillation. Circulation. 1995;91(5):1588–1595.

3 Pang H, Ronderos R, Ricardo Perez-Riera A, Femenia F, Baranchuk A. Reverse atrial electrical remodeling: a systematic review. Cardiol J. 2011;18(6):625–631.

4 Mahnkopf C, Badger TJ, Burgon NS, Daccarett M, Haslam TS, Badger CT, et al. Evaluation of the left atrial

substrate in patients with lone atrial fibrillation using delayed-enhanced MRI: implications for disease progression and response to catheter ablation. Heart Rhythm. 2010;7(10):1475–1481.

5 Bosch RF, Zeng X, Grammer JB, Popovic K, Mewis C, Kuhlkamp V. Ionic mechanisms of electrical remodeling in human atrial fibrillation. Cardiovasc Res. 1999;44 (1):121–131.

6 Yue L, Feng J, Gaspo R, Li GR, Wang Z, Nattel S. Ionic remodeling underlying action potential changes in a canine model of atrial fibrillation. Circ Res. 1997;81(4):512–525.

7 Nattel S, Burstein B, Dobrev D. Atrial remodeling and atrial fibrillation: mechanisms and implications. Circ Arrhythm Electrophysiol. 2008;1(1):62–73.

8 Wetzel U, Boldt A, Lauschke J, Weigl J, Schirdewahn P, Dorszewski A, et al. Expression of connexins 40 and 43 in human left atrium in atrial fibrillation of different aetiologies. Heart. 2005;91(2):166–170.

9 Misier AR, Opthof T, van Hemel NM, Defauw JJ, de Bakker JM, Janse MJ, et al. Increased dispersion of "refractoriness" in patients with idiopathic paroxysmal atrial fibrillation. J Am Coll Cardiol. 1992;19(7): 1531–1535.

10 Redfearn DP, Lane J, Ward K, Stafford PJ. High-resolution analysis of the surface P wave as a measure of atrial electrophysiological substrate. Ann Noninvasive Electrocardiol. 2006;11(1):12–19.

11 Redfearn DP, Skanes AC, Lane J, Stafford PJ. Signal-averaged P wave reflects change in atrial electrophysiological substrate afforded by verapamil following cardioversion from atrial fibrillation. Pacing Clin Electrophysiol. 2006;29(10):1089–1095.

12 Schotten U, Ausma J, Stellbrink C, Sabatschus I, Vogel M, Frechen D, et al. Cellular mechanisms of depressed atrial contractility in patients with chronic atrial fibrillation. Circulation. 2001;103(5):691–698.

13 Schotten U, Greiser M, Benke D, Buerkel K, Ehrenteidt B, Stellbrink C, et al. Atrial fibrillation-induced atrial contractile dysfunction: a tachycardiomyopathy of a different sort. Cardiovasc Res. 2002;53(1):192–201.

14 Allessie M, Ausma J, Schotten U. Electrical, contractile and structural remodeling during atrial fibrillation. Cardiovasc Res. 2002;54(2):230–246.

15 Delangen CDJ, Tieleman RG, Vanderwoude HJ, Grandjean JG, Bel KJ, Wijffels M, et al. Delayed recovery of atrial refractoriness after atrial tachycardia in the goat. Circulation. 1995;92(8):3629.

16 Chalfoun N, Harnick D, Pe E, Undavia M, Mehta D, Gomes JA. Reverse electrical remodeling of the atria post cardioversion in patients who remain in sinus rhythm assessed by signal averaging of the P-wave. Pacing Clin Electrophysiol.. 2007;30(4):502–509.

17 Aytemir K, Ozer N, Atalar E, Sade E, Aksoyek S, Ovunc K, et al. P wave dispersion on 12-lead electrocardiography in patients with paroxysmal atrial fibrillation. Pacing Clin Electrophysiol. 2000;23(7):1109–1112.

18 Andrikopoulos GK, Dilaveris PE, Richter DJ, Gialafos EJ, Synetos AG, Gialafos JE. Increased variance of P wave duration on the electrocardiogram distinguishes patients

with idiopathic paroxysmal atrial fibrillation. Pacing Clin Electrophysiol. 2000;23(7):1127–1132.

19 Budeus M, Wieneke H, Sack S, Erbel R, Perings C. Long-term outcome after cardioversion of atrial fibrillation: prediction of recurrence with P wave signal averaged ECG and chemoreflexsensitivity. Int J Cardiol. 2006;112 (3):308–315.

20 Healey JS, Theoret-Patrick P, Green MS, Lemery R, Birnie D, Tang AS. Reverse atrial electrical remodelling following atrial defibrillation as determined by signal-averaged ECG. Can J Cardiol. 2004;20(3):311–315.

21 Guo XH, Gallagher MM, Poloniecki J, Yi G, Camm AJ. Prognostic significance of serial P wave signal-averaged electrocardiograms following external electrical cardioversion for persistent atrial fibrillation: a prospective study. Pacing Clin Electrophysiol. 2003;26 (1 Pt 2):299–304.

22 Yu WC, Lee SH, Tai CT, Tsai CF, Hsieh MH, Chen CC, et al. Reversal of atrial electrical remodeling following cardioversion of long-standing atrial fibrillation in man. Cardiovasc Res. 1999;42(2):470–476.

23 Raitt MH, Kusumoto W, Giraud G, McAnulty JH. Reversal of electrical remodeling after cardioversion of persistent atrial fibrillation. J Cardiovasc Electrophysiol. 2004;15 (5):507–512.

24 Khan A, Choi A, Musat D, Bangalore S, Mittal S, Steinberg JS, et al. Predicting pulmonary vein isolation responders by using P wave duration on surface ECG. Heart Rhythm. 2007;4:S137.

25 Ausma J, van der Velden HM, Lenders MH, van Ankeren EP, Jongsma HJ, Ramaekers FC, et al. Reverse structural and gap-junctional remodeling after prolonged atrial fibrillation in the goat. Circulation. 2003;107(15):2051–2058.

26 Everett TH 4th, Li H, Mangrum JM, McRury ID, Mitchell MA, Redick JA, et al. Electrical, morphological, and ultrastructural remodeling and reverse remodeling in a canine model of chronic atrial fibrillation. Circulation. 2000;102(12):1454–1460.

27 Manios EG, Kanoupakis EM, Kaleboubas MD, Mavrakis HE, Chlouverakis GI, Vardas PE. Changes in atrial electrical properties following cardioversion of chronic atrial fibrillation: relation with recurrence. Eur Heart J. 2000;21:471.

28 Khan A, Mittal S, Kamath GS, Garikipati NV, Marrero D, Steinberg JS. Pulmonary vein isolation alone in patients with persistent atrial fibrillation: an ablation strategy facilitated by antiarrhythmic drug induced reverse remodeling. J Cardiovasc Electrophysiol. 2011;22(2):142–148.

29 Rivard L, Hocini M, Rostock T, Cauchemez B, Forclaz A, Jadidi AS, et al. Improved outcome following restoration of sinus rhythm prior to catheter ablation of persistent atrial fibrillation: a comparative multicenter study. Heart Rhythm. 2012;9(7):1025–1030.

30 O'Neill MD, Jais P, Takahashi Y, Jonsson A, Sacher F, Hocini M, et al. The stepwise ablation approach for chronic atrial fibrillation: evidence for a cumulative effect. J Int Card Electrophysiol. 2006;16(3):153–167.

31 Ghanbari H, Oral H. Restoration of sinus rhythm prior to catheter ablation of persistent atrial fibrillation: reverse remodeling or patient selection? Heart Rhythm. 2012;9 (7):1031–1032.

32 Nakagawa H, Scherlag BJ, Patterson E, Ikeda A, Lockwood D, Jackman WM. Pathophysiologic basis of autonomic ganglionated plexus ablation in patients with atrial fibrillation. Heart Rhythm. 2009;6 (12 Suppl):S26–S34.

33 Patterson E, Lazzara R, Szabo B, Liu H, Tang D, Li YH, et al. Sodium–calcium exchange initiated by the Ca^{2+} transient: an arrhythmia trigger within pulmonary veins. J Am Coll Cardiol. 2006;47(6):1196–1206.

34 Katritsis DG, Giazitzoglou E, Zografos T, Pokushalov E, Po SS, Camm AJ. Rapid pulmonary vein isolation combined with autonomic ganglia modification: a randomized study. Heart Rhythm. 2011;8(5):672–678.

35 Zhou Q, Hou Y, Yang S. A meta-analysis of the comparative efficacy of ablation for atrial fibrillation with and without ablation of the ganglionated plexi. Pacing Clin Electrophysiol. 2011;34(12):1687–1694.

36 Pokushalov E, Romanov A, Katritsis DG, Artyomenko S, Shirokova N, Karaskov A, et al. Ganglionated plexus ablation vs linear ablation in patients undergoing pulmonary vein isolation for persistent/long-standing persistent atrial fibrillation: a randomized comparison. Heart Rhythm. 2013;10(9):1280–1286.

37 Konings KT, Smeets JL, Penn OC, Wellens HJ, Allessie MA. Configuration of unipolar atrial electrograms during electrically induced atrial fibrillation in humans. Circulation. 1997;95(5):1231–1241.

38 Lin J, Scherlag BJ, Zhou J, Lu Z, Patterson E, Jackman WM, et al. Autonomic mechanism to explain complex fractionated atrial electrograms (CFAE). J Cardiovasc Electrophysiol. 2007;18(11):1197–1205.

39 Nademanee K, McKenzie J, Kosar E, Schwab M, Sunsaneewitayakul B, Vasavakul T, et al. A new approach for catheter ablation of atrial fibrillation: mapping of the electrophysiologic substrate. J Am Coll Cardiol. 2004; 43(11):2044–2053.

40 Verma A, Novak P, Macle L, Whaley B, Beardsall M, Wulffhart Z, et al. A prospective, multicenter evaluation of ablating complex fractionated electrograms (CFEs) during atrial fibrillation (AF) identified by an automated mapping algorithm: acute effects on AF and efficacy as an adjuvant strategy. Heart Rhythm. 2008;5(2):198–205.

41 Allessie MA, de Groot NM, Houben RP, Schotten U, Boersma E, Smeets JL, et al. Electropathological substrate of long-standing persistent atrial fibrillation in patients with structural heart disease: longitudinal dissociation. Circ Arrhythm Electrophysiol. 2010;3(6):606–615.

42 Narayan SM, Krummen DE, Shivkumar K, Clopton P, Rappel WJ, Miller JM. Treatment of atrial fibrillation by the ablation of localized sources: CONFIRM (Conventional Ablation for Atrial Fibrillation With or Without Focal Impulse and Rotor Modulation) Trial. J Am Coll Cardiol. 2012;60(7):628–636.

CHAPTER 22

Long-standing persistent atrial fibrillation ablation

Luigi Di Biase,[1,2,3,8] Pasquale Santangeli,[1,3,4] Alessandro Paoletti Perini,[1,5] Francesco Santoro,[1,3] Rong Bai,[1] Javier E. Sanchez,[1] Rodney Horton,[1] John David Burkhardt,[1] & Andrea Natale[1,2,6,7]

[1]Texas Cardiac Arrhythmia Institute, St. David's Medical Center, Austin, TX, USA
[2]Department of Biomedical Engineering, University of Texas, Austin, TX, USA
[3]Department of Cardiology, University of Foggia, Foggia, Italy
[4]University of Pennsylvania, Philadelphia, USA
[5]Department of Heart and Vessel, University of Florence, Florence, Italy
[6]EP Services, California Pacific Medical Center, San Francisco, California, USA
[7]Dell Medical School, Austin, Texas, USA
[8]Albert Einstein College of Medicine at Montefiore Hospital, New York, USA

Introduction

Atrial fibrillation (AF) is the most common supraventricular arrhythmias in Western countries and represents one of the major causes of hospitalizations in the United States [1].

Randomized controlled trials show that catheter ablation is superior to antiarrhythmic drugs (AADs) therapy to achieve freedom from AF, improved symptoms, and quality of life [2–4] especially in the settings of paroxysmal AF.

Pulmonary vein electrical isolation (PVI) represents the most important end point in patients with AF [5].

Meta-analyses have demonstrated that PV's isolation is sufficient to achieve freedom from AF in the majority of patients with paroxysmal AF [6,7].

In the setting of nonparoxysmal AF and especially long-standing persistent atrial fibrillation (LSPAF), PVI alone has shown dismal success rate at follow-up [6–9].

Long-standing persistent atrial fibrillation is defined as continuous AF greater than 12 months' duration [10].

Therefore, in addition to PVs several targets such as complex fractionated atrial electrograms (CFAEs), ganglionated plexi, AF nest, rotors, and other non-PV triggers such as left atrial posterior wall (PW), coronary sinus (CS), left atrial septum, left atrial appendage (LAA), ligament of Marshall, and the superior vena cava (SVC) [9–11] have been proposed without a uniform consensus.

In addition, hybrid procedures combining surgical and electrophysiology expertise have been proposed to improve the outcomes with unsatisfactory results in the setting of LSPAF.

This chapter will summarize the ablation strategy approaches described in the literature for the treatment of long-standing persistent AF and more extensively the author's approach that we believe allows a better outcome at the long-term follow-up.

Lessons learned from the literature for the treatment of LSP AF

Pulmonary vein isolation (PVI) confirmed by a circular mapping catheter is a recommended step.

PVI alone has dismal success rate at 2 years follow-up not exceeding 25%.

Wider pulmonary vein isolation such as antrum isolation (verified with a circular mapping catheter) is

Practical Guide to Catheter Ablation of Atrial Fibrillation,
Second Edition. Edited by Jonathan S. Steinberg, Pierre Jaïs and Hugh Calkins.
© 2016 John Wiley & Sons, Ltd. Published 2016 by John Wiley & Sons, Ltd.

preferable to ostial ablation. Success rate does not increase with multiple procedures if the ablation is limited to PVI alone [9].

Complex fractionated atrial electrograms ablation alone has a dismal success rate at the long-term follow-up ranging from 64% in a single study down to 24 % at 18 months follow up [9].

CFAE ablation as an adjunct to PVI increases the outcome at 2 years up to 65%.

CFAEs are commonly localized at different left atrium areas such as posterior wall, roof, coronary sinus, septum, and left atrial appendage. Right atrial CFAEs ablation does not seem to influence the outcomes. Redo procedures increase the success rate up to 80% [9]. Stepwise procedures that include linear ablation in addition to PVI and CFAEs ablation does not seem superior to PVI plus CFAEs ablation [9]. Termination of AF during ablation does not correlate with the overall freedom from atrial arrhythmias at follow-up [12,13].

The approach that we believe is the most effective at the long-term follow-up includes in addition to PVI electrical isolation of the posterior wall, the roof, the coronary sinus, the left septum, and the left atrial appendage with or without CFAEs. In our experience, right atrial ablation does not seem to increase success with the exception of patients with severe sleep apnea or in older women especially in the presence of thyroid problems. Success rate at the long-term follow-up may increase to 88% with multiple procedures with the aim of achieving reisolation of all the above-mentioned areas [9].

Preprocedural and periprocedural management

AADs with the exception of amiodarone are discontinued 3 to 5 days prior to the procedure [10]. Patients on amiodarone are asked to discontinue the drug 4 to 6 months prior to the ablation due to its longer half-life. Switching to tikosin 5 days prior to the procedure represents a viable option. We prefer performing ablation off AADs for two main reasons: they may influence the termination of AF during ablation limiting the amount of "critical mass" ablated during the index procedure due to the AF termination and they may suppress or mask non-PV triggers responsible for AF. In both cases, in our experience, the success rate at the long-term follow-up is lower when procedures are performed while on AADs.

The preliminary results of the SPECULATE study (NCT01173809), a randomized multicenter trial enrolling patients with LSPAF who were randomized to amiodarone discontinuation 4–6 months before the procedure versus no amiodarone discontinuation [14]

showed that freedom from AF was significantly lower in the group of patients undergoing ablation without amiodarone discontinuation at the 6 months follow-up. It appears that amiodarone masks non-PV triggers, increases the chances of late recurrences. We do not routinely perform preoperative CT scan or MRI of the left atrium at the index procedure while they are always considered in patients undergoing "redo" procedures to exclude the presence of asymptomatic preprocedural PV stenosis. Postoperative CT or MRI scan is instead performed in all patients at the 3 months follow-up to exclude PV stenosis [15,16].

To reduce the risk of periprocedural TIA/stroke, procedures are performed under "therapeutic" INR.

All patients are required to undergo oral anticoagulation with warfarin for at least a month.

We do not discontinue warfarin before the procedure and we do not bridge with low weight molecular heparin.

Preprocedural transesophageal echocardiography (TEE) is not routinely performed unless patients are subtherapeutic the day of the procedure. If the preprocedural INR is above 3.5, one or two units of fresh frozen plasma are utilized immediately before the procedure to reduce the INR value.

All patients are type- and cross-matched before the procedure and fresh frozen plasma and red cell are easily available in case of perforation.

A bolus of unfractionated heparin (10,000 U in males and 8000 U in females) is administered before transseptal [17]. We reported that in 9% of the cases a soft thrombus forms on the right sheath immediately after sheath exchange and while tenting the fossa ovalis [18].

During the procedures, an activated clotting time (ACT) above 300 s is mandatory and 350 s is our goal.

Our sheaths are continuously infused with heparinized saline and care is taken to avoid air embolism.

The results of the COMPARE randomized trial (NCT01006876) clearly shows that in patients with nonparoxysmal AF performing the procedure without warfarin discontinuation is key to reduce the risk of periprocedural TIA/stroke [19].

Data on LSPAF ablation with the use of the newer anticoagulant are not widely available.

We showed that performing ablation on dabigatran increases the risk for TIA/stroke in patients with LSP [20]. We recently presented preliminary data of long-standing persistent AF ablation while on rivaroxaban showing that it is as safe as warfarin [21]. No data on apixaban and endoxaban are available yet.

All patients undergo ablation under general anesthesia. The anesthesia protocol utilized has been extensively described elsewhere. Muscular paralysis is avoided to detect diaphragmatic paralysis [22]. The use of general anesthesia adds several advantages since it improves catheter stability allowing a better lesion quality and improves the compliance of patients to redo procedures that in the setting of LSP are usually needed to achieve a long-term freedom from AF.

Left atrial instrumentation is achieved by double transseptal punctures; the circular mapping catheter is placed in all four pulmonary vein antrums, and along the posterior wall of the left atrium.

In cases of thickened or hypertrophied interatrial septum resistant to transseptal puncture and often during redo procedures, electrocautery is utilized to instrument the left atrium.

Catheter maneuverability in the left atrium depends on the way the LA is accessed.

The use of ICE is key because it allows the operator to choose a more posterior access to the left atrium than a fluoroscopic guided transseptal.

An esophageal probe is inserted in all patients to monitor esophageal temperature during ablation in area in close proximity to the esophagus such as the posterior wall. This probe is moved as the circular mapping catheter and the ablation catheter move to a different location [23].

Ablation protocol

The circular mapping catheter under fluoroscopic guidance confirmed by ICE is maneuvered around the antrum of all pulmonary veins.

The target for ablation is represented by PV potentials recorded by the circular mapping catheter. Abolition of all PV antrum electrograms is the primary end point. We target the left PVs first and then the ablation catheter encompasses the entire posterior wall guided by the circular mapping catheter that is dragged around each vein and the posterior wall to achieve electrical isolation.

Entry block is determined when no PV potentials can be recorded along the antrum or inside the vein by the circular mapping catheter. In some cases, the presence of dissociated firing from the left atrium allows exit block verification as well.

In the setting of long-standing persistent AF, electrical isolation of all pulmonary vein antrum and the entire posterior wall down to the coronary sinus is always achieved. In addition, the ablation is extended to the left side of the septum and to the left atrial roof. Ablation of CFAEs in the left atrium and in the coronary sinus is also performed if fragmented potential are found. The coronary sinus is targeted endocardially first and epicardially later. If after extensive ablation termination cannot be achieved, cardioversion is performed [12,23] (also see Figure 1).

At our institution, procedural termination of AF is not sought as an end point [12].

Elayi et al. in a prospective study on 306 patients with long-standing persistent AF showed that after a mean follow-up of 25 ± 6.9 months had no differences in terms of tachyarrhythmia recurrences between

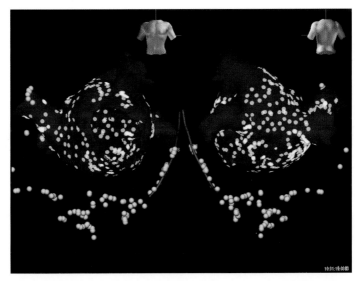

Figure 1 Typical *lesion set performed in long-standing persistent AF patients*. Left panel shows anteroposterior right panel and posteroanterior view of a 3D electroanatomic left atrial map (Navs, St Jude Medical). White dots indicate lesions at the level of the pulmonary vein antra, the left septum, the posterior wall down to the endocardial coronary sinus and the left atrial appendage. Lesions within the epicardial CS, the right atrium, and the SVC are shown with yellow dots.

patients who had procedural termination/organiza-
tion of AF during the procedure and those who
remained in AF and received cardioversion [12].

After a stable sinus rhythm is achieved either during
ablation or after cardioversion, and after PVs, posterior wall, roof and left atrial septum are confirmed
electrically silent, isoproterenol infusion up to 30 mcg/
min for 15–20 min is given to all patients to discover
any non-PV triggers or tachycardia and to look for
acute reconnections [23]. Figures 2–4 show firing
from different structures such as posterior wall, proximal coronary sinus, and left atrial appendage.

Radiofrequency energy is delivered with a maximum temperature setting of 41 °C and a power of 40–
45 W (35 W in the posterior wall and in the coronary
sinus) with a flow rate of 15 cc/min with the
ThermoCool® SF Catheter with Surround Flow technology (Biosense Webster, Diamond Bar, California,
USA). This catheter allows a more uniform cooling of
the entire catheter tip with at least half the fluid
administered to the patients compared to the old-
generation ThermoCool catheter. The infusion of less
fluid is extremely important to reduce postprocedure
fluid overload since the amount of tissue that is
burned in the left atrium is higher compared to
paroxysmal patients.

Energy delivery is discontinued when the temperature of esophageal probe increase and/or reaches 39 °C.

To avoid esophageal damage, we limit each radiofrequency application to 20 s per site.

Mapping of PACs and or tachycardia during isoproterenol challenge is guided by our standard catheter
positioning that includes the circular mapping catheter
at the ostium of the left superior PV, the ablation
catheter at the ostium of the right superior PV, and
the duodecapolar catheter introduced in the right
atrium from the internal jugular vein with 20 poles
that cover the right atrium and the coronary sinus. This
catheter placement allows us to identify the site of origin
of any significant ectopic atrial activity and/or tachycardia, by comparing the activation sequence of the
sinus beat with the one of the ectopic beat.

In case triggers from either the coronary sinus or
the left atrial appendage are seen, electrical isolation of
these structures and not focal ablation achieves the
best results.

In all cases, before ending the procedures, the
circular mapping catheter is positioned at the level
of the SVC under ICE guidance and isolation of the
SVC is performed [24].

High-voltage pacing (at least 30 mA) is used to
check phrenic nerve capture at the lateral level of
the SVC prior to deliver radiofrequency to prevent
phrenic nerve palsy [23,24].

At the end of the procedure, systemic anticoagulation
with heparin is partially reversed with protamine and
sheaths are removed when the ACT is ≤200 s.

Isolation of the coronary sinus is usually performed
first along the left atrium endocardial aspect (and after
epicardially within the coronary sinus [25]).

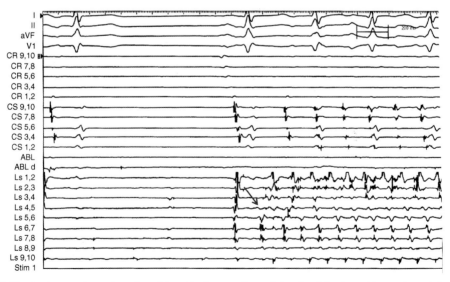

Figure 2 The circular mapping catheter is positioned in the posterior wall showing firing from this area (arrow). From top
to bottom: surface ECG leads, I, II, aVF, and V1; right atrium crista (RA) from proximal (9–10) to distal (1–2); CS catheter
from proximal (9–10) to distal (1–2); ablation catheter (ABL) from proximal (p) to distal (d); and circular catheter (Ls) from
1–2 to 9–10 of the LA.

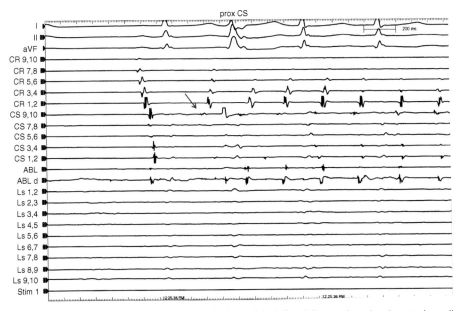

Figure 3 The circular mapping catheter is positioned at the base of the left atrial appendage showing a tachycardia originating from this structure (arrow). From top to bottom: Surface ECG leads: I, II, aVF, and V1; right atrium crista (RA) from proximal (9–10) to distal (1–2); CS catheter from proximal (9–10) to distal (1–2); ablation catheter (ABL) from proximal (p) to distal (d); and circular catheter (Ls) from 1–2 to 9–10 of the LA.

Endocardially, the ablation usually starts from the distal coronary sinus and progresses to the septal area anterior to the right PVs. At the level of the right PV, continuous monitoring of the PR interval is advisable to avoid AV block since leftward extensions of the AV node could be in close proximity to this area. Continuous movement of the ablation catheter along the CS, limiting the ablation to 20 s per site, reduces potential

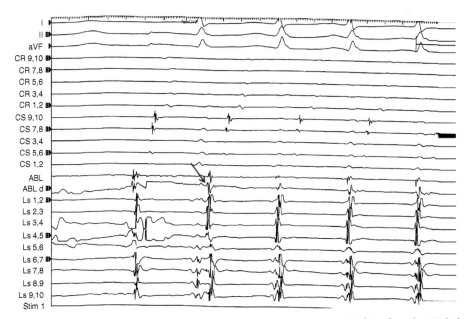

Figure 4 The circular mapping catheter is positioned at the base of the LAA. A tachycardia firing from the LAA is shown (solid black arrow). From top to bottom: Surface ECG leads, I, II, and aVF; right atrium crista (RA) from proximal (9–10) to distal (1–2); CS catheter from proximal (9–10) to distal (1–2); and ablation catheter (ABL) from proximal (p) to distal (d); and circular catheter (Ls) from 1–2 to 9–10 of the LA.

complications such as perforation and coronary artery damages.

We should always take into account that long-standing persistent AF is characterized by significant changes in atrial substrate, so we believe that non-PV sites play a significant role in triggering and maintaining the arrhythmia supporting the dismal success reported in these patients when PVAI alone is performed [26].

Although initially the ablation of the left atrial appendage as an additional trigger source for AF was limited to redo cases, we now routinely isolate the appendage in these patients in case of firing from this structure. LAA isolation is performed similar to PV isolation. The circular mapping catheter is positioned at the ostium of the LAA guided by ICE. Radiofrequency applications are delivered targeting the earliest electrical activation on the circular mapping catheter. Since the LAA has a thin wall, caution should be taken when isolating this structure to avoid high contact pressure.

During AF, it is hard to identify the earliest activation on the circular mapping catheter, thus often resulting in ineffective LAA isolation. On the contrary, in sinus rhythm, the earliest activation is easily recognized and the LAA isolation is relatively easier.

In our experience, although electrically isolated the LAA shows a preserved contractility during the 6 months TEE in 35–40% of the patients due to LAA reconnection or a passive contraction of the LAA. In case of limited or absent contraction and in patients who would like to avoid long-term oral anticoagulation, an appendage closure device could be considered.

The "BELIEF" study (NCT01362738) randomizing patients with long-standing persistent atrial fibrillation to empirical LAA isolation plus standard approach versus standard approach without LAA isolation will clarify the relevance of the LAA isolation in patients with LSP. In many case outside the belief trial, the empirical left atrial appendage isolation has the capability in our experience to improve the success rate of catheter ablation of long-standing persistent atrial fibrillation after a single procedure [27].

Postprocedural management and follow-up

Patients are usually discharged on their previously ineffective AADs with the exception of amiodarone during the blanking period (12 weeks) and then are discontinued.

In cases of recurrences after the blanking period, patients are first given their previously ineffective AADs and then considered for a redo procedure [23].

The follow-up is performed at 3, 6, 9, and 12 months after the procedure and every 6 months thereafter, with a 12-lead electrocardiogram (ECG), and 7-day Holter monitoring.

Patients are also given event recorder for 5 months after ablation, and they are asked to transmit their rhythm every time they have symptoms compatible with arrhythmias and at least twice a week even if asymptomatic. Any episode of AF/AT longer than 30 s is considered as a recurrence.

At our institution, dedicated nurses are in charge of the preprocedure education and the postprocedure follow-up of all patients.

Patients are asked to contact their assigned nurse and to seek medical attention in case of complications [23].

Conflict of interest

Dr Di Biase is a consultant for Biosense Webster, Hansen Medical, and St Jude Medical.

Dr Natale has received consultant fees or honoraria from Biosense Webster, Boston Scientific, Medtronic, and St Jude Medical.

References

1 Miyasaka Y, Barnes ME, Gersh BJ, et al. Secular trends in incidence of atrial fibrillation in Olmsted County, Minnesota, 1980 to 2000, and implications on the projections for future prevalence. Circulation. 2006;114:119–125.

2 Calkins H, Reynolds MR, Spector P, Sondhi M, Xu Y, Martin A, Williams CJ, Sledge I. Treatment of atrial fibrillation with antiarrhythmic drugs or radiofrequency ablation: two systematic literature reviews and meta-analyses. Circ Arrhythm Electrophysiol. 2009;2:349–361.

3 Wilber DJ, Pappone C, Neuzil P, et al. Comparison of antiarrhythmic drug therapy and radiofrequency catheter ablation in patients with paroxysmal atrial fibrillation: a randomized controlled trial. JAMA. 2010;303:333–340.

4 Bhargava M, Di Biase L, Mohanty P, et al. Impact of type of atrial fibrillation and repeat catheter ablation on long-term freedom from atrial fibrillation: results from a multicenter study. Heart Rhythm. 2009;6:1403–1412.

5 Haissaguerre M, Jais P, Shah DC, et al. Spontaneous initiation of atrial fibrillation by ectopic beats originating in the pulmonary veins. N Engl J Med. 1998;339:659–666.

6 Li WJ, Bai YY, Zhang HY, Tang RB, Miao CL, Sang CH, Yin XD, Dong JZ, Ma CS. Additional ablation of complex fractionated atrial electrograms after pulmonary vein isolation in patients with atrial fibrillation: a meta-analysis. Circ Arrhythm Electrophysiol. 2011;4:143–148.

7 Hayward RM, Upadhyay GA, Mela T, Ellinor PT, Barrett CD, Heist EK, Verma A, Choudhry NK, Singh JP. Pulmonary vein isolation with complex fractionated atrial electrogram ablation for paroxysmal and nonparoxysmal

atrial fibrillation: a meta-analysis. Heart Rhythm. 2011;8:9944–1000.

8 Calkins H. Catheter ablation to maintain sinus rhythm. Circulation. 2012;125:1439–1445.

9 Brooks AG, Stiles MK, Laborderie J, Lau DH, Kuklik P, Shipp NJ, Hsu LF, Sanders P. Outcomes of long-standing persistent atrial fibrillation ablation: a systematic review. Heart Rhythm. 2010;7:835–846.

10 Calkins H, Kuck KH, Cappato R, Brugada J, Camm AJ, Chen SA, Crijns HJ, Damiano RJ Jr, Davies DW, DiMarco J, Edgerton J, Ellenbogen K, Ezekowitz MD, Haines DE, Haissaguerre M, Hindricks G, Iesaka Y, Jackman W, Jalife J, Jais P, Kalman J, Keane D, Kim YH, Kirchhof P, Klein G, Kottkamp H, Kumagai K, Lindsay BD, Mansour M, Marchlinski FE, McCarthy PM, Mont JL, Morady F, Nademanee K, Nakagawa H, Natale A, Nattel S, Packer DL, Pappone C, Prystowsky E, Raviele A, Reddy V, Ruskin JN, Shemin RJ, Tsao HM, Wilber D; Heart Rhythm Society Task Force on Catheter and Surgical Ablation of Atrial Fibrillation. 2012 HRS/EHRA/ECAS Expert Consensus Statement on Catheter and Surgical Ablation of Atrial Fibrillation: recommendations for patient selection, procedural techniques, patient management and follow-up, definitions, endpoints, and research trial design: a report of the Heart Rhythm Society (HRS) Task Force on Catheter and Surgical Ablation of Atrial Fibrillation. Developed in partnership with the European Heart Rhythm Association (EHRA), a registered branch of the European Society of Cardiology (ESC) and the European Cardiac Arrhythmia Society (ECAS); and in collaboration with the American College of Cardiology (ACC), American Heart Association (AHA), the Asia Pacific Heart Rhythm Society (APHRS), and the Society of Thoracic Surgeons (STS). Endorsed by the governing bodies of the American College of Cardiology Foundation, the American Heart Association, the European Cardiac Arrhythmia Society, the European Heart Rhythm Association, the Society of Thoracic Surgeons, the Asia Pacific Heart Rhythm Society, and the Heart Rhythm Society. Heart Rhythm. 2012;9:632–696.

11 Di Biase L, Burkhardt JD, Mohanty P, Sanchez J, Mohanty S, Horton R, Gallinghouse GJ, Bailey SM, Zagrodzky JD, Santangeli P, Hao S, Hongo R, Beheiry S, Themistoclakis S, Bonso A, Rossillo A, Corrado A, Raviele A, Al-Ahmad A, Wang P, Cummings JE, Schweikert RA, Pelargonio G, Dello Russo A, Casella M, Santarelli P, Lewis WR, Natale A. Left atrial appendage: an underrecognized trigger site of atrial fibrillation. Circulation. 2010;122:109–118.

12 Elayi CS, Di Biase L, Barrett C, Ching CK, al Aly M, Lucciola M, Bai R, Horton R, Fahmy TS, Verma A, Khaykin Y, Shah J, Morales G, Hongo R, Hao S, Beheiry S, Arruda M, Schweikert RA, Cummings J, Burkhardt JD, Wang P, Al-Ahmad A, Cauchemez B, Gaita F, Natale A. Atrial fibrillation termination as a procedural endpoint during ablation in long-standing persistent atrial fibrillation. Heart Rhythm. 2010;7:1216–1223.

13 O'Neill MD, Wright M, Knecht S, et al. Long-term follow-up of persistent atrial fibrillation ablation using

termination as a procedural endpoint. Eur Heart J. 2009;30:1105–1112.

14 Mohanty S, Di Biase L, Mohanty P, Trivedi C, Santangeli P, Bai R, Burkhardt JD, Gallinghouse JG, Horton R, Sanchez JE, Hranitzky PM, Zagrodzky J, Al-Ahmad A, Pelargonio G, Lakkireddy D, Reddy M, Forleo G, Rossillo A, Themistoclakis S, Hongo R, Beheiry S, Casella M, Dello Russo A, Tondo C, Natale A. Effect of periprocedural amiodarone on procedure outcome in patients with long-standing persistent atrial fibrillation undergoing extended pulmonary vein antrum isolation: results from a randomized study (SPECULATE). Heart Rhythm. 2015;12:477–83. Erratum in: Heart Rhythm. 2015;12:1100.

15 Di Biase L, Fahmy TS, Wazni OM, Bai R, Patel D, Lakkireddy D, Cummings JE, Schweikert RA, Burkhardt JD, Elayi CS, Kanj M, Popova L, Prasad S, Martin DO, Prieto L, Saliba W, Tchou P, Arruda M, Natale A. Pulmonary vein total occlusion following catheter ablation for atrial fibrillation: clinical implications after long-term follow-up. J Am Coll Cardiol. 2006;48:2493–2499.

16 Barrett CD, Di Biase L, Natale A. How to identify and treat patient with pulmonary vein stenosis post atrial fibrillation ablation. Curr Opin Cardiol. 2009;24:42–49.

17 Di Biase L, Burkhardt JD, Mohanty P, et al. Periprocedural stroke and management of major bleeding complications in patients undergoing catheter ablation of atrial fibrillation: the impact of periprocedural therapeutic international normalized ratio. Circulation. 2010;121:2550–2556.

18 Di Biase L, Mohanty P, Sanchez J, Horton R, Mohanty S, Bai R, Gallinghouse GJ, Themistoclakis S, Raviele A, Hao S, Hongo R, Beheiry S, Lewis WR, Natale A. Abstract 17354: Prevalence of right atrial thrombus on the transseptal sheaths detected by intracardiac echocardiography during catheter ablation for atrial fibrillation while on therapeutic Coumadin. Circulation. 2010;122:A17354.

19 Di Biase L, Burkhardt JD, Santangeli P, Mohanty P, Sanchez JE, Horton R, Gallinghouse GJ, Themistoclakis S, Rossillo A, Lakkireddy D, Reddy M, Hao S, Hongo R, Beheiry S, Zagrodzky J, Rong B, Mohanty S, Elayi CS, Forleo G, Pelargonio G, Narducci ML, Dello Russo A, Casella M, Fassini G, Tondo C, Schweikert RA, Natale A. Periprocedural stroke and bleeding complications in patients undergoing catheter ablation of atrial fibrillation with different anticoagulation management: results from the Role of Coumadin in Preventing Thromboembolism in Atrial Fibrillation (AF) Patients Undergoing Catheter Ablation (COMPARE) randomized trial. Circulation. 2014;129:2638–44.

20 Lakkireddy D, Reddy YM, Di Biase L, Vanga SR, Santangeli P, Swarup V, Pimentel R, Mansour MC, D'Avila A, Sanchez JE, Burkhardt JD, Chalhoub F, Mohanty P, Coffey J, Shaik N, Monir G, Reddy VY, Ruskin J, Natale A. Feasibility and safety of dabigatran versus warfarin for periprocedural anticoagulation in patients undergoing radiofrequency ablation for atrial fibrillation: results from a multicenter prospective registry. J Am Coll Cardiol. 2012;59:1168–1174.

21 R Lakkireddy D, Reddy M, Swarup V, Bakdunes W, Mansour M, Chaloub F, Ruskin J, Di Biase L, Vallakatti

A, Janga P, Umbarger L, Sanchez J, Burkhardt D, Horton R, Reddy V, D'Avila A, Atkins D, Bommana S, Natale A. Uninterrupted rivaroxaban vs. warfarin for periprocedural anticoagulation during atrial fibrillation ablation: a multicenter experience. Heart Rhythm. 2013;10(5S):S74 [AB33-01].

22 Di Biase L, Conti S, Mohanty P, Bai R, Sanchez J, Walton D, John A, Santangeli P, Elayi CS, Beheiry S, Gallinghouse GJ, Mohanty S, Horton R, Bailey S, Burkhardt JD, Natale A. General anesthesia reduces the prevalence of pulmonary vein reconnection during repeat ablation when compared with conscious sedation: results from a randomized study. Heart Rhythm. 2011;8:368–372.

23 Di Biase L, Santangeli P, Natale A. How to ablate longstanding persistent atrial fibrillation? Curr Opin Cardiol. 2013;28:26–35.

24 Arruda M, Mlcochova H, Prasad SK, Kilicaslan F, Saliba W, Patel D, Fahmy T, Morales LS, Schweikert R, Martin D, Burkhardt D, Cummings J, Bhargava M, Dresing T, Wazni O, Kanj M, Natale A. Electrical isolation of the superior vena cava: an adjunctive strategy to pulmonary vein antrum isolation improving the outcome of AF ablation. Cardiovasc Electrophysiol. 2007;18:1261–1266.

25 Di Biase L, Bai R, Mohanty P, Sanchez JE, Mohanty S, Burkhardt JD, Horton R, Bailey S, Zagrodzky J, Gallinghouse GJ, Santangeli P, Dello Russo A, Casella M, Pelargonio G, Riva S, Fassini G, Hongo R, Beheiry S, Lakkireddy D, Vanga SR, Schweikert RA, Gibson D, Lewis WR, Tondo C, Natale A. Atrial fibrillation triggers from the coronary sinus: comparison between isolation versus focal ablation. Heart Rhythm. 2011;8(5S):S78 [AB35-2].

26 Elayi CS, Verma A, Di Biase L, Ching CK, Patel D, Barrett C, Martin D, Rong B, Fahmy TS, Khaykin Y, Hongo R, Hao S, Pelargonio G, Dello Russo A, Casella M, Santarelli P, Potenza D, Fanelli R, Massaro R, Arruda M, Schweikert RA, Natale A. Ablation for longstanding permanent atrial fibrillation: results from a randomized study comparing three different strategies. Heart Rhythm. 2008;5:1658–1664.

27 Di Biase L, Santangeli P, Mohanty P, Bai R, Mohanty S, Pump A, Yan R, Sanchez JE, Gallinghouse GJ, Zagrodsky J, Bailey S, Horton R, Hongo R, Beheiry S, Burkhardt JD, Natale A. Empirical left atrial appendage isolation improves the success rate of catheter ablation of long standing persistent atrial fibrillation after a single procedure: results from a prospective multicenter study. Heart Rhythm. 2012;9(5S):S126 PO1-103.

CHAPTER 23

Mapping and ablation of left atrial flutter

Matthew Daly, Yuki Komatsu, & Pierre Jaïs

CHU de Bordeaux, Hopital Cardiologique Haut Leveque, Pessac, France
Université de Bordeaux, IHU LIRYC, Bordeaux, France

Introduction

Stepwise or substrate ablation is frequently performed in addition to pulmonary vein isolation for persistent atrial fibrillation (AF). It is much more common for AF to terminate to atrial tachycardia (AT) rather than directly to sinus rhythm. When AF is terminated by ablation at the index procedure, recurrence is more likely to be AT than AF [1–4]. If linear lesions are unsuccessfully attempted, AT is likely to occur in the future. AT may be either macroreentrant or focal.

There are three major forms of macroreentrant AT or atrial flutter [5], each with a distinct anatomical "anchor." The circuit of perimitral flutter revolves around the mitral annulus. Roof-dependent flutter rotates around the left or right veins using the left atrial (LA) roof as the critical isthmus. Peritricuspid, or "common" flutter, revolves around the tricuspid annulus. In each case, the circuit may revolve in either direction.

Principle

AT is an organized atrial rhythm with stable morphology and activation sequence. A greater than 15% variation in cycle length strongly suggests a focal AT, which is described elsewhere (Figures 1 and 2). Where there is a less than 15% variation, a focal AT is not ruled out; however, it is reasonable to first perform a map looking for a macroreentrant AT, as this may be

performed more rapidly and easily [6]. Occasionally, ATs may alternate; that is, morphology, activation, and cycle length may alternate. A combination of roof-dependent and perimitral flutter is possible.

Macroreentry is defined as a circuit involving more than three atrial segments, usually greater than 2 cm in diameter and in which more than 75% of the circuit is mapped.

The first step to diagnose macroreentrant AT is activation mapping. It is reasonable to use a decapolar catheter in the coronary sinus (CS). This shows the activation pattern of the inferior LA continuously, and will alert the operator of changes to the AT. It provides a stable reference from which activation timing may be measured. With a roving catheter, the following questions should be answered: Is activation low-to-high or high-to-low on the posterior and anterior LA walls? Is activation septal to lateral or lateral to septal on the anterior LA wall? What is the direction of activation around the tricuspid annulus? A highly detailed map is not required, just enough points (at least two) to establish the global direction of activation. The general principle is that activation fronts heading in opposite directions on opposite atrial segments are compatible with macroreenty involving those segments. With this information, it should be apparent if a macroreentrant tachycardia is possible, and if it is not, focal mapping should be performed.

The next step to confirm a macroreentrant AT is entrainment mapping [7,8]. If possible, this should be done from a site with distinct high-amplitude signals at 20 ms less than the tachycardia cycle length (TCL). Once entrainment is confirmed, the postpacing interval (PPI) is measured. Ideally, there should be three points within the suspected circuit with a

---

Practical Guide to Catheter Ablation of Atrial Fibrillation,
Second Edition. Edited by Jonathan S. Steinberg, Pierre Jaïs
and Hugh Calkins.

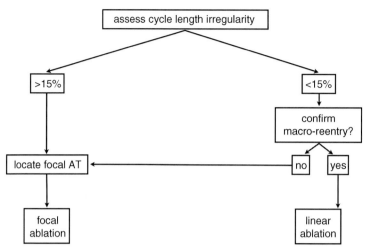

Figure 1 Atrial tachycardia mapping strategy. Deductive steps for mapping and ablation of atrial tachycardia postablation of persistent atrial fibrillation.

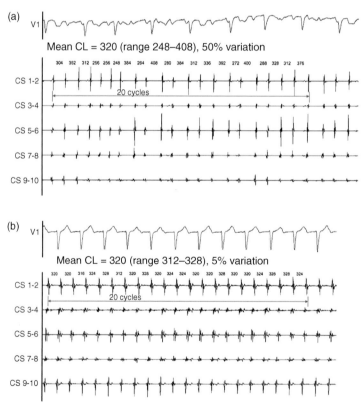

Figure 2 Cycle length variation. Where there is a greater than 15% variation in cycle length (a) a focal atrial tachycardia is more likely. Where there is a less than 15% variation in cycle length (b) both macroreentry and focal atrial tachycardia are possible; it is reasonable to first perform a map looking for a macroreentrant AT, as this may be performed more rapidly and easily.

PPI-TCL of less than 30 ms. If there has been an extensive ablation or if there is significant fibrosis, the PPI-TCL may be longer, even when pacing within the circuit. This is especially problematic when pacing from an ablated coronary sinus. If this situation is suspected, entrainment should be repeated in a different location within the circuit. If PPI is good from multiple locations, a significant distance apart, for instance, in two opposite segments of the atrium, focal AT has been ruled out; the mechanism must be macroreentrant.

The combination of activation and entrainment mapping is very powerful and compensates for the potential limitations of either method when used in isolation.

As a rule, diagnosis of macroreentry is easy, particularly when this systematic approach is used.

Perimitral flutter

The characteristic feature of perimitral flutter is that the inferior and anterior LA walls activate in opposite directions, that is, lateral-to-septal in the one and septal-to-lateral in the other. Opposite sides of the annulus must not activate simultaneously, and the entire cycle length should be covered around the annulus.

Viewed from the apex, it may be clockwise or counterclockwise. In clockwise perimitral flutter, activation in the CS is distal-to-proximal, that is, lateral-to-septal in the inferior part of the mitral annulus. The roving catheter should find septal-to-lateral activation in the anterosuperior part of the mitral annulus. Counterclockwise perimitral flutter is the reverse, with proximal-to-distal activation in the CS and lateral-to-septal activation in the anterosuperior part of the annulus.

In both cases, posterior and anterior walls should activate low to high. Where there has been extensive ablation within the CS, its activation may be less reliable, and the activation of the inferior LA should be assessed with the roving catheter as well [9].

For entrainment mapping, the proximal and distal CS is often used, provided prior ablation has not been too extensive and there is no CS disconnection. A site at either the anteroseptal, anterolateral or lateral LA is used as well.

Roof-dependent flutter

The characteristic feature of roof-dependent flutter is that the anterior and posterior walls activate in opposite directions, that is, high to low in the one and low to high in the other. The anterior and posterior walls must not activate simultaneously at any point and the entire cycle length should be covered along the anterior and posterior walls. CS activation is nonspecific, but most frequently is a chevron or reverse chevron pattern when the posterior wall is activated high to low or low to high (Figure 3).

To confirm with entrainment mapping, it is important to demonstrate a good PPI on the posterior and anterior walls. Theoretically, this might be dependent on the shape of the circuit. Roof-dependent flutter may revolve around the right or left pulmonary veins or both. PPI should be shorter near the circuit or longer away from it. For instance, for a circuit around the left veins, PPI-TCL might be slightly longer if entrainment is performed from an anteroseptal region than from an anterolateral position. In practice, however, this is rarely an issue; the most important feature is that opposite sides of the atria, that is, the posterior and anterior walls, activate in opposite directions and both are "in the circuit" as demonstrated by a good PPI.

Peritricuspid flutter

Although it is the most common atrial tachycardia in clinical practice, peritricuspid flutter is least frequently encountered in the postpersistent AF ablation AT patient population. One might expect it to be the easiest to identify, based on the surface ECG; however, prior extensive ablation may render this unreliable [10]. Peritricuspid flutter should be considered irrespective of the surface ECG appearances.

The CS activation should be proximal to distal. The timing of the F wave may be helpful in suggesting a right-sided circuit, that is, the peak of the F wave in lead V1 should precede the CS sequence rather than activate simultaneously [11]. Generally, the LA is activated septal to lateral in both the anterior and the posterior walls. The entire tachycardia circuit should be contained within the right atrium (RA) and its septal and lateral walls should not be activated simultaneously.

Entrainment is performed in the lateral RA, the RA septum, and in the cavo-tricuspid "isthmus." There are reports that the PPI-TCL may be a little longer than 30 ms when pacing from the peritricuspid circuit, depending on cycle length variability and pacing location [12]. The superior part of the RA may be particularly problematic for entrainment. Of course, a PPI-TCL of a little over 30 ms when entraining from the lateral RA would be very unlikely to occur in the setting of an LA macroreentrant circuit, and should be considered suggestive of peritricuspid flutter.

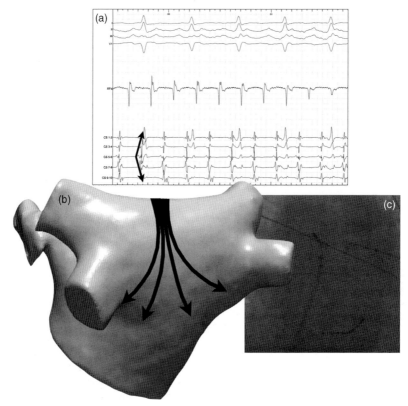

Figure 3 Chevron pattern in the coronary sinus. Signal descending the posterior wall leads to a centrifugal activation of the coronary sinus and a chevron pattern.

Simultaneous macroreentrant tachycardia

Rarely, a double-loop flutter will occur. In its most common form, this consists of a tachycardia encircling the mitral valve in a counterclockwise direction, that is, the CS activates in a proximal-to-distal sequence and the anterosuperior part of the annulus activates in a lateral-to-septal direction, and the tachycardia also rotates around the pulmonary veins, so that the anterior LA activates low to high while the posterior wall activates high to low (instead of the low-to-high activation anterior and posterior in "normal" perimitral flutter). Entrainment with a good PPI is possible along both circuits. Typically, the return cycle will not exceed the TCL by more than 50 ms in the second loop.

If the roof line ablation is performed first, the tachycardia will convert to a perimitral flutter with ablation, and vice versa. This is usually heralded by a prolongation in the cycle length. Ultimately, both a mitral and roof line will usually need to be performed.

Other tachycardias

Two other mechanisms may be encountered. The arrhythmia may be truly focal or due to localized reentry. In both cases, the activation is centrifugal and the PPI equals the TCL only at the site of the arrhythmia. The PPI increases with increasing distance from the arrhythmia source. Therefore, if the PPI exceeds the TCL by 100 ms or more, one may need to investigate the other atrium! As a rule, localized reentry is more frequent than focal AT.

The most troublesome mimic of macroreentrant AT is focal AT or localized reentry originating near a blocked linear lesion. For example, if an AT were to originate anterior to a blocked LA roofline, activation would be high to low anteriorly, low to high posteriorly, and the CS sequence would probably be in a "reverse chevron" pattern. This would be identical to the findings in a roof-dependent flutter. This underscores the importance of entrainment mapping. The PPI-TCL is likely to be less than 30 ms with entrainment performed immediately anterior to the roof line, but crucially would be long if performed from the posterior wall and even longer if performed immediately posterior to the roof line. This phenomenon is important as it is relatively common, it may lead to unnecessary ablation of an already-blocked line, and, if recognized, it gives a strong hint to the location of the tachycardia source.

An unusual potential confounder is the occurrence of incarcerated focal AT. With extensive ablation, it is possible to electrically isolate segments of the atria, most commonly the pulmonary veins, the left atrial appendage, coronary sinus or posterior LA. Rarely, there may be a focal tachycardia within the isolated segment, which is unable to propagate to the remainder of the heart, and can continue independent of the rhythm in the rest of the atria [13]. These segments are generally recognized as their activation timing varies when measured against a reference, and, on closer inspection, they are found to have a different cycle length to the rest of the atria. Interestingly, conduction often recovers once the TCL prolongs upon restoration of sinus rhythm.

Three-dimensional (3D) electroanatomic mapping

Advanced 3D mapping systems are now widely available and frequently used for complex ablation. For atrial tachycardia diagnosis, an activation map is used. A reference is carefully selected, usually a coronary sinus bipole, free of confusing far-field components, and in a stable position. The window of interest is set to include the entire TCL and timing is recorded from various parts of the atrium.

The key to a good quality picture, however, is a little understanding of the circuit before mapping is actually performed. While most ATs originate in the LA, they may also arise from the RA. It is reasonable to perform some form of analysis, such as entrainment, to ensure the correct chamber is assessed. One should be sure to acquire points along the length of the suspected or potential active circuits. Often, during point acquisition, one encounters double potentials; distinct electrograms separated by an isoelectric interval. These occur where the catheter detects activation on both sides of a line of block or conduction delay. Simply taking the earliest potential will lead to a misleading activation sequence;

with a little movement of the catheter one should determine which potential is local and which is far-field from the opposite side of the line of block. If this cannot be determined, it is preferable to mark a point as "double potential, location only." Likewise, the timing of "near-field" versus "far-field" signals within fractionated potentials may be difficult to establish. It is particularly important to correctly annotate double or fractionated signals near linear lesions. More complex, multipotential signals are not rare and may be impossible for automatic annotation of local activation time (LAT). In this setting, we typically acquire several further neighboring points and manually set the LAT from the earliest to the latest components of the complex electrogram.

The characteristic feature of macroreentrant AT on an activation map is "early-meets-late" activation, that is, the area of the latest activation is adjacent to the area of the earliest activation. In general, to achieve this, one must map around 90% of the TCL. Concentric or centrifugal activation suggests a focal tachycardia. If less than 50% of the cycle length has been covered, one needs to consider the possibility that the active circuit may be in the contralateral atrium.

The main disadvantage of this method of diagnosis is that the tachycardia must remain stable for the significant amount of time it takes to accurately complete a map. It is common to encounter multiple ATs in a postpersistent AF ablation patient; each would require a separate activation map, which can become a time-consuming affair. In some patients, ATs may change every few minutes, which can make for a particularly frustrating time where one relies on 3D electroanatomic mapping alone. The use of simultaneous high-density multielectrode mapping may significantly increase the speed of point acquisition [14]. A similar concept is proposed by the new Rhythmia™ (Boston Scientific, Natick, MA) mapping system.

Once the activation map has been completed, selective entrainment mapping should be performed, as previously described.

Noninvasive mapping

While the surface 12-lead ECG can provide valuable hints to identify ATs [15], a number of high-density, surface ECG-based systems have been used to improve diagnostic accuracy. A recent report describes the use of one such system for producing a 3D map of epicardial activation from a single beat of an atrial tachycardia noninvasively [16]. Using invasive mapping as a gold standard, the diagnostic accuracy was 100% in *de novo* ablations and 83% in patients with prior AF ablation. The system was more accurate in cases of centrifugal AT compared to macroreentrant AT, particularly perimitral flutter. Although extensive prior ablation may make interpretation more difficult, the potential for very rapid (single beat) mapping makes this system very promising.

Ablation

The subject of linear ablation is discussed in detail in a separate chapter. In brief, perimitral flutter requires a line of lesions between the mitral annulus and, usually, the isolated left veins; roof-dependent flutter requires a line of lesions between the isolated right and left superior veins; and peritricuspid flutter requires a line of lesions between the tricuspid annulus and the inferior vena cava, that is the cavo-tricuspid isthmus [17,18].

It may be challenging to achieve tachycardia termination and bidirectional block across the significant distances and complex anatomy of the LA. The creation of contiguous transmural lesions remains difficult with current ablation catheter technology. Although 3D mapping packages are widely available, and are an excellent tool for marking lesion location, the gap in a line may be in an area of previous incomplete ablation. Furthermore, some patients have already undergone linear ablation; where possible it is better to target the gap in the line, rather than repeat a full line of lesions. Although these gaps may be identified by their narrow split potentials or continuous fractionation, acute edema from ablation may make their low amplitude signals difficult to detect.

It is possible to use some of the information obtained from mapping to help identify gaps in a line.

For instance, after establishing that a patient with prior mitral isthmus ablation is in a counter-clockwise perimitral flutter, it would be reasonable to first measure timing just lateral to the mitral line of ablation, looking for the earliest "breakthrough" point. In clockwise flutter, the earliest point on the septal side of the line should be sought. In a patient with prior roofline ablation and roof-dependent flutter, the "breakthrough" point may be sought from anterior to the line where the posterior wall activates low to high and on the posterior side when activation is high to low. Thus, one may establish whether the gap is on the septal or lateral side, for

example. As previously discussed, PPI may be shorter near the circuit, and, in particular, the gap in a line set, than further away.

In an ideal world, upon successful atrial tachycardia termination, we ought to be rewarded with sinus rhythm. In the real world, however, this is not always the case. Often, when one tachycardia is eliminated another immediately replaces it. While this can usually be easily recognized because of a change in the coronary sinus activation sequence and a prolongation in the cycle length, the change may be very subtle. This is especially true in the context of extensive ablation with linear lesions. Sometimes, the only sign of a change in tachycardia will be a change in F-wave morphology or timing on the surface ECG. If in doubt, a quick activation map or entrainment from the suspected circuit may show a new sequence and prevent unnecessary ablation.

The following *case study* will illustrate this point: A 47-year-old man underwent his third catheter ablation for persistent atrial fibrillation. Previously, pulmonary vein isolation, complex-fractionated electrogram ablation, and left atrial roof and mitral isthmus lines were performed. At baseline, he was in a stable atrial tachycardia with a cycle length of 275 ms.

Activation was proximal to distal in the coronary sinus and lateral to septal in the anterior left atrium (Figure 4), therefore compatible with a

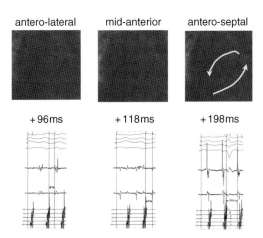

antero-lateral	mid-anterior	antero-septal
+96 ms	+118 ms	+198 ms

Figure 4 Case study. Activation timing anterior is earlier lateral (96 ms after the reference) than septal (198 ms after the reference), that is, lateral-to-septal. Activation posteriorly is proximal-to-distal, that is, septal-to-lateral, and covers the remainder of the cycle length. This is consistent with anticlockwise perimitral flutter.

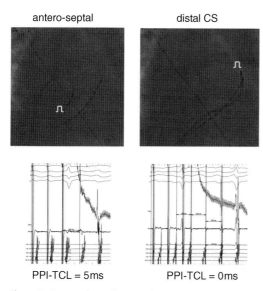

antero-septal	distal CS
PPI-TCL = 5ms	PPI-TCL = 0ms

Figure 5 Case study. During entrainment mapping, the postpacing interval in the distal coronary sinus was equal to the tachycardia cycle length, and only 5 ms longer in the septum. The fact that distant sites are both "in circuit" is consistent with a macroreentrant tachycardia and in this instance is consistent with perimitral flutter.

counterclockwise perimitral circuit. Entrainment mapping found a good PPI on both the LA septum and in the distal coronary sinus (Figure 5), that is, confirming a perimitral flutter. However,

further entrainment mapping demonstrated a good PPI in the high anterior and low posterior LA, that is, consistent with a double-loop tachycardia (Figure 6).

Ablation was started on the roof line, at a fragmented site. There was cycle length prolongation with no change to the coronary sinus sequence or the F-wave morphology (Figure 7). Repeat entrainment was performed from the low posterior LA (Figure 8) that was now long. A quick activation map was consistent with a perimitral circuit.

Ablation was delivered at a fragmented site on the mitral isthmus. This time, during ablation there was no alteration in cycle length or coronary sinus activation; however, F-wave morphology clearly changed (Figure 9). A quick activation map now showed septal-to-lateral activation in the anterior wall. The coronary sinus continued to show proximal-to-distal activation in the posterior wall. Activation was septal to lateral in the right atrium. That is, this was not consistent with a macroreentrant tachycardia; it was suggestive of a focal tachycardia, possibly near the septum.

Using the proximal coronary sinus as a reference, the site of the earliest activation was found in the high septum. Note the sharp, low amplitude potential recorded by the ablation catheter (RF D) just before the high amplitude component. This is frequently seen and often predicts a successful ablation, as in this case (Figure 10).

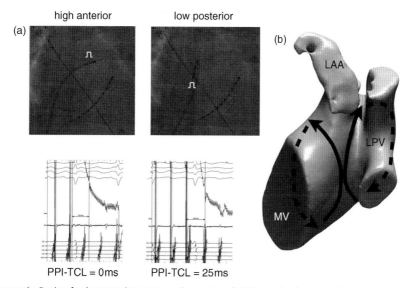

high anterior	low posterior	
(a)		(b)
PPI-TCL = 0ms	PPI-TCL = 25ms	

Figure 6 Case study. During further entrainment mapping, a "good" PPI was also found on the high anterior and low posterior LA (a), suggesting a concomitant roof-dependent circuit. In this double-loop flutter, the circuit revolves around the mitral annulus in a counterclockwise direction, and around the left pulmonary veins. From this angle (b), it is easy to see why they are often called a "figure-of-eight" circuit.

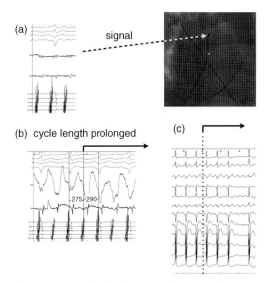

(a)

signal

(b) cycle length prolonged

(c)

275 290

Figure 7 Case study. Ablation was performed at the roof line at a site with fragmented signal (a). Shortly after ablation start, there was a cycle length prolongation (b). However, there was no change to the F-wave morphology on the surface ECG (c).

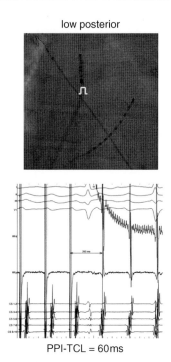

low posterior

PPI-TCL = 60ms

Figure 8 Case study. Repeat entrainment from the low posterior wall found a postpacing interval 60 ms longer than the tachycardia cycle length. The tachycardia is now only perimitral; the roof-dependent component has been successfully terminated.

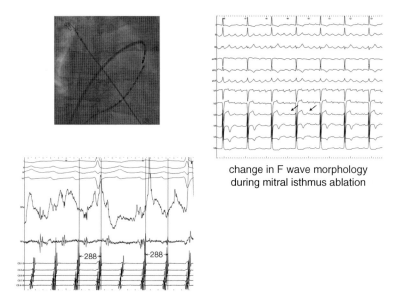

change in F wave morphology
during mitral isthmus ablation

288   288

Figure 9 Case study. During mitral isthmus ablation, there was no change in either the cycle length or the coronary sinus activation. However, there was a clear change in F-wave morphology during ablation.

high septal

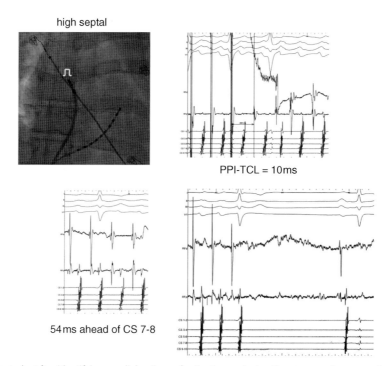

PPI-TCL = 10ms

54 ms ahead of CS 7-8

Figure 10 Case study. After identifying a radial pattern of activation and using the coronary sinus as a reference, this high septal site was found to have the earliest activation and a "good" PPI. Ablation here restored sinus rhythm.

Summary

Macroreentrant atrial tachycardia is frequently encountered in the setting of ablation for persistent atrial fibrillation. By understanding their circuits, they may be readily diagnosed and successfully ablated.

Abbreviations

3D	three-dimensional
AF	atrial fibrillation
AT	atrial tachycardia
CS	coronary sinus
ECG	electrocardiogram
LA	left atrium
LAT	local activation time
PPI	postpacing interval
RA	right atrium
TCL	tachycardia cycle length

References

1 Haïssaguerre M, Sanders P, Hocini M, et al. Catheter ablation of long-lasting persistent atrial fibrillation: critical structures for termination. J Cardiovasc Electrophysiol. 2005;16:1125–1137.

2 O'Neill MD, Wright M, Knecht S, et al. Long-term follow-up of persistent atrial fibrillation ablation using termination as a procedural endpoint. Eur Heart J. 2009; 30:1105–1112.

3 Knecht S, Hocini M, Wright M, et al. Left atrial linear lesions are required for successful treatment of persistent atrial fibrillation. Eur Heart J. 2008;29:2359–2366.

4 Ammar S, Hessling G, Reents T, et al. Arrhythmia type after persistent atrial fibrillation ablation predicts success of the repeat procedure. Circ Arrhythm Electrophysiol. 2011;4:609–614.

5 Saoudi N, Cosio F, Waldo A, et al. A classification of atrial flutter and regular atrial tachycardia according to electrophysiological mechanisms and anatomical bases; a Statement from a Joint Expert Group from the Working Group of Arrhythmias of the European Society and the North American Society of Pacing and Electrophysiology. Eur Heart J. 2001;22:1162–1182.

6 Jaïs P, Matsuo S, Knecht S, et al. A deductive mapping strategy for atrial tachycardia following atrial fibrillation ablation: importance of localized reentry. J Cardiovasc Electrophysiol. 2009;20:480–491.

7 Cosio FG, Lopez Gil M, Arribas F, et al. Mechanisms of entrainment of human common flutter studied with multiple endocardial recordings. Circulation. 1994;89: 2117–2125.

8 Santucci PA, Varma N, Cytron J, et al. Electroanatomic mapping of post pacing intervals clarifies the complete active circuit and variants in atrial flutter. Heart Rhythm. 2009;6:1586–1595.

9 Pascale P, Shah AJ, Roten L, et al. Disparate activation of the coronary sinus and inferior left atrium during atrial tachycardia after persistent atrial fibrillation ablation: prevalence, pitfalls, and impact on mapping. J Cardiovasc Electrophysiol. 2012;23:697–707.

10 Chugh A, Latchamsetty R, Oral H, et al. Characteristics of cavotricuspid isthmus-dependent atrial flutter after left atrial ablation of atrial fibrillation. Circulation. 2006;113 (5):609–615.

11 Pascale P, Shah A, Roten L, et al. Pattern and timing of the coronary sinus activation to guide rapid diagnosis of atrial tachycardia after atrial fibrillation ablation. Circ Arrhythm Electrophysiol. 2013;6:481–490.

12 Vollmann D, Stevenson WG, Luthje L, et al. Misleading long post-pacing interval after entrainment of typical atrial flutter from the cavo-tricuspid isthmus. J Am Coll Cardiol. 2012;59:819–824.

13 Miyazaki S, Shah AJ, Haïssaguerre M, et al. Multiple atrial tachycardias after atrial fibrillation ablation: the importance of careful mapping and observation. Circ Arrhythm Electrophysiol. 2011;4(2):251–254.

14 Patel AM, d'Avila A, Neuzil P, et al. Atrial tachycardia after ablation of persistent atrial fibrillation: identification of the critical isthmus with a combination of multi-electrode activation mapping and targeted entrainment mapping. Circ Arrhythm Electrophysiol. 2008;1(1): 14–22.

15 Gerstenfeld EP, Dixit S, Bala R, et al. Surface electro-cardiogram characteristics of atrial tachycardias occurring after pulmonary vein isolation. Heart Rhythm. 2007;4(9):1136–1143.

16 Shah AJ, Hocini M, Xhaet O, et al. Validation of novel 3D electrocardiographic mapping of atrial tachycardias by invasive mapping and ablation: a multicenter study. J Am Coll Cardiol. 2013;62(10):889–897.

17 Hocini M, Jaïs P, Sanders P, et al. Techniques, evaluation, and consequences of linear block at the left atrial roof in paroxysmal atrial fibrillation: a prospective randomized study. Circulation. 2005;112:3688–3696.

18 Jaïs P, Hocini M, Hsu LF, et al. Technique and results of linear ablation at the mitral isthmus. Circulation. 2004; 110:2996–3002.

CHAPTER 24

Follow-up after ablation: assessing success, symptom status, and recurrent arrhythmias

Simon Kircher, Charlotte Eitel, & Gerhard Hindricks

Department of Electrophysiology, University of Leipzig, Heart Center Leipzig, Germany

Introduction

Whilst standardized procedural endpoints have been established for different atrial fibrillation (AF) ablation approaches, a uniform definition of *ablation success* is lacking. *Ablation success* may be clinically defined as the absence of any AF-related symptoms during the follow-up period. This definition, however, is limited by the lack of specificity of reported symptoms, the high incidence of silent arrhythmia recurrence after ablation, and the need for a more precise rhythm assessment in certain subsets of patients. Freedom from arrhythmia recurrence as evidenced by different electrocardiogram (ECG) recording strategies usually is applied as a more objective outcome measure. The diagnostic yield of different strategies, however, varies greatly with intensity and duration of rhythm monitoring. This chapter will summarize and discuss clinically relevant aspects of currently applied follow-up strategies after AF ablation and their implications for *ablation success*.

Limitations of symptom-based follow-up strategies

A postinterventional follow-up strategy purely based on symptom reporting may be considered sufficient to define *ablation success* since AF ablation primarily

Practical Guide to Catheter Ablation of Atrial Fibrillation,
Second Edition. Edited by Jonathan S. Steinberg, Pierre Jaïs and Hugh Calkins.
© 2016 John Wiley & Sons, Ltd. Published 2016 by John Wiley & Sons, Ltd.

aims at the elimination of AF-associated symptoms and the improvement of quality of life [1,2]. Additionally, full disclosure of rhythm outcome may not be required since long-term anticoagulation should be guided by the individual stroke risk rather than by the absence of arrhythmia recurrences [1,2]. A more objective rhythm assessment, however, based on regularly scheduled or even continuous ECG monitoring may be advantageous in both clinical care and clinical research trials for several reasons:

First, a follow-up strategy solely based on symptom reporting is considerably limited by the high incidence of asymptomatic arrhythmia recurrences after ablation (see below) and a poor symptom–arrhythmia correlation, respectively (Figures 1 and 2) [3–10]. Palpitations resulting from extrasystoles or sinus tachycardia, for instance, may be falsely classified as AF in a substantial proportion of patients. This lack of specificity of reported symptoms has been demonstrated in several patient cohorts [3–7]. Israel et al. reported that 44 out of 110 patients (40%) with a history of AF and a permanent pacemaker experienced AF-related symptoms, while standard ECG recordings and device interrogations proved the absence of AF at the time of symptom occurrence [3]. In a study by Quirino et al. including 89 pacemaker patients with paroxysmal AF, perceived symptoms could be attributed to device-stored AF in only 240 out of 1141 (21%) reported episodes [4]. A subgroup analysis of the "Mode Selection Trial" (MOST) including 312 pacemaker recipients revealed a sensitivity of symptom reporting of 82.4%, whereas specificity and positive predictive value measured only 38.3% and 58.7%, respectively, when symptom data and device-stored "atrial high

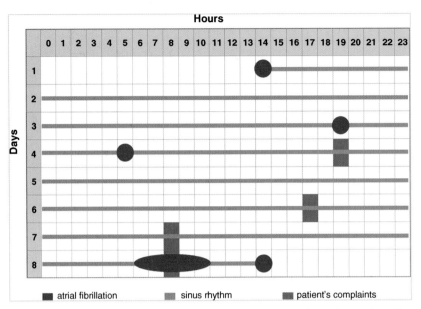

Figure 1 Schematic representation of a "complaints table" derived from a patients' log during a 7-day Holter recording period. This example demonstrates the poor correlation between reported symptoms (blue) and documented episodes of AF recurrence (red). *Source:* Arya et al., Pacing Clin Electrophysiol 2007;30:458–462. Reproduced with permission of Wiley.

rate events" were analyzed [5]. Similar data were reported from clinical trials investigating the diagnostic value of symptom reporting after catheter ablation for AF [6,7]. Neumann et al. reported that 9 out of 80 patients (11%) experienced symptoms suggestive of arrhythmia recurrences without any corresponding ECG documentation during repetitive rhythm monitoring using an external event recorder [6]. In another study using an implantable loop recorder (ILR) with automated AF detection for continuous rhythm monitoring, false positive symptom reporting was observed in 13 out of 45 patients (29%) without arrhythmia recurrence with the sensitivity of symptom reporting being only 53% [7].

Second, valid rhythm surveillance is a prerequisite for the comparison of different rhythm control interventions in both clinical practice and research trials [11]. Third, detection of asymptomatic AF or atrial tachycardia episodes in the early postablation period may help to identify patients who are at a higher risk of long-term treatment failure since early recurrences have been shown to independently predict late recurrences [12,13]. And finally, a more reliable assessment of rhythm outcome may help to guide decision making in certain clinical scenarios, for example, discontinuation of antithrombotic therapy in patients with a low to moderate stroke risk according to currently applied clinical risk stratification schemes.

Asymptomatic arrhythmia recurrence after catheter ablation

It is well established that *silent* or *asymptomatic* AF occurs frequently in the general AF population and that *real* AF burden may be grossly underestimated [14,15]. It is appreciated that at least one third of AF patients have subclinical arrhythmia episodes [16]. Additionally, there is growing evidence that asymptomatic AF confers a relevant risk for thromboembolic events [17,18]. Patients who are selected for AF ablation predominantly constitute a highly symptomatic subgroup among AF patients. Thus, AF-related symptoms theoretically may provide a valid surrogate parameter to detect arrhythmia recurrences after ablation. This concept, however, is not only limited by the low specificity of symptom reporting but also by the observation that AF may recur without any clinical signs or symptoms in a substantial proportion of patients [7–10]. Klemm et al. followed 80 patients after catheter ablation for paroxysmal AF using daily and symptom-activated transtelephonic ECG transmissions [8]. After 6 months of follow-up, 752 out of 1398 (54%) transmitted AF episodes were clinically silent with approximately 9% of patients with documented AF recurrence being completely asymptomatic. In another study including 114 highly symptomatic patients undergoing AF

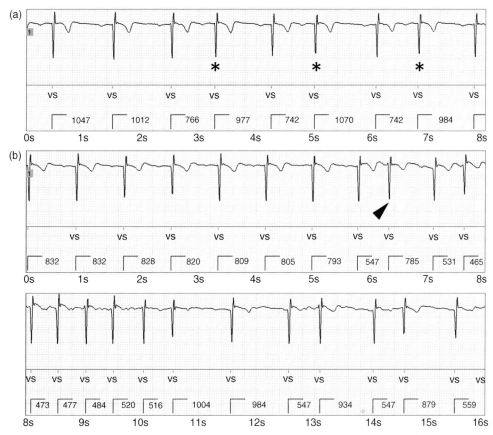

Figure 2 Two examples of device-stored electrograms derived from an implantable loop recorder. In Figure 2a, electrogram storage was manually triggered by the patient due to palpitations suggestive of atrial fibrillation. Analysis of the stored electrogram, however, revealed frequent premature atrial contractions (*), but no atrial fibrillation. Figure 2b displays the initiation (black arrow) of a clinically silent atrial fibrillation episode that was automatically stored and correctly classified by the implantable loop recorder.

catheter ablation, rhythm monitoring consisted of serial 7-day Holter ECG recordings performed prior to the ablation procedure, immediately after ablation and after 3, 6, and 12 months of follow-up [9]. Prior to the procedure, exclusively asymptomatic AF was observed in 5 out of 92 patients (5%) with AF episodes. After ablation, the proportion of patients with entirely silent AF recurrence significantly increased to 38%, 37%, and 36% after 3, 6, and 12 months of follow-up, respectively (Figure 3). These results were confirmed by the "Discerning Symptomatic and Asymptomatic Episodes Pre and Post Radiofrequency Ablation of Atrial Fibrillation" (DISCERN AF) trial [10]. In this prospective, multicenter trial including 50 patients undergoing AF ablation, an ILR was used for continuous rhythm monitoring. The proportion of asymptomatic arrhythmia episodes significantly increased from 52% before to 79% after ablation ($p = 0.002$) with the ratio of silent to

symptomatic AF episodes rising from 1.1 before to 3.7 after ablation. Exclusively asymptomatic arrhythmia recurrences were observed in 12% of patients during the 18-month follow-up period. In a study by Tondo et al. using the same ILR, almost half of the patients with arrhythmia recurrences (21 out of 46 patients) experienced entirely silent recurrence beyond a 3-month blanking period [7]. Potential explanations for this modified arrhythmia perception may be changes in arrhythmia pattern (e.g., shorter duration of recurrences, lower heart rate variability during arrhythmia episodes), an ablation-induced modulation of the autonomic nervous system, the effect of postinterventional antiarrhythmic drug therapy, and a placebo effect that has been previously observed after other invasive procedures [9,10,19]. Verma et al. described a time-dependent pattern in the occurrence of silent arrhythmia relapses in 86 patients with a permanent pacemaker allowing

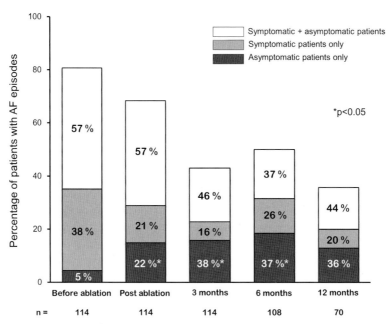

Figure 3 Rhythm outcome and atrial fibrillation perception before and after catheter ablation. After circumferential pulmonary vein ablation and placement of linear lesions at the left atrial roof and at the mitral isthmus line, respectively, patients were followed by serial 7-day Holter ECG recordings. The inferior part of each bar (*dark gray*) represents the percentage of patients with exclusively asymptomatic AF episodes among all patients with AF documentation on Holter ECG. *Source:* Hindricks et al., 2005 [9], Circulation 2005;112:307–313. Reproduced with permission of Lippencott, Williams & Wilkins.

for continuous rhythm surveillance [20]. During the first 3 months after ablation, 21 out of 66 (32%) asymptomatic patients had mode-switch episodes indicating arrhythmia recurrence. Beyond that period, this percentage significantly declined with only 2 out of 66 (3%) asymptomatic patients having silent recurrences until 9 months of follow-up.

Tools for postablation rhythm monitoring

In clinical practice, follow-up is usually based on *intermittent* or *noncontinuous* rhythm monitoring technologies including scheduled and symptom-triggered standard ECGs, Holter ECG recordings (24 h to 7 days), external loop recorders, and event recorders [1]. Some technologies provide repetitive *snapshots* of cardiac rhythm (e.g., standard ECGs, event recorders) whereas others allow for continuous rhythm surveillance during a predefined time window (e.g., Holter ECG recordings, external loop recorders). Choice of either method and the intensity of follow-up depend upon the clinical impact of arrhythmia recognition and the patient's compliance that may be negatively affected by a more complex monitoring strategy [21]. Event recorders are used

for scheduled (e.g., daily) and patient-initiated ECG recordings with a recording duration of 30 to 60 s [22]. Recorded ECGs may be transmitted via telephone or internet to a service center or may be stored on a memory card for further analyses. As the device is not permanently attached to the skin, this technology may be used for extended follow-up periods. The diagnostic yield of this technology, however, is limited by the lack of information concerning the duration of the detected arrhythmia episodes. ECG loop recorders (external and implantable) are equipped with a retrospective memory function allowing for continuous ECG recording and deletion. ECG storage is activated either automatically in the event of arrhythmia episodes detected by incorporated algorithms or manually by the patient when arrhythmia-related symptoms are perceived (Figure 2). As opposed to event recorders, external loop recorders require permanent attachment of adhesive electrodes on the skin leading to discomfort and lifestyle restrictions that have been shown to impair patient's adherence [22]. Thus, this tool is restricted to highly motivated individuals for a limited period of time (usually 1 to 4 weeks).

Continuous rhythm monitoring is largely based on implantable cardiac devices allowing for permanent

(a)

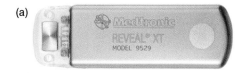

(b)

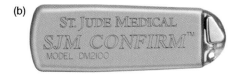

(c)

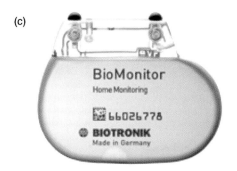

Figure 4 Examples of commercially available implantable loop recorders. From top to bottom: The REVEAL® XT (Medtronic Inc., Minneapolis, USA), the Confirm™ (St Jude Medical Inc., St Paul, USA), and the BioMonitor (Biotronik SE, Berlin, Germany). This list is not intended to be exhaustive.

arrhythmia detection irrespective of episode duration or associated symptoms. Permanent pacemakers and implantable cardioverter-defibrillators equipped with an atrial lead and capable of arrhythmia detection, storage, and quantification provide highly accurate rhythm surveillance [23]. By nature, these technologies are confined to a small group of patients with a standard indication for device therapy. More recently, subcutaneous leadless ILRs have been introduced as new diagnostic tools to enable uninterrupted long-term rhythm monitoring without the need for intracardiac ECG recording (Figure 4). These ILRs have been incorporated into current guidelines as diagnostic tools for the work-up of patients with unexplained syncope [24]. The Reveal XT Performance Trial (XPECT) prospectively validated the performance of an ILR equipped with dedicated AF detection capabilities in 247 patients with paroxysmal AF [25]. The AF detection algorithm analyzes the irregularity and incoherence of R–R intervals within a 2-min time window. Comparison of the automated AF detection algorithm of the ILR with simultaneously acquired 46-h Holter ECG recordings demonstrated a sensitivity, specificity, positive predictive value, and negative predictive value of 96.1%,

85.4%, 79.3%, and 97.4%, respectively, for detecting patients with any AF episode. False-positive classification by the detection algorithm was due to frequent premature atrial or ventricular complexes, oversensing of myopotentials, sinus arrhythmias, R-wave undersensing, and other atrial arrhythmias. Major shortcomings of currently available ILR technologies include storage overflow, the high proportion of non-diagnostic device interrogations, and the exclusion of short-lasting AF episodes [26]. These limitations may be successfully approached by software modifications, individual device programming and remote device interrogation aiming at reducing the risk of storage exhaustion.

Intensity of ECG monitoring and rhythm outcome

The wide range of reported *success rates* after catheter ablation is not only related to differences in patient cohorts, ablation strategies, definitions of arrhythmia recurrences, patients' AF burden, blanking periods, and the use of concomitant antiarrhythmic treatment but also to the intensity of postinterventional rhythm monitoring [27–35]. The positive correlation between the intensity of follow-up and the arrhythmia detection rate has been consistently demonstrated in several clinical studies investigating the diagnostic yield of different ECG monitoring technologies (Figure 5, Table 1). In a study by Kottkamp et al. the rate of AF recurrences detected by 7-day Holter ECG monitoring was significantly higher both immediately after ablation and at 3 and 6 months follow-up compared to a conventional approach using 24-h Holter ECG recordings in 100 patients with paroxysmal or persistent AF (Figure 6) [30]. These data were confirmed by Dagres et al. who assessed the impact of different Holter ECG durations on recurrence rate in 215 patients at 6 months after catheter ablation [31]. Extending the duration of Holter ECG recording substantially enhanced the sensitivity for arrhythmia detection with any Holter ECG duration equal to or lower than 5 days missing a statistically significant percentage of patients with recurrence when compared to the complete 7-day Holter monitoring period. Senatore et al. followed 72 patients by 12-lead ECGs and conventional 24-h Holter ECG recordings performed 1 and 4 months after ablation and by daily plus symptom-initiated 30-s transtelephonic ECG transmissions applied during a 3-month period [32]. During the follow-up period, transtelephonic ECG monitoring identified significantly more patients with AF recurrence, thereby decreasing short-term *success rate* from 86 to 72% ($p = 0.001$). In a

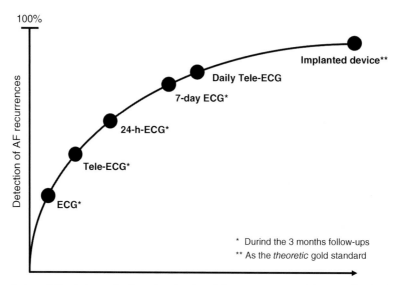

Figure 5 Estimated correlation between the intensity of a given follow-up strategy and the rate of arrhythmia detection after radiofrequency catheter ablation. *Source:* Arya et al., Pacing Clin Electrophysiol 2007;30:458–462. Reproduced with permission of Wiley.

study by Piorkowski et al., serial 7-day Holter ECG recordings and regularly scheduled (i.e. every 2 days) plus symptom-driven transtelephonic ECG transmissions were equally effective in detecting AF recurrence (50 and 45% of patients, respectively) during a follow-up period of 6 months [33]. The additive benefit of continuous rhythm monitoring has been demonstrated in clinical studies using cardiac devices for rhythm monitoring. In the DISCERN AF study, the absence of arrhythmia recurrence could be found in 56% of patients if follow-up was based on symptom reporting and intermittent ECG recordings using standard ECGs and 48-h Holter monitoring performed every 3 months [10]. *Procedural success*, however, decreased to 46% when arrhythmia episodes detected by the ILR were considered. In the prospective "Assessing Arrhythmia Burden after Catheter Ablation of Atrial Fibrillation Using an Implantable Loop Recorder" (ABACUS) trial, 44 patients undergoing AF ablation received an ILR and conventional monitoring consisting of twice daily pulse rate assessment by the patient and three 30-day transtelephonic monitors at discharge, at 5 months, and at 11 months postablation [34]. During the initial 6 months of the study period after ablation, significantly more patients with AF recurrence were identified by the ILR in comparison to *conventional* monitoring (47% versus 18%; $p = 0.002$). Martinek et al. followed 14 patients with a permanent pacemaker capable of arrhythmia detection and storage for 41.4 ± 15.1 months [35]. Ablation success was defined as a reduction of atrial tachyarrhythmia burden to less than 10 min per day.

This *response rate* decreased from 71% when follow-up was solely based on symptom reporting to 57% when simulated 7-day Holter recordings were analyzed. The *success rate* further dropped to 43% when outcome was assessed by pacemaker interrogations with only 21% of patients being free from any arrhythmia recurrence.

Duration of the follow-up period and long-term success

Another major determinant of *arrhythmia recurrence rate* is the duration of the entire follow-up period. The inverse relationship between rhythm outcome and follow-up duration has been described in clinical studies that demonstrated a successive decline of arrhythmia-free survival over a time span of several years [36–38]. Even in highly experienced centers less than one third of patients were free from arrhythmia recurrence after a single ablation procedure during long-term follow-up lasting up to 6 years [36,37]. In a study by Weerasooriya et al., 100 patients with paroxysmal or persistent AF were followed by serial 24-h Holter ECGs and symptom-triggered ECG recording [36]. After a single catheter ablation procedure, the absence of any AF or atrial tachycardia recurrence lasting at least 30 s was achieved in 40%, 37%, and 29% of patients at 1, 2, and 5 years, respectively. In a retrospective observational study by Bertaglia et al. 177 patients who were considered free from any atrial arrhythmia recurrence during the first year after a single catheter ablation procedure were followed for another 49.7 ± 13.3 months [38]. During

Table 1 This table demonstrates the relationship between different methods of rhythm follow-up and the ablation success in a sample of clinical trials that evaluated the diagnostic yield of different rhythm monitoring tools.

Writing group	No. of patients	Type of AF	Definition of ablation success	Method of arrhythmia recurrence detection	Follow-up duration (months)	Success rate (%)
Vasamreddy et al. [21]	19	PAF/ PsAF	Absence of symptomatic and asymptomatic AF	Symptom reporting	6	70
				External loop recorder		50
Kottkamp et al. [30]	100	PAF/ PsAF	Freedom from AF recurrences >30 s	24-h Holter monitoring	12	78*
				7-day Holter monitoring		63*
Senatore et al. [32]	72	PAF/ PsAF	Atrial arrhythmia recurrences	24-h Holter monitoring plus 12-lead ECGs	4	86
				Daily and symptom-triggered TT ECG recordings		72
				Symptom reporting	6	70
Piorkowski et al. [33]	30	PAF/ PsAF	Freedom from AF recurrences >30 s	7-day Holter monitoring		50
				Regularly scheduled (i.e. every 2 days) plus symptom-triggered TT ECG recordings		45
Verma et al. [10]	50	PAF/ PsAF	Freedom from AF/AFL/ AT recurrence ≥2 min	Symptom reporting	18	58
				Symptom reporting plus 48-h Holter monitoring plus ECGs		56
				ILR		46
Kapa et al. [34]	44	PAF/ PsAF	Absence of AF/OAT recurrence	Twice daily pulse rate assessment plus two 30-day TT monitor periods	6	82
				ILR		53
Martinek et al. [35]	14	PAF/ PsAF	Reduction of ATB to less than 10 min per day	Symptom reporting	41.4 ± 15.1	72
				24- or 48-h Holter monitoring		64
				7-day Holter ECG monitoring		57
				Permanent pacemaker		43

Notably, there is no uniform definition of *arrhythmia recurrence*. Abbreviations: AF, atrial fibrillation; AFL, atrial flutter; AT, atrial tachycardia; ATB, atrial tachyarrhythmia burden; ECG, electrocardiogram; ILR, implantable loop recorder; OAT, organized atrial tachycardia; PAF, paroxysmal atrial fibrillation; PsAF, persistent atrial fibrillation; TT, transtelephonic.
*Reported rhythm outcome was assessed during the Holter monitoring period at 12 months.

that follow-up period, arrhythmia recurrences defined as any atrial tachyarrhythmia lasting longer than 30 s could be detected in approximately 42% of these patients. These very late arrhythmia recurrences emphasize the need for prolonged rhythm surveillance even in those patients who appear to be successfully treated after 12 months of follow-up. Factors that may contribute to the development of late recurrence include resumption of pulmonary vein conduction, the emergence of non-pulmonary vein triggers, and a dynamic substrate related to the progression of an underlying fibrotic atrial cardiomyopathy and to the permanent influence of associated clinical conditions (e.g., arterial hypertension and aging), respectively [39,40].

Practical considerations and definition of ablation success

The optimal outcome of any rhythm control strategy would be complete freedom from any atrial

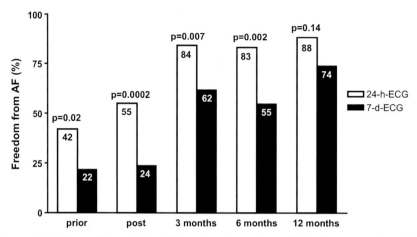

Figure 6 Diagnostic yield of two different Holter ECG durations after catheter ablation for paroxysmal atrial fibrillation. As compared to 24-h Holter ECG recordings (open bars), 7-day Holter ECGs (closed bars) identified significantly more patients with AF episodes prior to ablation, immediately after ablation, and at 3 and 6 months, respectively. *Source:* Kottkamp et al., 2004 [30], J Am Coll Cardiol 2004;44(4):869–77. Reproduced with permission of Elsevier.

arrhythmia recurrence. This global definition of *ablation success*, however, does not withstand reality, which is related to methodological limitations of conventionally applied postinterventional intermittent rhythm monitoring strategies to reliably detect all arrhythmia episodes. Whilst full disclosure of rhythm outcome would be desirable in clinical research trials to assess the efficacy of different rhythm control strategies irrespective of symptomatology, a more differentiated appraisal is required to assess the value and the practicability of available rhythm monitoring methods in clinical practice. Expert consensus recommends that all patients should be followed with repetitive ECGs at a minimum of 3 months after the ablation and subsequently every 6 months for at least 2 years [1]. A more intense follow-up should be mainly driven by the clinical relevance of arrhythmia detection. Currently, clinical follow-up is largely based on symptom reporting, symptom-triggered ECG recording, and intermittent ECG monitoring (e.g., 24-h to 7-day Holter recordings). Repetitive 7-day Holter ECG recordings or routine daily plus symptom-initiated event recordings are estimated to capture approximately 70% of AF recurrences [1,41]. Regularly scheduled ECG recordings help to detect asymptomatic arrhythmia episodes, which is particularly important in patients who are prone to AF-related complications (e.g., thromboembolic events or tachycardia-induced cardiomyopathy). As described above, however, noncontinuous ECG monitoring fails to disclose arrhythmia recurrence in a substantial proportion of patients. The clinical impact of this limited sensitivity has to be judged on an individual basis. Elimination or attenuation of

arrhythmia-related symptoms may be an acceptable therapeutic success in patients with entirely silent AF or minimally symptomatic, short-lasting episodes of arrhythmia recurrence. Additionally, rhythm control by means of previously ineffective antiarrhythmic drugs may be considered a successful treatment. These *clinical definitions* of ablation success are supported by data indicating a significant improvement in quality of life in patients with asymptomatic arrhythmia recurrence after ablation [42]. Conversely, highly accurate rhythm surveillance may be needed to guide clinicians' decision making in certain subgroups of patients. A more comprehensive monitoring strategy may be advisable for rhythm–symptom correlation in patients who report arrhythmia-related symptoms outside the monitoring window. Furthermore, discontinuation of oral anticoagulation might be considered in selected patients with a low-to-moderate stroke risk and freedom from any arrhythmia recurrence as evidenced by a rhythm monitoring strategy allowing for reliable conclusions about rhythm control. In a retrospective analysis by Botto et al. including 568 patients with a history of AF and permanent pacemaker implantation, the combination of the CHADS$_2$ score with the duration of AF episodes derived from device memory was associated with a more precise characterization of the individual risk for thromboembolic events [43]. It has to be emphasized that there is no generally accepted recommendation for anticoagulant therapy after apparently successful ablation that is related to a lack of randomized, clinical studies investigating the safety of anticoagulation discontinuation [1,2]. Extended ECG monitoring may add valuable information to postprocedural treatment in the event of arrhythmia recurrences or in case of uncertainties concerning rhythm control. In the ABACUS trial, continuous monitoring with an ILR was associated with a significantly higher rate of antiarrhythmic drug and rate control agent discontinuation compared to conventional monitoring using transtelephonic ECG transmission [34]. These differences were attributed to a lack of rhythm–symptom correlation in conventionally monitored patients in the event of symptom perception and the detection of clinically relevant non-AF arrhythmias (bradycardias and ventricular tachycardias) in the ILR group.

Conclusions

The definition of *ablation success* after ablation for AF remains controversial, which is primarily related to the limited diagnostic yield of currently applied postinterventional rhythm monitoring strategies. The lacking specificity of symptom reporting and the high incidence of asymptomatic arrhythmia recurrences have been clearly demonstrated in clinical trials. The accuracy of detecting arrhythmia recurrences depends chiefly upon the intensity and duration of follow-up. In clinical practice, the choice of either ECG monitoring strategy should be based on the clinical impact of arrhythmia detection. In certain subgroup of patients, a precise and sufficiently long rhythm monitoring may be required to guide individual clinical decision making. Recently, a leadless ILR has been validated in a clinical trial demonstrating a high sensitivity and overall accuracy for detecting AF. Uninterrupted rhythm monitoring provided by ILRs may allow for the development of new follow-up standards for both clinical care and scientific purposes.

References

1 Calkins H, Kuck KH, Cappato R, et al. 2012 HRS/EHRA/ECAS Expert Consensus Statement on Catheter and Surgical Ablation of Atrial Fibrillation: Recommendations for Patient Selection, Procedural Techniques, Patient Management and Follow-up, Definitions, Endpoints, and Research Trial Design. Europace. 2012;14:528–606.

2 Camm JA, Cappato R, Ann Chen S, et al. Venice Chart international consensus document on atrial fibrillation ablation: 2011 update. J Cardiovasc Electrophysiol. 2012;23:890–923.

3 Israel CW, Grönefeld G, Ehrlich JR, et al. Longterm risk of recurrent atrial fibrillation as documented by an implantable monitoring device: implications for optimal patient care. J Am Coll Cardiol. 2004;43:47–52.

4 Quirino G, Giammaria M, Corbucci G, et al. Diagnosis of paroxysmal atrial fibrillation in patients with implanted pacemakers: relationship to symptoms and other variables. Pacing Clin Electrophysiol. 2009;32:91–98.

5 Glotzer TV, Hellkamp AS, Zimmerman J, et al. Atrial high rate episodes detected by pacemaker diagnostics predict death and stroke: report of the Atrial Diagnostics Ancillary Study of the MOde Selection Trial (MOST). Circulation. 2003;107:1614–1619.

6 Neumann T, Erdogan A, Dill T, et al. Asymptomatic recurrences of atrial fibrillation after pulmonary vein isolation. Europace. 2006;8:495–498.

7 Tondo C, Tritto M, Landolina M, et al. Rhythm–symptom correlation in patients on continuous monitoring after catheter ablation of atrial fibrillation. J Cardiovasc Electrophysiol. 2014;25:154–160.

8 Klemm HU, Ventura R, Rostock T, et al. Correlation of symptoms to ECG diagnosis following atrial fibrillation ablation. J Cardiovasc Electrophysiol. 2006;17:146–150.

9 Hindricks G, Piorkowski C, Tanner H, et al. Perception of atrial fibrillation before and after radiofrequency catheter ablation: relevance of asymptomatic arrhythmia recurrence. Circulation. 2005;112:307–313.

10 Verma A, Champagne J, Sapp J, et al. Discerning the incidence of symptomatic and asymptomatic episodes of atrial fibrillation before and after catheter ablation (DISCERN AF): a prospective, multicenter study. JAMA Intern Med. 2013;173:149–156.

11 Kirchhof P, Bax J, Blomstrom-Lundquist C, et al. Early and comprehensive management of atrial fibrillation: proceedings from the 2nd AFNET/EHRA consensus conference on atrial fibrillation entitled "research perspectives in atrial fibrillation." Europace. 2009;11:860–885.

12 Arya A, Hindricks G, Sommer P, et al. Long-term results and the predictors of outcome of catheter ablation of atrial fibrillation using steerable sheath catheter navigation after single procedure in 674 patients. Europace. 2010;12:173–180.

13 Oral H, Knight BP, Ozaydin M, et al. Clinical significance of early recurrences of atrial fibrillation after pulmonary vein isolation. J Am Coll Cardiol. 2002;40:100–104.

14 Rho RW, Page RL. Asymptomatic atrial fibrillation. Prog Cardiovasc Dis. 2005;48:79–87.

15 Ziegler PD, Koehler JL, Mehra R. Comparison of continuous versus intermittent monitoring of atrial arrhythmias. Heart Rhythm. 2006;3:1445–1452.

16 Savelieva I, Camm AJ. Clinical relevance of silent atrial fibrillation: prevalence, prognosis, quality of life, and management. J Interv Card Electrophysiol. 2000;4:369–382.

17 Flaker GC, Belew K, Beckman K, et al. Asymptomatic atrial fibrillation: demographic features and prognostic information from the Atrial Fibrillation Follow-up Investigation of Rhythm Management (AFFIRM) study. Am Heart J. 2005;149:657–663.

18 Healey JS, Connolly SJ, Gold MR, et al. Subclinical atrial fibrillation and the risk of stroke. N Engl J Med. 2012;366:120–129.

19 Saririan M, Eisenberg MJ. Myocardial laser revascularization for the treatment of end-stage coronary artery disease. J Am Coll Cardiol. 2003;41:173–183.

20 Verma A, Minor S, Kilicaslan F, et al. Incidence of atrial arrhythmias detected by permanent pacemakers (PPM) post-pulmonary vein antrum isolation (PVAI) for atrial fibrillation (AF): correlation with symptomatic recurrence. J Cardiovasc Electrophysiol. 2007;18:601–606.

21 Vasamreddy CR, Dalal D, Dong J, et al. Symptomatic and asymptomatic atrial fibrillation in patients undergoing radiofrequency catheter ablation. J Cardiovasc Electrophysiol. 2006;17:134–139.

22 Brignole M, Vardas P, Hoffman E, et al. Indications for the use of diagnostic implantable and external ECG loop recorders. Europace. 2009;11:671–687.

23 Kircher S, Hindricks G, Sommer P. Long-term success and follow-up after atrial fibrillation ablation. Curr Cardiol Rev. 2012;8:354–361.

24 Moya A, Sutton R, Ammirati F, et al. Guidelines for the diagnosis and management of syncope (version 2009). Eur Heart J. 2009;30:2631–2671.

25 Hindricks G, Pokushalov E, Urban L, et al. Performance of a new leadless implantable cardiac monitor in detecting and quantifying atrial fibrillation: results of the XPECT trial. Circ Arrhythm Electrophysiol. 2010;3:141–147.

26 Eitel C, Husser D, Hindricks G, et al. Performance of an implantable automatic atrial fibrillation detection device: impact of software adjustments and relevance of manual episode analysis. Europace. 2011;13:480–485.

27 Wazni OM, Marrouche NF, Martin DO, et al. Radiofrequency ablation vs. antiarrhythmic drugs as first-line treatment of symptomatic atrial fibrillation: a randomized trial. JAMA. 2005;293:2634–2640.

28 Pappone C, Augello G, Sala S, et al. A randomized trial of circumferential pulmonary vein ablation versus antiarrhythmic drug therapy in paroxysmal atrial fibrillation: the APAF Study. J Am Coll Cardiol. 2006;48:2340–2347.

29 Jaïs P, Cauchemez B, Macle L, et al. Catheter ablation versus antiarrhythmic drugs for atrial fibrillation: the A4 study. Circulation. 2008;118:2498–2505.

30 Kottkamp H, Tanner H, Kobza R, et al. Time courses and quantitative analysis of atrial fibrillation episode number and duration after circular plus linear left atrial lesions: trigger elimination or substrate modification: early or delayed cure? J Am Coll Cardiol. 2004;44(4): 869–877.

31 Dagres N, Kottkamp H, Piorkowski C, et al. Influence of the duration of Holter monitoring on the detection of arrhythmia recurrences after catheter ablation of atrial fibrillation: implications for patient follow-up. Int J Cardiol. 2010;139:305–306.

32 Senatore G, Stabile G, Bertaglia E, et al. Role of transtelephonic electrocardiographic monitoring in detecting short-term arrhythmia recurrences after radiofrequency ablation in patients with atrial fibrillation. J Am Coll Cardiol. 2005;45:873–876.

33 Piorkowski C, Kottkamp H, Tanner H, et al. Value of different follow-up strategies to assess the efficacy of circumferential pulmonary vein ablation for the curative treatment of atrial fibrillation. J Cardiovasc Electrophysiol. 2005;16:1286–1292.

34 Kapa S, Epstein AE, Callans DJ, et al. Assessing arrhythmia burden after catheter ablation of atrial fibrillation using an implantable loop recorder: the ABACUS study. J Cardiovasc Electrophysiol. 2013;24:875–881.

35 Martinek M, Aichinger J, Nesser HJ, et al. New insights into long-term follow-up of atrial fibrillation ablation: full disclosure by an implantable pacemaker device. J Cardiovasc Electrophysiol. 2007;18:818–823.

36 Weerasooriya R, Khairy P, Litalien J, et al. Catheter ablation for atrial fibrillation: are results maintained at 5 years of follow-up? J Am Coll Cardiol. 2011;57:160–166.

37 Sorgente A, Tung P, Wylie J, et al. Six year follow-up after catheter ablation of atrial fibrillation: a palliation more than a true cure. Am J Cardiol. 2012;109:1179–1186.

38 Bertaglia E, Tondo C, De Simone A, et al. Does catheter ablation cure atrial fibrillation? Single-procedure outcome of drug refractory atrial fibrillation ablation: a 6-year multicentre experience. Europace. 2010;12: 181–187.

39 Shah AN, Mittal S, Sichrovsky TC, et al. Long-term outcome following successful pulmonary vein isolation: pattern and prediction of very late recurrence. J Cardiovasc Electrophysiol. 2008;19:661–667.

40 Kottkamp H. Human atrial fibrillation substrate: towards a specific fibrotic atrial cardiomyopathy. Eur Heart J. 2013;34:2731–2738.

41 Arya A, Piorkowski C, Sommer P, et al. Clinical implications of various follow up strategies after catheter ablation of atrial fibirllation. Pacing Clin Electrophysiol. 2007;30:458–462.

42 Pontoppidan J, Nielsen JC, Poulsen SH, et al. Symptomatic and asymptomatic atrial fibrillation after pulmonary vein ablation and the impact on quality of life. Pacing Clin Electrophysiol. 2009;32:717–726.

43 Botto GL, Padeletti L, Santini M, et al. Presence and duration of atrial fibrillation detected by continuous monitoring: crucial implications for the risk of thromboembolic events. J Cardiovasc Electrophysiol. 2009;20: 241–248.

CHAPTER 25

How to strategize the "redo" ablation procedure

Jeffrey S. Arkles & David J. Callans
Cardiology Division, Hospital of the University of Pennsylvania, Philadelphia, PA, USA

Introduction

With our current understanding of AF and technology to ablate it, repeat or redo AF ablation is a reality for many patients. Although constantly improving, progress has been incremental rather than exponential toward a goal of single ablation AF control for all patients [1]. In 2010, a worldwide registry reported an average of 1.3 procedures per patient to achieve AF control [2]. In nonparoxysmal patients, with larger and more abnormal atria more ablation procedures are required for control of AF [2–5]. One recent series reported an average of 2.3 ablations per nonparoxysmal patient to achieve AF control [6]. Therefore, "redo" ablation is a reality and one that the patient and practitioner should be comfortable with. Practically, strategizing the redo ablation begins when first meeting the patient. Patients should be honestly informed about the potential need for redo ablation to avoid frustration if there is recurrence. Those patients with a higher likelihood for recurrence should be made very aware that it may require two or more procedures to achieve AF control. If a patient recurs with no improvement in symptoms and will not undergo redo ablation due to discouragement, they will have yielded little benefit for the risk they were exposed to.

Preprocedural factors associated with recurrence

Characteristics of patients likely to experience recurrence after ablation have been described in many

Practical Guide to Catheter Ablation of Atrial Fibrillation, Second Edition. Edited by Jonathan S. Steinberg, Pierre Jaïs and Hugh Calkins.
© 2016 John Wiley & Sons, Ltd. Published 2016 by John Wiley & Sons, Ltd.

studies [7–9]. However, the many of the identified variables are highly confounded and correlate strongly with one another. Left atrial dilation, hypertension, and structural heart disease, including left ventricular and mitral valvular dysfunction, all predict AF recurrence but when controlled for persistence and duration of AF their independent value is lessened [10]. Age and gender are not strong independent predictors of AF when other factors are appropriately controlled [10]. The most consistent, preprocedural patient characteristics are persistence and duration of AF, left atrial size, and presence of structural heart disease. Practically, persistence of AF can be used as a rough guide for estimating the overall risk of recurrence with all other variables refining that risk.

Promising results from different imaging modalities have been shown to predict success and risk of recurrence after AF ablation. A proprietary method of quantification of delayed enhanced MRI (DE-MRI) with atrial specific protocols can predict response to ablation by giving a score related to atrial scar [11]. Intuitively, patients with highly scarred atria are more likely to recur compared to patients with less scar and healthier atria. Subsequent work coregistering atrial voltage maps to areas of DE-MRI supports the validity of DE-MRI-based scar detection in the atria [12]. Echo strain imaging has also been correlated with persistence of AF and degree of atrial scar determined by DE-MRI [13]. Although these imaging techniques show great potential, they have not entered our routine clinical practice.

In our patient population, obstructive sleep apnea is common and often underdiagnosed. The efficacy of AF ablation with obstructive sleep apnea is reduced when compared to patients without sleep disordered breathing even after other comorbidites have been controlled for [14–16]. Treatment of sleep apnea can improve prognosis after AF ablation [14]. Occasionally, we have initiated sleep apnea therapy while inpatient after ablation to speed the process.

Procedural factors and issues related to recurrence and redo ablation

The ablation strategy employed as well as information from initial and subsequent ablations can be useful in predicting future AF recurrence. Antral PVI alone is generally associated with a low burden of organized left atrial tachycardias. A strategy employing linear lesions or substrate-based ablation is at greater risk for the development of left atrial tachycardias [17,18].

Procedure records should be studied to note where ablation may have been limited due to poor contact or limited power delivery because of potential phrenic or esophageal damage. Sites of acute reconnection do not necessarily predict sites of chronic reconnection at redo [19]. When careful assessment of acute reconnection is made and reisolation is performed, acute reconnection does not predict recurrence [20].

Voltage mapping to determine area and extent of scar is useful to determine the likelihood of recurrence [21]. Intuitively, the area and extent of scarring generally correlates with the persistence of AF [22]. Coregistration of DE-MRI scar and voltage map derived areas of scar has shown agreement supporting the validity of both modalities [12].

Postprocedural characteristics of recurrence related to redo ablation

Detailed follow up of the timing and nature arrhythmia recurrence is critical to determining the prognosis and management after ablation. For patients with persistent AF, the type of arrhythmia recurrence can predict the success of the second procedure. Formerly persistent patients with recurrent paroxysmal AF had the best second procedural success, followed by organized atrial tachycardia, and finally persistent AF had the least second procedural success [23].

Early atrial arrhythmias, occurring within 3 months of ablation, are a unique situation. Early recurrences when compared to late or very late recurrence confer a worse prognosis for long-term arrhythmia control [24,25]. Late or very late recurrences are more often to be sporadic and more likely to be manageable with antiarrhythmic drug therapy [26]. However, early atrial arrhythmias after ablation sometimes remit and the long-term prognosis can improve [24,27–29].

The mechanism of these arrhythmias can vary from inflammation-mediated automaticity to proarrhythmia from ablation as well as unmasking of other arrhythmogenic foci.

The majority of recurrences will happen during the first 6–12 months after ablation; however, very late recurrence does also occur. Even in patients with many years of freedom from arrhythmia, there is a 5–6% per year rate of recurrence [30,31].

Non-AF recurrence

Many patients will not recur with AF but rather atrial tachycardias, typical or atypical flutters. Frequently, patients are more symptomatic with a rapidly conducted atrial tachycardia than with their AF. Less commonly other arrhythmias can present that may not have been detected prior to ablation.

Typical right atrial flutter is, of course, associated with AF that can occur after AF ablation. Whenever observed clinically, an appropriate ablation line across the cavo-tricuspid isthmus should be created. However, it is not always diagnosed prior to or during the procedure [32]. There is a reported association in patients with prior cardiac surgery undergoing AF ablation who recur with typical atrial flutter [33].

AVNRT can also seen after AF ablation. Generally, patients with AVNRT as a trigger for AF are younger with a lesser degree of structural heart disease [34]. Although relatively uncommon, it is important not to miss this easily treatable trigger for AF.

The most common non-AF arrhythmias after AF ablation are broadly referred to as "left atrial" tachycardias. Three separate mechanisms, namely, macro-reentry, local re-entry, and focal automaticity are responsible for these arrhythmias [35–37]. The ECG characteristics of these arrhythmias have been reported and can be useful to guide ablation [38]. The incidence of these arrhythmias varies and is often determined by the type of initial ablation. Antral pulmonary vein isolation alone has a reported rate of left atrial flutter of 3–4%, whereas linear lesions are associated with greater risk [17,18].

Macroreentrant atypical flutters are common after ablation. These flutters utilize physical barriers in the left atrium such as the mitral isthmus as well as scar from ablation lesions to create circuits of reentry. Linear ablation lesions with gaps serve as substrate by creating a critical isthmus for slow conduction to occur [18]. Although, many different types of flutters have been documented, they frequently involve reentry around the mitral annulus or reentry around pulmonary veins [35]. The mapping and ablation

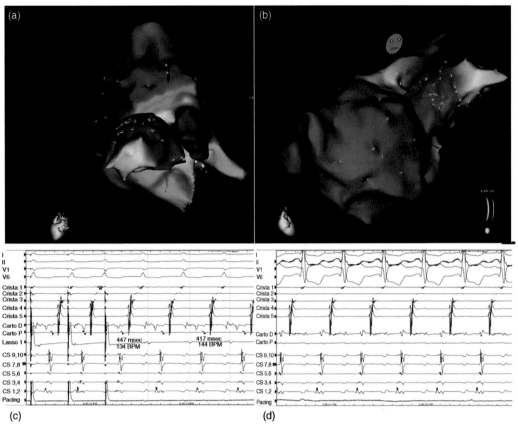

Figure 1 Localized reentry along the LSPV after PVI. The patient presented with a persistent atrial arrhythmia after AF ablation. Entrainment from the proximal and distal coronary sinus was "out" with long return cycle. Activation emanated from the near ridge and LSPV (a) and (b). Entrainment from the LSPV was <30 ms (c). A continuous diastolic potential was noted on the ridge with LSPV and appendage signals present (d). Ablation at this site terminated the tachycardia and isolated the LSPV.

of these arrhythmias are discussed in detail in Chapter 22.

Focal reentrant and nonreentrant atrial tachycardias are also commonly encountered after AF ablation. Focal reentrant tachycardias can be seen at the edges of ablation lesions, for example, between the LSPV and the left atrial appendage [39] (Figure 1). Nonreeentrant focal tachycardias are most commonly seen in the pulmonary veins; however, they can be seen from many other areas of the heart including the crista or coronary sinus [18,39].

Patient selection

For the majority of patients with recurrence, selection is little different from the initial patient selection process. Generally, there is no significant increase in risk with a second or third ablation compared to the first. With each ablation, a thorough evaluation of

the patient's symptoms and arrhythmia burden is required. Significant changes in the health and status of comorbidities can occur in the interim between procedures and a thorough reevaluation should be performed. Hypertension should be adequately controlled, mitral valvular disease should be reassessed for progression, and heart failure should be treated with optimal medical therapy. Not infrequently, patients will receive stents for coronary disease necessitating concurrent dual antiplatelet therapy that may make postponement of ablation for several months prudent. To summarize, there are no shortcuts in patient selection for the redo.

Timing reablation

Early after ablation the atrium is in flux, with forces of inflammation and remodeling taking hold. Although early recurrence has a negative prognostic value and does predict the need for future ablation, many in this group will improve and not require further ablation. Early redo ablation has been shown to increase the overall number of follow-up procedures without improving long-term results [25]. We agree with the guidelines recommending a 3-month blanking period before repeat ablation is performed [28]. Infrequently, patients may present with incessant and refractory organized atrial arrhythmias that are difficult to control such as a one-to-one flutter. In those cases, early redo ablation may be necessary.

Transseptal puncture

Thickening and scarring of the interatrial septum can occur after repeat procedures making transseptal puncture difficult in some patients [40,41]. The use of cautery of specialized or traditional needles has also been useful in select circumstances [42].

Practically, it is rare that repeat transseptal puncture is significantly difficult or requires the use of specialized needles or cautery. Frequently, the greater difficulty is with sheath crossing rather than the transseptal puncture itself. A stiff wire or ablator positioned in the LSPV as rail can safely guide the sheath to the left atrium. In some cases, either upgrade or downgrade in caliber of sheath is required to cross. It is important to note that intracardiac echocardiography (ICE) is used in almost all cases at our institution, and results may differ without ICE or transesophageal echo guidance [43,44].

Radiation exposure

The risks associated with radiation exposure are both stochastic and cumulative. Patients who undergo multiple procedures are particularly at risk for cumulative effects. In our laboratory, electroanatomic mapping and intracardiac echocardiography are used for nearly all AF ablations. Electroanatomic mapping and intracardiac echocardiography can significantly reduce the use of fluoroscopy [45,46]. To further mitigate the risk of radiation exposure, we downscale the fluoroscopy frame rate to 4 frames per second after transseptal puncture to minimize the dose of radiation delivered. Another important source of radiation is from CT scanning. Although CT has better spatial resolution, MRI is sufficient to describe left atrial geometry and assess pulmonary vein stenosis and is a good alternative free of ionizing radiation [47].

Pulmonary vein stenosis

Modern wide-area circumferential AF ablation rarely results in pulmonary vein stenosis. In our recent redo ablations, we rarely encounter pulmonary vein stenosis and do not routinely order 3D imaging to assess for PV stenosis. However, in cases where there was ablation further into the ostia or vein, pulmonary vein stenosis should be assessed. Similarly, in redo patients where the initial procedure was performed outside of our own institution, we prefer preprocedural pulmonary vein assessment. We prefer imaging with CT or MRI for accurate noninvasive measurements in patients we suspect or are at risk for stenosis [47,48]. However, ICE is also useful in assessing pulmonary veins stenosis and is performed routinely on all patients before and after ablation [49].

Electrophysiologic issues related to the reablation procedure

The strategy of the prior ablation predicts much of what will be seen at redo. For example, there are more organized atrial arrhythmias with substrate and linear ablation compared to PVI alone. The most frequent and consistent finding at redo ablation is reconnection of the pulmonary veins [50–52]. Electrical reisolation of pulmonary veins is, therefore, the cornerstone of redo ablation. The recurrence of AF does not necessitate the use of empiric linear lesions [52]. The general strategy employed when mapping pulmonary vein chronic reconnection is not significantly different from the initial procedure. Statistically, some sites around the pulmonary veins are at greater risk of reconnection including along the appendage vein border of the left veins and the septal border of the right veins [19,50].

When pulmonary veins appear chronically isolated at redo ablation, it is important to assess for nonpulmonary vein triggers as well as dormant pulmonary vein conduction. Adenosine can uncover a dormant pulmonary vein connection [53] and is superior to isopreteronol for that purpose [54]. Assessment and elimination of nonpulmonary vein triggers is also routinely performed. Isoproterenol is titrated with phenylephrine to support blood pressure. Burst pacing is performed from sites in the right and left atrium to expose non-PV triggers that are then targeted.

When linear ablation has been performed, it is critical to prove bidirectional block across the line. Slow conduction through the line may be difficult to distinguish from complete block. Activation mapping can be a useful tool to achieve this. Meticulous ablation needs to be performed to ensure that proarrhythmia does not result from linear lesions [55].

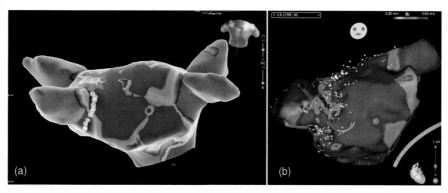

Figure 2 Multipolar mapping chronic reconnections during redo ablations. An Ensite/NavX™ map showing an area of normal voltage extending into the RSPV (a). In a separate procedure, a Carto3 MEM™ map showing an isolated area of normal voltage extending into the RSPV. In both procedures, ablation targeted to this area resulted in isolation of the vein.

Multipolar left atrial voltage mapping

Both the EnSite NavX (St Jude Medical, MN, USA) and Carto 3 with MEM technology (Biosense Webster, CA, USA) allow for rapid acquisition of left atrial voltage acquired with a circular Lasso or other multipolar catheters. Especially in redo procedures, these maps are useful in quickly identifying arrhythmogenic regions and visualizing prior ablation. Focal gaps in contiguous ablations are detected as areas of relatively increased or more normal voltage adjacent to areas of low voltage or scar (Figure 2). Distal coronary sinus pacing or pacing from near the vein in question is often useful to separate pulmonary vein potentials from left atrial potentials. A comprehensive voltage map can be collected in a few minutes with multipolar mapping (Figure 3).

Antiarrhythmic drug therapy

Medical therapy may be more or less efficacious after ablation depending on the type of atrial arrhythmia recurrence. Based on prospective randomized results, we generally maintain patients on antiarrhythmic drugs for the short term after ablation while periprocedural inflammation rescinds resulting in fewer cardioversion and hospitalization [56]. Late or very late recurrence is more likely to respond to medical therapy than patients with early recurrence [26].

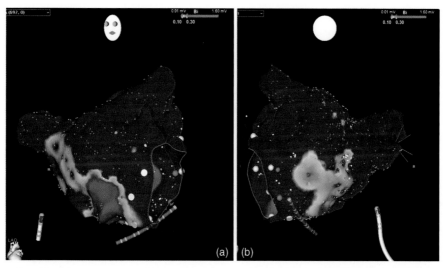

Figure 3 Left atrial voltage map created with Lasso multipolar mapping and Carto 3 MEM™. Dense areas of low voltage and sparse areas of greater voltage in a patient presenting with a left atrial tachycardia after 2 prior AF ablations.

When to not redo

There is no absolute number of ablations a patient can undergo and the decision to reablate is always individualized. As mentioned previously, if a rigorous assessment of symptoms and arrhythmia is found to correlate, it makes sense to treat the arrhythmia in an effective manner. Any unchecked comorbidities must be treated before proceeding. The risks of repeat ablation are minimal over initial ablation and constantly improving. If a patient is unlikely to have sustained benefit from redo ablation, it is best not to offer it even if patient desires it.

Conclusions

Ablation therapy for atrial fibrillation is constantly evolving and improving. The safety of the procedure continues to improve as well, allowing electrophysiologists to more easily recommend multiple procedures to patients who need them. Patients with persistent atrial fibrillation are more likely to require multiple procedures to achieve AF control. All patients and especially those likely to experience recurrence need to understand this at the onset to avoid frustration and fruitless efforts. Until technology and our understanding of AF improve, redo ablation remains an inconvenient truth. It is crucial to strategize redo AF ablations to maximize success.

References

1 Hutchinson MD, Garcia FC, Mandel JE, Elkassabany N, Zado ES, Riley MP, et al. Efforts to enhance catheter stability improve atrial fibrillation ablation outcome. Heart Rhythm. 2013;10(3):347–353.

2 Cappato R, Calkins H, Chen S-A, Davies W, Iesaka Y, Kalman J, et al. Updated worldwide survey on the methods, efficacy, and safety of catheter ablation for human atrial fibrillation. Circ Arrhythm Electrophysiol. 2010; 3(1):32–38.

3 Seow S-C, Lim T-W, Koay C-H, Ross DL, Thomas SP. Efficacy and late recurrences with wide electrical pulmonary vein isolation for persistent and permanent atrial fibrillation. Europace. 2007;9(12):1129–1133.

4 O'Neill MD, Wright M, Knecht S, Jaïs P, Hocini M, Takahashi Y, et al. Long-term follow-up of persistent atrial fibrillation ablation using termination as a procedural endpoint. Eur Heart J. 2009;30(9):1105–1112.

5 Ganesan AN, Shipp NJ, Brooks AG, Kuklik P, Lau DH, Lim HS, et al. Long-term outcomes of catheter ablation of atrial fibrillation: a systematic review and meta-analysis. J Am Heart Assoc. 2013;2(2):e004549.

6 Rostock T, Salukhe TV, Steven D, Drewitz I, Hoffmann BA, Bock K, et al. Long-term single- and multiple-procedure outcome and predictors of success after catheter ablation for persistent atrial fibrillation. Heart Rhythm. 2011;8(9):1391–1397.

7 Vasamreddy CR, Lickfett L, Jayam VK, Nasir K, Bradley DJ, Eldadah Z, et al. Predictors of recurrence following catheter ablation of atrial fibrillation using an irrigated-tip ablation catheter. J Cardiovasc Electrophysiol. 2004; 15(6):692–697.

8 Berruezo A, Tamborero D, Mont L, Benito B, Tolosana JM, Sitges M, et al. Pre-procedural predictors of atrial fibrillation recurrence after circumferential pulmonary vein ablation. Eur Heart J. 2007;28(7):836–841.

9 Lee S-H, Tai C-T, Hsieh M-H, Tsai C-F, Lin Y-K, Tsao H-M, et al. Predictors of early and late recurrence of atrial fibrillation after catheter ablation of paroxysmal atrial fibrillation. J Interv Card Electrophysiol. 2004;10(3): 221–226.

10 Balk EM, Garlitski AC, Alsheikh-Ali AA, Terasawa T, Chung M, Ip S. Predictors of atrial fibrillation recurrence after radiofrequency catheter ablation: a systematic review. J Cardiovasc Electrophysiol. 2010;21(11):1208–1216.

11 Oakes RS, Badger TJ, Kholmovski EG, Akoum N, Burgon NS, Fish EN, et al. Detection and quantification of left atrial structural remodeling with delayed-enhancement magnetic resonance imaging in patients with atrial fibrillation. Circulation. 2009;119(13):1758–1767.

12 Spragg DD, Khurram I, Zimmerman SL, Yarmohammadi H, Barcelon B, Needleman M, et al. Initial experience with magnetic resonance imaging of atrial scar and co-registration with electroanatomic voltage mapping during atrial fibrillation: success and limitations. Heart Rhythm. 2012;9(12):2003–2009.

13 Kuppahally SS, Akoum N, Burgon NS, Badger TJ, Kholmovski EG, Vijayakumar S, et al. Left atrial strain and strain rate in patients with paroxysmal and persistent atrial fibrillation: relationship to left atrial structural remodeling detected by delayed-enhancement MRI. Circ Cardiovasc Imaging. 2010;3(3):231–239.

14 Fein AS, Shvilkin A, Shah D, Haffajee CI, Das S, Kumar K, et al. Treatment of obstructive sleep apnea reduces the risk of atrial fibrillation recurrence following catheter ablation. J Am Coll Cardiol. 2013;62(4).

15 Dimitri H, Ng M, Brooks AG, Kuklik P, Stiles MK, Lau DH, et al. Atrial remodeling in obstructive sleep apnea: implications for atrial fibrillation. Heart Rhythm. 2012; 9(3):321–327.

16 Matiello M, Nadal M, Tamborero D, Berruezo A, Montserrat J, Embid C, et al. Low efficacy of atrial fibrillation ablation in severe obstructive sleep apnoea patients. Europace. 2010;12(8):1084–1089.

17 Wasmer K, Mönnig G, Bittner A, Dechering D, Zellerhoff S, Milberg P, et al. Incidence, characteristics, and outcome of left atrial tachycardias after circumferential antral ablation of atrial fibrillation. Heart Rhythm. 2012; 9(10):1660–1666.

18 Chugh A, Oral H, Lemola K, Hall B, Cheung P, Good E, et al. Prevalence, mechanisms, and clinical significance of macroreentrant atrial tachycardia during and following left atrial ablation for atrial fibrillation. Heart Rhythm. 2005;2(5):464–471.

19 Rajappan K, Kistler PM, Earley MJ, Thomas G, Izquierdo M, Sporton SC, et al. Acute and chronic pulmonary vein reconnection after atrial fibrillation ablation: a prospective characterization of anatomical sites. Pacing Clin Electrophysiol. 2008;31(12):1598–1605.

20 Sauer WH, McKernan ML, Lin D, Gerstenfeld EP, Callans DJ, Marchlinski FE. Clinical predictors and outcomes associated with acute return of pulmonary vein conduction during pulmonary vein isolation for treatment of atrial fibrillation. Heart Rhythm. 2006;3(9):1024–1028.

21 Verma A, Wazni OM, Marrouche NF, Martin DO, Kilicaslan F, Minor S, et al. Pre-existent left atrial scarring in patients undergoing pulmonary vein antrum isolation: an independent predictor of procedural failure. J Am Coll Cardiol. 2005;45(2):285–292.

22 Teh AW, Kistler PM, Lee G, Medi C, Heck PM, Spence SJ, et al. Electroanatomic remodeling of the left atrium in paroxysmal and persistent atrial fibrillation patients without structural heart disease. J Cardiovasc Electrophysiol. 2012;23(3):232–238.

23 Ammar S, Hessling G, Reents T, Fichtner S, Wu J, Zhu P, et al. Arrhythmia type after persistent atrial fibrillation ablation predicts success of the repeat procedure. Circ Arrhythm Electrophysiol. 2011;4(5):609–614.

24 Leong-Sit P, Roux J-F, Zado E, Callans DJ, Garcia F, Lin D, et al. Antiarrhythmics after ablation of atrial fibrillation (5A Study): six-month follow-up study. Circ Arrhythm Electrophysiol. 2011;4(1):11–14.

25 Lellouche N, Jaïs P, Nault I, Wright M, Bevilacqua M, Knecht S, et al. Early recurrences after atrial fibrillation ablation: prognostic value and effect of early reablation. J Cardiovasc Electrophysiol. 2008;19(6):599–605.

26 Gaztañaga L, Frankel DS, Kohari M, Kondapalli L, Zado ES, Marchlinski FE. Time to recurrence of atrial fibrillation influences outcome following catheter ablation. Heart Rhythm. 2013;10(1):2–9.

27 Bertaglia E, Stabile G, Senatore G, Zoppo F, Turco P, Amellone C, et al. Predictive value of early atrial tachyarrhythmias recurrence after circumferential anatomical pulmonary vein ablation. Pacing Clin Electrophysiol. 2005;28(5):366–371.

28 Calkins H, Kuck KH, Cappato R, Brugada J, Camm AJ, Chen S-A, et al. 2012 HRS/EHRA/ECAS Expert Consensus Statement on Catheter and Surgical Ablation of Atrial Fibrillation: Recommendations for Patient Selection, Procedural Techniques, Patient Management and Follow-Up, Definitions, Endpoints, and Research Trial Design. Europace. 2012;14(4):528–606.

29 Pokushalov E, Romanov A, Corbucci G, Bairamova S, Losik D, Turov A, et al. Does atrial fibrillation burden measured by continuous monitoring during the blanking period predict the response to ablation at 12-month follow-up? Heart Rhythm. 2012;9(9):1375–1379.

30 Weerasooriya R, Khairy P, Litalien J, Macle L, Hocini M, Sacher F, et al. Catheter ablation for atrial fibrillation: are results maintained at 5 years of follow-up? J Am Coll Cardiol. 2011;57(2):160–166.

31 Tzou WS, Marchlinski FE, Zado ES, Lin D, Dixit S, Callans DJ, et al. Long-term outcome after successful

catheter ablation of atrial fibrillation. Circ Arrhythm Electrophysiol. 2010;3(3):237–242.

32 Scharf C, Veerareddy S, Ozaydin M, Chugh A, Hall B, Cheung P, et al. Clinical significance of inducible atrial flutter during pulmonary vein isolation in patients with atrial fibrillation. J Am Coll Cardiol. 2004;43(11): 2057–2062.

33 Kilicaslan F, Verma A, Yamaji H, Marrouche NF, Wazni O, Cummings JE, et al. The need for atrial flutter ablation following pulmonary vein antrum isolation in patients with and without previous cardiac surgery. J Am Coll Cardiol. 2005;45(5):690–696.

34 Sauer WH, Alonso C, Zado E, Cooper JM, Lin D, Dixit S, et al. Atrioventricular nodal reentrant tachycardia in patients referred for atrial fibrillation ablation: response to ablation that incorporates slow-pathway modification. Circulation. 2006;114(3):191–195.

35 Gerstenfeld EP, Callans DJ, Dixit S, Russo AM, Nayak H, Lin D, et al. Mechanisms of organized left atrial tachycardias occurring after pulmonary vein isolation. Circulation. 2004;110(11):1351–1357.

36 Patel AM, d'Avila A, Neuzil P, Kim SJ, Mela T, Singh JP, et al. Atrial tachycardia after ablation of persistent atrial fibrillation: identification of the critical isthmus with a combination of multielectrode activation mapping and targeted entrainment mapping. Circ Arrhythm Electrophysiol. 2008;1(1):14–22.

37 Oral H, Knight BP, Morady F. Left atrial flutter after segmental ostial radiofrequency catheter ablation for pulmonary vein isolation. Pacing Clin Electrophysiol. 2003;26(6):1417–1419.

38 Gerstenfeld EP, Dixit S, Bala R, Callans DJ, Lin D, Sauer W, et al. Surface electrocardiogram characteristics of atrial tachycardias occurring after pulmonary vein isolation. Heart Rhythm. 2007;4(9):1136–1143.

39 Gerstenfeld EP, Callans DJ, Sauer W, Jacobson J, Marchlinski FE. Reentrant and nonreentrant focal left atrial tachycardias occur after pulmonary vein isolation. Heart Rhythm. 2005;2(11):1195–1202.

40 Tomlinson DR, Sabharwal N, Bashir Y, Betts TR. Interatrial septum thickness and difficulty with transseptal puncture during redo catheter ablation of atrial fibrillation. Pacing Clin Electrophysiol. 2008;31(12):1606–1611.

41 Marcus GM, Ren X, Tseng ZH, Badhwar N, Lee BK, Lee RJ, et al. Repeat transseptal catheterization after ablation for atrial fibrillation. J Cardiovasc Electrophysiol. 2007; 18(1):55–59.

42 Babaliaros VC, Green JT, Lerakis S, Lloyd M, Block PC. Emerging applications for transseptal left heart catheterization old techniques for new procedures. J Am Coll Cardiol. 2008;51(22):2116–2122.

43 Capulzini L, Paparella G, Sorgente A, de Asmundis C, Chierchia GB, Sarkozy A, et al. Feasibility, safety, and outcome of a challenging transseptal puncture facilitated by radiofrequency energy delivery: a prospective single-centre study. Europace. 2010;12(5):662–667.

44 Bayrak F, Chierchia G-B, Namdar M, Yazaki Y, Sarkozy A, de Asmundis C, et al. Added value of transoesophageal echocardiography during transseptal puncture performed

by inexperienced operators. Europace. 2012;14(5): 661–665.

45 Stabile G, Scaglione M, del Greco M, De Ponti R, Bongiorni MG, Zoppo F, et al. Reduced fluoroscopy exposure during ablation of atrial fibrillation using a novel electroanatomical navigation system: a multicentre experience. Europace. 2012;14(1):60–65.

46 Ferguson JD, Helms A, Mangrum JM, Mahapatra S, Mason P, Bilchick K, et al. Catheter ablation of atrial fibrillation without fluoroscopy using intracardiac echocardiography and electroanatomic mapping. Circ Arrhythm Electrophysiol. 2009;2(6):611–619.

47 Dong J, Vasamreddy CR, Jayam V, Dalal D, Dickfeld T, Eldadah Z, et al. Incidence and predictors of pulmonary vein stenosis following catheter ablation of atrial fibrillation using the anatomic pulmonary vein ablation approach: results from paired magnetic resonance imaging. J Cardiovasc Electrophysiol. 2005;16(8): 845–852.

48 Ghaye B, Szapiro D, Dacher J-N, Rodriguez L-M, Timmermans C, Devillers D, et al. Percutaneous ablation for atrial fibrillation: the role of cross-sectional imaging. Radiographics. 2003;23(Spec. No.):S19–33; discussion S48–S50.

49 Ren J-F, Marchlinski FE, Callans DJ, Zado ES. Intracardiac Doppler echocardiographic quantification of pulmonary vein flow velocity: an effective technique for monitoring pulmonary vein ostia narrowing during focal atrial fibrillation ablation. J Cardiovasc Electrophysiol. 2002;13(11):1076–1081.

50 Ouyang F, Antz M, Ernst S, Hachiya H, Mavrakis H, Deger FT, et al. Recovered pulmonary vein conduction as a dominant factor for recurrent atrial tachyarrhythmias after complete circular isolation of the pulmonary veins: lessons from double Lasso technique. Circulation. 2005;111(2):127–135.

51 Verma A, Kilicaslan F, Pisano E, Marrouche NF, Fanelli R, Brachmann J, et al. Response of atrial fibrillation to pulmonary vein antrum isolation is directly related to resumption and delay of pulmonary vein conduction. Circulation. 2005;112(5):627–635.

52 Callans DJ, Gerstenfeld EP, Dixit S, Zado E, Vanderhoff M, Ren J-F, et al. Efficacy of repeat pulmonary vein isolation procedures in patients with recurrent atrial fibrillation. J Cardiovasc Electrophysiol. 2004;15(9): 1050–1055.

53 Miyazaki S, Kuwahara T, Kobori A, Takahashi Y, Takei A, Sato A, et al. Adenosine triphosphate exposes dormant pulmonary vein conduction responsible for recurrent atrial tachyarrhythmias: importance of evaluating the dormant conduction during the re-do ablation procedure. Circulation. 2009;73(6):1160–1162.

54 Datino T, Macle L, Chartier D, Comtois P, Khairy P, Guerra PG, et al. Differential effectiveness of pharmacological strategies to reveal dormant pulmonary vein conduction: a clinical-experimental correlation. Heart Rhythm. 2011;8(9):1426–1433.

55 Jaïs P, Hocini M, O'Neill MD, Klein GJ, Knecht S, Sheiiro M, et al. How to perform linear lesions. Heart Rhythm. 2007;4(6):803–809.

56 Roux J-F, Zado E, Callans DJ, Garcia F, Lin D, Marchlinski FE, et al. Antiarrhythmics after ablation of atrial fibrillation (5A Study). Circulation. 2009;120(12): 1036–1040.

CHAPTER 26

Periprocedural care for catheter ablation of atrial fibrillation

Chirag Barbhaiya, Justin Ng, & Gregory F. Michaud

Shapiro Cardiovascular Center, Brigham and Women's Hospital, Boston, MA, USA

Procedural considerations to avoid acute complications and improve efficacy

Catheter ablation of atrial fibrillation (AF) has rapidly evolved in the last 10–15 years and is now a commonly performed ablation procedure at many medical centers. However, AF ablation remains a complex procedure and is associated with a higher incidence of complications compared to conventional ablation procedures [1]. Many investigators have studied the risks of major complications related to AF ablation, and these risks have remained essentially unchanged over time despite improvements in understanding and technology (Table 1) [2–6].

Periprocedural anticoagulation

Patients have elevated thromboembolic risk during and after ablation procedures for AF, which mandates a careful periprocedural anticoagulation management [7,8]. Thrombus can form on catheters and sheaths placed in the left atrium and RF ablation lesions can be thrombogenic, thus patients undergoing AF ablation are at elevated risk for stroke [9–11]. The intensity of anticoagulation is determined by balancing prevention of thrombus formation against minimizing complications such as pericardial tamponade and vascular complications [2,12,13].

Current guidelines for AF ablation suggest an approach to anticoagulation and transesophageal echocardiography (TEE) screening that is to guide

Practical Guide to Catheter Ablation of Atrial Fibrillation, Second Edition. Edited by Jonathan S. Steinberg, Pierre Jaïs and Hugh Calkins.

patients undergoing electrical or pharmacologic conversion of AF. Briefly, 3 weeks of therapeutic anticoagulation or a TEE to rule out left atrial appendage thrombus is required if the patient has been in continuously for more than 48 h or for an unknown duration. Some experts recommend routine TEE prior to AF ablation for all patients, although in our opinion, if the patient has a CHADS$_2$-VASc score of 0 or 1, has been appropriately anticoagulated for more than 3 weeks, and presents in sinus rhythm, we do not routinely order a screening TEE. Following AF ablation, patients should be anticoagulated systemically, usually orally, for at least 2 months postablation [14]. Intracardiac echocardiography and preprocedure CT or MRI imaging lack sufficient sensitivity and specificity for routine screening of LA thrombi in patients with elevated stroke risk [15–17].

Uninterrupted warfarin

For patients anticoagulated with warfarin, discontinuation of warfarin and a strategy of "bridging" with unfractionated or low molecular weight heparin result in an increased risk of bleeding complications, primarily at vascular access sites [18]. More importantly, stroke risk appears to be higher among patients in whom a bridging strategy is employed. The COMPARE study randomized patients to a bridging strategy with LMW heparin versus uninterrupted warfarin with target INR of 2.5 [19]. The bridging strategy led to a ninefold increase in periprocedural stroke (4.5% versus 0.5%), and was worse for patients with persistent AF. Experienced centers routinely perform AF ablation in patients who are continuously and therapeutically anticoagulated with warfarin [20–22]. Latchamsetty et al. showed that pericardial tamponade occurring in the presence of a therapeutic INR was not

Table 1 Reported AF ablation complication rates over time.

	Cappato et al. [2] (n = 8745)	Spragg et al. JCE 2008 (n = 641)	Cappato et al. [3] (n = 20,825)	Aldhoon et al. [6] (n = 1192)	Shah et al. [4] (n = 4156)
Any complication	5.9%	5%	4.5%	3.4%	5.1%
Vascular complication	1.0%	1.7%	1.5%	2.2%	2.6%
Perforation/tamponade	1.2%	1.2%	1.3%	0.3%	2.5%
Stroke/TIA	0.9%	1.1%	0.9%	0.4%	0.3%
Pneumothorax/ hemothorax	0.2%	0.3%	0.2%	0.1%	0.1%
Phrenic nerve paralysis	0.11%	Not reported	0.17%	0.08%	Not reported
Esophageal fistula	Not reported	0%	0.04%	0%	Not reported

more severe or difficult to manage than in patients in whom warfarin had been discontinued [23]. Kim et al. found that the optimal INR range for the procedure was 2.1–2.4, although a steep rise in vascular complications was observed with INR > 3.5 [24].

Despite a therapeutic INR, it is necessary to give patients unfractionated heparin during an AF procedure. Ren et al. showed that an activated clotting time (ACT) >300 s decreased the risk of thrombus detected in the left atrium (LA) by intracardiac echocardiography (ICE), particularly in patients who demonstrated spontaneous echo contrast [25]. In our center, for patients with a normal INR, 120 units/kg body weight is necessary to achieve a target ACT >350 s versus 80 units/kg for patients with a therapeutic INR [18]. Hummel and coworkers recently published a useful nomogram incorporating body weight and INR to decide the proper unfractionated heparin bolus necessary to achieve a target ACT >300 s [26]. The timing of heparin administration is important since transseptal sheaths that dwell for a significant time in the right atrium can form thrombus prior to transseptal puncture, even with a therapeutic INR. Bruce et al. found a higher incidence of thrombus detected in the left atrium by ICE when heparin was delayed [27]. For this reason, we recommend heparin administration immediately following vascular sheath insertion.

Protamine can be administered for persistent bleeding or cardiac tamponade if a patient is anticoagulated with heparin. For acute reversal of anticoagulation with warfarin, one may consider administration of Fresh frozen plasma, prothrombin complex concentrates, or recombinant activated factor VII [28].

Management of newer oral anticoagulants

Periablation anticoagulation strategies incorporating newer oral anticoagulants, such as dabigatran, a direct thrombin inhibitor, or the Factor Xa inhibitors rivaroxaban and apixaban, require more study to determine safety relative to uninterrupted warfarin. These agents are attractive because they obviate the need for routine coagulation monitoring due to their predictable pharmacological profile and rapid onset of activity [29]. Thrombin time can be measured to determine the effect of dabigatran, and chromogenic antifactor Xa assays can be used to monitor the effect of rivaroxaban and apixaban; however, these tests are not widely available [30].

For patients with CHA_2DS_2-VASc score ≥2, we will transition from a newer oral anticoagulant to uninterrupted warfarin for 3 weeks prior to the procedure. For low-risk patients taking dabigatran, apixaban, or rivaroxaban, discontinuation 36 h prior to the procedure and reinitiation 12–24 h postablation is reasonable, but untested [31]. This purported strategy includes bridging with an unfractionated heparin drip starting 4 h after sheath removal.

In recent case–control studies, dabigatran discontinued approximately 24 h prior to AF ablation and resumed shortly after vascular hemostasis was as safe and effective a method as uninterrupted warfarin, although this needs to be studied in a greater number of patients before it can be widely recommended. Of note, patients on dabigatran prior to ablation were found to require higher doses of heparin in order to achieve therapeutic ACTs intraprocedurally [32,33]. Dabigatran discontinuation within 12 h of the procedure was associated with higher bleeding rates. Given the shorter half-life of rivaroxaban (5–9 h), some operators have begun using uninterrupted rivaroxaban, taken the night before the procedure, but data is limited as to the safety of this approach [34].

In the event of clinically significant bleeding, reversal of anticoagulation for newer anticoagulants is not well understood, but includes prothrombin complex concentrate for rivaroxaban and apixaban, and recombinant factor VIIa and hemodialysis for dabigatran [30,35,36].

Vascular access

Procedural strategies that have been shown to decrease the risk of vascular complications include the use of a micropuncture needle and avoiding femoral arterial access for hemodynamic monitoring [37]. The use of direct visualization with a vascular ultrasound probe can be considered in patients felt to be at high risk for vascular complications. This strategy has not been studied for routine use. The routine use of fluoroscopy to target femoral venous puncture at the level of the lower half of the femoral head can be used to avoid access above the inguinal ligament, increasing the risk of retroperitoneal bleeding, and below the bifurcation of the saphenous vein, increasing the risk of aneurysm and fistula formation.

After establishment of vascular access, careful sheath management, particularly after transseptal puncture, is essential in order to avoid air embolization and thrombus formation on sheaths. In addition to anticoagulation strategies discussed above, continuous flushing of the transseptal sheath through an air filter should be strongly considered, particularly if the sheath remains in the left atrium. Continuous flushing should be interrupted during catheter exchanges so as to avoid entrainment of air into the sheath. Whether certain ablation technologies carry a higher risk of stroke or asymptomatic cerebral microembolization is an ongoing area of investigation. Sauren et al. have reported increased risk of cerebral microemboli with the use of nonirrigated RF ablation catheters compared to irrigated RF ablation and cryoballoon ablation catheters [38], but more recent unpublished results from the ERACE study show this risk can be greatly mitigated.

Intravenous protamine at the conclusion of an ablation procedure may be used to reverse the heparin anticoagulation effect and allow for expedited vascular sheath removal. Alternatively, some operators choose to and wait for the ACT to fall below 180–220 s prior to sheath removal without protamine [14]. Protamine has been reported to be associated with a ~1% risk of an idiosyncratic drug reaction, which can result in profound hypotension [39], although in our experience this happens more rarely. As a result, a 5-mg test dose should be administered prior to administration of the full reversal dose.

General anesthesia versus conscious sedation

AF ablation is commonly performed with general anesthesia or conscious sedation, depending on patient characteristics, availability of qualified anesthetists and operator preference. Conscious sedation with fentanyl and midazolam can be performed safely; however, during general anesthesia, the patient is immobile, respirations are regular and predictable, and thoracic excursions are reduced, all of which are likely to improve catheter stability and mapping system accuracy.

In a randomized clinical trial comparing conscious sedation with general anesthesia in patients undergoing catheter ablation of paroxysmal atrial fibrillation, the use of general anesthesia was associated with a reduced rate of intermediate-term recurrence of AF, a reduced number of reconnected pulmonary veins in patients with AF recurrence, and few adverse events related to general anesthesia. Improved catheter stability has also been observed with general anesthesia during robotic AF ablation [40,41].

Increased catheter stability provided by general anesthesia may increase the risk of esophageal damage as assessed by capsule endoscopy, but the mechanism is not clear. Precautions such as esophageal temperature monitoring and limitation of power and duration of posterior wall lesions may mitigate the risk of esophageal injury [42].

Positive outcomes have been reported for high-frequency jet ventilation during general anesthesia for AF ablation [43]. Jet ventilation, however, has unique risks in addition to those of standard mechanical ventilation, including a requirement for the use of paralytic agents, which prevents assessment of phrenic nerve injury during ablation [44]. We routinely employ short periods of apnea (30 s to 3 min) during RF applications in locations that are adversely affected by respiration, such as the ridge between the LSPV and the LAA, as well as the left atrial dome [45]. Figures 1–3 illustrate the impact of respiration and apnea during RF ablation. A respiratory depressant such as remifentanil can be used to allow apnea for limited periods without the need for paralytic agents.

Cardiac tamponade

Cardiac tamponade occurs in approximately 1% of patients undergoing AF ablation and is the most common cause of death related to AF ablation [3]. We routinely use intracardiac echocardiography to guide transseptal puncture and assess for the presence of intrapericardial fluid prior to sheath removal; fluoroscopy screening is a simple tool to diagnose cardiac tamponade. The lateral heart border will no longer move with systolic contractions in the presence of a significant pericardial effusion and this finding usually precedes hypotension [46]. A proportion of patients will develop cardiac tamponade hours after sheath removal [47]. Urgent transthoracic echocardiography should be obtained for unexplained postprocedure

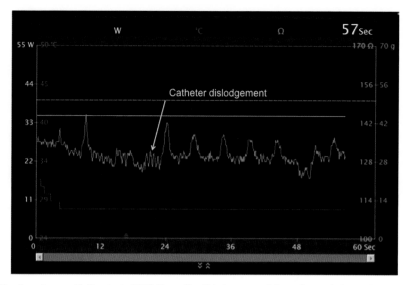

Figure 1 Falling impedance with the start of RF followed by dislodgement of the catheter tip by respiratory movement and no further decrease in impedance.

hypotension and personnel with proficiency in pericardiocentesis should be immediately available.

In some cases of cardiac tamponade, particularly related to steam pop perforations, percutaneous drainage may be inadequate and surgical drainage and repair is needed [48]. If this is the case, continuous aspiration of blood from the pericardial space following pericardiocentesis and reinfusion into a femoral vascular sheath with large volume syringes can be performed for a short time as a temporizing measure pending availability of red cell transfusions and surgical intervention.

In-patient monitoring

Recent multicenter registries have reported a major complication rate of approximately 5% for patients following catheter ablation of atrial fibrillation [3–6]. Adequate in-patient postprocedure monitoring,

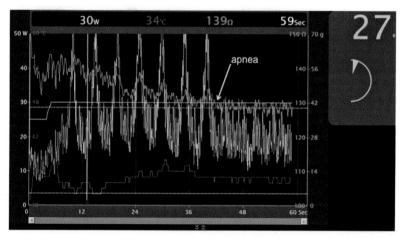

Figure 2 Large, phasic variations in contact force related to respiratory movement on the LA roof with stabilization of contact force with apnea measured using a novel force-sensing ablation catheter.

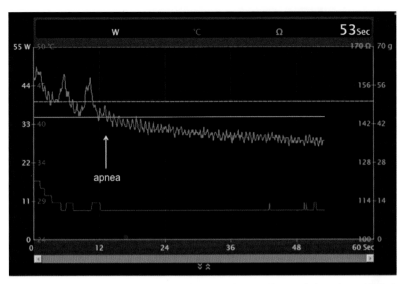

Figure 3 Respirophasic impedance variation at the start of ablation followed by steady-impedance fall during apnea.

typically for 18–24 h, including telemetry and frequent assessment of vital signs and venipuncture sites, is essential for the early recognition and management of these complications. In recent studies, TIA and stroke are reported to occur in approximately 1% of patients following AF ablation [3]. Neurologic status should be assessed immediately following the procedure and at frequent intervals thereafter. An immediate head CT or MRI and neurologic consultation should be obtained if there is evidence of a neurologic deficit suggesting stroke. Headache is a common associated symptom after AF ablation, particularly in those with a history of migraine headaches and can be a confounding symptom [49].

Chest discomfort is common following AF ablation and is most typically related to a transient pericarditis, minor esophageal injury, or alterations in gastric motility that are self-limited and can be managed conservatively. Patients should be counseled prior to discharge to directly contact the physician who performed the AF ablation procedure in the event of severe or unrelenting chest discomfort or odynophagia, in order to facilitate early detection and management of a life-threatening atrioesophageal fistula.

Postprocedural shortness of breath should raise concern for phrenic nerve injury. Ablation anterior to the right PVs with RF or the cryoballoon catheter may result in transient or permanent phrenic nerve injury. Pacing at potential RF ablation sites anterior to

the right PVs should be performed to rule out the phrenic capture prior to lesion delivery. A phrenic nerve map can be incorporated on to the electroanatomic map to serve as a guide (Figure 4). During ablation of the right PVs with the cryoballoon catheter, the phrenic nerve should be continually paced from the SVC, cranial to the ablation site, and ablation discontinued for the loss of phrenic capture or diminution of phrenic capture. In cases of phrenic nerve injury, an upright chest X-ray will show an elevated right hemidiaphragm, and chest fluoroscopy will show paralysis of the right hemidiaphragm.

The most common complication of AF ablation is vascular injury related to sheath access. Patients should have strict bed rest for 4–6 h following sheath removal to facilitate hemostasis. A vascular ultrasound can be obtained if there is concern for arterial–venous fistula or pseudoaneurysm formation. Patients should be instructed to avoid strenuous physical activity for approximately 1 week following ablation in order to prevent delayed vascular complications.

The use of open irrigated ablation catheters can result in administration of significant amounts of IV fluid during AF ablation. Intraprocedure fluid balance should be closely monitored with consideration of empiric diuresis in patients with left ventricular dysfunction.

Table 2 provides a brief summary of procedural considerations for the avoidance and management of periprocedural complications.

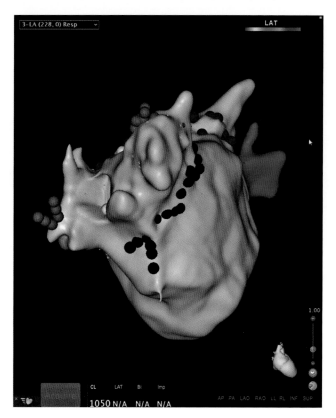

Figure 4 Right lateral view of left atrial electroanatomic map in a patient undergoing RF ablation of atrial fibrillation. Black dots represent areas of phrenic capture anterior the right pulmonary veins.

Table 2 Avoidance and management of major complications.

Major complication	Procedural considerations for avoidance/management
Perforation/tamponade	• Use of ICE for transseptal puncture
	• Power limitation/avoidance of "pops"
	• Reversal of procedural anticoagulation with protamine
	• Availability of stat TTE
	• Availability of pericardiocentesis and cardiac surgery
Vascular complications	• Micropuncture kit for femoral access
	• Vascular ultrasound guidance
	• Fluoroscopy of femoral head prior to puncture
Esophageal injury	• Esophageal temperature monitoring
	• Esophageal mapping with ICE or preprocedure imaging
	• Posterior wall power limitation
	• Postprocedure PPI/H2 blocker
TIA/stroke	• Uninterrupted pre- and postprocedure anticoagulation with warfarin
	• Consider newer anticoagulation agents in low-risk patients
	• Aggressive anticoagulation prior to transseptal puncture
	• Continuous flushing of transseptal sheaths with bubble traps
Phrenic nerve injury	• Pacing of ablation sites anterior to right PVs prior to RF ablation
	• Diaphragmatic pacing during right PV ablation with cryoballoon

Periprocedural arrhythmia management

Preprocedure arrhythmia monitoring

Arrhythmia monitoring is important to confirm that a patient's symptoms result from AF and to determine whether a patient has paroxysmal or persistent AF that may be useful in planning ablation strategy [14]. Assessment of rate control adequacy is important in patients with depressed left ventricular function who may have a reversible tachycardia-mediated cardiomyopathy since left ventricular function can be expected to improve following ablation [50].

Preprocedure arrhythmia monitoring may also be useful to determine if a patient has a regular supraventricular tachycardia as a triggering mechanism that degenerates to AF and can be targeted solely or in combination with PVI during ablation [51].

Postprocedure arrhythmia monitoring

The frequency of recurrent AF during the first few days postablation is variable and up to 15% of patients will complain of more frequent episodes than preablation [52]. Of note, the absence of early AF recurrence during the initial 6-week period after ablation was found to be a strong independent predictor of 6-month freedom from AF (84% without early recurrences versus 38% with early recurrences) [53]; however, nearly 60% of patients who experience early recurrence of AF after catheter ablation remain free of AF following a 3-month "blanking period" for at least one year. Thus, early recurrence should not prompt immediate reablation attempts, and routine outpatient rhythm monitoring is not recommended immediately following AF ablation [54].

Periprocedural AADs

It is standard practice at many institutions to continue antiarrhythmic medication (AADs) prior to and up to 3 months following catheter ablation of AF. The rationale for this is to prevent early recurrence of AF during the immediate postprocedure period. Both a retrospective observational study and a prospective, randomized clinical trial recently demonstrated a decrease in short-term AF recurrence rates, including hospitalization and cardioversion, but no difference in intermediate-term AF recurrence rates in ablations performed with patients remaining on AADs [53,55]. Antiarrhythmic choices were based on the absence or presence of structural heart disease: (1) normal left ventricular (LV) function with no obstructive coronary artery disease (CAD), propafenone 150 mg TID or flecainide 100 mg BID; (2) normal LV function with CAD, sotalol 80 mg BID; and (3) abnormal LV function, sotalol 80 mg BID or dofetilide 500 g BID [53].

Postablation inflammation

Proinflammatory processes caused by ablation therapy have been implicated in early AF recurrence [56]. A corticosteroid regimen of IV hydrocortisone 2 mg/kg immediately after the procedure followed by oral prednisone 0.5 mg/kg/day for three days after AF ablation may be effective and safe for preventing immediate and mid-term AF recurrences after PVI [57]. Prophylactic corticosteroids are used routinely by <10% of Guideline Committee members due to concerns related to common comorbidities in AF ablation patients and the lack of supportive corroborative data [14].

More recently, colchicine 0.5 twice a day for 3 months following catheter ablation of AF has been shown to significantly reduce intermediate-term AF recurrence and reduce serum inflammatory marker levels [58]. Our practice includes routine use of colchicine in patients who have undergone extensive left atrial ablation both for prevention of AF recurrence and for treatment of symptoms of pericarditis.

Postdischarge follow-up and prevention of late complications

Following AF ablation, patients should be seen in follow-up at a minimum of 3 months following the ablation procedure, and then every 6 months for at least 2 years [14]. The development of atrial esophageal fistula following catheter ablation of atrial fibrillation is a rare, but often fatal, complication that has been reported following AF ablation with multiple energy sources, including the commonly used irrigated tip ablation catheter and cryoballoon catheter [59,60]. Early detection is essential for effective management, so we pay particular attention to teaching patients the potential early signs and symptoms of esophageal damage and ask to be contacted directly with any patient concerns, particularly within the first month after ablation when most AEFs occur.

Compared to the low rate of atrio-esophageal fistula, there is a high prevalence of esophageal mucosal changes following left atrial posterior wall ablation [61,62]. Gastroesophageal reflux aggravating mucosal injury may play a key role in fistula formation as suggested by several case reports that identified the esophagus as the initial site of perforation [63,64]. Proton pump inhibitors (PPI) are known to effectively reduce esophageal pH and have an excellent safety profile. Given this, despite the lack of supportive clinical trial data, short-term PPI use following catheter ablation of atrial fibrillation is reasonable for the prevention of progressive esophageal injury.

Optimal periprocedural care for patients undergoing AF ablation requires meticulous attention to detail and a team approach. Such protocols should be developed within an institution for best practices and a database maintained to understand procedural efficacy and to identify and mitigate potential safety issues.

References

1 Bohnen M, Stevenson WG, Tedrow UB, et al. Incidence and predictors of major complications from contemporary catheter ablation to treat cardiac arrhythmias. Heart Rhythm. 2011;8(11):1661–1666.

2 Cappato R, Calkins H, Chen SA, et al. Worldwide survey on the methods, efficacy, and safety of catheter ablation for human atrial fibrillation. Circulation. 2005;111 (9):1100–1105.

3 Cappato R, Calkins H, Chen SA, et al. Updated worldwide survey on the methods, efficacy, and safety of catheter ablation for human atrial fibrillation. Circ Arrhythm Electrophysiol. 2010;3: 32–38.

4 Shah RU, Freeman JV, Shilane D, Wang PJ, Go AS, Hlatky MA. Procedural complications, rehospitalizations, and repeat procedures after catheter ablation for atrial fibrillation. J Am Coll Cardiol. 2012;59: 143–149.

5 Spragg DD, Dalal D, Cheema A, et al. Complications of catheter ablation of atiral fibrillation: incidence and predictors. J Cardiovsc Electrophysiol. 2008;19: 627–631.

6 Aldhoon B, Wichterle D, Peichl P, Cihak R, Kautzner J. Complications of cateter ablation for atrial fibrillation in a high-volume center with the use of intracardiac echocardiography. Europace. 2013;15: 24–32.

7 Scherr D, Sharma K, Dalal D, et al. Incidence and predictors of periprocedural cerebrovascular accident in patients undergoing catheter ablation of atrial fibrillation. J Cardiovasc Electrophysiol. 2009;20(12):1357–1363.

8 Vazquez SR, Johnson SA, Rondina MT. Peri-procedural anticoagulation in patients undergoing ablation for atrial fibrillation. Thromb Res. 2010;126(2):e69–e77.

9 Manolis AS, Melita-Manolis H, Vassilikos V, et al. Thrombogenicity of radiofrequency lesions: results with serial D-dimer determinations. J Am Coll Cardiol. 1996;28: 1257–1261.

10 Dorbala S, Cohen AJ, Hutchinson LA, Menchavez-Tan E, Steinberg JS. Does radiofrequency ablation induce a prethrombotic state? Analysis of coagulation system activation and comparison to electrophysiologic study. J Cardiovasc Electrophysiol. 1998;9: 1152–1160.

11 Anfinsen OG, Gjesdal K, Brosstad F, et al. The activation of platelet function, coagulation, and fibrinolysis during radiofrequency catheter ablation in heparinized patients. J Cardiovasc Electrophysiol. 1999;10: 503–512.

12 Abhishek F, Heist EK, Barrett C, et al. Effectiveness of a strategy to reduce major vascular complications from catheter ablation of atrial fibrillation. J Interv Card Electrophysiol. 2011;30(3):211–215.

13 Hoyt H, Bhonsale A, Chilukuri K, et al. Complications arising from catheter ablation of atrial fibrillation: temporal trends and predictors. Heart Rhythm. 2011.

14 Calkins H, Kuck KH, Cappato R, et al. 2012 HRS/EHRA/ ECAS Expert Consensus Statement on Catheter and Surgical Ablation of Atrial Fibrillation: Recommendations for Patient Selection, Procedural Techniques, Patient Management and Follow-up, Definitions, Endpoints, and Research Trial Design. Heart Rhythm. 2012;9: 632–696.

15 Gottlieb I, Pinheiro A, Brinker JA, et al. Diagnostic accuracy of arterial phase 64-slice multidetector CT angiography for left atrial appendage thrombus in patients undergoing atrial fibrillation ablation. J Cardiovasc Electrophysiol. 2008;19(3):247–251.

16 Saksena S, Sra J, Jordaens L, et al. A prospective comparison of cardiac imaging using intracardiac echocardiography with transesophageal echocardiography in patients with atrial fibrillation: the intracardiac echocardiography guided cardioversion helps interventional procedures study. Circ Arrhythm Electrophysiol. 2010;3 (6):571–577.

17 Patel A, Au E, Donegan K, et al. Multidetector row computed tomography for identification of left atrial appendage filling defects in patients undergoing pulmonary vein isolation for treatment of atrial fibrillation: comparison with transesophageal echocardiography. Heart Rhythm. 2008;5(2):253–260.

18 Gautam S, John RM, Stevenson WG, et al. Effect of therapeutic INR on activated clotting times, heparin dosage, and bleeding risk during ablation of atrial fibrillation. J Cardiovasc Electrophysiol. 2011;22 (3):248–254.

19 Di Biase L, Burkhardt JD, Santangeli P, et al. Periprocedural stroke and bleeding complications in patients undergoing catheter ablation of atrial fibrillation with different anticoagulation management: results from the Role of Coumadin in Preventing Thromboembolism in Atrial Fibrillation (AF) Patients Undergoing Catheter Ablation (COMPARE) randomized trial. Circulation. 2014 Jun 24;129(25):2638-44. doi: 10.1161/CIRCULATIONAHA.113.006426. Epub 2014 Apr 17.

20 Di Biase L, Burkhardt JD, Mohanty P, et al. Periprocedural stroke and management of major bleeding complications in patients undergoing catheter ablation of atrial fibrillation: the impact of periprocedural therapeutic international normalized ratio. Circulation. 2010;121 (23):2550–2556.

21 Hakalahti A, Uusimaa P, Ylitalo K, Raatikainen MJ. Catheter ablation of atrial fibrillation in patients with therapeutic oral anticoagulation treatment. Europace. 2011;13(5):640–645.

22 Kwak JJ, Pak HN, Jang JK, et al. Safety and convenience of continuous warfarin strategy during the periprocedural period in patients who underwent catheter ablation of atrial fibrillation. J Cardiovasc Electrophysiol. 2010;21 (6):620–625.

23 Latchamsetty R, Gautam S, Bhakta D, et al. Management and outcomes of cardiac tamponade during atrial

fibrillation ablation in the presence of therapeutic anti-coagulation with warfarin. Heart Rhythm. 2011;8: 805–808.

24 Kim JS, Jongnarangsin K, Latchamsetty R, et al. The optimal range of international normalized ratio for radiofrequency catheter ablation of atrial fibrillation during therapeutic anticoagulation with warfarin. Circ Arrhythm Electrophysiol. 2013;6(2):302–309. doi: 10.1161/CIRCEP.112.000143. Epub 2013 Feb 26.

25 Ren JF, Marchlinski FE, Callans DJ, et al. Increased intensity of anticoagulation may reduce risk of thrombus during atrial fibrillation ablation procedures in patients with spontaneous echo contrast. J Cardiovasc Electro-physiol. 2005;16: 474–477.

26 Hamam I, Daoud EG, Zhang J, Kalbfleisch SJ, Augostini R, Winner M, Tsai S, Rhodes TE, Houmsse M, Liu Z, Love CJ, Tyler J, Sachdev M, Weiss R, Hummel JD. Impact of international normalized ratio and activated clotting time on unfractionated heparin dosing during ablation of atrial fibrillation. Circ Arrhythm Electrophysiol. 2013;6 (3):491–496. Epub 2013 May 17.

27 Bruce CJ, Friedman PA, Narayan O, et al. Early heparin-ization decreases the incidence of left atrial thrombi detected by intracardiac echocardiography during radio-frequency ablation for atrial fibrillation. J Interv Card Electrophysiol. 2008;22: 211–219.

28 Majeed A, Eelde A, Agren A, Schulman S, Holmstrom M. Thromboembolic safety and efficacy of prothrombin complex concentrates in the emergency reversal of war-farin coagulopathy. Thromb Res. 2011.

29 Winkle RA, Mead RH, Engel G, Kong MH, Patrawala RA. The use of dabigatran immediately after atrial fibrillation ablation. J Cardiovasc Electrophysiol. 2011, doi: 10.1111/ j.1540-8167.2011.02175.x.

30 Miyares MA, Davis K. Newer oral anticoagulants: a review of laboratory monitoring options and reversal agents in the hemorrhagic patient. Am J Health Syst Pharm. 2012;69: 1473–1484.

31 Knight BP, Bhave PD. Optimal strategies including use of newer anticoagulantsfor prevention of stroke and bleeding complications before, during, and after catheter ablation of atrial fibrillation and atrial flutter. Cur Treat Option Cardiovasc Med. DOI 10.1007/s11936-013-0242-9.

32 Kim JS, She F, Jongnarangsin K, Chugh A, Latchamsetty R, Ghanbari H, et al. Dabigatran vs warfarin for radio-frequency catheter ablation of atrial fibrillation. Heart Rhythm. 2013;10: 483–489.

33 Bassiouny M, Saliba W, Rickard J, et al. Use of dabigatran for peri-procedural anticoagulation in patients under-going catheter ablation for atrial fibrillation. Circ Arrhythm Electrophysiol. Published online April 3, 2013. DOI: 10.1161/CIRCEP.113.000320.

34 Lakkireddy DR, Reddy YM, Di Biasi L, et al. Feasibility and safety of uninterrupted rivaroxaban for periprocedural anti-coagulation in patients undergoing radiofrequency ablation for atrial fibrillation: results from a multicenter prospective registry. J Am Coll Cardiol. 2014 Mar 18;63(10):982-8. doi: 10.1016/j.jacc.2013.11.039. Epub 2014 Jan 8.

35 Eerenberg ES, Kamphuisen PW, Sijpkens MK, Meijers JC, Buller HR, Levi M. Reversal of rivaroxaban and dabiga-tran by prothrombin complex concentrate: a randomized, placebo–controlled, crossover study in healthy subjects. Circulation. 2011;124: 1573–1579.

36 Warkentin TE, Margetts P, Connolly SJ, Lamy A, Ricci C, Eikelboom JW. Recombinant factor VIIa (rFVIIa) and hemodialysis to manage massive dabigatran-associated postcardiac surgery bleeding. Blood. 2012;119: 2172–2174.

37 Abhishek F, Heist EK, Barrett C, et al. Effectiveness of a strategy to reduce major vascular complications from catheter ablation of atrial fibrillation. J Interv Card Electrophysiol. 2011;30: 211–215.

38 Sauren LD, Van Belle Y, De Roy L, et al. Transcranial measurement of cerebral microembolic signals during endocardial pulmonary vein isolation: comparison of three different ablation techniques. J Cardiovasc Electrophysiol. 2009;20: 1102–1107.

39 Chilukuri K, Henrikson CA, Dalal D, et al. Incidence and outcomes of protamine reactions in patients undergoing catheter ablation of atrial fibrillation. J Interv Card Electrophysiol. 2009;25: 175–181.

40 Di Biasi L, Conti S, Mohanty P, Bai R, et al. General anesthesia reduces the prevalence of pulmonary vein reconnection during repeat ablation when compared with conscious sedation: results from a randomized study. Heart Rhythm. 2011;8: 368–372.

41 Malcolme-Lawes LC, Lim PB, Koa-Wing M, Whinnett ZI, Jamil-Copley S, Hayat S, Francis DP, Kojodojo P, Davies DW, Peters NS, Kangaratnam P. Robotic assist-ance and general anaesthesia improve catheter stability and increase signal attenuation during atrial fibrillation ablation. Europace. 2013;15: 41–47.

42 Di Biase L, Saenz LC, Burkhardt JD, et al. Esophageal capsule endoscopy after radiofrequency catheter ablation for atrial fibrillation: documented higher risk of luminal esophageal damage with general anesthesia as compared with conscious sedation. Circ Arrhythmia Electrophysiol. 2009;2: 108–112.

43 Goode JS, Taylor RL, Buffington CW, Klain MM, Schwartzman D. High frequency jet ventilation: utility in posterior left atrial catheter ablation. Heart Rhythm. 2006;3: 13–19.

44 Jaquet Y, Monnier P, Van Melle G, et al. Complications of different ventilation strategies in endoscopic laryngeal surgery. A 10 year review. Anesthesiology. 2006;104: 52–59.

45 Kumar S, Morton JB, Halloran K, Spence SJ, Lee G, Wong WCG, Kistler PM, Kalman JM. Effect of respiration on catheter-tissue contact force during ablation of atrial arrhythmias. Heart Rhythm. 2012;9: 1041–1047.

46 McElderry HT, Yamada T. How to diagnose and treat cardiac tamponade in the electrophysiology laboratory. Heart Rhythm. 2009;6: 1531–1535.

47 Cappato R, Calkins H, Chen SA, Icsaka Y, Kalman J, Kim YH, et al. Delayed cardiac tamponade after radiofre-quency catheter ablation of atrial fibrillation. JACC. 2011;58(25):2696–2697.

48 Bunch TJ, Asirvatham SJ, Friedman PA, et al. Outcomes after cardiac perforation during radiofrequency ablation of the atrium. J Cardiovasc Electrophysiol. 2005;16 (11):1172–1179.

49 Noheria A, Roshan J, Kapa S, Srivathsan K, Packer DL, Asirvatham SJ. Migraine headaches following catheter ablation for atrial fibrillation. J Interv Card Electrophysiol. 2011;30: 227–232.

50 Gentlesk PJ, Sauer WH, Gerstenfeld EP, et al. Reversal of left ventricular dysfunction following ablation of atrial fibrillation. J Cardiovasc Electrophysiol. 2007;18(1):9–14.

51 Sauer WH, Alonso C, Zado E, et al. Atrioventricular nodal reentrant tachycardia in patients referred for atrial fibrillation ablation: response to ablation that incorporates slow-pathway modification. Circulation. 2006;114 (3):191–195.

52 Oral H, Knight BP, Ozaydin M, et al. Clinical significance of early recurrences of atrial fibrillation after pulmonary vein isolation. J Am Coll Cardiol. 2002;40(1):100–104.

53 Leong-Sit P, Roux JF, Zado E, et al. Antiarrhythmics after ablation of atrial fibrillation (5A Study): six-month follow-up study. Circ Arrhythm Electrophysiol. 2011;4(1):11–14.

54 O'Donnell D, Furniss SS, Dunuwille A, Bourke JP. Delayed cure despite early recurrence after pulmonary vein isolation for atrial fibrillation. Am J Cardiol. 2003;91 (1):83–85.

55 Dukes JW, Chilukuri K, Scherr D, Marine JE, Berger RD, Nazarian S, Cheng A, Spragg DD, Calkins H, Henrickson CA. The effect of antiarrhythmic medication management on atrial fibrillation ablation outcomes. J Cardiovasc Electrophysiol. 2013 Aug;24(8):882-7. doi: 10.1111/jce.12147. Epub 2013 Apr 11.

56 Koyama T, Sekiguchi Y, Tada H, et al. Comparison of characteristics and significance of immediate versus early versus no recurrence of atrial fibrillation after catheter ablation. Am J Cardiol. 2009;103: 1249–1254.

57 Koyama T, Tada H, Sekiguchi Y, et al. Prevention of atrial fibrillation recurrence with corticosteroids after radiofrequency catheter ablation: a randomized controlled trial. J Am Coll Cardiol. 2010;56: 1463–1472.

58 Deftereos S, Giannopoulos G, Kossyvakis C, et al. Colchicine for prevention of early atrial fibrillation recurrence after pulmonary vein isolation: a randomized control study. J Am Coll Cardiol. 2012;60: 1790–1796.

59 Pappone C, Oral H, Santinelli V, Vicedomini G, Lang CC, Manguso F, et al. Atrio-esophageal fistula as a complication of percutaneous transcatheter ablation of atrial fibrillation. Circulation. 2004;109: 2724–2726.

60 Zellerhoff S, Lenze F, Schulz R, Eckardt L. Fatal course of esophageal stenting of an atrioesophageal fistula after atrial fibrillation ablation. Heart Rhythm. 2011;8: 624–626.

61 Schmidt M, Nölker G, Marschang H, et al. Incidence of oesophageal wall injury post-pulmonary vein antrum isolation for treatment of patients with atrial fibrillation. Europace. 2008;10: 205–209.

62 Halm U, Gaspar T, Zachäus M, et al. Thermal esophageal lesions after radiofrequency catheter ablation of left atrial arrhythmias. Am J Gastroenterol. 2010;105: 551–556.

63 Martinek M, Hassanein S, Bencsik G, et al. Acute development of gastroesophageal reflux after radiofrequency catheter ablation of atrial fibrillation. Heart Rhythm. 2009;6: 1457–1462.

64 Grubina R, Cha Y-M, Bell MR, Sinak LJ, Asirvatham SJ. Pneumopericardium following radiofrequency ablation for atrial fibrillation: insights into the natural history of atrial esophageal fistula formation. J Cardiovasc Electrophysiol. 2010;21: 1046–1049.

CHAPTER 27

Complications: early and late after ablation

Antonio Sorgente[1] & Riccardo Cappato[2]

[1]Heart & Vascular Institute, Cleveland Clinic Abu Dhabi, Abu Dhabi, UAE
[2]Arrhythmia & Electrophysiology Research Center, IRCCS Humanitas Research Hospital, Rozzano, Milan, Italy

Catheter-based pulmonary vein isolation (PVI) is a well-established option for the treatment of both paroxysmal and persistent atrial fibrillation (AF) [1]. The lack of new effective antiarrhythmic drugs and the side effects linked to the acute and chronic use of the older ones have encouraged the development and the implementation of AF catheter ablation, which nowadays can be pursued with different strategies and/or technologies [1].

From its first foray in the world of cardiology at the end of the last century [2], catheter ablation of AF has increased in popularity. Despite encouraging results, complications associated with this procedure are still present. The various complications associated with AF ablation and their management have been previously well described [1]. Here, we discuss the complications of AF ablation and possible strategies to reduce their incidence and limiting harm to patients.

A recent worldwide survey focusing on the methods, efficacy, and safety of AF catheter ablation [3] revealed that its clinical indications have progressively widened. Nowadays, AF ablation is increasingly offered to larger patient populations presenting with greater degrees of comorbidity. This could explain the lower than expected procedural success rates but similar complication rates despite improvements in techniques and operators' experience.

Complications of AF ablation may range from local (mostly related to the percutaneous access that

precedes catheter ablation) to life-threatening conditions. According to the most recent international guidelines on AF ablation [1], "a major complication is defined as a complication that results in permanent injury or death, requires intervention for treatment, or prolongs or requires hospitalization."

In the above-mentioned worldwide survey, major complications were reported to occur in 4.5% of patients: death accounted for 0.15%, whereas atrio-esophageal fistula for 0.04%. Among the other major complications, cardiac tamponade accounted for 1.31%, stroke for 0.23%, transient ischemic attack for 0.71%, and PV stenosis requiring surgical or percutaneous dilation for another 0.29% of all procedures. Femoral pseudo-aneurysms occurred in 0.93% of all interventions whereas artero-venous fistulae were reported to take place in 0.54% of all procedures.

Shah et al. [4] recently reported on the safety of AF ablation in the real world. Out of about 4000 patients undergoing a first AF ablation procedure between 2005 and 2008 in the State of California, 5% experienced periprocedural complications, which were mostly vascular, with 9% requiring readmission within 30 days. Elderly, females, and patients who had already experienced hospitalization for AF were more prone to develop a complication compared to the remainder of the population. There was also a higher probability of complications in centers with less experience. Overall, there was a high rate of all-cause and arrhythmia-related hospitalizations (38.5% and 21.7%, respectively).

Complications of AF ablation can be classified as "early," when they occur during the procedure itself and "late" if they occur within 30 days thereafter [5].

Practical Guide to Catheter Ablation of Atrial Fibrillation, Second Edition. Edited by Jonathan S. Steinberg, Pierre Jaïs and Hugh Calkins.
© 2016 John Wiley & Sons, Ltd. Published 2016 by John Wiley & Sons, Ltd.

Early complications

Death

Death is a rare complication of AF catheter ablation. According to a recent report [6], the incidence of periprocedural death was similar to that of patients undergoing catheter ablation of supraventricular tachycardias [7,8].

There are several factors that can lead to death during or after AF ablation. These include the need for a transseptal puncture to approach the left atrium, catheter manipulation in the left atrium, deployment of radiofrequency lesions in the left atrium, and high levels of procedural anticoagulation. In recent animal studies, the probability of cardiac perforation was reported to be related to the contact force exerted by the ablation catheter on the cardiac wall [9,10]. New ablation catheters that are able to detect beat-by-beat contact force are now available. Their use may help in understanding the impact of catheter manipulation on cardiac tissues and therefore limiting the risk of cardiac perforation [11,12].

According to the worldwide AF ablation survey, cardiac tamponade was found to be the most common fatal complication leading to cardiac arrest during or after AF ablation. Other causes included atrio-esophageal fistula, cerebral ischemia or cardiac embolism, extrapericardial bleeding, and postoperative massive pneumonia. Also reported were conditions such as torsade de pointes, sudden respiratory failure or acute respiratory distress syndromes in the postoperative context.

The strategy adopted to perform PVI (e.g., CARTO-guided versus Lasso-guided or irrigated tip ablation versus 4-mm-tip ablation) does not appear to influence mortality rates during or after AF catheter ablation [13].

Hemorrhagic complications

Hemorrhagic complications involve major and minor bleeding. Major bleeding comprises any hematoma that requires intervention, the need for blood transfusions, massive hemoptysis, hemothorax, and retroperitoneal bleeding. Minor bleeding includes any kind of hematoma or bleeding that does not require intervention or is asymptomatic. Femoral pseudo-aneurysms and femoral arterovenous fistulas are included in hemorrhagic complications and could cause, depending on their extent, major or minor bleeding.

Different physiopathologic mechanisms lead to cardiac tamponade during and after PVI. Two of the main contributing factors are the transseptal puncture [14] and ablation-related damage to the left atrium [1].

Transseptal puncture carries an inherent risk for procedural complications. Current techniques have hardly evolved from those used in the 1950s [15]. Safety of transseptal puncture lies in the recognition of the right atrial anatomy and, in particular, the fossa ovalis. In a recent study, Sy et al. (ref) provided an overview on this and proposed a "problem-based stepwise approach" [16]. The study highlighted the utility of intracardiac or transesophageal echocardiography in cases where right atrial anatomy is unusual or engagement of the fossa ovalis proves difficult. However, transesophageal echocardiography is often poorly tolerated and requires deep sedation or general anesthesia while intracardiac echocardiography is associated with increased costs and requires expertise. Mitchell-Heggs et al. have recently proposed another transseptal technique that uses an intracardiac echocardiography probe positioned intranasally into the esophagus [17].

Left atrial linear ablation is also associated with an increased risk of cardiac tamponade [18]. Hsu and coworkers found a significant correlation between cardiac tamponade and "popping," a well-known physical phenomenon related to the sudden boiling of the endocardial tissue and its consequent rupture, when exposed to high levels of radiofrequency energy [19]. However, radiofrequency energy is not the only cause of cardiac rupture. Contact force is another relevant cofactor and many studies conducted in the preclinical field corroborated this finding [9,10,20]. Yokoyama et al. [20] developed an open irrigated ablation catheter able to measure the contact force at ablation target sites. Notably, the authors found that lesion size, steam pop, and thrombus incidence are all related to the degree of contact force exerted by the ablation catheter at the interface with cardiac tissue. In the TOCCATA study [11], Kuck and coworkers demonstrated that perforations might occur not only during application of radiofrequency energy but also during catheter manipulation. The authors reported a case of cardiac tamponade 20 s after a single recording of a contact force of 137 g during mapping of the left atrium.

Speaking more generally about AF ablation-related bleeding, an increasing amount of data has been produced in the last few years to clarify the optimal anticoagulation management before and after PVI. Significant contributions in this field come from the same group of investigators, who had initially demonstrated that periprocedural administration of warfarin was safe and efficacious [21] and may reduce thromboembolic events without increasing the risk of hemorrhagic complications (both major and minor bleeding) [22]. Future randomized international multicenter trials should confirm if the standard protocol of anticoagulation (which usually includes discontinuation of warfarin 3–5 days before the procedure and bridging with low molecular weight heparin before and after the procedure along with restoration of warfarin) should be modified. With the recent introduction of novel oral anticoagulants, the feasibility and safety of AF catheter ablation in patients taking these drugs (mainly dabigratan) have been tested, with contradictory results [23–25].

Thromboembolic events

Many studies have investigated the incidence of thromboembolic events (including transient ischemic attacks and major strokes) during or after AF catheter ablation. The introduction of open irrigated catheters and the use of early and aggressive heparinization have significantly reduced the risk of cerebrovascular events related to the procedure [26–28], although it remains unclear whether the benefit has shifted more toward late cerebrovascular events than periprocedural ones. Even though Scherr et al. [29] showed an incidence of 1.4% of periprocedural thromboembolic events using an open irrigated catheter, more robust data are needed to demonstrate a benefit of these catheters over the nonirrigated 4-mm ones. On the other hand, a multicenter retrospective study examined rates of stroke after catheter ablation of AF and, surprisingly, over a follow-up of about two-and-a-half years, no differences in thromboembolic events were noted between patients who withdrew oral anticoagulation and patients who continued to be anticoagulated [30].

As evidenced in studies using intracardiac echocardiography [26–28], an activated clotting time of more than 300 s and high-flow perfusion of the transseptal sheath are mandatory to reduce thromboembolic complications during AF catheter ablation. Furthermore, as already stated above [22], continuous administration of warfarin throughout the procedure without low molecular weight heparin bridging could help in reducing the incidence of stroke and transient ischemic attacks with little effect on the number of bleeding complications.

To complicate matters further, studies by Lickfett and colleagues [31] as well as Gaita et al. [32] not only reported an incidence of clinically apparent thromboembolic events comparable to what was already demonstrated in previous studies (0.4%) but also showed that clinically silent embolic lesions were found in 10–14% of patients who had undergone AF catheter ablation by using pre- and postprocedural cerebral magnetic resonance imaging. The degree of anticoagulation and the use of electrical or pharmacological cardioversions during the procedure correlated significantly with silent cerebral embolism.

Furthermore, contradictory and insufficient data have been produced on the thromboembolic risk associated with "one-size-fits-all" devices such as the cryoballoon, the laser balloon, the Mesh™ ablator or the Ablation Frontiers™ ablator. In this regard, the MACPAF study compared the efficacy and safety of cryoballoon ablation versus Mesh ablation in patients with drug-refractory paroxysmal AF [33]. A very high incidence of silent cerebral ischemic lesions (41%) was found in the immediate follow-up period, with only 18% of these lesions being confirmed at medium term follow-up (9 months). Fortunately, no detrimental effects on the patients' cognitive function were observed.

Finally, it is still unknown if a therapeutic INR, which has been demonstrated to reduce the incidence of periprocedural stroke [22], could completely replace intraprocedural heparinization.

Phrenic nerve injury

Phrenic nerve injury is another well-described complication of AF ablation. Sacher et al. [34] first examined rates of phrenic injury in 3755 consecutive patients who had undergone AF ablation at five different centers between 1997 and 2004. Phrenic nerve injury occurred in 0.48% of cases, with the right phrenic nerve affected more frequently than the left. Right phrenic nerve injury was commonly associated with the electrical isolation of the right superior pulmonary vein or of the superior vena cava. Conversely, left phrenic nerve injury occurred mainly after ablation of the left atrial appendage. Phrenic nerve palsy might be asymptomatic, but may also be associated with dyspnea, cough, or hiccups; and in the worst cases it may result in pneumonia, atelectasis, pleural effusions and respiratory failure. Diagnosis is usually made on a chest X-ray showing diaphragmatic elevation. Prognosis of phrenic nerve injury is usually very good. Bai et al. have described complete recovery after an average follow-up of about 9 months [35].

Phrenic nerve injury has also been described as a consequence of AF catheter ablation that employ different technologies. Among these, cryoballoon ablation seems to be exposed to a higher incidence of right phrenic nerve injury. For example, in the STOP-AF trial [36], the incidence of right phrenic nerve palsy was 11.2% with complete resolution noted in more than 80% of cases. This technology is indeed based on the delivery of cryothermal energy through a balloon catheter introduced in the left atrium with a 15 Fr outer diameter sheath (Flexcath, Medtronic, Minneapolis, MN). The inflation of the balloon at the ostium of the right pulmonary veins, which might be very close to the right phrenic nerve course, might explain this finding. Anecdotal case reports have reported phrenic nerve injury during PVI using the Ablation Frontiers pulmonary vein ablation catheter [37], during PVI using a novel endoscopic ablation system [38] or during PVI obtained with a forward directed, high-intensity focused ultrasound balloon catheter [39].

Attempts to avoid this complication can be made using high output "pace mapping" in the areas of presumable contact with phrenic nerves (usually right superior pulmonary vein, superior vena cava, and the roof of left atrial appendage) before delivery of any type of energy. Recently, Horton et al. reported a novel method of localizing the anatomy of the phrenic nerve with cardiac computed tomography and found that a distance between the right pericardionephric artery and the right superior pulmonary vein of <10 mm exposes patients to higher risks of phrenic nerve palsy when using a balloon-based ablation system [40].

Late complications

Late complications of AF catheter ablation should be considered as any adverse event, which usually happens after the procedure, occurring within a temporal frame of 30 days or is clearly related to the procedure. These complications are frequently underrecognized or misinterpreted because specialists other than electrophysiologists often evaluate them. It is, therefore, advisable to inform patients and their general practitioner on the characteristics and modalities of potential complications that may arise in order to reduce any delay in recognition and treatment.

Esophageal injury/atrio-esophageal fistula

Atrio-esophageal fistula is a very rare complication of AF catheter ablation. Described for the first time in two very experienced centers in 2004 [41,42], this is the most dreadful and lethal complication related to AF catheter ablation. Its clinical presentation is extremely variable; patients with an atrio-esophageal fistula could present with a variety of signs and symptoms such as chest pain, heartburn, dysphagia, anorexia, and hematemesis immediately after or more often late after the index procedure. Usually, death occurs because of cerebral or myocardial air embolism, endocarditis, massive gastrointestinal bleeding, and septic shock [43–45]. Surgical repair is mandatory to increase survival in these patients; therefore, a rapid diagnosis is highly desirable. The diagnostic investigation of choice would be cardiac computed

tomography while endoscopy should be avoided due to the high risk of worsening the damage to the esophageal wall. Interestingly, Bunch et al. [46] have suggested that inserting temporary esophageal stents may be a possible nonsurgical treatment for this complication, allowing for complete healing of the damaged esophageal wall.

However, the ideal management is to prevent the formation of atrio-esophageal fistulas in the first place. In this regard, a lot of studies have sought to investigate the physiopathologic mechanism underlying this complication. As demonstrated by computed tomography [47], cardiac magnetic resonance [48] and intracardiac echocardiography [49], and the close anatomic relationship between the left atrium and the esophagus together with the delivery of radiofrequency energy on the posterior wall of the left atrium are the principal causes leading to the occurrence of atrio-esophageal fistula or, more generally, of esophageal injury. Interestingly, Meng et al. have demonstrated that new esophageal late gadolinium enhancement is present in almost one-third of patients after PVI and this finding is irrespective of the type of catheter ablation (irrigated versus nonirrigated tip) used during the procedure, the ablation time, the anatomical location of the esophagus compared to the left atrium, the size of the left atrial cavity, or the timing of cardiac magnetic resonance study after PVI [50].

Different strategies can be adopted in order to avoid or reduce the incidence of this dreadful complication. First of all, localization of the region of contact between left atrium and esophagus can be obtained before the procedure itself by means of computed tomography, a barium swallow, magnetic resonance after a barium plus gadolinium diglutamate swallow [51], or during the ablation procedure with intracardiac echocardiography [52]. Moreover, electroanatomical mapping systems such as CARTO^{TM} (Biosense Webster, Diamond Bar, CA, USA) and NavX^{TM} (St Jude Medical, Sylmar, CA, USA) allow the superimposition of the esophageal imaging obtained with the Carto SoundStar^{TM} probe or with the NavX^{TM} itself with the real-time electroanatomical map of the left atrium [53,54]. Second, it is strongly advisable to avoid delivery of high levels of radiofrequency energy on the posterior wall of the left atrium or on the posterior aspect of the PV antra, which are usually areas of presumed contact with the esophagus. To this aim, since radiofrequency energy theoretically increases local temperature, it is common practice in many centers to monitor the esophageal temperature with an esophageal probe [55,56] and to titrate the radiofrequency energy application at the areas of greatest risk for esophageal injury with immediate cessation of energy delivery when a rapid elevation of the esophageal internal temperature is recorded. In centers that do not perform cardiac computed tomography or cardiac magnetic resonance before the procedure, the use of an esophagram with water-soluble contrast may represent a valuable tool to avoid ablation on portions of the left atrium that are in close vicinity to the esophagus.

However, the main issue related to this practice is the lack of knowledge of what should be the "safest" amount of radiofrequency energy. Indeed, the accuracy of esophageal luminal temperature monitoring in predicting the extent of esophageal injury is uncertain [57]. Poor correlation between esophageal internal temperature and total radiofrequency energy delivery has been demonstrated in initial clinical studies [54,58]. Inter-individual variability in esophageal and posterior left atrial wall thickness may explain this finding along with a presumable lack of fidelity of the luminal probe in measuring the heating of the esophageal wall. Furthermore, as brilliantly evidenced by Nakagawa et al. [59], esophageal tissue heating and consequent injury seem to be related more to the catheter tip–tissue contact force rather than to the total amount of radiofrequency energy delivered for PVI.

There is no compelling evidence to suggest that any of the popular strategies employed in current practice successfully reduces or even avoids this complication. The most common measures adopted in this context are reducing the power and the duration of radiofrequency energy delivery near or over the esophagus (25 W is usually considered safe) as well as monitoring the esophageal temperature by means of an endoscopic probe. Another very simple and intuitive option is to avoid any radiofrequency delivery at the posterior left atrial wall; as to the best of our knowledge, there is no conclusive evidence that linear lesions in this region would improve late outcomes compared to accurate, stable (i.e. long-lasting) PV isolation in whichever form of AF (i.e., paroxysmal, persistent, and permanent). There is also the empirical use of proton-pump inhibitors after ablation to mitigate reflux, which has been observed in many cases and correlated with pH studies [60]. There is also the questionable clinical utility of a cooled saline-irrigated balloon inside the esophageal lumen during AF catheter ablation [61]. Although cooling the internal lumen of the esophagus may limit the transmural rise of temperature, inflation of a balloon device inside the esophagus could increase the area of contact with the left atrium, enhancing paradoxically heat transfer and the chance of thermal injury.

The majority of atrio-esophageal fistulas described in the literature have been related to radiofrequency energy delivery. A possible and well-known alternative to radiofrequency is cryothermal energy. Used initially for the surgical treatment of ventricular arrhythmias and then later for endocardial treatment of specific supraventricular arrhythmias, very recently cryothermal energy indications have widened to also include atrial fibrillation or left atrial tachycardias [57]. Cryothermal energy can be delivered focally through traditional deflectable ablation catheters or circumferentially through innovative inflatable balloons with proven efficacy [1]. Unfortunately, as with radiofrequency energy, cryothermal energy induces a conductive heat transfer on the esophagus, resulting in an equivalent amount of esophageal injury compared to radiofrequency [62]. There is evidence in animal models that cryothermal ablation could result in transmural injury of the esophagus but, unlike radiofrequency energy that produces necrosis and ulcers, it preserves the architecture of the cells that greatly reduces the probability of a fistula or of ulceration [62]. However, a very recent report has revealed that an atrio-esophageal fistula had developed after cryoballoon ablation [63].

Overall, even though conflicting data exist on the risk of esophageal ulcerations after cryoballoon ablation [64,65], cryothermal energy could still represent a valid alternative to radiofrequency energy when ablation of the posterior wall is needed and hybrid approaches to AF catheter ablation has already been proposed [66].

PV stenosis

Occurring in 1–3% of cases, PV stenosis after AF catheter ablation was first described in 2000 [67]. As stated in the guidelines [1], "according to the percentage reduction of the luminal diameter, the severity of PV stenosis is generally defined as mild (<50%), moderate (50–70%), or severe (>70%)." The real incidence of PV stenosis has further decreased to below 1%, thanks to the progressive shift of the site of ablation from the internal portion of the veins toward the PV antrum and also to the great improvement in spatial accuracy of the most frequently used mapping systems [68]. Conversely, the introduction to the market of "one-size-fits-all" devices may yet contribute to an increase in the incidence PV narrowing. Very recently, De Greef et al. demonstrated that PV isolation obtained by means of the pulmonary vein ablation catheter (PVAC, Medtronic, Inc, MN) is associated with not so a negligible rate (15%) of PV narrowing at the level of the ostium, with an unpredictable probability to evolve toward clinical PV stenosis [69].

PV stenoses are often clinically silent; symptoms are extremely variegated and may include cough, dyspnea, chest pain, hemoptysis and recurrent respiratory infections [68]. Severity of the clinical presentation relies on the nature of the stenosis and the number of PVs involved [70]. Since the clinical picture associated with PV stenosis is extremely variable, PV stenosis should be suspected in every patient presenting with one of the above clinical symptoms after an AF catheter ablation. Cardiac computed tomography and cardiac magnetic resonance are the diagnostic tools commonly used to make the diagnosis; transthoracic or transesophageal echocardiography could help only partially but might be useful to assess pulmonary vein flows [70]. Radionuclide ventilation/perfusion imaging may also serve as a screening tool in symptomatic patients and help to clarify the hemodynamic significance of PV stenosis [71].

Optimal treatment for PV stenosis is still unknown. Balloon angioplasty alone or in association with stent implantation seems to be efficacious in the acute setting but is also associated with restenosis in 30–50% of patients [70]. Bearing this in mind, prevention of PV stenosis is mandatory and warrants widening the encircling of PVs to include the PV antra. There is also intense scientific debate that is ongoing on the possibility that different sources of energy, such as cryothermal energy applied through cryoballoon technology, could reduce the risk of PV stenosis. Even though theoretically cryothermal energy should avoid the development of fibrosis and/or stenosis, concerns have been raised recently after the publication of the results of the STOP-AF trial, where cryoballoon therapy was associated with a 3.1% incidence of PV stenosis.

Left atrial tachyarrhythmias

Left atrial tachycardias or left atrial flutters are the most common "electrophysiological" complications of AF catheter ablation. Occurring in up to 31% of patients undergoing this procedure [72], these arrhythmias are often more symptomatic than AF itself because they are frequently associated with fast regular ventricular responses. Usually caused by triggered activity originating from the ostia of reconnected PVs or by macroreentry around large functional or anatomical barriers (such as the mitral annulus or previously isolated PVs), these tachycardias are strictly connected to the type of AF ablation previously performed. Several studies have confirmed that PVI obtained with an anatomic approach (simple encircling of the PVs without confirmation of

electrical isolation) is associated with a higher incidence of atrial tachyarrhythmias compared to a segmental approach (consisting of PVI guided only by a circular mapping catheter) [73,74]. A possible explanation of this finding is that the substrate for AF ablation is often associated with electrical gaps and electrical gaps are usually the primary cause for both triggered and/or reentrant tachycardias [75]. Clinical management of these arrhythmias should be first of all conservative (rate control and cardioversion are both suitable options), since about one-third resolve spontaneously. For tachycardia persisting long after ablation, a redo procedure should be performed using one of the available 3D mapping systems.

Delayed tamponade

Some warning should be raised about the occurrence of the so-called delayed cardiac tamponade (DCT). A very recent report from Cappato et al. has deepened our knowledge on this topic [76], defining it as any "hypotension or cardiogenic shock requiring pericardial drainage or causing death due to documented pericardial effusion occurring at least 1 h post-procedurally but attributable to the ablation procedure." DCT had occurred in 0.2% of patients in this multicenter registry, which included 27,921 procedures in 21,478 patients. The median time frame from the index procedure to its occurrence was 12 days, with patients presenting with a cohort of nonspecific symptoms such as constant thoracic pain, neck or back pain, pain during breathing, dyspnea, dizziness, nausea, fever, peripheral or global edema, impending sense of doom or death, nausea, fever, or general malaise. Of the patients who experienced this complication 5% died; the majority of cases were treated by means of pericardial drainage but surgical intervention was needed in about 5% of cases. Predictors of DCT included large volume of patients treated (odds ratio: 5.03), use of irrigation catheter (odds ratio: 2.77), and treatment of paroxysmal AF only (odds ratio: 3.97).

Conclusions

Even though catheter ablation is a safe treatment for symptomatic drug-refractory AF, complications can still occur with sometimes very unpredictable outcomes. Awareness of such complications is as important as the knowledge of the procedural technique itself because, in this circumstance more than in any other clinical context, "prevention is better than cure." Hopefully, as worldwide experience increases and we learn from current evidence [3], the overall incidence of complications continues to fall, thus allowing for a better outcome in the future. Patient's safety is paramount and is the most important rule electrophysiologists (especially if young or inexperienced) need to respect in the context of AF ablation. To aid this ethos, we firmly believe that knowledge of guidelines is helpful and highly recommended. Finally and most importantly, we should not forget that "patient's safety begins in the office and not in the electrophysiology lab."

References

1 Calkins H, Kuck KH, Cappato R, Brugada J, Camm AJ, Chen SA, Crijns HJ, Damiano RJ, Jr., Davies DW, DiMarco J, Edgerton J, Ellenbogen K, Ezekowitz MD, Haines DE, Haissaguerre M, Hindricks G, Iesaka Y, Jackman W, Jalife J, Jais P, Kalman J, Keane D, Kim YH, Kirchhof P, Klein G, Kottkamp H, Kumagai K, Lindsay BD, Mansour M, Marchlinski FE, McCarthy PM, Mont JL, Morady F, Nademanee K, Nakagawa H, Natale A, Nattel S, Packer DL, Pappone C, Prystowsky E, Raviele A, Reddy V, Ruskin JN, Shemin RJ, Tsao HM, Wilber D. 2012 HRS/EHRA/ECAS Expert Consensus Statement on Catheter and Surgical Ablation of Atrial Fibrillation: Recommendations for Patient Selection, Procedural Techniques, Patient Management and Follow-Up, Definitions, Endpoints, and Research Trial Design. Europace. 2012;14(4):528–606.
2 Haissaguerre M, Jais P, Shah DC, Takahashi A, Hocini M, Quiniou G, Garrigue S, Le MA, Le MP, Clementy J. Spontaneous initiation of atrial fibrillation by ectopic beats originating in the pulmonary veins. N Engl J Med. 1998;339:659–666.
3 Cappato R, Calkins H, Chen SA, Davies W, Iesaka Y, Kalman J, Kim YH, Klein G, Natale A, Packer D, Skanes A, Ambrogi F, Biganzoli E. Updated worldwide survey on the methods, efficacy, and safety of catheter ablation for human atrial fibrillation. Circ Arrhythm Electrophysiol. 2010;3:32–38.
4 Shah RU, Freeman JV, Shilane D, Wang PJ, Go AS, Hlatky MA. Procedural complications, rehospitalizations, and repeat procedures after catheter ablation for atrial fibrillation. J Am Coll Cardiol. 2012;59:143–149.
5 Hoyt H, Bhonsale A, Chilukuri K, Alhumaid F, Needleman M, Edwards D, Govil A, Nazarian S, Cheng A, Henrikson CA, Sinha S, Marine JE, Berger R, Calkins H, Spragg DD. Complications arising from catheter ablation of atrial fibrillation: temporal trends and predictors. Heart Rhythm. 2011;8(12):1869–1874.
6 Cappato R, Calkins H, Chen SA, Davies W, Iesaka Y, Kalman J, Kim YH, Klein G, Natale A, Packer D, Skanes A. Prevalence and causes of fatal outcome in catheter ablation of atrial fibrillation. J Am Coll Cardiol. 2009;53:1798–1803.
7 Hindricks G. The Multicentre European Radiofrequency Survey (MERFS): complications of radiofrequency catheter ablation of arrhythmias. The Multicentre European Radiofrequency Survey (MERFS) investigators of the Working Group on Arrhythmias of the European Society of Cardiology. Eur Heart J. 1993;14:1644–1653.
8 Calkins H, Yong P, Miller JM, Olshansky B, Carlson M, Saul JP, Huang SK, Liem LB, Klein LS, Moser SA, Bloch DA, Gillette P, Prystowsky E. Catheter ablation of accessory pathways, atrioventricular nodal reentrant tachycardia, and the atrioventricular junction: final results of a prospective, multicenter clinical trial. The Atakr Multicenter Investigators Group. Circulation. 1999;99:262–270.
9 Perna F, Heist EK, Danik SB, Barrett CD, Ruskin JN, Mansour M. Assessment of the catheter tip contact force resulting in cardiac perforation in the swine atria using the force sensing technology. Circ Arrhythm Electrophysiol. 2011;4(2):218–224.
10 Shah D, Lambert H, Langenkamp A, Vanenkov Y, Leo G, Gentil-Baron P, Walpoth B. Catheter tip force required for mechanical perforation of porcine cardiac chambers. Europace. 2011;13:277–283.
11 Reddy VY, Shah D, Kautzner J, Schmidt B, Saoudi N, Herrera C, Jaïs P, Hindricks G, Peichl P, Yulzari A, Lambert H, Neuzil P, Natale A, Kuck KH. The relationship between contact force and clinical outcome during radiofrequency catheter ablation of atrial fibrillation in the TOCCATA study. Heart Rhythm. 2012;9:1789–1795.
12 Neuzil P, Reddy VY, Kautzner J, Petru J, Wichterle D, Shah D, Lambert H, Yulzari A, Wissner E, Kuck KH. Electrical reconnection after pulmonary vein isolation is contingent on contact force during initial treatment: results from the EFFICAS I Study. Circ Arrhythm Electrophysiol. 2013;6:327–333.
13 Cappato R, Calkins H, Chen SA, Davies W, Iesaka Y, Kalman J, Kim YH, Klein G, Natale A, Packer D, Skanes A. Prevalence and causes of fatal outcome in catheter ablation of atrial fibrillation. J Am Coll Cardiol. 2009;53:1798–1803.
14 De Ponti R, Cappato R, Curnis A, Della Bella P, Padeletti L, Raviele A, Santini M, Salerno-Uriarte JA. Trans-septal catheterization in the electrophysiology laboratory: data from a multicenter survey spanning 12 years. J Am Coll Cardiol. 2006;47:1037–1042.
15 Ross J, Jr., Braunwald E, Morrow AG. Transseptal left atrial puncture: new technique for the measurement of left atrial pressure in man. Am J Cardiol. 1959;3:653–655.
16 Sy RW, Klein GJ, Leong-Sit P, Gula LJ, Yee R, Krahn AD, Skanes AC. Troubleshooting difficult transseptal catheterization. J Cardiovasc Electrophysiol. 2011;22(6):723–727.
17 Mitchell-Heggs L, Lellouche N, Deal L, Elbaz N, Hamdaoui B, Castanié JB, Dubois-Randé JL, Guéret P, Lim P. Transseptal puncture using minimally invasive echocardiography during atrial fibrillation ablation. Europace. 2010;12:1435–1438.
18 Jaïs P, Shah DC, Haïssaguerre M, Takahashi A, Lavergne T, Hocini M, Garrigue S, Barold SS, Le Métayer P, Clémenty J. Efficacy and safety of septal and left-atrial linear ablation for atrial fibrillation. Am J Cardiol. 1999;84(9A):139R–146R.
19 Hsu LF, Jaïs P, Hocini M, Sanders P, Scavée C, Sacher F, Takahashi Y, Rotter M, Pasquie JL, Clémenty J, Haïssaguerre M. Incidence and prevention of cardiac

tamponade complicating ablation for atrial fibrillation. Pacing Clin Electrophysiol. 2005;28 (Suppl. 1):S106–S109.

20 Yokoyama K, Nakagawa H, Shah DC, Lambert H, Leo G, Aeby N, Ikeda A, Pitha JV, Sharma T, Lazzara R, Jackman WM. Novel contact force sensor incorporated in irrigated radiofrequency ablation catheter predicts lesion size and incidence of steam pop and thrombus. Circ Arrhythm Electrophysiol. 2008;1:354–362.

21 Wazni OM, Beheiry S, Fahmy T, Barrett C, Hao S, Patel D, Di Biase L, Martin DO, Kanj M, Arruda M, Cummings J, Schweikert R, Saliba W, Natale A. Atrial fibrillation ablation in patients with therapeutic international normalized ratio: comparison of strategies of anticoagulation management in the periprocedural period. Circulation. 2007;116:2531–2534.

22 Di Biase L, Burkhardt JD, Mohanty P, Sanchez J, Horton R, Gallinghouse GJ, Lakkireddy D, Verma A, Khaykin Y, Hongo R, Hao S, Beheiry S, Pelargonio G, Dello Russo A, Casella M, Santarelli P, Santangeli P, Wang P, Al-Ahmad A, Patel D, Themistoclakis S, Bonso A, Rossillo A, Corrado A, Raviele A, Cummings JE, Schweikert RA, Lewis WR, Natale A. Periprocedural stroke and management of major bleeding complications in patients undergoing catheter ablation of atrial fibrillation: the impact of periprocedural therapeutic international normalized ratio. Circulation. 2010;121:2550–2556.

23 Lakkireddy D, Reddy YM, Di Biase L, Vanga SR, Santangeli P, Swarup V, Pimentel R, Mansour MC, D'Avila A, Sanchez JE, Burkhardt JD, Chalhoub F, Mohanty P, Coffey J, Shaik N, Monir G, Reddy VY, Ruskin J, Natale A. Feasibility and safety of dabigatran versus warfarin for periprocedural anticoagulation in patients undergoing radiofrequency ablation for atrial fibrillation: results from a multicenter prospective registry. J Am Coll Cardiol. 2012;59:1168–1174.

24 Maddox W, Kay GN, Yamada T, Osorio J, Doppalapudi H, Plumb VJ, Gunter A, McElderry HT. Dabigatran versus warfarin therapy for uninterrupted oral anticoagulation during atrial fibrillation ablation. J Cardiovasc Electrophysiol. 2013;24(8):861–865.

25 Bassiouny M, Saliba W, Rickard J, Shao M, Sey A, Diab M, Martin DO, Hussein A, Khoury M, Abi-Saleh B, Alam S, Sengupta J, Borek PP, Baranowski B, Niebauer M, Callahan T, Varma N, Chung M, Tchou PJ, Kanj M, Dresing T, Lindsay BD, Wazni O. Use of dabigatran for periprocedural anticoagulation in patients undergoing catheter ablation for atrial fibrillation. Circ Arrhythm Electrophysiol. 2013; 6(3):460–466. doi: 10.1161/CIRCEP.113.000320. Epub 2013 Apr 3. Erratum in: Circ Arrhythm Electrophysiol. 2013;6(5):e79.

26 Kanj MH, Wazni O, Fahmy T, Thal S, Patel D, Elay C, Di Biase L, Arruda M, Saliba W, Schweikert RA, Cummings JE, Burkhardt JD, Martin DO, Pelargonio G, Dello Russo A, Casella M, Santarelli P, Potenza D, Fanelli R, Massaro R, Forleo G, Natale A. Pulmonary vein antral isolation using an open irrigation ablation catheter for the treatment of atrial fibrillation: a randomized pilot study. J Am Coll Cardiol. 2007;49:1634–1641.

27 Ren JF, Marchlinski FE, Callans DJ, Gerstenfeld EP, Dixit S, Lin D, Nayak HM, Hsia HH. Increased intensity of

anticoagulation may reduce risk of thrombus during atrial fibrillation ablation procedures in patients with spontaneous echo contrast. J Cardiovasc Electrophysiol. 2005;16:474–477.

28 Bruce CJ, Friedman PA, Narayan O, Munger TM, Hammill SC, Packer DL, Asirvatham SJ. Early heparinization decreases the incidence of left atrial thrombi detected by intracardiac echocardiography during radiofrequency ablation for atrial fibrillation. J Interv Card Electrophysiol. 2008;22:211–219.

29 Scherr D, Sharma K, Dalal D, Spragg D, Chilukuri K, Cheng A, Dong J, Henrikson CA, Nazarian S, Berger RD, Calkins H, Marine JE. Incidence and predictors of periprocedural cerebrovascular accident in patients undergoing catheter ablation of atrial fibrillation. J Cardiovasc Electrophysiol. 2009;20:1357–1363.

30 Themistoclakis S, Corrado A, Marchlinski FE, Jais P, Zado E, Rossillo A, Di Biase L, Schweikert RA, Saliba WI, Horton R, Mohanty P, Patel D, Burkhardt DJ, Wazni OM, Bonso A, Callans DJ, Haissaguerre M, Raviele A, Natale A. The risk of thromboembolism and need for oral anticoagulation after successful atrial fibrillation ablation. J Am Coll Cardiol. 2010;55:735–743.

31 Lickfett L, Hackenbroch M, Lewalter T, Selbach S, Schwab JO, Yang A, Balta O, Schrickel J, Bitzen A, Lüderitz B, Sommer T. Cerebral diffusion-weighted magnetic imaging: a tool to monitor the thrombogenicity of left atrial catheter ablation. J Cardiovasc Electrophysiol. 2006;17:1–7.

32 Gaita F, Caponi D, Pianelli M, Scaglione M, Toso E, Cesarani F, Boffano C, Gandini G, Valentini MC, De Ponti R, Halimi F, Leclercq JF. Radiofrequency catheter ablation of atrial fibrillation: a cause of silent thromboembolism? Magnetic resonance imaging assessment of cerebral thromboembolism in patients undergoing ablation of atrial fibrillation. Circulation. 2010;122: 1667–1673.

33 Haeusler KG, Koch L, Herm J, Kopp UA, Heuschmann PU, Endres M, Schultheiss HP, Schirdewan A, Fiebach JB. 3 Tesla MRI-detected brain lesions after pulmonary vein isolation for atrial fibrillation: results of the MACPAF study. J Cardiovasc Electrophysiol. 2013: 24:14–21.

34 Sacher F, Monahan KH, Thomas SP, Davidson N, Adragao P, Sanders P, Hocini M, Takahashi Y, Rotter M, Rostock T, Hsu LF, Clémenty J, Haïssaguerre M, Ross DL, Packer DL, Jaïs P. Phrenic nerve injury after atrial fibrillation catheter ablation: characterization and outcome in a multicenter study. J Am Coll Cardiol. 2006;47:2498–2503.

35 Bai R, Patel D, Di Biase L, Fahmy TS, Kozeluhova M, Prasad S, Schweikert R, Cummings J, Saliba W, Andrews-Williams M, Themistoclakis S, Bonso A, Rossillo A, Raviele A, Schmitt C, Karch M, Uriarte JA, Tchou P, Arruda M, Natale A. Phrenic nerve injury after catheter ablation: should we worry about this complication? J Cardiovasc Electrophysiol. 2006;17:944–948.

36 Packer DL, Kowal RC, Wheelan KR, Irwin JM, Champagne J, Guerra PG, Dubuc M, Reddy V, Nelson L, Holcomb RG, Lehmann JW, Ruskin JN; STOP AF Cryoablation Investigators. Cryoballoon Ablation of

Pulmonary Veins for Paroxysmal Atrial Fibrillation: First Results of the North American Arctic Front (STOP AF) Pivotal Trial. J Am Coll Cardiol. 2013;61(16):1713–1723.

37 Ahsan SY, Flett AS, Lambiase PD, Segal OR. First report of phrenic nerve injury during pulmonary vein isolation using the Ablation Frontiers pulmonary vein ablation catheter. J Interv Card Electrophysiol. 2010;29:187–190.

38 Schmidt B, Metzner A, Chun KR, Leftheriotis D, Yoshiga Y, Fuernkranz A, Neven K, Tilz RR, Wissner E, Ouyang F, Kuck KH. Feasibility of circumferential pulmonary vein isolation using a novel endoscopic ablation system. Circ Arrhythm Electrophysiol. 2010;3:481–488.

39 Nakagawa H, Antz M, Wong T, Schmidt B, Ernst S, Ouyang F, Vogtmann T, Wu R, Yokoyama K, Lockwood D, Po SS, Beckman KJ, Davies DW, Kuck KH, Jackman WM. Initial experience using a forward directed, high-intensity focused ultrasound balloon catheter for pulmonary vein antrum isolation in patients with atrial fibrillation. J Cardiovasc Electrophysiol. 2007;18:136–144.

40 Horton R, Di Biase L, Reddy V, Neuzil P, Mohanty P, Sanchez J, Nguyen T, Mohanty S, Gallinghouse GJ, Bailey SM, Zagrodzky JD, Burkhardt JD, Natale A. Locating the right phrenic nerve by imaging the right pericardio-phrenic artery with computerized tomographic angiography: implications for balloon-based procedures. Heart Rhythm. 2010;7:937–941.

41 Pappone C, Oral H, Santinelli V, Vicedomini G, Lang CC, Manguso F, Torracca L, Benussi S, Alfieri O, Hong R, Lau W, Hirata K, Shikuma N, Hall B, Morady F. Atrio-esophageal fistula as a complication of percutaneous transcatheter ablation of atrial fibrillation. Circulation. 2004;109:2724–2726.

42 Scanavacca MI, Davila A, Parga J, Sosa E. Left atrial-esophageal fistula following radiofrequency catheter ablation of atrial fibrillation. J Cardiovasc Electrophysiol. 2004;15:960–962.

43 Doll N, Borger MA, Fabricius A, Stephan S, Gummert J, Mohr FW, Hauss J, Kottkamp H, Hindricks G. Esophageal perforation during left atrial radiofrequency ablation: is the risk too high? J Thorac Cardiovasc Surg. 2003;125:836–842.

44 Aryana A, Arthur A, O'Neill PG, D'Avila A. Catastrophic manifestations of air embolism in a patient with atrioesophageal fistula following minimally invasive surgical ablation of atrial fibrillation. J Cardiovasc Electrophysiol. 2013;24(8):933–934.

45 Rivera GA, David IB, Anand RG. Successful atrioesophageal fistula repair after atrial fibrillation ablation. J Am Coll Cardiol. 2013;61(11):1204.

46 Bunch TJ, Nelson J, Foley T, Allison S, Crandall BG, Osborn JS, Weiss JP, Anderson JL, Nielsen P, Anderson L, Lappe DL, Day JD. Temporary esophageal stenting allows healing of esophageal perforations following atrial fibrillation ablation procedures. J Cardiovasc Electrophysiol. 2006;17:435–439.

47 Lemola K, Sneider M, Desjardins B, Case I, Han J, Good E, Tamirisa K, Tsemo A, Chugh A, Bogun F, Pelosi F, Jr., Kazerooni E, Morady F, Oral H. Computed tomographic analysis of the anatomy of the left atrium and the

esophagus: implications for left atrial catheter ablation. Circulation. 2004;110:3655–3660.

48 Badger TJ, Adjei-Poku YA, Burgon NS, Kalvaitis S, Shaaban A, Sommers DN, Blauer JJ, Fish EN, Akoum N, Haslem TS, Kholmovski EG, MacLeod RS, Adler DG, Marrouche NF. Initial experience of assessing esophageal tissue injury and recovery using delayed-enhancement MRI after atrial fibrillation ablation. Circ Arrhythm Electrophysiol. 2009;2:620–625.

49 Ren JF, Marchlinski FE. Utility of intracardiac echocardiography in left heart ablation for tachyarrhythmias. Echocardiography 2007;24:533–540.

50 Meng J, Peters DC, Hsing JM, Chuang ML, Chan J, Fish A, Josephson ME, Manning WJ. Late gadolinium enhancement of the esophagus is common on cardiac MR several months after pulmonary vein isolation: preliminary observations. Pacing Clin Electrophysiol. 2010;33:661–666.

51 Pollak SJ, Monir G, Chemoby MS, Elenberger CD. Novel imaging techniques of the esophagus enhancing safety of left atrial ablation. J Cardiovasc Electrophysiol. 2005;16:245–248.

52 Ren JF, Lin D, Marchlinski FE, Callans DJ, Patel V. Esophageal imaging and strategies for avoiding injury during left atrial ablation for atrial fibrillation. Heart Rhythm. 2006;3:1156–1161.

53 Piorkowski C, Hindricks G, Schreiber D, Tanner H, Weise W, Koch A, Gerds-Li JH, Kottkamp H. Electroanatomic reconstruction of the left atrium, pulmonary veins, and esophagus compared with the "true anatomy" on multislice computed tomography in patients undergoing catheter ablation of atrial fibrillation. Heart Rhythm. 2006;3:317–327.

54 Cummings JE, Schweikert RA, Saliba WI, Burkhardt JD, Brachmann J, Gunther J, Schibgilla V, Verma A, Dery M, Drago JL, Kilicaslan F, Natale A. Assessment of temperature, proximity, and course of the esophagus during radiofrequency ablation within the left atrium. Circulation. 2005;112:459–464.

55 Redfearn DP, Trim GM, Skanes AC, Petrellis B, Krahn AD, Yee R, Klein GJ. Esophageal temperature monitoring during radiofrequency ablation of atrial fibrillation. J Cardiovasc Electrophysiol. 2005;16:589–593.

56 Perzanowski C, Teplitsky L, Hranitzky PM, Bahnson TD. Real-time monitoring of luminal esophageal temperature during left atrial radiofrequency catheter ablation for atrial fibrillation: observations about esophageal heating during ablation at the pulmonary vein ostia and posterior left atrium. J Cardiovasc Electrophysiol. 2006;17:166–170.

57 Bahnson TD. Strategies to minimize the risk of esophageal injury during catheter ablation for atrial fibrillation. Pacing Clin Electrophysiol. 2009;32:248–260.

58 Teplitsky L, Perzanowski C, Durrani S, Berman AE, Hranitzky P, Bahnson TD. Radiofrequency catheter ablation for atrial fibrillation produces delayed and long lasting elevation of luminal esophageal temperature independent of lesion duration and power. Heart Rhythm. 2005;2:S8–S9.

59 Nakagawa H. Role of contact force in esophageal injury during left atrial radiofrequency ablation. Heart Rhythm. 2008;5:S317–S317.

60 Martinek M, Hassanein S, Bencsik G, Aichinger J, Schoefl R, Bachl A, Gerstl S, Nesser HJ, Purerfellner H. Acute development of gastroesophageal reflux after radiofrequency catheter ablation of atrial fibrillation. Heart Rhythm. 2009;6:1457–1462.

61 Tsuchiya T, Ashikaga K, Nakagawa S, Hayashida K, Kugimiya H. Atrial fibrillation ablation with esophageal cooling with a cooled water-irrigated intraesophageal balloon: a pilot study. J Cardiovasc Electrophysiol. 2007;18:145–150.

62 Teplitsky L, Hegland DD, Bahnson TD. Catheter based cryoablation and radiofrequency ablation for atrial fibrillation results in conductive heat transfer from and to the esophagus. Heart Rhythm. 2006;3:S242–S242.

63 Stöckigt F, Schrickel JW, Andrié R, Lickfett L. Atrioesophageal fistula after cryoballoon pulmonary vein isolation. J Cardiovasc Electrophysiol. 2012;23:1254–1257.

64 Neumann T, Vogt J, Schumacher B, Dorszewski A, Kuniss M, Neuser H, Kurzidim K, Berkowitsch A, Koller M, Heintze J, Scholz U, Wetzel U, Schneider MA, Horstkotte D, Hamm CW, Pitschner HF. Circumferential pulmonary vein isolation with the cryoballoon technique results from a prospective 3-center study. J Am Coll Cardiol. 2008;52:273–278.

65 Ahmed J, D'avila A, Neuzil P, Ruskin JN, Reddy VY. Esophageal damage after PV isolation with cryoballoon catheter. Heart Rhythm. 2008;5:S46–S46.

66 Mansour M, Forleo GB, Pappalardo A, Barrett C, Heist EK, Avella A, Bencardino G, Dello Russo A, Casella M, Ruskin JN, Tondo C. Combined use of cryoballoon and focal open-irrigation radiofrequency ablation for treatment of persistent atrial fibrillation: results from a pilot study. Heart Rhythm. 2010;7:452–458.

67 Scanavacca MI, Kajita LJ, Vieira M, Sosa EA. Pulmonary vein stenosis complicating catheter ablation of focal atrial fibrillation. J Cardiovasc Electrophysiol. 2000;11: 677–681.

68 Takahashi A, Kuwahara T, Takahashi Y. Complications in the catheter ablation of atrial fibrillation: incidence and management. Circ J. 2009;73:221–226.

69 De Greef Y, Tavernier R, Raeymaeckers S, Schwagten B, Desurgeloose D, De Keulenaer G, Stockman D, De Buyzere M, Duytschaever M. Prevalence, characteristics, and predictors of pulmonary vein narrowing after isolation using the pulmonary vein ablation catheter. Circ Arrhythm Electrophysiol. 2012;5:52–60.

70 Holmes DR, Jr., Monahan KH, Packer D. Pulmonary vein stenosis complicating ablation for atrial fibrillation: clinical spectrum and interventional considerations. JACC Cardiovasc Interv. 2009;2:267–276.

71 Nanthakumar K, Mountz JM, Plumb VJ, Epstein AE, Kay GN. Functional assessment of pulmonary vein stenosis using radionuclide ventilation/perfusion imaging. Chest. 2004;126:645–651.

72 Deisenhofer I, Estner H, Zrenner B, Schreieck J, Weyerbrock S, Hessling G, Scharf K, Karch MR, Schmitt C. Left atrial tachycardia after circumferential pulmonary vein ablation for atrial fibrillation: incidence, electrophysiological characteristics, and results of radiofrequency ablation. Europace. 2006;8:573–582.

73 Pappone C, Manguso F, Vicedomini G, Gugliotta F, Santinelli O, Ferro A, Gulletta S, Sala S, Sora N, Paglino G, Augello G, Agricola E, Zangrillo A, Alfieri O, Santinelli V. Prevention of iatrogenic atrial tachycardia after ablation of atrial fibrillation: a prospective randomized study comparing conventional pulmonary vein ablation with a modified approach. Circulation. 2004;110: 3036–3042.

74 Karch MR, Zrenner B, Deisenhofer I, Schreieck J, Ndrepepa G, Dong J, Lamprecht K, Barthel P, Luciani E, Schomig A, Schmitt C. Freedom from atrial tachyarrhythmias after catheter ablation of atrial fibrillation: a randomized comparison between 2 current ablation strategies. Circulation. 2005;111:2875–2880.

75 Gerstenfeld EP, Marchlinski FE. Mapping and ablation of left atrial tachycardias occurring after atrial fibrillation ablation. Heart Rhythm. 2007;4:S65–S72.

76 Cappato R, Calkins H, Chen SA, Davies W, Iesaka Y, Kalman J, Kim YH, Klein G, Natale A, Packer D, Ricci C, Skanes A, Ranucci M. Delayed cardiac tamponade after radiofrequency catheter ablation of atrial fibrillation: a worldwide report. J Am Coll Cardiol. 2011;58(25): 2696–2697.

CHAPTER 28

Charting long-term success and the challenge of monitoring outcomes

Isabel Deisenhofer

German Heart Center Munich, Department for Electrophysiology, Technische Universität München, München, Germany

Charting what we do: how to evaluate (long-term) success in atrial fibrillation ablation

Over the last decade, catheter ablation of atrial fibrillation (AF) has become an established therapeutic approach that has the potential to "cure" this most common human arrhythmia [1–6]. Despite the worldwide use of this technique, it is still very difficult to estimate the "true" effectiveness of AF ablation, with a wide range of success rates being reported [1].

This difficulty is in part due to the varying definitions of ablation success and the even more disperse methods to evaluate ablation outcome. Additionally, a variety of different ablation techniques as shown in the previous chapters of this book with different timelines of effectiveness have to be considered.

Possible end points of AF ablation trials include ECG-based "rhythm" end points or focus on the clinical improvement of the patient or the quality of life [1,7,8]. "Rhythm" end points comprise freedom of any atrial tachyarrhythmia, freedom of atrial fibrillation only (atrial tachycardia other than AF would be counted as success), and/or reduction of AF burden. Possible "nonrhythm" end points of AF ablation may be improvement of (1) NYHA heart failure class, (2) echocardiographic parameters such as left ventricular ejection fraction or left atrial size, or (3) quality of life assessed with standard or especially designed questionnaires. Sinus rhythm with or without antiarrhythmic

Practical Guide to Catheter Ablation of Atrial Fibrillation, Second Edition. Edited by Jonathan S. Steinberg, Pierre Jaïs and Hugh Calkins.

drug therapy (often with a previously ineffective drug) and with one or more ablation procedure as well as blanking periods immediately after ablation and total time of follow-up are additional variables that should be discussed.

Taking all this into consideration it might turn out to be quite difficult to compare atrial fibrillation ablation trials, as they generally differ in at least one of these variables.

Despite recommendations of the societies, criteria for AF ablation follow-up [1] and especially ablation success are not always used in currently published trials. Thus, we try to give an overview of currently used definitions of success, follow-up methods, and follow-up timeframes.

The "rhythm" end points

Freedom of any kind of atrial tachyarrhythmia is the strongest end point of AF ablation, but the most difficult to prove. AF ablation is generally performed in patients suffering from symptoms during AF. Especially at the beginning of the AF ablation era, only highly symptomatic patients with paroxysmal AF were included in AF ablation trials [2–6]. When screening for AF recurrence, clinical evaluation of patients' symptoms seemed to be sufficient. However, it was observed that even previously highly symptomatic patients experienced asymptomatic episodes of AF after ablation. This seemed to occur independently of the chosen ablation technique [7,8]. The percentage of patients who experienced no AF symptoms after ablation despite occurrence of AF episodes ranges between 20 and 70% [9–11].

The reasons for this loss of symptoms are not clear. One might be a placebo effect merely due to the invasive procedure. Another could be an ablation-induced modification of the intrinsic cardiac nervous system by damaging (as a "side effect") mixed ganglionated plexus. A third interesting one is the suspicion that also before ablation asymptomatic AF episodes occurred. The latter has been demonstrated by Hindricks and coworkers [9] using 7-day Holter ECG before AF ablation and by several investigators [14–17] using the arrhythmia Holter of implanted devices before and after AF ablation. The disappearance of symptoms after ablation is obviously not linked to a lower heart rate during AF or an ablation-mediated more regularized conduction of AF to the ventricles [12]. In the DISCERN trial [13], these findings were confirmed using an implanted loop recorder (ILR) 3 months before and 18 months after ablation:

1 Before ablation, 52% of all AF episodes were asymptomatic.

2 This increased to 79% of all AF episodes being asymptomatic after ablation and episodes had a 3 fold risk to be asymptomtic after ablation.

3 12% of patients had only asymptomatic AF episodes after ablation, that were undetected by conventional 24 hour Holter ECG.

The lesson from all these observations is that freedom of atrial tachyarrhythmia should be *documented* rather than to be assumed by patients' symptoms.

Assessment of complete freedom from any atrial tachyarrhythmia

Complete freedom from any atrial tachyarrhythmia can be proven only with a "permanent" Holter ECG documenting any atrial high rate episode [14]. Implanted devices like pacemakers or ICDs could provide these data, provided that the atrial sensing is (close to) "infallible" [14–17]. In some AF ablation studies, a considerable proportion of included patients had already received an implantable device and thus the optimal monitoring tool, but this is rather the exception than the rule [14–17].

Since implantable loop recorders have been developed, their use in AF trials has been discussed. The possible advantage is that with these small devices, which are implanted only subcutaneously and have no lead, any kind of device-related complication, for example, pocket bleeding, infection, endocarditis, or lead fracture, is virtually excluded. On the other hand, the rhythm assessment is done by evaluating a two-point surface ECG derived from the two ends of the lighter-shaped device. Thus, there is no intracardiac recording of atrial activity, but AF detection algorithms mostly use heart rate (changes) and variability

of R–R intervals to detect AF. It has been reported that using only these two parameters, a sensitivity of 95%, but a specificity of only 85%, could be reached compared to a 48-h Holter recording [17]. The main issue was frequent VPC or APC events. Since only the latest 10 episodes are stored together with an ECG, whereas all earlier episodes of automatically detected arrhythmias are simply listed, the results of the loop recorder can be misleading in both directions; or it can lead to an overestimation of AF burden, since, for example, of 800 listed episodes only the latest 9 are AF, whereas all 791 are in fact VPCs, but without ECG recordings. On the other hand, underestimation of AF can occur if the stored ECG of the most recent 8 out of 800 episodes show only ventricular bigeminus, whereas, in fact, 791 would have shown AF.

In patients without an implanted device, there are mainly two methods of intensive, long-term rhythm monitoring: repetitive long-term Holter ECG recordings like 7-day Holter ECG or event monitoring (with *daily* ECG recordings and *additional* recording in case of symptoms). Both have been used in AF ablation studies [8–11,19–22] and have been found to be comparable regarding the sensitivity of AF episodes detection. Strikingly, both revealed that approximately 70% of AF episodes are "missed" with a conventional 24 h Holter ECG, which is the most commonly used rhythm assessment tool [19]. As pointed out before, another interesting finding is that approximately 20–70% of recurrences of AF seem to be asymptomatic [8–11,19,20]. Thus, ECG event monitor recordings performed only in the moment of symptoms are obviously not sufficient for a dense follow-up of rhythm after AF ablation.

With both methods, the frequency of ECG recordings or the duration of regular telemetric ECG transmissions is very important. The general rule that the more intensive the screening the more clinical events (i.e., episodes of AF) are found is true for AF in the same way as for other clinical entities. One main problem from a practical aspect is the quantity of follow-up ECG data that have to be analyzed by medically trained persons and stored in a comprehensive manner [8,13,19]. The other is patients' compliance regarding the daily transmission or even weekly transmission of ECGs. To have a sufficiently reliable database, it is absolutely necessary to obtain at least 80% of the planned ECG recordings [1], which is hard to achieve.

Regardless of the chosen monitoring tool, the question still remains how long AF has to last to be named "AF recurrence." Looking at Holter ECGs, investigators have not reached a consensus what is "sustained AF" after an AF ablation. The range comprises

AF episodes lasting more than 30 s, 5 min, or 30 min [2–6,9–11,19–22]. Nademanee et al. chose the longest period with episodes lasting more than 24 h, but their patient cohort included many patients with persistent or permanent AF [18]. A solution might be to take into account the length of the average AF episode in the individual patient before and after ablation. In paroxysmal AF, the aim of the procedure is to eliminate all AF episodes, even those lasting only for seconds. To render AF trials comparable, the HRS/ EHRA/ECAS recommendations stick to the (arbitrary, but accepted) end point of AF lasting more than 30 s [1].

Regular atrial tachycardias after AF ablation

As mentioned before, the freedom of *any kind* of atrial tachyarrhythmia is the strongest end point in AF ablation. The significance of postablation *regular* atrial tachycardia like (atypical) atrial flutter instead of AF is not yet clear [23–27]. These tachycardias might be considered as (partial) AF ablation success since the atria are not able to fibrillate any more. In this view, atrial tachycardia would not represent a recurrence of AF and a patient suffering from this kind of tachycardia would be counted as a successful ablation patient. Many studies dealing with the stepwise ablation approach for persistent AF support this view, since the patients with a mere recurrence of AF have a much worse outcome of repeat ablations than those who experience "only" AT recurrence. On the other hand, these tachycardias could represent last "remnants" of AF or be interpreted as a proarrhythmic effect of ablation. The fact is that it requires some experience to map and ablate successfully these tachycardias. Whatever flipside of the coin you want to look at, it has to be kept in mind that anticoagulation is still necessary in patients with persistent atrial tachycardia, even if it is regular.

AF burden

This term has been mainly used by studies evaluating the effect of pacemaker stimulation algorithms on the frequency and duration of AF episodes. It represents the percentage of total recording time that a patient is actually in AF [14–18]. This makes sense by definition only in patients with an implantable device. In patients monitored only with repetitive 7-day Holter ECG, the assessment of AF burden is much more difficult. If the decrease of AF burden is the end point of data analysis, a valuable preablation AF burden assessment has to be performed, again preferentially with a device – and much less accurate with a 7-day Holter ECG [10,12]. The measurement of AF burden

turns into a statistical hazard in patients with few AF episodes. Recording a 7-day Holter ECG seems not enough to assess the frequency and duration of AF before and after ablation if patients experience only monthly AF episodes [8,12]. Even in patients with a (continuously recording) device, AF burden remains a "surrogate" end point in AF ablation as the aim should be total elimination of AF.

Clinical evaluation

The clinical evaluation of ambulatory patients with questionnaires or standard ECG documentation is insufficient to prove freedom from AF. Nevertheless, some important information might be gained from a simple routine 12-lead ECG like accelerated or decreased sinus rate at rest, change of P-wave morphology during sinus rhythm (indicating intra-atrial conduction disturbance), frequent premature atrial contractions or prolonged PQ or QT interval (e.g., due to antiarrhythmic medication). Clinical evaluation of all patients after AF ablation (e.g., at 1, 3, 6, and 12 months) can provide interesting and important information even though it might be time-consuming and costly [7,11]. Regular clinical visits after AF ablation are clearly more popular in Europe, probably because of the shorter distances between clinic and patients' homes [2,5,6,11,16–18,23–25]. In the United States, the mean distances between clinic and patients' residences render clinical visits more difficult [4,26–28]. As an alternative, transmissions of local ECG recordings to the clinic are proposed [24,29]. This seems a fairly good way to monitor patient outcomes. It is in any way preferable to telephonic follow-up or no follow-up at all.

The confounding variables of rhythm end points

Blanking periods

Clinical reality has shown that in a large proportion of patients with early AF recurrence, these episodes are followed by total arrhythmia freedom during follow-up [6,9–11,19–22]. The mechanisms of this "delayed cure" are supposed to be related to a pronounced postablation inflammatory reaction and thus might be increased with more extensive ablation approaches, for example, circumferential instead of segmental PVI. Another factor that needs some time to fully develop its effects is the "reverse atrial remodeling" [34–36]. In analogy to the atrial remodeling process released with AF [37,38] and the resulting undesirable promotion of even more AF ("atrial fibrillation begets atrial fibrillation"), a reverse atrial remodeling is promoted by sinus rhythm, that is, "sinus rhythm begets sinus rhythm." Since this process needs time, a "blanking period" immediately after ablation makes sense.

Another explanation of the late success of AF ablation might be the "maturation" of lesions. Especially atrial linear lesions seem to be subject to this late effect, which might lead to spontaneous disappearance of early occurring atrial tachycardias [11,19–22]. This time effect has been reported by several groups, describing the spontaneous disappearance of secondary arrhythmias within the first 3 months after AF ablation.

From these observations, it has been suggested to install a "blanking period" after AF ablation. This avoids taking into account transient effects when assessing the efficacy of an AF ablation method [9–10,19–22,28,29]. There is no general consensus how long this blanking period should last. In most studies, 4 weeks up to 3 months are chosen, but exact data on the time course of the delay of cure are lacking. Moreover, not all investigators have observed this improvement over time [3,4,22]. However, there is now the general recommendation that a blanking period of at least 1 month should be observed until ablation lesion-related inflammation has cooled down [1].

The discussion about blanking periods and time effect on AF ablation outcome is important from a practical standpoint when thinking about the timing of a repeat ablation. In other words: should a repeat ablation be scheduled at the time of the first AF recurrence or should we wait for the beneficial late effects of the ablation? If yes, how long is enough?

It seems that AF ablation outcome is unique regarding the relevance of recurrences. Most other ablation procedures (e.g., WPW ablation) provide a "success" or "failure" result after ablation. In AF ablation, there is often no such easy "black and white" answer to the patients' question about ablation efficacy. Even knowing this, it is sometimes difficult for the patient and the operator to adopt a "time will tell" attitude after ablation. However, early (in the first 4 weeks) reablation has been widely given up, later (after >3 months) reablation being the accepted proceeding [1].

Additional medication

In many AF ablation trials, one prerequisite for inclusion is that antiarrhythmic drugs have been shown to be ineffective prior to ablation. The desired ablation effect is that no antiarrhythmic medication has to be used anymore to achieve stable sinus rhythm. However, in some cases, the freedom of arrhythmia after AF ablation is possible only with additional antiarrhythmic medication. Several studies point out that the medication effective after ablation was ineffective

before in suppressing AF or that the effective dosage is substantially reduced [20,21,32,33]. This is regarded as a positive ablation effect or even a "surrogate success." It has to be remembered that AF ablation was promoted because other AF treatment strategies were ineffective in long-term (cardioversion) or – in the case of antiarrhythmic drugs – only moderately effective in mid-term with possible side-effects. To treat a patient with a combination of AF ablation (with possible complications) and afterward still ongoing antiarrhythmic drugs is at least a very weak definition of a "successful therapeutic concept."

This might be different for transient pharmacological support of sinus rhythm after ablation of persistent or permanent AF. In these cases, antiarrhythmic medication is often given for a short time to stabilize sinus rhythm in order to give the reverse remodeling time to take place [18,25,26].

Amiodarone with its long half-life merits a special consideration in this context. If it is given, for example, for 4 months after ablation, and the rhythm outcome is assessed 6 months after ablation, the resulting rhythm outcome will reflect the combined effect of ablation and amiodarone treatment. In this case, the true result of ablation needs to be evaluated at a sufficient time interval after stopping amiodarone treatment.

Repeat ablations

Repeat AF ablation procedures are necessary in approximately 10–30% of patients with paroxysmal AF and up to 80% of patients with persistent AF to achieve complete freedom of arrhythmia [9–11,18–26,28,33–36,45–50]. Despite this rather high percentage, repeat ablations have not gained much attention. The majority of reablations are performed 1–6 months after the first ablation, in early studies even only few days after the first procedure [3,7,11,18–22,32–36,45–50]. In most studies, the follow-up period starts with the initial ablation date, and the rhythm outcome of the patient is evaluated at fixed intervals after the initial ablation procedure (e.g., 1, 3, 6, and 12 months). Most studies do not break down the results with and without repeat ablation. The interval between the repeat ablation and the fixed follow-up date is often not given – but it will be of course shorter than the interval to the initial ablation. Thus, duration of follow-up after the *last* ablation is mostly not known and for sure overestimated.

The intervals between initial and repeat ablation were getting longer starting from 2005 on because of the increasing acceptance of the reverse remodeling concept. Consecutively, the discrepancy between follow-up duration since first ablation procedure and follow-up duration since reablation are nowadays mostly between 3–6 months and should be given separately.

Clinical improvement and quality of life

The target of AF ablation is the restoration of sinus rhythm. Therefore, the classic measure for AF ablation outcome is the resulting rhythm – sinus rhythm or arrhythmia. This refers mainly to patients presenting with symptomatic, mostly paroxysmal AF [2,4,7,11] in whom the problem is the arrhythmia itself together with the resulting symptoms (palpitations, decreased physical performance, and dyspnoea). Nowadays AF ablation is increasingly performed in patients (most of them with persistent or permanent AF) who suffer not so much from palpitations but more from "side effects" of AF like heart failure. In these patients, the measure for successful AF ablation has been adjusted to the aimed effect. It is not so much the will to eliminate AF but to improve atrial and ventricular function and thus the patients mid- and long-term prognosis regarding morbidity and mortality. The ideal measure for AF ablation outcome would thus be a comparison of left ventricular ejection fraction (invasive or noninvasive), performance at exercise testing, and improvement in functional NYHA class [7].

Improvement of left ventricular function in patients with heart failure and AF

There are only few data about the improvement of left ventricular (LV) function after AF ablation, most of these in patients with congestive heart failure or NYHA class 2–3. Most studies report about results of consecutive echocardiographic measurements of LV ejection fraction (LVEF) or LV fractional shortening [51–56]. It seems that patients who are mostly in sinus rhythm can profit from AF ablation in terms of LVEF increase [51,52] and reduction of heart chamber diameter (especially the diameter of the left atrium [LA]) [50–52]. These data, however, have not been confirmed by larger trial results. A more technical but nevertheless important detail is that echocardiographic data at baseline and at follow-up are sometimes not acquired during the same rhythm. LVEF and LA diameter at baseline are measured during AF. These data might always be worse than those obtained during sinus rhythm in the same patient, even if sinus rhythm is present only for a very short time (e.g., after cardioversion). Regarding LA size and transport function after AF ablation, discrepant data have been published. Several studies describe

a decrease in left atrial size after ablation, which seems to be present in all patients but more pronounced in patients who remain in stable SR. On the other hand, there are few data suggesting deterioration in LA transport function due to extensive left atrial ablation [55–57]. A new and quite disturbing finding is the so-called syndrome of the "stiff left atrium" that occurs after extensive (repeated) left atrial ablations with extensive scarring and fibrosis due to ablation lesions [58]. These patients suffer from postcapillary pulmonary hypertension despite good LV function because of a left atrial diastolic dysfunction.

The best end point in AF ablation trials would be cardiac mortality and morbidity due to AF and the occurrence of stroke [1,8,52], which would require a large scale multicenter trial. The CABANA trial is such a large-scale, multicenter, prospective randomized trial trying to assess the effect of AF ablation on mortality and morbidity in a follow-up of 3 years.

Quality of life

Apart from its association with morbidity and mortality, AF leads to substantial impairment of health-related quality of life (QOL). The monitoring of patients' QOL has gained for some years in the late 2000 years increasing interest, maybe because the evaluation of "rhythm only" end points seemed so variable and incomparable.

The well-accepted SF 36 questionnaire, the "WHO five well-being" and other standard measures of QOL, as well as specifically designed "AF QOL" questionnaires were used routinely to assess the impact of AF and of AF ablation on QOL. Studies have found that the reduction in quality of life before ablation is correlated neither to the extent of AF-induced individual symptoms nor to the actual severity of AF such as AF frequency, AF duration, and concomitant morbidity [59–62]. In two independent studies that did QOL comparisons before and after AF ablation, there were strong indications that AF ablation might produce, in part, a placebo effect: in both large-scale trials, a sustainable significant increase in all QOL measures was found, with no relation to the ablation success. Reassuringly, in both studies, patients after successful AF ablation had a significantly higher increase in QOL in AF-specific measures [30,31].

Unsolved problems

The ablation of AF started as an experimental treatment strategy and as such was in constant need for justification: A complete chain of evidence proving the long-term efficacy with success rates >60% has yet to be established. This includes studies in large patient populations to assess that this approach is safe, easily feasible, and effective also in the long-term.

Small patients' series

Published data about AF ablation most commonly stem from single-center studies with small-to-moderate patient numbers. There are only few studies in AF ablation exceeding a number of 500 included patients, and this did not change too much over the last decade [2–6,9–11,17–26,32–36,46–50,52–57]. Fortunately, there are now an increasing number of controlled randomized studies and even meta-analysis of the different ablation approaches both for paroxysmal AF and for persistent AF. This is mostly due to the fact that AF ablation moved from an experimental, challenging procedure to a routinely performed ablation with clear-cut procedural end points and comprehensive complication prevention and management.

Follow-up

Another problem has already been addressed in part: the heterogeneous follow-up methods. Some studies even lack simple information about follow-up methods (e.g., rhythm assessed with normal resting ECG or with Holter ECG) [23].) The sheer follow-up duration is another problem. AF ablation is – even more than 15 years after the groundbreaking publication of Haissaguerre et al., a relatively "young" treatment option and there are still only extremely few data beyond the first 5 years of follow-up [68–70]. Most studies report a follow-up of less than a year. There are two quite disturbing publications regarding the 5-year results after AF ablation: in a long-term observation of a mixed paroxysmal and persistent AF population by the Bordeaux group [69], single procedure success after a single procedure was only about 30%, whereas it increased to over 60% with multiple ablation procedures (but then follow-up after the last ablation was not 5 years anymore).

In a study that observed the long-term outcome in patients with persistent AF only, the Hamburg group of Kuck [70] found that only 20% were in stable sinus rhythm after one procedure, this increased to 40% with multiple ablations. In a study by our group, yearly late recurrence rate was approximately 3% per year, if patients were in sinus rhythm for the first year after ablation.

Another question that gained increasing interest was the question of the "natural course" of this disease in our patients. This will be addressed at least in part by the CABANA trial.

Results and complications

Enthusiasm was the prevailing feeling at the beginning of the AF ablation era. Mostly "good to excellent" results were published and problematic cases were neglected. This led to a dramatic overestimation of achievable success rates and an equally dramatic (but extremely dangerous) underestimation of complications [1,65]. In 2005, a "worldwide survey on the methods, efficacy, and safety of catheter ablation for human atrial fibrillation" was published. This survey resumes the (anonymous) answers of 118 centers worldwide who performed AF ablation from 1995–2002 to a detailed questionnaire [66]. In total, 8745 patients had undergone AF ablation with 27% requiring more than one procedure. Overall efficacy in respect to freedom of symptoms (!) off drugs was 52% (varying from 14.5 to 76.5%). Another 24% of patients became asymptomatic after ablation using previously ineffective drugs during a mean follow-up of 11.6 ± 7.7 months. Disquietingly, the mean rate of major complications was 6%, with four cases of death (0.05%). Major complications included cardiac tamponade in 1.3% of patients, severe pulmonary vein stenosis in 1.5%, and stroke or TIA in 0.28 and 0.66% of patients, respectively. Therefore, the authors urged operators to inform patients about all possible complications and to carefully select patients eligible for AF ablation.

Fortunately, a repeat survey in 2010 showed that complication rates decreased to 4.5% [67].

In conclusion, monitoring the outcome of AF catheter ablation may be a challenging and sometimes cumbersome task – but it is an indispensable step in establishing AF ablation as a standard procedure.

References

1 Calkins H, Kuck KH, Cappato R, Brugada J, Camm AJ, Chen SA, Crijns HJ, Damiano RJ, Jr., Davies DW, DiMarco J, Edgerton J, Ellenbogen K, Ezekowitz MD, Haines DE, Haissaguerre M, Hindricks G, Iesaka Y, Jackman W, Jalife J, Jais P, Kalman J, Keane D, Kim YH, Kirchhof P, Klein G, Kottkamp H, Kumagai K, Lindsay BD, Mansour M, Marchlinski FE, McCarthy PM, Mont JL, Morady F, Nademanee K, Nakagawa H, Natale A, Nattel S, Packer DL, Pappone C, Prystowsky E, Raviele A, Reddy V, Ruskin JN, Shemin RJ, Tsao HM, Wilber D. Heart Rhythm Society Task Force on Catheter and Surgical Ablation of Atrial Fibrillation. 2012 HRS/EHRA/ECAS Expert Consensus Statement on Catheter and Surgical Ablation of Atrial Fibrillation: Recommendations for Patient Selection, Procedural Techniques, Patient Management and Follow-Up, Definitions, Endpoints, and Research Trial Design: a report of the Heart Rhythm Society (HRS) Task Force on Catheter and Surgical Ablation of Atrial Fibrillation. Developed in partnership with the European Heart Rhythm

Association (EHRA), a registered branch of the European Society of Cardiology (ESC) and the European Cardiac Arrhythmia Society (ECAS); and in collaboration with the American College of Cardiology (ACC), American Heart Association (AHA), the Asia Pacific Heart Rhythm Society (APHRS), and the Society of Thoracic Surgeons (STS). Endorsed by the governing bodies of the American College of Cardiology Foundation, the American Heart Association, the European Cardiac Arrhythmia Society, the European Heart Rhythm Association, the Society of Thoracic Surgeons, the Asia Pacific Heart Rhythm Society, and the Heart Rhythm Society. Heart Rhythm. 2012;9(4): 632–696.

2 Haissaguerre M, Jais P, Shah DC, Takahashi A, Hocini M, Quiniou G, Garrigue S, LeMouroux A, Le Metayer P, Clementy J. Spontaneous initiation of atrial fibrillation by ectopic beats originating in the pulmonary veins. N Engl J Med. 1998;339:659–666.

3 Pappone C, Oreto G, Rosanio S, Vicedomini G, Tocchi M, Gugliotta F, Salvati A, Dicandia C, Calabro MP, Mazzone P, Ficarra E, Di Gioia C, Gulletta S, Nardi S, Santinelli V, Benussi S, Alfieri O. Atrial electroanatomic remodeling after circumferential radiofrequency pulmonary vein ablation: efficacy of an anatomic approach in a large cohort of patients with atrial fibrillation. Circulation. 2001;104:2539–2544.

4 Oral H, Knight BP, Tada H, Ozaydin M, Chugh A, Hassan S, Scharf C, Lai SW, Greenstein R, Pelosi F, Jr., Strickberger SA, Morady F. Pulmonary vein isolation for paroxysmal and persistent atrial fibrillation. Circulation. 2002;105:1077–1081.

5 Arentz T, von Rosenthal J, Blum T, Stockinger J, Burkle G, Weber R, Jander N, Neumann FJ, Kalusche D Feasibility and safety of pulmonary vein isolation using a new mapping and navigation system in patients with refractory atrial fibrillation. Circulation. 2003;108:2484–2490.

6 Deisenhofer I, Schneider MA, Bohlen-Knauf M, Zrenner B, Ndrepepa G, Schmieder S, Weber S, Schreieck J, Weyerbrock S, Schmitt C. Circumferential mapping and electric isolation of pulmonary veins in patients with atrial fibrillation. Am J Cardiol. 2003;91:159–163.

7 Wyse DG. Selection of endpoints in atrial fibrillation studies. J Cardiovasc Electrophysiol. 2002;13:S47–S52.

8 Prystowsky EN. Assessment of rhythm and rate control in patients with atrial fibrillation. J Cardiovasc Electrophysiol. 2006;17(Suppl. 2):S7–S10.

9 Kottkamp H, Tanner H, Kobza R, Schirdewahn P, Dorszewski A, Gerds-Li JH, Carbucicchio C, Piorkowski C, Hindricks G. Time courses and quantitative analysis of atrial fibrillation episode number and duration after circular plus linear left atrial lesions: trigger elimination or substrate modification: early or delayed cure? J Am Coll Cardiol. 2004;44(4):869–877.

10 Hindricks G, Piorkowski C, Tanner H, Kobza R, Gerds-Li JH, Carbucicchio C, Kottkamp H. Perception of atrial fibrillation before and after radiofrequency catheter ablation: relevance of asymptomatic arrhythmia recurrence. Circulation. 2005;112:307–313.

11 Karch MR, Zrenner B, Deisenhofer I, Schreieck J, Ndrepepa G, Dong J, Lamprecht K, Barthel P, Luciani E, Schomig A, Schmitt C. Freedom from atrial tachyarrhythmias after catheter ablation of atrial fibrillation: a randomized comparison between 2 current ablation strategies. Circulation. 2005;111:2875–2880.

12 Darbar, D, Roden M. Symptomatic burden as an endpoint to evaluate interventions in patients with atrial fibrillation. Heart Rhythm. 2005;2:544–549.

13 Verma A, Champagne J, Sapp J, Essebag V, Novak P, Skanes A, Morillo CA, Khaykin Y, Birnie D. Discerning the incidence of symptomatic and asymptomatic episodes of atrial fibrillation before and after catheter ablation (DISCERN AF): a prospective, multicenter study. JAMA Intern Med. 2013;173(2):149–156.

14 Hohnloser SH, Capucci A, Fain E, Gold MR, van Gelder IC, Healey J, Israel CW, Lau CP, Morillo C, Connolly SJ. Asymptomatic atrial fibrillation and Stroke Evaluation in pacemaker patients and the atrial fibrillation Reduction atrial pacing Trial (ASSERT). Am Heart J. 2006;152: 442–447.

15 Israel CW, Groenefeld G, Ehrlich JR, Li YG, Hohnloser SH. Long-term risk of recurrent atrial fibrillation as documented by an implantable monitoring device: implications for optimal patient care. JACC. 2004;43:47–52.

16 Purerfellner H, Aichinger J, Martinek M, Nesser HJ, Ziegler P, Koehler J, Warman E, Hettrick D. Quantification of atrial tachyarrhythmia burden with an implantable pacemaker before and after pulmonary vein isolation. Pacing Clin Electrophysiol. 2004;27:1277–1283.

17 Hindricks G, Pokushalov E, Urban L, Taborsky M, Kuck KH, Lebedev D, Rieger G, Pürerfellner H; XPECT Trial Investigators. Performance of a new leadless implantable cardiac monitor in detecting and quantifying atrial fibrillation: results of the XPECT trial. Circ Arrhythm Electrophysiol. 2010;3(2):141–147.

18 Nademanee K, McKenzie J, Kosar E, Schwab M, Sunsaneewitayakul B, Vasavakul T, Khunnawat C, Ngarmukos T. A new approach for catheter ablation of atrial fibrillation: mapping of the electrophysiologic substrate. J Am Coll Cardiol. 2004;43:2044–2053.

19 Piorkowski C, Kottkamp H, Tanner H, Kobza R, Nielsen JC, Arya A, Hindricks G. Value of different follow-up strategies to assess the efficacy of circumferential pulmonary vein ablation for the curative treatment of atrial fibrillation. J Cardiovasc Electrophysiol. 2005;16 (12):1286–1292.

20 Stabile G, Bertaglia E, Senatore G, De Simone A, Zoppo F, Donnici G, Turco P, Pascotto P, Fazzari M, Vitale DF. Catheter ablation treatment in patients with drug-refractory atrial fibrillation: a prospective, multi-centre, randomized, controlled study (Catheter Ablation For the Cure of Atrial Fibrillation Study). Eur Heart J. 2006;27: 216–221.

21 Pappone C, Augello G, Sala S, Gugliotta F, Vicedomini G, Gulletta S, Paglino G, Mazzone P, Sora N, Greiss I, Santagostino A, LiVolsi L, Pappone N, Radinovic A, Manguso F, Santinelli V. A randomized trial of circumferential pulmonary vein ablation versus antiarrhythmic drug therapy in paroxysmal atrial fibrillation: the APAF Study. J Am Coll Cardiol. 2006;48(11):2340–2347.

22 Ouyang F, Antz M, Ernst S, Hachiya H, Mavrakis H, Deger FT, Schaumann A, Chun J, Falk P, Hennig D, Liu X, Bansch D, Kuck KH. Recovered pulmonary vein conduction as a dominant factor for recurrent atrial tachyarrhythmias after complete circular isolation of the pulmonary veins: lessons from double Lasso technique. Circulation. 2005;111:127–135.

23 Deisenhofer I, Estner H, Zrenner B, Schreieck J, Weyerbrock S, Hessling G, Scharf K, Karch MR, Schmitt C. Left atrial tachycardia after circumferential pulmonary vein ablation for atrial fibrillation: incidence, electrophysiological characteristics and results of radiofrequency ablation. Europace. 2006;8(8):572–583.

24 Chugh A, Oral H, Lemola K, Hall B, Cheung P, Good E, Tamirisa K, Han J, Bogun F, Pelosi, F, Jr., Morady F. Prevalence, mechanisms, and clinical significance of macroreentrant atrial tachycardia during and following left atrial ablation for atrial fibrillation. Heart Rhythm. 2005;2:464–471.

25 O'Neill MD, Wright M, Knecht S, Jaïs P, Hocini M, Takahashi Y, Jönsson A, Sacher F, Matsuo S, Lim KT, Arantes L, Derval N, Lellouche N, Nault I, Bordachar P, Clémenty J, Haissaguerre M. Long-term follow-up of persistent atrial fibrillation ablation using termination as a procedural endpoint. Eur Heart J. 2009;30(9):1105–1112.

26 Rostock T, Salukhe TV, Steven D, Drewitz I, Hoffmann BA, Bock K, Servatius H, Müllerleile K, Sultan A, Gosau N, Meinertz T, Wegscheider K, Willems S. Long-term single- and multiple-procedure outcome and predictors of success after catheter ablation for persistent atrial fibrillation. Heart Rhythm. 2011;8(9):1391–1397.

27 Ammar S, Hessling G, Reents T, Paulik M, Fichtner S, Schön P, Dillier R, Kathan S, Jilek C, Kolb C, Haller B, Deisenhofer I. Importance of sinus rhythm as endpoint of persistent atrial fibrillation ablation. J Cardiovasc Electrophysiol. 2013;24(4):388–395.

28 Vasamreddy CR, Lickfett L, Jayam VK, Nasir K, Bradley DJ, Eldadah Z, Dickfeld T, Berger R, Calkins H. Predictors of recurrence following catheter ablation of atrial fibrillation using an irrigated-tip ablation catheter. J Cardiovasc Electrophysiol. 2004;15:692–697.

29 Oral H, Scharf C, Chugh A, Hall B, Cheung P, Good E, Veerareddy S, Pelosi F, Jr., Morady F. Catheter ablation for paroxysmal atrial fibrillation: segmental pulmonary vein ostial ablation versus left atrial ablation. Circulation. 2003;108:2355–2360.

30 Wokhlu A, Monahan KH, Hodge DO, Asirvatham SJ, Friedman PA, Munger TM, Bradley DJ, Bluhm CM, Haroldson JM, Packer DL. Long-term quality of life after ablation of atrial fibrillation the impact of recurrence, symptom relief, and placebo effect. J Am Coll Cardiol. 2010;55(21):2308–2316.

31 Fichtner S, Deisenhofer I, Kindsmüller S, Dzijan-Horn M, Tzeis S, Reents T, Wu J, Luise Estner H, Jilek C, Ammar S, Kathan S, Hessling G, Ladwig KH. Prospective assessment of short- and long-term quality of life after ablation for atrial fibrillation. J Cardiovasc Electrophysiol. 2012;23(2):121–127.

32 Vasamreddy CR, Dalal D, Eldadah Z, Dickfeld T, Jayam VK, Henrickson C, Meininger G, Dong J, Lickfett L, Berger R, Calkins H. Safety and efficacy of circumferential pulmonary vein catheter ablation of atrial fibrillation. Heart Rhythm. 2005;2:42–48.

33 Marrouche NF, Martin DO, Wazni O, Gillinov AM, Klein A, Bhargava M, Saad E, Bash D, Yamada H, Jaber W, Schweikert R, Tchou P, Abdul-Karim A, Saliba W, Natale A. Phased-array intracardiac echocardiography monitoring during pulmonary vein isolation in patients with atrial fibrillation: impact on outcome and complications. Circulation. 2003;107:2710–2716.

34 Hocini M, Sanders P, Deisenhofer I, Jais P, Hsu LF, Scavee C, Weerasoriya R, Raybaud F, Macle L, Shah DC, Garrigue S, Le Metayer P, Clementy J, Haissaguerre M. Reverse remodeling of sinus node function after catheter ablation of atrial fibrillation in patients with prolonged sinus pauses. Circulation. 2003;108(10):1172–1175.

35 Lo LW, Tai CT, Lin YJ, Chang SL, Wongcharoen W, Chen SA. Reverse atrial electrical remodeling after catheter ablation of persistent atrial fibrillation. J Cardiovasc Electrophysiol. 2006;17(7):798–799.

36 Cheema A, Vasamreddy CR, Dalal D, Marine JE, Dong J, Henrikson CA, Spragg D, Cheng A, Nazarian S, Sinha S, Halperin H, Berger R, Calkins H. Long-term single procedure efficacy of catheter ablation of atrial fibrillation. J Interv Card Electrophysiol. 2006;15(3):145–155.

37 Wijffels MC, Kirchhof CJ, Dorland R, Allessie MA. Atrial fibrillation begets atrial fibrillation. A study in awake chronically instrumented goats. Circulation. 1995;92:1954–1968.

38 Schotten U, Duytschaever M, Ausma J, Eijsbouts S, Neuberger HR, Allessie M. Electrical and contractile remodeling during the first days of atrial fibrillation go hand in hand. Circulation. 2003;107:1433–1439.

39 Oral H, Chugh A, Good E, Sankaran S, Reich SS, Igic P, Elmouchi D, Tschopp D, Crawford T, Dey S, Wimmer A, Lemola K, Jongnarangsin K, Bogun F, Pelosi F, Jr., Morady F. A tailored approach to catheter ablation of paroxysmal atrial fibrillation. Circulation. 2006;113(15):1824–1831.

40 Scherlag BJ, Nakagawa H, Jackman WM, Yamanashi YM, Patterson E, Po S, Lazzara R. Electrical stimulation to identify neural elements on the heart: their role in atrial fibrillation. J Interv Cardiac Electrophysiol. 2005;13:37–42.

41 Tse HF, Reek S, Timmermans C, Lee KL, Geller JC, Rodriguez LM, Ghaye B, Ayers GM, Crijns HJ, Klein HU, Lau CP. Pulmonary vein isolation using transvenous catheter cryoablation for treatment of atrial fibrillation without risk of pulmonary vein stenosis. J Am Coll Cardiol. 2003;42:752–758.

42 Kocheril AG, Calkins H, Sharma AD, Cher D, Stubbs HA, Block JE. Hybrid therapy with right atrial catheter ablation and previously ineffective antiarrhythmic drugs for the management of atrial fibrillation. J Interv Card Electrophysiol. 2005;3:189–197.

43 Tojo H, Kumagai K, Noguchi H, Ogawa M, Yasuda T, Nakashima H, Zhang B, Miura S, Saku K. Hybrid therapy with pilsicainide and pulmonary vein isolation for atrial fibrillation. Circ J. 2005;69(12):1503–1507.

44 Hersi A, Wyse DG. Management of atrial fibrillation. Curr Probl Cardiol. 2005;4:175–233. Review.

45 Haissaguerre M, Hocini M, Sanders P, Sacher F, Rotter M, Takahashi Y, Rostock T, Hsu LF, Bordachar P, Reuter S, Roudaut R, Clementy J, Jais P. Catheter ablation of long-lasting persistent atrial fibrillation: clinical outcome and mechanisms of subsequent arrhythmias. J Cardiovasc Electrophysiol. 2005;16:1138–1147.

46 Ouyang F, Ernst S, Chun J, Bansch D, Li Y, Schaumann A, Mavrakis H, Liu X, Deger FT, Schmidt B, Xue Y, Cao J, Hennig D, Huang H, Kuck KH, Antz M. Electrophysiological findings during ablation of persistent atrial fibrillation with electroanatomic mapping and double Lasso catheter technique. Circulation. 2005;112: 3038–3048.

47 Sanders P, Hocini M, Jais P, Sacher F, Hsu LF, Takahashi Y, Rotter M, Rostock T, Nalliah CJ, Clementy J, Haissaguerre M. Complete isolation of the pulmonary veins and posterior left atrium in chronic atrial fibrillation. Long-term clinical outcome. Eur Heart J. 2007.

48 Mesas CE, Augello G, Lang CC, Gugliotta F, Vicedomini G, Sora N, De Paola AA, Pappone C. Electroanatomic remodeling of the left atrium in patients undergoing repeat pulmonary vein ablation: mechanistic insights and implications for ablation. J Cardiovasc Electrophysiol. 2006;12:1279–1285.

49 Rostock T, O'Neill MD, Sanders P, Rotter M, Jais P, Hocini M, Takahashi Y, Sacher F, Jonsson A, Hsu LF, Clementy J, Haissaguerre M. Characterization of conduction recovery across left atrial linear lesions in patients with paroxysmal and persistent atrial fibrillation. J Cardiovasc Electrophysiol. 2006;17(10):1106–1111.

50 Cheema A, Dong J, Dalal D, Vasamreddy CR, Marine JE, Henrikson CA, Spragg D, Cheng A, Nazarian S, Sinha S, Halperin H, Berger R, Calkins H. Long-term safety and efficacy of circumferential ablation with pulmonary vein isolation. J Cardiovasc Electrophysiol. 2006;17(10): 1080–1085.

51 Stevenson WG, Tedrow U. Management of atrial fibrillation in patients with heart failure. Heart Rhythm. 2007;4 (3S):S28–S30. Epub 2006 Dec 6.

52 Pappone C, Rosanio S, Augello G, Gallus G, Vicedomini G, Mazzone P, Gulletta S, Gugliotta F, Pappone A, Santinelli V, Tortoriello V, Sala S, Zangrillo A, Crescenzi G, Benussi S, Alfieri O. Mortality, morbidity, and quality of life after circumferential pulmonary vein ablation for atrial fibrillation: outcomes from a controlled non-randomized long-term study. J Am Coll Cardiol. 2003;42:185–197.

53 Chen MS, Marrouche NF, Khaykin Y, Gillinov AM, Wazni O, Martin DO, Rossillo A, Verma A, Cummings J, Erciyes D, Saad E, Bhargava M, Bash D, Schweikert R, Burkhardt D, Williams-Andrews M, Perez-Lugones A, Abdul-Karim A, Saliba W, Natale A. Pulmonary vein isolation for the treatment of atrial fibrillation in patients with impaired systolic function. J Am Coll Cardiol. 2004;43:1004–1009.

54 Hsu LF, Jais P, Sanders P, Garrigue S, Hocini M, Sacher F, Takahashi Y, Rotter M, Pasquie JL, Scavee C, Bordachar P, Clementy J, Haissaguerre M. Catheter ablation for atrial fibrillation in congestive heart failure. N Engl J Med. 2004;351:2373–2383.

55 Lemola K, Sneider M, Desjardins B, Case I, Chugh A, Hall B, Cheung P, Good E, Han J, Tamirisa K, Bogun F, Pelosi F, Jr., Kazerooni E, Morady F, Oral H: effects of left atrial ablation of atrial fibrillation on size of the left atrium and pulmonary veins. Heart Rhythm. 2004;1:576–581.

56 Lemola K, Desjardins B, Sneider M, Case I, Chugh A, Good E, Han J, Tamirisa K, Tsemo A, Reich S, Tschopp D, Igic P, Elmouchi D, Bogun F, Pelosi JF, Kazerooni E, Morady F, Oral H: effect of left atrial circumferential ablation for atrial fibrillation on left atrial transport function. Heart Rhythm. 2005;2:923–928.

57 Verma A, Kilicaslan F, Adams JR, Hao S, Beheiry S, Minor S, Ozduran V, Elayi S, Martin DO, Schweikert RA, Saliba W, Thomas JD, Garcia M, Klein A, Natale A: extensive ablation during pulmonary vein antrum isolation has no adverse impact on left atrial function: an echocardiography and cine computed tomography analysis. J Cardiovasc Electrophysiol. 2006;17: 741–746.

58 Gibson DN, Di Biase L, Mohanty P, Patel JD, Bai R, Sanchez J, Burkhardt JD, Heywood JT, Johnson AD, Rubenson DS, Horton R, Gallinghouse GJ, Beheiry S, Curtis GP, Cohen DN, Lee MY, Smith MR, Gopinath D, Lewis WR, Natale A. Stiff left atrial syndrome after catheter ablation for atrial fibrillation: clinical characterization, prevalence, and predictors. Heart Rhythm. 2011; 8(9):1364–1371.

59 Thrall G, Lane D, Carroll D, Lip GY. Quality of life in patients with atrial fibrillation: a systematic review. Am J Med. 2006;119(5):448–467.

60 Newman D. Quality of life as an endpoint for atrial fibrillation research: pitfalls and practice. Heart Rhythm. 2004;1:20–26.

61 Coyne K, Margolis MK, Grandy S, Zimetbaum P, The state of patient-reported outcomes in atrial fibrillation. Pharmacoeconomics. 2005;23:687–708.

62 Dorian P, Jung W, Newman D, et al. The impairment of health-related quality of life in patients with intermittent atrial fibrillation: implications for the assessment of investigational therapy. J Am Coll Cardiol. 2000;36: 1303–1309.

63 Bauer A, Deisenhofer I, Schneider R, Zrenner B, Barthel P, Karch M, Wagenpfeil S, Schmitt C, Schmidt G. Effects of circumferential or segmental pulmonary vein ablation for paroxysmal atrial fibrillation on cardiac autonomic function. Heart Rhythm. 2006;3(12):1428–1435.

64 Brand FN, Abbott RD, Kennel WB, et al. Characteristics and prognosis of lone atrial fibrillation. JAMA. 1985;254: 3449–3453.

65 Wellens HJJ. Pulmonary vein ablation in atrial fibrillation: hype or hope? Circulation. 2000;102:2562–2564.

66 Cappato R, Calkins H, Chen SA, Davies W, Iesaka Y, Kalman J, Kim YH, Klein G, Packer D, Skanes A. Worldwide survey on the methods, efficacy, and safety of catheter ablation for human atrial fibrillation. Circulation. 2005;111:1100–1105.

67 Cappato R, Calkins H, Chen SA, Davies W, Iesaka Y, Kalman J, Kim YH, Klein G, Natale A, Packer D, Skanes A, Ambrogi F, Biganzoli E. Updated worldwide survey on the methods, efficacy, and safety of catheter ablation for human atrial fibrillation. Circ Arrhythm Electrophysiol. 2010;3(1):32–38.

68 Fichtner S, Czudnochowsky U, Hessling G, Reents T, Estner H, Wu J, Jilek C, Ammar S, Karch MR, Deisenhofer I. Very late relapse of atrial fibrillation after pulmonary vein isolation: incidence and results of repeat ablation. Pacing Clin Electrophysiol. 2010;33(10): 1258–1263.

69 Weerasooriya R, Khairy P, Litalien J, Macle L, Hocini M, Sacher F, Lellouche N, Knecht S, Wright M, Nault I, Miyazaki S, Scavee C, Clementy J, Haissaguerre M, Jais P. Catheter ablation for atrial fibrillation: are results maintained at 5 years of follow-up? J Am Coll Cardiol. 2011;57 (2):160–166.

70 Tilz RR, Rillig A, Thum AM, Arya A, Wohlmuth P, Metzner A, Mathew S, Yoshiga Y, Wissner E, Kuck KH, Ouyang F. Catheter ablation of long-standing persistent atrial fibrillation: 5-year outcomes of the Hamburg Sequential Ablation Strategy. J Am Coll Cardiol. 2012;60(19):1921–1929.

Index

Practical Guide to Catheter Ablation of Atrial Fibrillation,
Second Edition. Edited by Jonathan S. Steinberg, Pierre Jaïs
and Hugh Calkins.
© 2016 John Wiley & Sons, Ltd. Published 2016 by
John Wiley & Sons, Ltd.